MW00806215

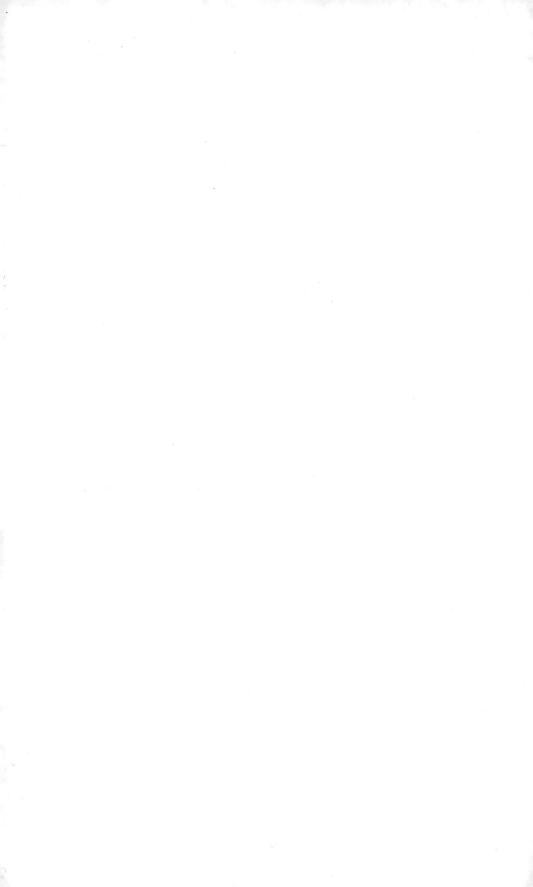

EEG—fMRI

Christoph Mulert • Louis Lemieux (Eds.)

EEG–fMRI

Physiological Basis, Technique and Applications

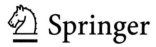 Springer

PD Dr. Christoph Mulert
Universitätsklinikum München
Psychiatrische Klinik Ludwig-Maximilians-
Universität München (LMU)
Nußbaumstr. 7
80336 München
Germany
Christoph.Mulert@med.uni-muenchen.de

Louis Lemieux, PhD
UCL Institute of Neurology
Department of Clinical and Experimental
Epilepsy
University College London
Queen Square
London
United Kingdom WC1N 3BG
l.lemieux@ion.ucl.ac.uk

ISBN: 978-3-540-87918-3   e-ISBN: 978-3-540-87919-0

DOI: 10.1007/978-3-540-87919-0

Springer Heidelberg Dordrecht London New York

Library of Congress Control Number: 2009926259

Cover design: eStudioCalamar Figueres/Berlin

Printed on acid-free paper

Springer is part of Springer Science+Business Media (www.springer.com)

Foreword

It is a great pleasure to write a preface for this book, which I see as the first comprehensive treatment of human brain mapping using multimodal approaches. The content and ambitions addressed in these pages represent some of the most challenging and advanced applications in imaging neuroscience. Since the inception of modern brain mapping two decades ago, there has been an implicit hope that different measurements of brain activity might be integrated to provide an unprecedented and multilateral view of its structure and function. This book provides a compelling review of this integrative approach and reflects the excitement of those working in the field.

Until the introduction of positron emission tomography (PET) and functional magnetic resonance imaging (fMRI), the principal way of measuring brain activity noninvasively was by measuring electrical signals from the brain using electroencephalography. In the late 1980s and early 1990s, PET and fMRI heralded a new era in imaging neuroscience; allowing scientists to pinpoint the metabolic and haemodynamic correlates of electrical activity, anywhere in the brain. Over the past decade, much thought has been given to combining electromagnetic and haemodynamic measurements to look at aspects of functional anatomy that could not be seen with one modality alone. An analogy for this multimodal approach is the ability to perceive depth with binocular vision, compared to using one eye alone. To harness multimodal perspectives on brain dynamics, people thought that we would need underlying generative models of neuronal activity that could explain both electromagnetic and haemodynamic signals. From this emerged the notion of multimodal fusion, in which sense could be made of multimodal data by reference to a common generative model. Perhaps rather surprisingly, this line of thinking has proved much less fruitful than exploring the relationships between electromagnetic and haemodynamic signals directly. This relationship can go in one of two directions. One can use the spatial deployment of haemodynamic signals, across the brain, to predict or constrain the sources of electromagnetic activity. Conversely, one can look for the physiological correlates of electromagnetic signals using fMRI. Although technically very challenging, the latter approach has furnished the greatest insights into the relationship between fast neuronal dynamics and their spatially resolved haemodynamic correlates. It is this relationship that is studied with EEG–fMRI and is the subject of this book.

There has been an enormous interest in the relationship between electrophysiological and brain mapping signals. This relationship has been addressed invasively and noninvasively with multimodal or conjoint recordings. It is of great importance, not only for our basic understanding of brain mapping signals per se, but it also has profound implications for understanding the functional anatomy of epilepsy and related disorders. It is interesting to note that it was the epilepsy community that advanced the noninvasive side of this endeavour more than any other field in neuroimaging. They have overcome some profound technical difficulties, entailed by having to acquire minuscule electromagnetic signals in the context of a magnetic resonance imaging environment. Furthermore, they have had to deal with the confounding effects of artefacts and data modelling that far exceed the challenges usually incurred by conventional brain mapping. It is therefore of no surprise that many of the contributors to this book have been pioneers not only in neuroimaging but also in MRI physics and its clinical applications.

Karl Friston

Preface

This book is about a measurement technique commonly called "EEG–fMRI", or EEG-correlated functional MRI to give it its full name, which is designed to capture the electrophysiological and haemodynamic manifestations of brain activity synchronously. The chapters attempt to provide a thorough overview of the state of EEG–fMRI in all its aspects through the compositions of acknowledged experts in their respective field.

The technique's origin, albeit in a very specific and restricted field of neuroscience, is worth discussing in detail, as it highlights important aspects of the motivation for combining the two modalities.

EEG–fMRI emerged from the field of epilepsy imaging, soon after the development of fMRI, when John Ives and colleagues wheeled their EEG machine into the scanner room at the Beth Israel Hospital in Boston, USA. This action was doubtless driven by the desire to map epileptic brain activity. The reason is simple: the need for noninvasive imaging of the epileptic focus. Even today, EEG source estimation during seizures remains a formidable challenge, and while in some cases structural imaging reveals abnormal brain regions, which for all practical purposes correspond to the focus, this is not the rule—even with current MRI. The same could be said for "functional" imaging techniques such as PET and SPECT. Epilepsy is a condition defined by perturbed brain activity. Techniques that can record changes in brain activity between two states—normal and epileptic for example—thus have an immediate appeal. The time scale of these perturbations ranges from 10 ms to minutes or even hours (the bandwidth extending into the tens of Hz), hence the crucial role of EEG, with its exquisite temporal resolution, in the study of epilepsy. The most common EEG abnormality observed in patients with epilepsy is the interictal epileptiform discharge, commonly called "epileptic spike", which has a duration of 100 ms; their relative abundance and often close relationship between their generator and the focus makes them scientifically and clinically attractive. Although a great deal of effort has been dedicated to estimating the generators of spikes, electrical source imaging suffers from the well-known intractability of the EEG inverse problem. What about imaging spikes? Spikes occur without any external manifestation, in contrast to seizures, and are considered a purely EEG phenomenon. Furthermore, they occur spontaneously, which means that producing images of the "spike state" requires the recording of EEG. The temporal resolution of fMRI, which is somewhere between that of EEG and that of PET/SPECT, makes it uniquely suitable for the study of the haemodynamic correlates of individual spikes noninvasively and throughout the brain. In epilepsy, we therefore have an ideal application of this multimodal approach: the "EEG" in "EEG–fMRI applied to epilepsy" is simply a necessity if one is interested in mapping the haemodynamic correlates of spikes. The same can be said of the study of spontaneous (paradigm-free) brain activity, such as natural variations in EEG background (alpha rhythm), wakefulness, or activity in the default mode network.

Apart from the study of EEG and fMRI correlation in the resting state, what can EEG–fMRI bring to the neuroscience table? Another way of expressing the conditions under which simultaneous multimodal acquisitions are necessary is the need to eliminate potential intersession bias. In the case of interictal epileptic activity and the study of spontaneous variations in brain rhythms, for example, there is no way of guaranteeing matched datasets without simultaneous EEG. In the field of cognitive neuroscience, and the study of evoked responses in particular, simultaneous acquisitions are also a means of eliminating the potential effects of habituation, learning, attention, fatigue, anxiety, etc., across sessions.

Once this has been achieved, and the resulting data can be guaranteed to relate to the same brain activity, one has the possibility of studying the variance that is left once the experimental, deterministic factors have been taken into account, since averaged effects can be studied offline (in the absence of systematic intersession bias). For example, we will see how EEG–fMRI can been used to study the relationship between response latency and BOLD signal change and the the relationship between spontaneous variations in local field potential and the BOLD signal, leading to improved understanding of the electrophysiological substrate of the BOLD signal.

Therefore, simultaneous EEG–fMRI is the technique of choice to guarantee matched EEG and fMRI datasets, and is necessary for the study of the unpredictable parts of the signals.

An unfortunate aspect of the way EEG–fMRI is perceived is the often-stated claim that it combines the advantages of EEG (high temporal resolution) with those of fMRI (better spatial coverage), while of course the experimentalist soon realises that it also suffers from the limitations of both (EEG's spatial sensitivity bias and fMRI's sluggish relationship to neuronal events).

In cognitive neuroscience, research has been performed for decades using EEG and ERP to describe the neural basis of cognitive processes. ERPs such as the P300 potential, the N100 or the ERN have been used successfully to better understand brain function involved in target detection, selective attention or error processing. In addition, specific oscillation patterns have been identified as being associated with cognition (e.g. theta or gamma oscillations). However, for most of these potentials or oscillation patterns, discussions concerning their generation have continued and several lines of information have been used to get the desired knowledge (intracranial recordings, studies in patients with lesions, animal studies, EEG source localisation). All of these strategies have their limitations, and therefore imaging techniques such as fMRI represent an attractive alternative to get reliable information on neuroanatomical structures related to cognitive processes.

EEG–fMRI therefore may be a strategy that can make use of the high temporal resolution of EEG to achieve goals such as "mental chronometry" (describing the timeline of brain activity in relation to cognitive processing) and to specify the role of distinct oscillation patterns in combination with reliable information about the neuroanatomical structures involved. While this can be seen as the ultimate goal of EEG–fMRI in cognitive neuroscience, there are a number of pitfalls in terms of basic physiology, study design, artefacts and analysis techniques that have to be taken into account to avoid misguided data acquisition strategies or oversimplified interpretations of EEG–fMRI findings.

As the reader new to the field will soon discover, EEG–fMRI has mainly been used as an imaging technique: a special form of fMRI. In most applications, EEG is used as either an epoch (image) categorisation device or as a supplier of potential explanatory variables for the BOLD model. This bias or asymmetry in its use and interpretation is probably a reflection of the intrinsic visual instinct of humans, the associated need for explanations for numerous EEG observations made over the last 80 years, and also the perceived weakness of EEG-derived localisation. We believe that this represents a form of underachievement and a challenge. Success will doubtless come from discoveries on the nature of the relationship between electrical and MR signals, and it is our hope that this book will provide some of the required motivation.

We would like to thank all of the contributors for their hard work and patience throughout the editing and production process. We are particularly grateful to Dr Ute Heilmann of Springer for giving us the opportunity to realise this book.

Louis Lemieux and Christoph Mulert

Contents

Contributors

Philip J. Allen
Department of Clinical Neurophysiology,
The National Hospital for Neurology and
Neurosurgery, Queen Square, London
WC1N 3BG, UK

Andrew P. Bagshaw
School of Psychology, University of
Birmingham, Birmingham B15 2TT, UK

Robert Becker
Department of Neurology, Charité
Universitätsmedizin, Charitéplatz 1,
10117 Berlin, Germany

Christian-G. Bénar
INSERM, Université de la Méditerranée,
27 Bd Jean Moulin, 13385 Marseille
Cedex 05, France

Hal Blumenfeld
Yale Departments of Neurology,
Neurobiology, and Neurosurgery,
333 Cedar Street, New Haven,
CT 06520-8018, USA

Giorgio Bonmassar
AbiLab, Athinoula A. Martinos Center
for Biomedical Imaging, Massachusetts
General Hospital, Charlestown,
MA, USA

Andre Brechmann
Leibniz-Institute for Neurobiology,
Brenneckestr. 6, 39118 Magdeburg,
Germany

David Carmichael
UCL Institute of Neurology
Department of Clinical and
Experimental Epilepsy, University College
London, London WC1N 3BG, UK

Patrick Carney
Brain Research Institute, Austin Health,
Florey Neuroscience Institutes,
University of Melbourne, Melbourne,
Australia

Umair J. Chaudhary
University College London,
Institute of Neurology, Queen Square,
London WC1N 3BG, UK

Michael Czisch
Max Planck Institute of Psychiatry,
Kraepelinstr. 2-10, 80804 Munich,
Germany

Jean Daunizeau
University College London
Wellcome Trust for Neuroimaging,
Institute of Neurology, 12 Queen Square,
London, WC1N 3BG, UK

Stefan Debener
Medical Research Council
Institute of Hearing Research,
Royal South Hants Hospital,
Southampton SO14 0YG, UK

Ralf Deichmann
University Hospital, Brain Imaging Center,
Haus 95H, Schleusenweg 2-16,
60528 Frankfurt-Main, Germany

Francois Dubeau
Montreal Neurological Hospital and
Institute, Department of Neurology
and Neurosurgery, McGill University,
Montreal, QC, Canada

Damien J. Ellens
Yale Departments of Neurology,
Neurobiology, Neurosurgery,
Yale University School of Medicine,
333 Cedar Street, New Haven,
CT 06520, USA

Fabrizio Esposito
Department of Cognitive Neuroscience,
Maastricht University, MD Maastricht,
The Netherlands

Frank Freyer
Department of Neurology,
Charité Universitätsmedizin Berlin,
Charitéplatz 1, 10117 Berlin,
Germany

Karl J. Friston
The Wellcome Centre for Neuroimaging,
University College London
12 Queen Square, London,
WC1N 3BG, UK

Rainer Goebel
Department of Cognitive Neuroscience
Maastricht University,
MD Maastricht, The Netherlands

Ingmar Gutberlet
Brain Products GmbH, Zeppelinstrasse 7,
82205 Gilching, Germany

Christoph S. Herrmann
Department of Biological Psychology,
Otto-von-Guericke-University of
Magdeburg, 39016 Magdeburg, Germany

Giandomenico D. Iannetti
Department of Physiology, Anatomy
and Genetics, University of Oxford,
South Parks Road, Oxford OX1 3QX, UK

Graeme Jackson
Brain Research Institute, Austin Health,
Heidelberg West, Australia

Susanne Karch
Functional Brain Imaging Branch,
Klinik für Psychiatrie und Psychotherapie
der LMU München, Nussbaumstr 7,
80336 München, Germany

James M. Kilner
The Wellcome Trust Centre for
Neuroimaging, UCL Institute of Neurology, 12 Queen Square, London WC1N
3BG, UK

Cornelia Kranczioch
Department of Psychology, University of
Portsmouth, Portsmouth, PO1 2DY, UK

Helmut Laufs
Department of Neurology and Brain
Imaging Center, Johann Wolfgang
Goethe-Universität, Theodor-Stern-Kai 7,
60590 Frankfurt am Main, Germany

Gregor Leicht
Department of Psychiatry and
Psychotherapy, Clinical Neurophysiology
and Functional Brain Imaging,
Ludwig-Maximilians-University Munich,
Nußbaumstr. 7, 80336 Munich, Germany

Louis Lemieux
UCL Institute of Neurology, Department
of Clinical and Experimental Epilepsy,
University College London, Queen Square,
London WC1N 3BG, UK

MRI Unit, National Society for Epilepsy,
Chesham Lane, Chalfont St Peter, Buckinghamshire SL9 0RJ, UK

Fernando Lopes da Silva
Center of NeuroSciences, Swammerdam
Institute for Life Sciences, University
of Amsterdam, Kruislaan 320,
1098 SM Amsterdam, The Netherlands

André Mouraux
Department of Clinical Neurology,
University of Oxford, South Parks Road,
Oxford OX1 3QX, UK

Christoph Mulert
Functional Brain Imaging Branch,
Department of Psychiatry and Psychotherapy LMU Munich, Nussbaumstrasse 7,
80336 Munich, Germany

Karen J. Mullinger
Sir Peter Mansfield Magnetic Resonance
Centre, School of Physics and Astronomy,
University of Nottingham, University
Park, Nottingham, NG7 2RD, UK

Ulrike Nöth
Helmholtz Center Munich, German
Research Center for Environmental
Health (GmbH), Neuherberg,
Germany

Petra Ritter
Deptartment of Neurology, Charité
Universitätsmedizin Berlin, Charitéplatz 1,
10117 Berlin, Germany

Henning Scheich
Leibniz-Institute for Neurobiology,
Brenneckestr. 6, 39118 Magdeburg,
Germany

Amir Shmuel
Montreal Neurological Institute,
McGill University, Montreal, QC,
Canada

Michael Siniatchkin
University Hospital of Pediatric
Neurology, Christian-Albrechts-University
of Kiel, Schwanenweg 20, 24105 Kiel,
Germany

Arno Villringer
Berlin NeuroImaging Center and Charité,
Universitätsmedizin Berlin, Berlin,
Germany

Department of Cognitive Neurology, Max Planck Institute for Human
Cognitive and Brain Sciences,
Stephanstrasse 1A, 04103 Leipzig,
Germany

Matthew C. Walker
UCL Institute of Neurology, Department
of Clinical and Experimental Epilepsy,
University College London, Queen Square,
London WC1N 3BG, UK

Renate Wehrle
Max Planck Institute of Psychiatry,
Kraepelinstr. 2-10, 80804 Munich,
Germany

Nikolaus Weiskopf
UCL Institute of Neurology, Wellcome
Trust Centre for Neuroimaging,
University College London,
London, UK

Part I

Background

Principles of Multimodal Functional Imaging and Data Integration

1

Arno Villringer, Christoph Mulert, and Louis Lemieux

1
Introduction

In a system as complex as the human brain, one cannot conceive of meaningful events involving a change in a single observable (physiological parameter). Therefore, achieving the ultimate aim of a complete understanding of brain events and brain activity in general will require the integration of a variety of observations related to these events. Multimodal imaging, or more generally measurements whereby data from various types of instruments are brought together, has arisen partly from this realisation, partly because some events are best observed in one modality and the investigator is interested in another (e.g. a more recently developed modality), and to be honest sometimes as a response to the technical challenge of combining modalities for simultaneous observations. Fundamentally, multimodal imaging should allow the investigator to address the question: what happens to brain observable Z when observable X changes (or event Y occurs)?

In the second half of the twentieth century, and particularly since the 1990s, a rapid development of noninvasive functional and structural brain imaging methods has occurred. While some of these developments have resulted from gradual improvements in some methods, other developments have led to completely new approaches for measuring brain activity, affording new types of information about the brain. In the former case, the older methods were eventually replaced [e.g. scintigraphic methods by positron emission tomography (PET), and SPECT or low-field MRI (magnetic resonance imaging) by higher field MRI]. In the latter case, however, newer developments have not replaced older ones; rather, they have been added to an ever-larger orchestra of functional and structural neuroimaging methods consisting of techniques that offer complementary information about the brain. Table 1 gives an overview of currently available methods for noninvasive brain imaging and the principle that each exploits.

A. Villringer (✉)
Department of Cognitive Neurology, Max Planck Institute for Human Cognitive and Brain Sciences, Stephanstrasse 1A, 04103, Leipzig, Germany
e-mail: Villringer@cbs.mpg.de

C. Mulert and L. Lemieux (eds.), *EEG–fMRI*
DOI: 10.1007/978-3-540-87919-0_1, © Springer Verlag Berlin Heidelberg 2010

Table 1 Noninvasive brain imaging methods

Method	Physical principle
Computerised tomography (CT)	Absorption of X-rays
Positron emission tomography (PET)	Emission/detection of positrons
Magnetic resonance imaging (MRI)	Nuclear magnetic resonance (NMR)
Optical imaging	Light absorption, scattering, fluorescence
Electroencephalography (EEG)	Electrical potentials
Magnetoencephalography (MEG)	Magnetic fields
Electrical impedance tomography (EIT)	Changes in electrical impedance
Functional transcranial Doppler sonography (fTCD)	Doppler effect in ultrasound

While in some instances combining multimodal measurements is a relatively straightforward task from a technical point of view [e.g. transcranial Doppler sonography/near-infrared optical spectroscopy (TCD/NIRS)], the combination of other methods poses major technical challenges (e.g. EEG–fMRI). Table 2 summarizes which imaging techniques have been combined successfully in order to perform simultaneous observations.

While the physical principles underlying each method are crucial to the feasibility of multimodal integration (Table 2), more subtle aspects of (or variations on) the basic principle (e.g. choice of pulse sequence in MRI, application of contrast agents in CT, MRI or ultrasound) determine the precise aspect of neurophysiology that can be captured in any given application (for an earlier review, see Villringer and Dirnagl 1995). From the standpoint of a neuroscientist, it seems more appropriate to categorise methods according to the neurophysiological processes that they reflect rather than according to physical principle. Table 3 illustrates how different modalities can provide complementary neurophysiological information that may allow neuroscientists to identify which combination is currently available and matches their interest. For example, in the assessment of brain activity for a certain cognitive task, it might be useful to combine the spatial resolution and relatively uniform spatial coverage of fMRI with evoked potentials measured using scalp electroencephalography (EEG) to a high temporal resolution (along with the large amount of knowledge on cognitive correlates accumulated over decades of research) in order to elucidate how the spatiotemporal haemodynamic and electrical patterns are correlated.

2
Modes of Data Integration

The integration of different measurement modalities can be achieved in a variety of ways, reflecting both the level of synchrony between the data acquired for each modality and the ways in which the data from each modality are used to analyse or interpret the findings. We refer to these as modes of integration.

Table 2   Technical feasibility of simultaneous multimodal imaging

Combination	References	Comments
EEG–MRI	Ives et al. (1993); Busch et al. (1995); Bonmassar et al. (1999, 2001); Allen et al. (1998, 2000), Lemieux et al. (1997, 2001), Goldman et al. (2000); Krakow et al. (2000)	Although the feasibility of this combination was shown a few years back, broad usage started with further developments in equipment, artefact elimination and analysis
NIRS–MRI	Kleinschmidt et al. (1996); Kida et al. (1996); Punwani et al. (1998); Toronov et al. (2001); Mehagnoul-Schipper et al. (2002); Strangman et al. (2002)	
TES–MRI	Brandt et al. (1996)	
MRI–MEG	Zotev et al. (2008)	
fTCD–MRI		Probably feasible, since combined ultrasound and MRI systems have been demonstrated (McDannold et al. 2003)
PET–NIRS	Villringer et al. (1997)	
PET–fTCD	Sabri et al. (2003)	
PET–EEG	Buchsbaum et al. (1984); Sadato et al. (1998); Barrington et al. (1998); Gamma et al. (2004)	
PET–MEG		Feasible in principle, but no example of a successful combination was found
PET–CT		Mainly used in clinical oncology (Beyer et al. 2000)
PET–MRI	Catana et al. (2008); Judenhofer et al. (2008)	
EEG–MEG	Salustri et al. (1989); Buchner et al. (1994)	
EEG–NIRS	Hoshi et al. (1994); Steinhoff et al. (1996); Kirkpatrick et al. (1998); Obrig et al. (2002)	
MEG–NIRS	Mackert et al. (2004)	
NIRS–TCD	Terborg et al. (2003)	

It goes almost without saying that the study of a given phenomenon using multiple modalities requires that all signals relate to the same phenomenon. However, the ways in which the data can be usefully acquired depend on what type of phenomenon and which aspect of the phenomenon one is interested in. For example, in experimental studies involving controlled tasks or stimuli, serial single-modality acquisitions may be adequate,

Table 3 Physiological parameters and noninvasive brain imaging methods

Physiological parameters	Technique	Method
Vascular/metabolic		
Cerebral blood flow	MRI	Arterial spin labelling (ASL)
		Bolus track MRI
	Positron emission tomography	H_2O PET
		Butanol-PET
	SPECT	ECD-SPECT
	Optical imaging	Bolus track near-infrared spectroscopy/imaging
Δ[deoxyhaemoglobin]	MRI	Blood oxygen level dependent (BOLD)
	Optical imaging	Near-infrared spectroscopy
Plasma volume	MRI	Bolus track MRI
	Optical	Bolus track optical imaging
Corpuscular volume	PET	CO-PET
	MRI	VASO
Glucose consumption	PET	Deoxyglucose PET
Oxygen consumption	PET	O_2 PET
	MRI	BOLD and CBF-MRI (calibrated with CO_2 challenge)
Electrophysiological markers of brain activity		
"Field potentials" (presumably reflecting synaptic activity)	EEG	Event-related evoked potentials
Action potentials (high-frequency bursts)	EEG	
Evoked fields (presumably reflecting synaptic activity)	MEG	Event-related evoked magnetic fields
Assessment of background rhythms and evoked rhythms	EEG, MEG	Assessment of occipital alpha rhythms
Molecular markers		
Various markers of energy metabolism containing phosphorus: ATP, ADP, creatinine phosphate	MR	P31 magnetic resonance spectroscopy
Various molecules in millimolar concentration range: lactate, N-acetylaspartate, glutamate, GABA, etc.	MR	H1 magnetic resonance spectroscopy
Other molecular markers at smaller concentrations	PET	PET of various positron-emitting tracers
	Optical	Fluorescence detection of various fluorescent/phosphorescent tracers
Brain morphology/volumetry		
Volumes of brain areas	MRI	Voxel-based morphometry (VBM)
Orientation of nerve fibres	MRI	Diffusion tensor imaging
Other		
Cell volume	MRI	Diffusion imaging
	Optical	Scattering

and it is less clear why it may be advantageous to combine methods in order to acquire the multimodal data simultaneously.

Similarly, a range of analytical strategies for multimodal datasets are available that are suited to different modes of acquisition and reflect varying degrees of sophistication of the underlying (integrative) model. For example, spatial coregistration of independently anal-ysed unimodal data represents one the simplest forms of integration—comparison, while the estimation of biophysical models of brain activity based on multimodal data must be one of the end-points of the multimodal integration project.

3
Multimodal Data Acquisition Strategies: Degree of Synchrony

In an ideal world, a single instrument would combine all imaging modalities and all brain imaging datasets would be multimodal. However, human brain imaging instruments are generally single modality, except for magnetoencephalography (MEG) systems, which often comprise an EEG recording system. Therefore, investigators interested in obtaining multimodal measurements must carefully consider the practical difficulties associated with simultaneous measurements in relation to the expected benefits for the data. These difficul-ties include: (a) higher costs (e.g. adaptation of instruments to the new environment; such as nonmagnetic materials for MR compatibility); (b) interactions between instruments that can lead to data quality degradation (e.g. EEG artefacts during MRI data acquisition) or increased health risks for subjects (higher risk of introducing magnetic material into the MR environment). These issues are discussed in greater detail in the chapters "EEG Instrumentation and Safety", "EEG Quality: Origin and Reduction of the EEG Cardiac-Related Artefact", "EEG Quality: The Image Acquisition Artefact", "Image Quality Issues" and "Specific Issues Related to EEG–fMRI at $B_0 > 3$ T".

Given satisfactory technical solutions to the above problems, there are clear theoretical benefits in performing simultaneous multimodal acquisitions, although their value will depend on the specific scientific questions being asked. The main consideration is whether one is confident that *the same thing* (brain activity) will happen if the experiment is repeated across modalities. Given that the human brain cannot be entirely controlled, a degree of interevent signal variability is inevitable (above and beyond any measurement uncertainty due to the instruments), and the issue boils down to whether one can guarantee that the parameters of interest would behave identically across sessions. This means that multimodal studies based on the parameterisation of individual events must be performed in a single session with simultaneous measurements from all modalities. According to the same reasoning, multimodal studies of unpredictable events (interevent timing variability) also require simultaneous data acquisitions. For studies of effects averaged over multiple events (such as traditional evoked response studies), intersession bias due to differences in the environment or possible learning effects (for example) must be avoided, and so the need for simultaneous acquisitions in a single session must be carefully considered. In all other circumstances, nonsimultaneous multimodal acquisitions may be adequate.

Note that while inferences made based on nonsimultaneously acquired multimodal data-sets can also be made based on simultaneously acquired datasets, the reverse is not true, given the loss of information on interevent variability in the former type of acquisition.

4
Multimodal Data Integration Strategies

Data from multiple modalities, and inferences made from them, can be brought together in various ways that can be characterised by the degree to which the relationship between the signals is incorporated into a model. At one end of the scale, modalities are simply compared in time or space and may be subjected to correlation analyses for example. At the other end of the scale we have methodologies that aim to model the multimodal signals from more fundamental building blocks, such as neuronal activity and biophysical forward models.

4.1
Spatial Coregistration

Cross-validation of measurements is one of the most common motivations for multimodal imaging. In this approach, information on the distribution of brain activity involved in a given process obtained independently from a number of modalities is compared, usually with the aim of assessing the value of a new localising technique. For example, the localising information provided by the relatively new technique of EEG-correlated fMRI regarding the generators of interictal spikes or event-related potentials has been compared to EEG source reconstruction, thus potentially validating the results from the former technique; however, there are many reasons for a possible lack of perfect spatial concordance, and the very notion of a gold standard is debatable in this specific context (Lemieux et al. 2001; Benar et al. 2003; Mulert et al. 2004) (see Table 4 for other examples).

The comparison of two independent measures of brain activity at a given location can increase our understanding of the mechanisms that give rise to the signals. For example, the mechanisms that lead to T2*-weighted fMRI during functional activation (Kwong et al. 1992; Ogawa et al. 1992; Frahm et al. 1992; Bandettini et al. 1992) were studied by comparing fMRI and NIRS, which relies on the differential light absorption of deoxy-Hb. It had been previously shown that the T2*-weighted MRI signal can change with

Table 4 Examples of cross-validation of EEG/MEG source estimation using tomographic functional brain imaging

Source estimation approach	Imaging validation method	References
MEG dipole source analysis	fMRI, PET, SPECT	Walter et al. (1992); Stefan et al. (1992)
EEG dipole source analysis	fMRI, PET	Menon et al. (1997); Grimm et al. (1998)
MEG linear source estimates		Not yet done
EEG linear source estimates	fMRI, PET	Gamma et al. (2004); Mulert et al. (2004)

Table 5   Examples of neurophysiological parameters studied using multimodal comparisons

Parameters measured for validation	Simultaneous combination of methods	References
[Deoxy-Hb]	fMRI and NIRS	Kleinschmidt et al. (1996); Kida et al. (1996); Punwani et al. (1998); Toronov et al. (2001); Mehagnoul-Schipper et al. (2002); Strangman et al. (2002)
Cerebral blood flow	H₂O- (or butanol)-PET and bolus-track MRI or ASL-MRI	Not yet done, but technically feasible and planned by a number of groups
Cerebral metabolic rate of oxygen (CMRO$_2$)	H₂O- (or butanol)- and O$_2$-PET and CMRO$_2$-MRI	Not yet done, but technically feasible and planned by a number of groups
Cerebral blood flow	Bolus track MRI and bolus track optical imaging	Feasible in principle, not yet done
Cerebral blood flow	Bolus track optical imaging (NIRS) and transcranial Doppler sonography (TCD)	Klaessens et al. (2005)
Corpuscular blood volume (total haemoglobin)	CO-PET and NIRS	Not yet done, although feasible in principle

haemoglobin oxygenation [the blood oxygen level dependent (BOLD) effect; Ogawa et al. 1990; Turner et al. 1991]; however, there are many other determinants of the T2* signal. Studies comparing the results of the two methods confirmed that T2*-weighted fMRI signal increases during functional activation correlate with local drops in [deoxy-Hb] (Kleinschmidt et al. 1996; Kida et al. 1996; Punwani et al. 1998; Toronov et al. 2001; Mehagnoul-Schipper et al. 2002; Strangman et al. 2002). Other examples of multimodal comparisons are given in Table 5.

4.2
Asymmetric Integration

A more advanced form of multimodal data integration than spatial comparison for validation or interpretation purposes is the use of data from one modality in the analysis of data from other modalities. This can be either spatially or temporally based. In the spatial domain, activated brain regions identified using PET or fMRI have been used as constraints or priors for the solution of the EEG/MEG inverse problem (Heinze et al. 1994; Liu et al. 1998; Daunizeau et al. 2006; Stancak et al. 2005; Babiloni et al. 2003).

Asymmetric integration in the temporal domain is commonly performed for the analysis of haemodynamic correlates of brain activity captured on EEG, and in particular in simultaneous acquisitions. For example, new insights into the relationship between neuronal activity and BOLD have been obtained by building models of BOLD change incorporating specific aspects of evoked responses measured at the single trial level in simultaneous EEG and fMRI acquisitions (Debener et al. 2005; Eichele et al. 2005; Mulert et al. 2008). A further variant is the assessment of evoked brain activity at different baseline states of the brain [e.g. sleep states (Portas et al. 2000), vigilance, attention, etc.], with the latter being identified by one method (often EEG) and the former by either the other method (e.g. fMRI) or again by a combination of the two (EEG–fMRI).

EEG usually provides the time or state marker in imaging studies of spontaneous brain activity: this is the EEG-derived hypothesis-driven approach to fMRI analysis. The paradigmatic example for the latter is the study of the haemodynamic correlates of epileptic spikes (Warach et al. 1996; Lemieux et al. 2001a, b; Krakow et al. 2001a, b). Again, one dataset (EEG) is used as a predictor of vascular changes in fMRI, PET or NIRS data. A similar situation is the assessment of vascular correlates of spontaneous changes in EEG rhythms, which can only be achieved by simultaneous studies (Goldman et al. 2002; Laufs et al. 2003; Moosmann et al. 2003). Examples are given in Table 6.

4.3
Symmetrical Data Fusion

The bias intrinsic to asymmetric data analysis strategies may reflect a preference on the part of the investigator, due to greater familiarity with, or better characterisation of (due to historical precedence for example), one of the signals of interest. As the relationship between signals from different modalities and the underlying generative mechanisms become better understood, this form of bias may diminish and more symmetric data integration strategies can emerge. For example, heuristic models of the relationship between EEG and BOLD can be integrated into joint source estimation schemes (Daunizeau et al. 2007; Brookings et al. 2009).

Some investigators have proposed a more fundamental approach to data integration aimed at creating biophysical models that relate the data from each modality within a unified framework in order to overcome current limitations in the interpretation of multimodal data and ultimately relate observations to the fundamental brain mechanisms. For example, while overlaying PET or NIRS activation maps with structural MRI can give an impression of a precise relationship between brain activity and structure, our understanding is ultimately limited by the lack of a proper model relating the two. This is also the case for the superposition of EP time courses at the millisecond time scale over fMRI activation sites that spatially coincide with electrical or magnetic source estimates. The spatial integration of EEG and fMRI is a much more complex issue than simply one offering another (independent) dimension to the other.

Data fusion at this neurophysiological level will require new computational models that link neuronal activity to haemodynamic, electrical, magnetic and other observables. This fundamental development represents the next frontier in neuroimaging, and will be discussed in the chapter "EEG–fMRI Information Fusion: Biophysics and Data Analysis".

Table 6 Examples of multimodal imaging that follows the principles of "adding complementary information" and "identifying and measuring"

Neurophysiological event	Measurement parameters	Combination of methods	References
Event-related brain activity under peripheral stimulation	Evoked potential (EEG), deoxy-Hb concentration changes (BOLD-fMRI)	EEG, MRI	Bonmassar et al. (1999, 2001); Allen et al. (2000); Goldman et al. (2000); Mulert et al. (2004, 2008); Becker et al. (2005)
	Evoked potential (EEG), deoxy-Hb and oxy-Hb concentration changes (BOLD-fMRI)	EEG, NIRS	Obrig et al. (2002); Horovitz and Gore (2004)
Variations in event-related brain activity under peripheral stimulation	Evoked potential (EEG), deoxy-Hb concentration changes (BOLD-fMRI)	EEG, MRI	Debener et al. (2005); Eichele et al. (2005); Benar et al. (2007); Mulert et al. (2008)
Alpha rhythms (background)	Occipital alpha rhythm (EEG), deoxy-Hb concentration changes (BOLD)	EEG, MRI	Goldman et al. (2002); Moosmann et al. (2003); Laufs et al. (2003)
	Occipital alpha rhythm (EEG), deoxy-Hb concentration changes (NIRS)	EEG, NIRS	Moosmann et al. (2003)
	Occipital alpha rhythm (EEG), cerebral blood flow (FDG-PET)	EEG, PET	Sheridan et al. (1988)
	Occipital alpha rhythm (EEG), cerebral blood flow (H_2O-PET)	EEG, PET	Sadato et al. (1998)
Epileptic brain activity	Epileptic spikes (EEG), deoxy-Hb concentration changes (BOLD-fMRI)	EEG, MRI	Warach et al. (1996); Lemieux et al. (2001a, b); Krakow et al. (2001a, b)
	Epileptic spikes (EEG), cerebral blood flow changes (flow-sensitive MRI)	EEG, MRI	Warach et al. (1994); Hamandi et al. (2008); Carmichael et al. (2008)
	Epileptic spikes (EEG), cerebral blood flow changes (Flow-sensitive MRI), deoxy-Hb concentration changes	EEG, MRI	Hamandi et al. (2008); Carmichael et al. (2008)
	Epileptic spikes (EEG), haemoglobin oxygenation changes (NIRS)	NIRS and EEG	Buchheim et al. (2004)
	Epileptic spikes (EEG), glucose metabolism (FDG-PET)	EEG, PET	Barrington et al. (1998)

(*continued*)

Table 6 (continued)

Neurophysiological event	Measurement parameters	Combination of methods	References
Evoked brain activity dependent on sleep state	Sleep stage (EEG), evoked potential (EEG), deoxy-Hb concentration changes (BOLD-fMRI)	EEG, MRI	Portas et al. (2000)
Pericentral alpha and beta rhythms	Pericentral rhythms (EEG), deoxy-Hb concentration changes (BOLD)	EEG and fMRI	Ritter et al. (2009)
Gamma band oscillation	40 Hz oscillation (EEG), deoxy-Hb concentration changes (BOLD-fMRI)	EEG, fMRI	Foucher et al. (2003)
Bursts of action potentials (spike bursts)	High frequency oscillations (600 Hz) in EEG, deoxy-Hb concentration changes (BOLD)	High-frequency EEG and fMRI	Ritter et al. (2008)
Evoked potentials (EEG) and evoked magnetic fields (MEG) (orthogonal to each other), both reflecting synaptic activity		MEG and EEG	Siedenberg et al. (1996)
Spreading depression	Cell swelling assessed by DWI and DC-EEG	MRI, EEG	Busch et al. (1995)
	Cell swelling assessed by DC-EEG, and changes in light scattering and haemoglobin oxygenation assessed by NIRS	MRI, NIRS	Kohl et al. (1998)
Slow neuronal events and vascular response	Slow neuronal depolarisation changes assessed by DC-MEG; changes in haemoglobin oxygenation assessed by NIRS	NIRS and MEG	Mackert et al. (2004, 2008)

5
Summary

Multimodal brain imaging is a key tool for gaining a comprehensive understanding of brain activity, since any single imaging method is limited to observing a limited aspect of brain function. We have noted that the validation of one imaging method using another has been a common reason for employing multimodal approaches over the last few years, and that various combinations of imaging methods may be useful, depending on the specific research questions that are being asked. However, the combination of information about the electrical activity of the brain with data on the corresponding haemodynamic changes, which offers superior spatial information, represents one of the most powerful examples of a multimodal imaging technique, and is one that is capable of providing new insights into brain function. While data acquired in separate sessions can be appropriate for some research questions, only simultaneous EEG–fMRI offers the opportunity to relate both modalities to actual brain events, an issue that is relevant to not only epilepsy but also numerous research questions in basic and cognitive neuroscience. In these cases, we believe that the extra effort required to deal with the specific practical problems of such a combination is easily outweighed by the potential new insights into human brain function that it offers. We hope to demonstrate this in the rest of this book.

References

Allen PJ, Josephs O, Turner R (2000) A method for removing imaging artifact from continuous EEG recorded during functional MRI. Neuroimage 12(2):230–9

Allen PJ, Polizzi G, Krakow K, Fish DR, Lemieux L (1998) Identification of EEG events in the MR scanner: the problem of pulse artifact and a method for its subtraction. Neuroimage 8(3): 229–39

Babiloni F, Babiloni C, Carducci F, Romani GL, Rossini PM, Angelone LM, Cincotti F (2003) Multimodal integration of high-resolution EEG and functional magnetic resonance imaging data: a simulation study. Neuroimage 19(1):1–15

Bandettini PA, Wong EC, Hinks RS, Tikofsky RS, Hyde JS (1992) Time course EPI of human brain function during task activation. Magn Reson Med 25(2):390–7

Barrington SF, Koutroumanidis M, Agathonikou A, Marsden PK, Binnie CD, Polkey CE, Maisey MN, Panayiotopoulos CP (1998) Clinical value of "ictal" FDG-positron emission tomography and the routine use of simultaneous scalp EEG studies in patients with intractable partial epilepsies. Epilepsia 39(7):753–66

Becker R, Ritter P, Moosmann M, Villringer A (2005) Visual evoked potentials recovered from fMRI scan periods. Hum Brain Mapp 26, 221–230

Benar C, Aghakhani Y, Wang Y, Izenberg A, Al Asmi A, Dubeau F, Gotman J (2003) Quality of EEG in simultaneous EEG-fMRI for epilepsy. Clin Neurophysiol 114, 569–580

Benar CG, Schon D, Grimault S, Nazarian B, Burle B, Roth M, Badier JM, Marquis P, Liegeois-Chauvel C, Anton JL (2007) Single-trial analysis of oddball event-related potentials in simultaneous EEG-fMRI. Hum Brain Mapp 28, 602–613

Beyer T, Townsend DW, Brun T, Kinahan PE, Charron M, Roddy R, Jerin J, Young J, Byars L, Nutt R (2000) A combined PET/CT scanner for clinical oncology. J Nucl Med 41(8):1369–79

Bonmassar G, Anami K, Ives J, Belliveau JW (1999) Visual evoked potential (VEP) measured by simultaneous 64-channel EEG and 3T fMRI. Neuroreport 10(9):1893–7

Bonmassar G, Schwartz DP, Liu AK, Kwong KK, Dale AM, Belliveau JW (2001) Spatiotemporal brain imaging of visual-evoked activity using interleaved EEG and fMRI recordings. Neuroimage 13(6 Pt 1):1035–43

Brandt SA, Davis TL, Obrig H, Meyer BU, Belliveau JW, Rosen BR, Villringer A (1996) Functional magnetic resonance imaging shows localized brain activation during serial transcranial stimulation in man. NeuroReport 7, 734–736

Brookings T, Ortigue S, Grafton S, Carlson J (2009) Using ICA and realistic BOLD models to obtain joint EEG/fMRI solutions to the problem of source localization. NeuroImage 44, 411–420

Buchheim K, Obrig H, v Pannwitz W, Müller A, Heekeren H, Villringer A, Meierkord H (2004) Decrease in haemoglobin oxygenation during absence seizures in adult humans. Neurosci Lett 354(2):119–22

Buchner H, Fuchs M, Wischmann HA, Dössel O, Ludwig I, Knepper A, Berg P (1994) Source analysis of median nerve and finger stimulated somatosensory evoked potentials: multichannel simultaneous recording of electric and magnetic fields combined with 3D-MR tomography. Brain Topogr 6(4):299–310

Busch E, Hoehn-Berlage M, Eis M, Gyngell ML, Hossmann KA (1995) Simultaneous recording of EEG, DC potential and diffusion-weighted NMR imaging during potassium induced cortical spreading depression in rats. NMR Biomed 8(2):59–64

Catana C, Procissi D, Wu Y, Judenhofer MS, Qi J, Pichler BJ, Jacobs RE, Cherry SR (2008) Simultaneous in vivo positron emission tomography and magnetic resonance imaging. Proc Natl Acad Sci USA 105(10):3705–10

Carmichael DW, Hamandi K, Laufs H, Duncan JS, Thomas DL, Lemieux L (2008) An investigation of the relationship between BOLD and perfusion signal changes during epileptic generalised spike wave activity. Magn Reson Imaging 26, 870–873

Daunizeau J, Grova C, Marrelec G, Mattout J, Jbabdi S, Pelegrini-Issac M, Lina JM, Benali H (2007) Symmetrical event-related EEG/fMRI information fusion in a variational Bayesian framework. NeuroImage 36, 69–87

Debener S, Ullsperger M, Siegel M, Fiehler K, von Cramon DY, Engel AK (2005) Trial-by-trial coupling of concurrent electroencephalogram and functional magnetic resonance imaging identifies the dynamics of performance monitoring. J Neurosci 25(50):11730–7

Eichele T, Specht K, Moosmann M, Jongsma ML, Quiroga RQ, Nordby H, Hugdahl K (2005) Assessing the spatiotemporal evolution of neuronal activation with single-trial event-related potentials and functional MRI. Proc Natl Acad Sci USA 102, 17798–17803

Foucher JR, Otzenberger H, Gounot D (2003) The BOLD response and the gamma oscillations respond differently than evoked potentials: an interleaved EEG-fMRI study. BMC Neurosci 4, 22

Frahm J, Bruhn H, Merboldt KD, Hänicke W (1992) Dynamic MR imaging of human brain oxygenation during rest and photic stimulation. J Magn Reson Imaging 2(5):501–5

Gamma A, Lehmann D, Frei E, Iwata K, Pascual-Marqui RD, Vollenweider FX (2004) Comparison of simultaneously recorded $[H_2^{15}O]$-PET and LORETA during cognitive and pharmacological activation. Hum Brain Mapp 22(2):83–96

Goldman RI, Stern JM, Engel J Jr, Cohen MS (2000) Acquiring simultaneous EEG and functional MRI. Clin Neurophysiol 111(11):1974–80

Goldman RI, Stern JM, Engel J Jr, Cohen MS (2002) Simultaneous EEG and fMRI of the alpha rhythm. Neuroreport 13(18):2487–92

Grimm Ch, Schreiber A, Kristeva-Feige R, Mergner Th, Hennig J, Lucking CH (1998) A comparison between electric source localisation and fMRI during somatosensory stimulation. Electroencephalogr-Clin-Neurophysiol 106, 22–29

Hamandi K, Laufs H, Noth U, Carmichael DW, Duncan JS, Lemieux L (2008) BOLD and perfusion changes during epileptic generalised spike wave activity. NeuroImage 39, 608–618

Heinze HJ, Mangun GR, Burchert W, Hinrichs H, Scholz M, Munte TF, Gos A, Scherg M, Johannes S, Hundeshagen H (1994) Combined spatial and temporal imaging of brain activity during visual selective attention in humans. Nature 372, 543–546

Horovitz SG, Gore JC (2004) Simultaneous event-related potential and near-infrared spectroscopic studies of semantic processing. Hum Brain Mapp 22(2):110–5

Hoshi Y, Mizukami S, Tamura M (1994) Dynamic features of hemodynamic and metabolic changes in the human brain during all-night sleep as revealed by near-infrared spectroscopy. Brain Res 652(2):257–62

Ives JR, Warach S, Schmitt F, Edelman RR, Schomer DL (1993) Monitoring the patient's EEG during echo planar MRI. Electroencephalogr Clin Neurophysiol 87:417–20

Judenhofer MS, Wehrl HF, Newport DF, Catana C, Siegel SB, Becker M, Thielscher A, Kneilling M, Lichy MP, Eichner M, Klingel K, Reischl G, Widmaier S, Röcken M, Nutt RE, Machulla HJ, Uludag K, Cherry SR, Claussen CD, Pichler BJ (2008) Simultaneous PET-MRI: a new approach for functional and morphological imaging. Nat Med 14(4):459–65

Kida I, Yamamoto T, Tamura M (1996) Interpretation of BOLD MRI signals in rat brain using simultaneously measured near-infrared spectrophotometric information. NMR Biomed 9(8): 333–8

Kirkpatrick PJ, Lam J, Al-Rawi P, Smielewski P, Czosnyka M (1998) Defining thresholds for critical ischemia by using near-infrared spectroscopy in the adult brain. J Neurosurg 89(3):389–94

Klaessens JH, Hopman JC, van Wijk MC, Djien Liem K, Thijssen JM (2005) Assessment of local changes of cerebral perfusion and blood concentration by near infrared spectroscopy and ultrasound contrast densitometry. Brain Dev 27(6):406–14

Kleinschmidt A, Obrig H, Requardt M, Merboldt KD, Dirnagl U, Villringer A, Frahm J (1996) Simultaneous recording of cerebral blood oxygenation changes during human brain activation by magnetic resonance imaging and near-infrared spectroscopy. J Cereb Blood Flow Metab 16(5):817–26

Kohl M, Lindauer U, Dirnagl U, Villringer A (1998) Separation of changes in light scattering and chromophore concentrations during cortical spreading depression in rats. Opt Lett 23(7): 555–7

Krakow K, Allen PJ, Symms MR, Lemieux L, Josephs O, Fish DR (2000) EEG recording during fMRI experiments: image quality. Hum Brain Mapp 10(1):10–5

Krakow K, Lemieux L, Messina D, Scott CA, Symms MR, Duncan JS, Fish DR (2001a) Spatiotemporal imaging of focal interictal epileptiform activity using EEG-triggered functional MRI. Epileptic Disord 3(2):67–74

Krakow K, Messina D, Lemieux L, Duncan JS, Fish DR (2001b) Functional MRI activation of individual interictal epileptiform spikes. Neuroimage 13(3):502–5

Kwong KK, Belliveau JW, Chesler DA, Goldberg IE, Weisskoff RM, Poncelet BP, Kennedy DN, Hoppel BE, Cohen MS, Turner R, Brady TJ, Rosen BR (1992) Dynamic magnetic resonance imaging of human brain activity during primary sensory stimulation. Proc Natl Acad Sci USA 89(12):5675–9

Laufs H, Kleinschmidt A, Beyerle A, Eger E, Salek-Haddadi A, Preibisch C, Krakow K (2003) EEG-correlated fMRI of human alpha activity. NeuroImage 19, 1463–1476

Lemieux L, Allen PJ, Franconi F, Symms MR, Fish DR (1997) Recording of EEG during fMRI experiments: patient safety. Magn Reson Med 38(6):943–52

Lemieux L, Krakow K, Fish DR (2001a) Comparison of spike-triggered functional MRI BOLD activation and EEG dipole model localization. Neuroimage 14(5):1097–104

Lemieux L, Salek-Haddadi A, Josephs O, Allen P, Toms N, Scott C, Krakow K, Turner R, Fish DR (2001b) Event-related fMRI with simultaneous and continuous EEG: description of the method and initial case report. Neuroimage 14(3):780–7

Liu AK, Belliveau JW, Dale AM (1998) Spatiotemporal imaging of human brain activity using functional MRI constrained magnetoencephalography data: Monte Carlo simulations. Proc-Natl-Acad-Sci-USA 95, 8945–8950

Mackert BM, Leistner S, Sander T, Liebert A, Wabnitz H, Burghoff M, Trahms L, Macdonald R, Curio G (2008) Dynamics of cortical neurovascular coupling analyzed by simultaneous DC-magnetoencephalography and time-resolved near-infrared spectroscopy. Neuroimage 39(3):979–86

Mackert BM, Wübbeler G, Leistner S, Uludag K, Obrig H, Villringer A, Trahms L, Curio G (2004) Neurovascular coupling analyzed non-invasively in the human brain. Neuroreport 15(1):63–6

McDannold N, Moss M, Killiany R, Rosene DL, King RL, Jolesz FA, Hynynen K (2003) MRI-guided focused ultrasound surgery in the brain: tests in a primate model. Magn Reson Med 49(6):1188–91

Mehagnoul-Schipper DJ, van der Kallen BF, Colier WN, van der Sluijs MC, van Erning LJ, Thijssen HO, Oeseburg B, Hoefnagels WH, Jansen RW (2002) Simultaneous measurements of cerebral oxygenation changes during brain activation by near-infrared spectroscopy and functional magnetic resonance imaging in healthy young and elderly subjects. Hum Brain Mapp 16(1):14–23

Menon V, Ford JM, Lim KO, Glover GH, Pfefferbaum A (1997) Combined event-related fMRI and EEG evidence for temporal-parietal cortex activation during target detection. NeuroReport 8, 3029–3037

Moosmann M, Ritter P, Krastel I, Brink A, Thees S, Blankenburg F, Taskin B, Obrig H, Villringer A (2003) Correlates of alpha rhythm in functional magnetic resonance imaging and near infrared spectroscopy. NeuroImage 20, 145–158

Mulert C, Jäger L, Schmitt R, Bussfeld P, Pogarell O, Möller HJ, Juckel G, Hegerl U (2004) Integration of fMRI and simultaneous EEG: towards a comprehensive understanding of localization and time-course of brain activity in target detection. Neuroimage 22(1):83–94

Mulert C, Seifert C, Leicht G, Kirsch V, Ertl M, Karch S, Moosmann M, Lutz J, Möller HJ, Hegerl U, Pogarell O, Jäger L (2008) Single-trial coupling of EEG and fMRI reveals the involvement of early anterior cingulate cortex activation in effortful decision making. Neuroimage 42(1):158–68

Obrig H, Israel H, Kohl-Bareis M, Uludag K, Wenzel R, Müller B, Arnold G, Villringer A (2002) Habituation of the visually evoked potential and its vascular response: implications for neurovascular coupling in the healthy adult. Neuroimage 17(1):1–18

Ogawa S, Lee TM, Kay AR, Tank DW (1990) Brain magnetic resonance imaging with contrast dependent on blood oxygenation. Proc Natl Acad Sci USA 87(24):9868–72

Ogawa S, Tank DW, Menon R, Ellermann JM, Kim SG, Merkle H, Ugurbil K (1992) Intrinsic signal changes accompanying sensory stimulation: functional brain mapping with magnetic resonance imaging. Proc Natl Acad Sci USA 89(13):5951–5

Portas CM, Krakow K, Allen P, Josephs O, Armony JL, Frith CD (2000) Auditory processing across the sleep-wake cycle: simultaneous EEG and fMRI monitoring in humans. Neuron 28(3):991–9

Punwani S, Ordidge RJ, Cooper CE, Amess P, Clemence M (1998) MRI measurements of cerebral deoxyhaemoglobin concentration [dHb]—correlation with near infrared spectroscopy (NIRS). NMR Biomed 11(6):281–9

Ritter P, Moosmann M, Villringer A (2009) Rolandic alpha and beta EEG rhythms' strengths are inversely related to fMRI-BOLD signal in primary somatosensory and motor cortex1. Hum Brain Mapp 30, 1168–1187

Sabri O, Owega A, Schreckenberger M, Sturz L, Fimm B, Kunert P, Meyer PT, Sander D, Klingelhöfer J (2003) A truly simultaneous combination of functional transcranial Doppler sonography and $H_2^{15}O$ PET adds fundamental new information on differences in cognitive activation between schizophrenics and healthy control subjects. J Nucl Med 44(5):671–81

Sadato N, Nakamura S, Oohashi T, Nishina E, Fuwamoto Y, Waki A, Yonekura Y (1998) Neural networks for generation and suppression of alpha rhythm: a PET study. Neuroreport 9(5):893–7

Salustri C, Chapman RM (1989) A simple method for 3-dimensional localization of epileptic activity recorded by simultaneous EEG and MEG. Electroencephalogr Clin Neurophysiol 73(6):473–8

Sheridan PH, Sato S, Foster N, Bruno G, Cox C, Fedio P, Chase TN (1988) Relation of EEG alpha background to parietal lobe function in Alzheimer's disease as measured by positron emission tomography and psychometry. Neurology 38(5):747–50

Siedenberg R, Goodin DS, Aminoff MJ, Rowley HA, Roberts TP (1996) Abstract comparison of late components in simultaneously recorded event-related electrical potentials and event-related magnetic fields. Electroencephalogr Clin Neurophysiol 99(2):191–4

Stancak A, Polacek H, Vrana J, Rachmanova R, Hoechstetter K, Tintra J, Scherg M (2005) EEG source analysis and fMRI reveal two electrical sources in the fronto-parietal operculum during subepidermal finger stimulation. NeuroImage 25, 8–20

Stefan H, Schneider S, Feistel H, Pawlik G, Schuler P, Abraham Fuchs K, Schlegel T, Neubauer U, Huk WJ (1992) Ictal and interictal activity in partial epilepsy recorded with multichannel magnetoelectroencephalography: correlation of electroencephalography/electrocorticography, magnetic resonance imaging, single photon emission computed tomography, and positron emission tomography findings. Epilepsia 33, 874–87

Steinhoff BJ, Herrendorf G, Kurth C (1996) Ictal near infrared spectroscopy in temporal lobe epilepsy: a pilot study. Seizure 5(2):97–101

Strangman G, Culver JP, Thompson JH, Boas DA (2002) A quantitative comparison of simultaneous BOLD fMRI and NIRS recordings during functional brain activation. Neuroimage 17(2): 719–31

Terborg C, Birkner T, Schack B, Weiller C, Röther J (2003) Noninvasive monitoring of cerebral oxygenation during vasomotor reactivity tests by a new near-infrared spectroscopy device. Cerebrovasc Dis 16(1):36–41

Toronov V, Webb A, Choi JH, Wolf M, Michalos A, Gratton E, Hueber D (2001) Investigation of human brain hemodynamics by simultaneous near-infrared spectroscopy and functional magnetic resonance imaging. Med Phys 28(4):521–7

Turner R, Le Bihan D, Moonen CT, Despres D, Frank J (1991) Echo-planar time course MRI of cat brain oxygenation changes. Magn Reson Med 22(1):159–66

Villringer A, Dirnagl U (1995) Coupling of brain activity and cerebral blood flow: basis of functional neuroimaging. Cerebrovasc Brain Metab Rev 7(3):240–76

Villringer K, Minoshima S, Hock C, Obrig H, Ziegler S, Dirnagl U, Schwaiger M, Villringer A (1997) Comparison of near infrared spectroscopy and positron emission tomography in the assessment of frontal brain activation in humans. Adv Exp Med Biol 413:149–153

Warach S, Ives JR, Schlaug G, Patel MR, Darby DG, Thangaraj V, Edelman RR, Schomer DL (1996) EEG-triggered echo-planar functional MRI in epilepsy. Neurology 47(1):89–93

Warach S, Levin JM, Schomer DL, Holman BL, Edelman RR (1994) Hyperperfusion of ictal seizure focus demonstrated by MR perfusion imaging. AJNR Am J Neuroradiol 15(5):965–8

Walter H, Kristeva R, Knorr U, Schlaug G, Huang Y, Steinmetz H, Nebeling B, Herzog H, Seitz RJ (1992) Individual somatotopy of primary sensorimotor cortex revealed by intermodal matching of MEG, PET, and MRI. Brain Topogr 5, 183–187

Zotev VS, Matlashov AN, Volegov PL, Savukov IM, Espy MA, Mosher JC, Gomez JJ, Kraus RH Jr (2008) Microtesla MRI of the human brain combined with MEG. J Magn Reson 194:115–20

EEG: Origin and Measurement

2

Fernando Lopes da Silva

1
Introduction to the Electrophysiology of the Brain

The existence of the electrical activity of the brain (i.e. the electroencephalogram or EEG) was discovered more than a century ago by Caton. After the demonstration that the EEG could be recorded from the human scalp by Berger in the 1920s, it made a slow start before it became accepted as a method of analysis of brain functions in health and disease. It is interesting to note that this acceptance came only after the demonstration by Adrian and Mathews (1934) that the EEG, namely the alpha rhythm, was likely generated in the occipital lobes in man, and was not artefactual. However, the neuronal sources of the alpha rhythm remained undefined until the 1970s, when we demonstrated, in dog, that the alpha rhythm is generated by a dipole layer cantered at layers IV and V of the visual cortex (Lopes da Silva and Storm van Leeuwen 1977). It may be not surprising that the mechanisms of generation and the functional significance of the EEG remained controversial for a relatively long time considering the complexity of the underlying systems of neuronal generators on the one hand and the rather involved transfer of signals from the cortical surface to the scalp due to the topological and electrical properties of the volume conductor (brain, cerebrospinal fluid, skull, scalp) on the other.

The EEG consists of the summed electrical activities of populations of neurons, with a modest contribution from glial cells. The neurons are excitable cells with characteristic intrinsic electrical properties, and their activity produces electrical and magnetic fields. These fields may be recorded by means of electrodes at a short distance from the sources (the local EEG or local field potentials, LFPs), or from the cortical surface (the electrocorticogram or ECoG), or at longer distances, even from the scalp (i.e. the EEG, in the most common sense). The associated MEG is usually recorded via sensors that are highly sensitive to changes in the very weak neuronal magnetic fields, which are placed at short distances around the scalp.

F. Lopes da Silva
Centre of NeuroSciences, Swammerdam Institute for Life Sciences, University of Amsterdam, Kruislaan 320, 1098, SM Amsterdam, The Netherlands
e-mail: silva@science.uva.nl

C. Mulert and L. Lemieux (eds.), *EEG– fMRI*
DOI: 10.1007/978-3-540-87919-0_2, © Springer Verlag Berlin Heidelberg 2010

2
Origin of EEG and MEG I: Cellular Sources

Neurons generate time-varying electrical currents when activated. These are ionic currents generated at the level of cellular membranes; in other words, they consist of transmembrane currents. We can distinguish two main forms of neuronal activation (Lopes da Silva and van Rotterdam 2005; Lopes da Silva 2002; Nunez (1995)): the fast depolarisation of the neuronal membranes, which results in the action potential mediated by the sodium and potassium voltage-dependent ionic conductances gNa and gK (DR), and the slower changes in membrane potential due to synaptic activation, as mediated by several neurotransmitter systems. The action potential consists of a rapid change in membrane potential such that the intracellular potential suddenly jumps from negative to positive, and quickly (in 1 or 2 ms) returns to the resting intracellular negativity. In this way, an impulse is generated that has the remarkable property of propagating along axons and dendrites without any loss of amplitude. Regarding the slower postsynaptic potentials, two main kinds have to be distinguished: the excitatory (EPSPs) and the inhibitory (IPSPs) potentials, which depend on the kind of neurotransmitter and corresponding receptor and their interactions with specific ionic channels and/or intracellular second messengers.

Generally speaking, at the level of a synapse in the case of the EPSP, the transmembrane current is carried by positive ions inwards (e.g. Na^+). In the case of the IPSP, it is carried by negative ions inwards (e.g. Cl^-) or positive ions (e.g. K^+) outwards. Thus, the positive electric current is directed to the extracellular medium in the case of an EPSP and is directed from the inside of the neuron to the outside in the case of an IPSP (Fig. 1).

As a consequence of these currents, an active sink is generated in the extracellular medium at the level of an excitatory synapse, whereas in the case of an inhibitory synapse an active source occurs. The flows of these compensating extracellularly currents depend on the electrical properties of the local tissue. Glial cells occupy an important part of the space between neurons and are coupled to one another by gap junctions. The conductivity of the latter is very sensitive to changes in pH and extracellular K^+ and Ca^{2+}, and can therefore be modulated under various physiological and pathological conditions (Huang et al. 2005). Furthermore, the volume of the extracellular space may change under various physiological and pathological conditions, which will also be reflected in changes in tissue conductivity.

Since there is no accumulation of charge anywhere in the medium, the transmembrane currents that flow in or out of the neuron at the active synaptic sites are compensated by currents that flow in the opposite direction elsewhere along the neuronal membrane. Consequently, in the case of an EPSP, besides the active sink at the level of the synapse, there are distributed passive sources along the soma-dendritic membrane. The opposite occurs in the case of an IPSP: besides the active source at the level of the synapse, distributed passive sinks are formed along the soma-dendritic membrane.

Therefore, we can state that synaptic activity at a given site of the soma-dendritic membrane of a neuron causes a sink–source configuration in the extracellular medium around the neurons. In the context of the present discussion, we have to take into consideration the geometry of the neuronal sources of electrical activity. Indeed, the neurons that mainly

Post-synaptic extra-cellular potentials

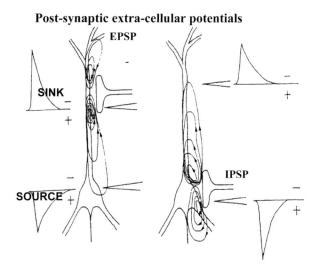

Fig. 1 Scheme of a cortical pyramidal cell showing the patterns of current flow caused by two modes of synaptic activation at an excitatory (*E*) and an inhibitory (*I*) synapse. Typically the apical dendrites of these cells are oriented toward the cortical surface. *EPSP*: current flow caused by the activation of an excitatory synapse at the level of the apical dendrite creates a *current sink* in the extracellular medium next to the synapse. The extracellularly recorded EPSP is drawn on the *left*. It has a negative polarity at the level of the synapse. At the soma there is a distributed passive *current source* resulting in an extracellular potential of positive polarity. *IPSP*: current flow caused by activation of an inhibitory synapse at the level of the soma creates an extracellular source at the level of the soma and a passive sink at the basal and apical dendrites. The IPSP recorded extracellularly at the level of the soma and of the apical dendrites is shown. Note that both cases show a dipolar source–sink configuration. (Adapted from Niedermeyer 2005; Lopes da Silva and van Rotterdam 2005)

contribute to the MEG or the EEG are those that form "open fields" according to the classic description of Lorente de Nó (1947), i.e. the pyramidal neurons of the cortex, since the latter are arranged in palisades with the apical dendrites aligned perpendicularly to the cortical surface. Pyramidal neurons, when activated with a certain degree of synchrony, generate coherent electric/magnetic fields. In this way, these neurons are akin to "current dipoles", the activity of which can be detected by electrodes placed at relatively small distances.

In quantitative terms, our current level of knowledge about the neuronal sources of EEG/MEG signals has benefited a great deal from recent model studies combining in vitro recordings and computational simulations, such as those proposed by the group of Yoshio Okada. These authors adapted the detailed compartmental models of Traub et al. (1994) and Traub and Miles (1991) and applied them to hippocampal slices kept in vitro, and also to the neocortex. Measured electric and magnetic activities were compared with the theoretical results of a computer model. The study of Murakami et al. (2006) in the neocortex is particularly relevant to the present discussion because it has yielded some results that may help to interpret EEG and MEG recordings from the scalp. These authors made a computer model, based on that proposed by Mainen and Sejnowski (1996), of the four main types of cortical neurons, taking into account their realistic shapes. Each neuron is described as a 3D compartmental model, where each compartment has its typical geometric dimensions, passive electrical properties (membrane capacitance and resistance, intracellular resistance), and five voltage-dependent ionic conductances; the quantitative values of these variables were taken from the literature. For example, the maximal sodium conductance gNa was assumed to be 40 pS μm^{-2} based on the measurements of Stuart and Sakman (1994), but several values were used in a trial and error way to reproduce experimental results. Neuronal activity was obtained by stimulating each neuron with an intracellular current injected at the soma. The intracellular current is represented by a vector quantity Q.

According to this model, the overall magnitude of Q for the activity of one pyramidal neuron of layers V and II/III is on the order of 0.29–0.90 pA, a value that is of the same order of magnitude as that estimated for hippocampal pyramidal neurons (Okada et al. 1997). Murakami et al. (2006) point out that, assuming a Q of 0.2 pA per cortical pyramidal neuron, a population of 50,000 synchronously active cells would generate a field with a magnitude of 10 nA, which corresponds precisely to the value measurable from the human cortex using the MEG according to Hämäläinen et al. (1993). According to the latter, the average value of the volume current density of the cerebral cortex is 175 nA/mm^2 (or nA mm/mm^3) for normal background activity. Assuming a cortical thickness of 3 mm, the average value of the corresponding surface current density is 525 nA/mm, and the average value of the dipole moment $m_i(t)$ associated with a neuronal population i of surface s_i is $M = s_i \times 525$ (nA mm). We will return to these concepts when discussing volume conduction and source estimation.

3
Main Types of Rhythmical EEG/MEG Activities: Phenomenology and Functional Significance

We do not consider all of the different types of rhythmical activities that can be recorded from the brain here, only some prominent activities that are frequently the object of neurocognitive studies, namely sleep rhythms, activities in the alpha frequency range and beta/gamma rhythms. A comprehensive, erudite and thoughtful analysis of these and other brain rhythms can be found in Buzsáki's (2006) monography *Rhythms of the Brain*.

3.1
Sleep EEG Phenomena

In the neurophysiology of sleep, two classic EEG phenomena have been established: the *spindles* or waves between 7 and 14 Hz, also called sleep or *sigma spindles*, which appear at sleep onset, and the *delta waves* (1–4 Hz), which are paradigmatic of deeper stages of sleep. Steriade and his group in Quebec (see Sect. 2) described another very slow oscillation (0.6–1 Hz) in animals that is able to modulate the occurrence of different typical EEG sleep events, such as delta waves, sleep spindles and even short, high-frequency bursts.

This very slow oscillation has now also been demonstrated in the human EEG and in the MEG, as indicated above.

The sleep spindles are generated in the thalamocortical circuits and result from the interplay between intrinsic membrane properties of the thalamocortical relay neurons (TCR) and of the GABAergic neurons of the reticular nucleus and the properties of the circuits to which these neurons belong. It is clear that the spindles are a collective property of the neuronal populations. Experimental evidence has demonstrated that the sleep spindle oscillations are generated in the thalamus since they can be recorded in this brain area after decortication and high brain stem transection. However, the very slow rhythm (0.6–1 Hz) is generated intracortically, since it survives thalamic lesions but it is disrupted by intracortical lesions. Interestingly, we may note that the rhythmicity of the very slow oscillation appears to be reflected in that of the typical K-complexes of human EEG during non-REM sleep (Amzica and Steriade 1997).

One question is: how are these oscillations controlled by modulating systems? It is well known that sleep spindles are under brain stem control. It is a well-known neurophysiological phenomenon that electrical stimulation of the brain stem can block thalamocortical oscillations, causing "EEG desynchronisation", as shown in classic studies by Moruzzi and Magoun (1949). This desynchronisation is caused mainly by the activation of cholinergic inputs arising from the mesopontine cholinergic nuclei, namely the pedunculopontine tegmental (PPT) and the laterodorsal tegmental (LTD) areas. Indeed, both the reticular nucleus and the TCR neurons receive cholinergic muscarinic synapses. Cholinergic activation of the reticular nucleus neurons elicits hyperpolarisation with an increase in K^+ conductance, which is mediated by an increase in a muscarinic-activated potassium current, and in contrast it causes depolarisation of TCR neurons. Furthermore, the reticular nucleus receives inputs from the basal forebrain that may be GABAergic and can also exert a strong inhibition on the reticular neurons, leading to the subsequent suppression of spindle oscillations. In addition, monoaminergic inputs from the brain stem, namely those arising at the mesopontine junction (i.e. from the noradrenergic neurons of the locus coeruleus and the serotoninergic neurons of the dorsal raphe nuclei) also modulate the rhythmic activities of the forebrain. These neuronal systems have only a weak thalamic projection but they have a diffuse projection to the cortex. Metabotropic glutamate receptors also appear to exert a modulating influence on the activation of thalamic circuits by descending corticothalamic systems.

Because this point is often misunderstood, we should emphasise that slow-wave sleep, characterised by typical EEG delta activity, does not correspond to a state where cortical neurons are inactive. On the contrary: in this sleep state cortical neurons can display mean rates of firing similar to those that they show during wakefulness and/or REM sleep. Regarding the neuronal firing patterns, the main difference between delta sleep on the one hand and wakefulness and REM sleep on the other is that, in the former, the neurons tend to display rather long bursts of spikes with relatively prolonged interburst periods of silence, whereas in the latter the firing pattern is more continuous. The functional meaning of these peculiar firing patterns of delta sleep has not yet been unravelled.

In general terms we can state that EEG signals co-vary strongly with different levels of arousal and consciousness. The changes in EEG with increasing levels of anaesthesia are typical examples of this property.

3.2
Alpha Rhythms of Neocortex and Thalamus

Alpha rhythms recorded from the occipital areas occur in relaxed awake animals and show a typical reactivity to closure of the eyes. Background illumination can result in decreased alpha rhythm amplitude (Paskewitz et al. 1973; Cram et al. 1977), while investigations of the suspected relationship between heart rate and alpha have not led to any firm conclusions (Stenett 1966; Surwillo 1965, 1967).

Although the frequency range of alpha rhythms overlaps that of sleep spindles, these two types of phenomena differ in a number of aspects. Namely, the behavioural states at which these types of oscillations occur are quite different, and their distributions over the thalamus and cortex also differ considerably, as exemplified by Fig. 2. The basic mechanisms responsible for alpha oscillations at the cellular level have not been described in detail. The reason for this is the inherent difficulty of studying a phenomenon that—by definition—occurs in the state of relaxed wakefulness, under conditions where measurement of the underlying membrane currents is not a simple task, since this cannot be done under anaesthesia. To overcome this difficulty, some researchers have assumed that spindles occurring under barbiturate anaesthesia are analogous to alpha rhythms. However, this analogy was challenged on experimental grounds because a comparative investigation of alpha rhythms obtained during restful wakefulness upon closure of the eyes, and spindles induced by barbiturates, recorded from the same sites over the visual cortex and lateral geniculate nuclei in dog, presented differences in frequency, spindle duration, topographic distribution and amount of coherence among different cortical and thalamic sites. Investigations combining multiple electrode arrays placed on the cortical surface, intracortical depth profiles and intrathalamic recordings from several thalamic nuclei unravelled a number of elementary properties of alpha rhythms (Lopes da Silva 1991):

- In the visual cortex, alpha waves are generated by a current dipole layer centred at the level of the somata and basal dendrites of the pyramidal neurons of layers IV and V
- The coherence between alpha waves recorded from neighbouring cortical sites is greater than any thalamocortical coherence
- The influence of alpha signals recorded from the pulvinar on cortical rhythms can be conspicuously large, depending on the cortical area, but intracortical factors play a significant role in establishing cortical domains of alpha activity

These experimental findings led to the conclusion that, in addition to the influence of some thalamic nuclei (mainly the pulvinar) on the generation of alpha rhythms in the visual cortex, there are systems of surface-parallel intracortical connections that are responsible for the propagation of alpha rhythms over the cortex. These oscillations appear to be generated in small patches of cortex that behave as epicentres, from which they propagate at relatively slow velocities, about 0.3 cm s^{-1}. This type of spatial propagation has been confirmed, in general terms, by experimental and model studies. A comprehensive study of alpha rhythms in the visual cortex of the cat (Rougeul-Buser and Buser 1997; Buser and Rougeul-Buser 2005) showed characteristics corresponding closely to those of alpha rhythms in man and in dog. It was found that this rhythmic

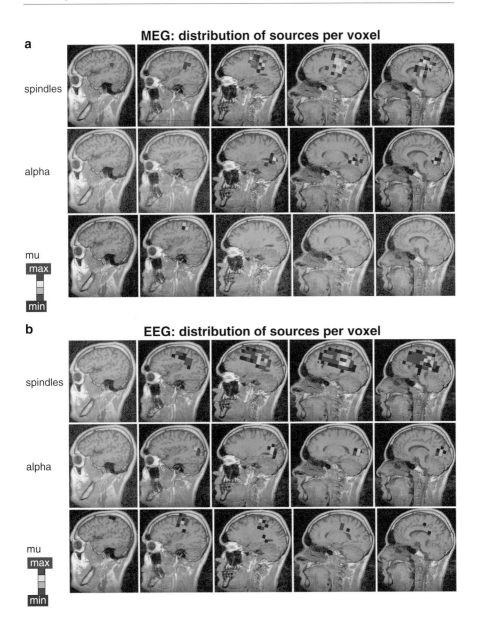

Fig. 2 a–b Dipole density plots of the MEG and EEG sleep spindles, alpha and mu rhythms of one subject. Voxels containing a relative high amount of dipoles are shown in *red. Blue* voxels contain relatively few dipoles. Voxels comprising less than 10% of the maximal amount of dipoles present in the red voxels are omitted for clarity. **a** MEG data: the "hot spots" for the MEG spindles are located in the centroposterior areas; **b** EEG data: the plots demonstrate that there is no overlap of the alpha and mu clusters. Furthermore, the "hot spot" of the alpha rhythm is located more superficially than those of the spindles, whereas the spindle cluster is more widespread than that of the alpha rhythm. The EEG sleep spindle dipoles spread to more frontal areas than the MEG data. (Adapted from Manshanden et al. 2002)

activity was localised to a limited part of the primary visual cortex area 18 and the border between 17 and 18. In this context, more insight into the sources of alpha rhythms in man was obtained using EEG and MEG recordings integrated with anatomical information obtained from magnetic resonance images (MRI), as shown in Fig. 2. Different sources of alpha rhythms were found to be mainly concentrated in the region around the calcarine fissure, with most sources occurring within 2 cm from the midline. In addition to the alpha rhythms of the visual cortex, rhythmic activities with about the same frequency range (in man: 8–13 Hz; in cat: 12–15 Hz) have been shown to occur in other cortical areas, namely in the somatosensory cortex (SI areas 1, 2 and 3). These activities are known as "rolandic *mu rhythms*", or "wicket rhythms" (named after the appearance of the records on the scalp in man), and have a typical reactivity, since they appear when the subject is at rest and are blocked by movement. The mu rhythm is particularly pronounced in the hand area of the somatosensory cortex, and it reacts typically to the movement of closing the fists. In the cat, there is no significant coherence between the mu rhythm of the SI cortex and the alpha rhythm of the visual cortex, which supports the general idea that these two types of rhythms are independent. Furthermore, mu rhythms of the SI area also differ from the alpha rhythms of the visual cortex recorded in the same animal, in that the former have systematically higher frequencies than the latter, the difference being about 2 Hz. Mu rhythms were also recorded in thalamic nuclei, namely in the ventropos-terior lateral nucleus. The mu rhythm has also been identified in MEG recordings over the Rolandic sulcus, particularly over the somatomotor hand area. In addition, another spon-taneous MEG activity, the so-called *tau rhythm*, was detected over the auditory cortex. This rhythmic activity was reduced by sound stimuli. This MEG tau rhythm, which was first described by the group of Hari (Hari et al. 1997; Lehtelä et al. 1997), is apparently similar to an EEG rhythm that was found using epidural electrodes over the midtemporal region by Niedermeyer (2005), who called it "third rhythm" or "independent temporal alphoid rhythm".

The cellular mechanisms responsible for the generation of alpha rhythms have recently been unveiled using in vitro preparations of thalamic nuclei. Hughes et al. (2004) showed that in the lateral geniculate nucleus, oscillations in the alpha frequency range can be gen-erated by the pharmacological activation of the metabotropic glutamate receptor (mGluR) mGluR1a. These oscillations display similarities with thalamic alpha rhythms recorded in the intact animal. Hughes and Crunelli (2005) discovered that the occurrence of these oscillations depends on the activity of a subset of thalamocortical (TC) neurons termed high-threshold (HT) bursting cells, which are interconnected via gap junctions. These in vitro thalamic alpha rhythms can slow down until the theta frequency range when the TC neuron population is less depolarised.

3.3
Beta/Gamma Activity of the Neocortex

The identification and characterisation of high-frequency rhythms in the neocortex has concentrated mainly on two neocortical areas, the visual cortex and the somatomotor cor-tex. Here we examine here some of the properties of the *beta/gamma* rhythmic activities for these two areas, although beta/gamma rhythmic activities have also been recorded in olfactory brain areas, particularly by Freeman (2005).

Commonly, the EEG of the *visual cortex* is associated with the alpha rhythm, with its typical reactivity upon closing and opening the eyes, as described above. However, other types of rhythmic activities can be present in the same cortical areas, namely within the beta frequency range. In the dog, we showed that the EEG spectral density was characterised by peaks within the beta/gamma frequency range while the animal was looking attentively at a visual stimulus (Lopes da Silva et al. 1970). Similarly, Freeman and van Dijk (1987) found in the visual cortex of a rhesus monkey that fast EEG rhythms (spectral peak of 30 ± 3.7 Hz) occurred during a conditioned task in response to a visual stimulus. A related finding is the discovery by the group of Charles Gray and Wolf Singer (Gray et al. 1989) and by Eckhorn et al. (1988) of oscillations within the beta/gamma frequency range (most commonly between 30 and 60 Hz) in the firing of individual neurons of the visual cortex in response to moving light bars. It was demonstrated using auto- and cross-correlation analyses that neurons tended to fire in synchrony, in an oscillatory mode, within cortical patches that could extend up to distances of about 7 mm. The oscillations in neuronal firing rate were correlated with those of the LFPs. The cortical oscillations are modulated by the activation of the mesencephalic reticular formation (MRF), but the stimulation of the MRF alone does not change the pattern of firing of the cortical neurons (Munk et al. 1996). However, MRF stimulation increases the amplitude and coherence of both the LFP and multiunit responses when applied jointly with a visual stimulus.

In the *somatomotor cortex*, beta/gamma oscillations of both neuronal firing and LFPs were also described in the awake cat by the group of Buser and Rougeul-Buser (2005), Bouyer et al. (1987) particularly when the animal was in a state of enhanced vigilance while watching an unreachable mouse. Also, fast oscillations were found in the somatomotor cortex in monkey during a state of enhanced attention (Rougeul et al. 1979). Oscillations of 25–35 Hz occurred in the sensorimotor cortex of awake, behaving monkeys in both LFPs and single-/multiunit recordings. They were particularly apparent during the performance of motor tasks that required fine finger movements and focussed attention. These oscillations were coherent over cortical patches extending up to at least 14 mm that included the cortical representation of the arm. Synchronous oscillations straddling the central sulcus were also found, so they may reflect the integration of sensory and motor processes. The LFP reversed polarity at about 800 μm under the cortical surface, indicating that the source of the LFP is in the superficial cortical layers. It is noteworthy that at least some of the cortical beta/gamma rhythmic activities appear to depend on projecting dopaminergic fibres arising in the ventral tegmental area, but the extent to which the beta rhythms of the somatomotor cortex are related to thalamic or other subcortical activities is not yet clear.

With respect to the origin of beta/gamma rhythmic activity, several experimental facts have led to the interpretation that these rhythmic activities are primarily generated in the cortex itself. These include the fact that oscillations in the beta/gamma frequency range were easily recorded from different cortical sites but not from simultaneously obtained recordings from thalamic electrodes; the observation that in the visual cortex there are neurons that show oscillatory firing rates with a phase difference of about a quarter cycle, which indicates that a local recurrent feedback circuit may be responsible for the oscillations; the finding of intrinsic oscillations in cortical neurons from layer IV of the frontal cortex of guinea pig in vitro. Nevertheless, it is possible that thalamic neuronal networks also contribute to the cortical beta/gamma rhythmic activity, since oscillatory (about 40 Hz) behaviour has been observed in neurons of the intralaminar centrolateral nucleus, which projects widely to the cerebral cortex, by Steriade et al. (1996). The question cannot be phrased as a simple alternative between a cortical or a thalamic rhythmic process, both considered to be exclusive mechanisms. As we have discussed in relation to other rhythmic activities of the mammalian brain, *both network- and membrane-intrinsic properties cooperate* in shaping the behaviour of the population, including its rhythmic properties and its ability to synchronise the neuronal elements. Recently, new observations made in vitro have shed light on the sources of these fast cortical rhythms. In an in vitro model of the cortex, the group of Whittington and Traub (Roopun et al. 2006) showed concurrent but independently generated gamma (30–70 Hz) rhythms in layer II/III and beta2 (20–30 Hz) rhythms in layer V somatosensory cortex. The beta2 rhythm occurred robustly in layer V intrinsically bursting (IB) neurons in the form of bursts admixed with spikelets, and single action potentials. It was blocked by reducing gap junction conductance with carbenoxolone, and was unaffected by the blockade of synaptic transmission sufficient to ablate the layer II/III gamma rhythm. It could also be seen in the absence of synaptic transmission with axonal excitability enhanced with 4-aminopyridine, suggesting a nonsynaptic rhythm mediated by axonal excitation. A network model based on the hypothesis of electrical coupling via axons, is consistent with this hypothesis. The frequency of this network beta2 rhythm appears to depend on the magnitude of the M current, a non-inactivating potassium current found in many neuronal cell types that can be modulated by a large array of receptor types, including muscarinic cholinergic receptors, in IB interneurons. These findings suggest the possibility that a normally occurring cortical network oscillation involved in motor control could be generated largely or entirely by nonsynaptic mechanisms. According to these authors, higher beta2 frequency oscillations occur mainly during the anticipatory period leading up to a movement in response to a sensory cue. Indeed, it was found that layer V pyramidal neurons and motor cortex LFPs displayed coherence at beta2 frequencies with hand and forearm EMG in monkeys performing a precision grip task (Baker et al. 1999). This group showed that the generation of beta2 in layer V stands in contrast to that of gamma rhythms in layers II/III, which may underlie corticocortical synchronisation. There are probably a variety of rhythmic activities in the beta/gamma range with different behavioural correlates, as discussed below with respect to event-related (de)synchronisation of EEG/MEG phenomena.

In this context it is interesting to consider changes in EEG/MEG phenomena, particularly in the beta and gamma frequency ranges, that are event-related and reflect a decrease or an increase in the synchrony of the underlying neuronal populations. The former is called event-related desynchronisation (ERD), and the latter event-related synchronisation (ERS) (Pfurtscheller and Lopes da Silva 1999). In relation to a hand movement, both the 10–12 Hz mu rhythm and the beta (around 20 Hz) display ERD, but with a different distribution over the scalp, although both activities are localised around the central sulcus. The mu rhythm ERD exhibits its maximum magnitude more posteriorly than the beta activity, indicating that it is generated mainly in the post-Rolandic somatosensory cortex, whereas the low beta activity is preferentially generated in the pre-rolandic motor area. In addition, after a voluntary movement, the central region exhibits a localised beta ERS that becomes evident in the first second after cessation of the movement, at a time where the rolandic mu rhythm still presents a desynchronised pattern. The exact frequency of this rebound beta ERS can vary considerably with the subject and type of movement. This beta ERS is observed not only after a real movement but also after an imagined movement. Furthermore. ERS in the gamma frequency band (around 36–40 Hz) can also be found over the central regions, preceding the execution of a movement, in contrast with the beta ERS, which has its maximum after the termination of the movement (Fig. 3).

Our understanding of the significance of ERS of the *beta* frequency range, which typically occurs after a movement, has been greatly enhanced by the observation that when this form of ERS occurs, the excitability of the corticospinal pathways decreases, as revealed by means of transcranial magnetic stimulation. This supports the hypothesis that the postmovement beta ERS corresponds to a deactivated state of the motor cortex. In contrast, the ERS in the *gamma* frequency band appears to reflect a state of active information processing.

From this perspective, it is important to note the likely connection between gamma oscillations and synaptic plasticity. As Buzsáki (2006) colourfully writes, the gamma oscillation may be considered the "buzz" that provides the central timing mechanism that is essential for modulating synaptic strength, and in this way it may stabilise the formation of neuronal assemblies in the cortex.

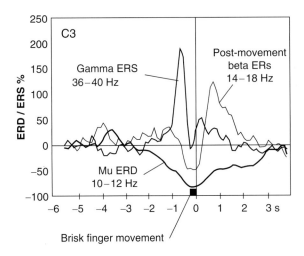

Fig. 3 Event-related desynchronisation (ERD) and event-related synchronisation (ERS) from one normal subject during self-paced voluntary movement. EEG recorded from C3. The results for three frequency bands are shown: alpha band (mu) 10–12 Hz ERD; beta 14–18 Hz ERD–ERS, and gamma 36–40 Hz ERS. The data analysis is triggered with respect to movement offset (vertical line at 0 s). Note that the ERDs or ERSs of different frequency bands have different dynamics: about 2 s before the movement the mu ERD appears, followed by a pre-movement beta ERD that changes to a postmovement ERS; a burst of gamma ERS appears just before the movement. (Adapted from Pfurtscheller et al. 1993)

3.4
DC

Is it possible to record DC on MEG or EEG? And if so, what is its physiological meaning? There are a lot of physical limitations (electrode impedances, electrode polarisation, skin/electrolyte junction) that do not allow EEG signals to be recorded down to 0 Hz, which would correspond to real DC, or "direct current". Also, environmental low-frequency noise imposes limitations on MEG with similar consequences. The point, however, is not to record down to the real DC level but to extend the effective frequency band to very low frequencies on the order of 0.1 Hz. (For a discussion of misconceptions of the meaning of "DC" in electroencephalography, see Niedermeyer's footnote in Speckmann and Elger 2005). The recording of ultraslow MEG/EEG signals can be achieved using appropriate techniques, as discussed, for example, for the EEG by Vanhatalo et al. 2005 and for the MEG by Burghoff et al. 2004. Phenomena such as the contingent negative variation (CNV) and the Bereitschaftspotential (readiness potential) are typical cases of very slow shifts of electric potential or magnetic fields that can be typically recorded using appropriate recording and analysis techniques. During slow-wave sleep, ultraslow-frequency components (around 0.5 Hz) have been recorded in the human EEG (Achermann and Borbély 1997; Amzica and Steriade 1997) and in MEG (Simon et al. 2000), which correspond to the ultraslow oscillations that can be recorded intracellularly from cortical neurons through layers II to VI, and consist of prolonged depolarising and hyperpolarising components, as have been analysed in detail by Steriade (2006).

4
Origin of the EEG/MEG II: Generators, Volume Conduction and Source Estimation

In order to take the next step towards an understanding of how EEG/MEG signals recorded outside the skull are generated, we have to take the folding of the cortex into consideration. The fact that the cortex is folded, forming gyri and sulci, implies that some populations of neurons have apical dendrites that are perpendicular to the overlying skull (i.e. those that are at the top of a gyrus), whereas others are parallel to the skull (i.e. those that are on the wall of a sulcus). The orientation of the neurons with respect to the skull is an important factor in the appearance of the EEG and MEG signals recorded outside the skull. This is particularly the case for the MEG, since the latter "sees" only those magnetic fields that are perpendicular to the skull due to the physical properties of magnetic fields, the way MEG is measured and the approximately spherical shape of the head. In effect, the observed magnetic fields are generated by neuronal currents that are oriented tangentially to the skull. In contrast, those that are oriented radially to the skull do not generate a magnetic field outside the head but contribute to the EEG.

The area of cortex within which the neuronal population must be synchronously active to produce a measurable EEG/MEG signal at the scalp is an important consideration when interpreting these signals. To address this problem, we must first point out some classical concepts about cortical organisation. The cortex is organised according to the columnar principle, as proposed in the 1970s by Mountcastle (see review from 1997), which means that the basic unit of the mature neocortex is the *minicolumn*: "a narrow chain of neurons extending vertically across the cellular layers II/VI, perpendicular to the pial surface", with a cross-section of diameter ~40–50 μm. A primate minicolumn contains about 80–100 neurons, although this number may vary between areas; in the striate cortex the cell density appears to be 2.5 times larger. Many minicolumns are bound together by short-range horizontal connections, and thus form what has been denominated *cortical columns* or cortical modules (Mountcastle 1997). One *column* in the somatic sensory cortex contains about 80 minicolumns and is roughly hexagonal with a width of about 300–400 μm (Favorov and Diamond 1990). These estimates can be used to give a rough answer to the question formulated above. Assuming that a minicolumn with a diameter of 40 μm contains 100 cells, the cortical surface corresponding to 50,000 cells should form a patch with a cross-sectional area of about 0.63 mm^2. If this cortical patch took a circular form, then its diameter would be about 0.88 mm. Buxhoeveden and Casanova (2002) noted that, from a functional perspective, cortical columns may exist in different dynamic states, and they coined the term "physiological macrocolumn" to indicate a set of cortical columns that cooperate in a given functional state or neural process. These physiological macrocolumns must be considered dynamic ensembles such that the number of columns contributing to a macrocolumn may vary as a function of time. It is important to note that neurons in separate columns can present synchronous oscillatory activities, as mediated by tangential and recurrent connections between different columns (Gray et al. 1989; Freiwald et al. 1995).

A basic problem in electroencephalography/magnetoencephalography is how to esti- mate the neuronal sources that are responsible for a certain distribution of electrical potentials or of magnetic fields recorded at the scalp. This is called the inverse problem of EEG/MEG, and is an ill-posed problem in the sense that it has no unique solution: there are an infinite number of possible source configurations that give rise to a given set of measured scalp potentials or magnetic fields (von Helmholtz 2004). Therefore, the estimation of EEG and MEG sources requires assumptions about the nature of the sources. The simplest source model is a current dipole, as indicated in the previous section. However, such a model does not imply that somewhere in the brain there is a point cur- rent dipole. Rather, it suggests that the EEG/MEG scalp distribution is best represented by an *equivalent* dipolar current source. This choice has been shown to be useful and accurate for certain types of activity, such as the event-related potentials (ERPs) and focal epileptic spikes. In such circumstances, the solution of the EEG/MEG inverse problem that is obtained based on the equivalent current dipole can be thought of as the centroid of the dipole layers that are active at a certain moment, in the statistical sense. An increase in the number of dipoles can easily lead to rather complex and ambiguous interpretations. Nevertheless, methods have been developed in order to obtain estimates of multiple dipoles using only the a priori criterion that they must be located at the surface of the cortex. An example of an algorithm that performs such an analysis is MUSIC (multiple signal classification). An alternative approach is to use linear estimation methods that apply the minimum norm constraint to estimate the sources within a given surface or volume of the brain.

The other main component of any estimation of EEG/MEG sources is the conduction problem, which allows the calculation of the field values given a postulated generator configuration (the so-called forward part of the inverse problem). A commonly used forward model is that of the three concentric conducting spheres, for which a convenient analytical expression for the surface potentials (or magnetic field) due to a dipole is available. However, realistically shaped volume conductor models derived from the individual subject's MRI images have been shown to improve the accuracy of the localisation of the sources, particularly in nonspherical parts of the head (Fuchs et al. 2007). Individual boundary element method (BEM) models derived from the subject's MRI represent the "gold standard" and have clear advantages over simplified spherical shell models. Anisotropic volume conduction properties of the bone layer or the white matter fibres can be modelled by the finite element method (FEM), but the latter require considerable computational power and are thus not used in daily applications. To reduce the computational effort, head models derived from an averaged MRI dataset have been proposed (Fuchs et al. 2007). New approaches are currently being explored that combine fMRI and EEG/MEG data in order to create more specific spatial constraints in order to reduce the solution space for the estimation of the underlying neuronal sources. This aspect of EEG and fMRI data fusion is addressed in more detail in the chapter "EEG–fMRI in Animal Models".

In general, the problems posed by the complexity of the volume conductor, including scalp, skull, cerebrospinal fluid layer and brain, are easier to solve in the case of the MEG than of the EEG, since these different media have different conductivities, which affects the EEG much more than the MEG. Therefore, a major advantage of MEG over EEG is the relative simplicity of the forward modelling and its consequences for source localisation. This means that when a dipole source algorithm is used on the basis of MEG recordings, a single homogeneous sphere model of the volume conductor can lead to a satisfactory solution.

The conductivity values that should be used for the different shells surrounding the sources, brain, cerebrospinal fluid, skull and scalp have been estimated in a number of studies, using both in vitro and in vivo measurements. In general, we can assume that the brain and scalp have the same conductivity. The conductivity of the skull is much lower than that of the brain, but the estimation of the ratio of the brain and skull conductivities has been a matter of debate. Our group (Gonçalves et al. 2003) estimated the conductivities in vivo using two different methods: electrical impedance tomography and a combined analysis of the evoked somatosensory cortical response, recorded simultaneously using MEG and EEG, since the former is not affected by the different conductivity of the skull, in contrast to the latter. The electrical impedance tomography results show a wide variation in the ratio of resistivities r_{skull}/r_{brain} among subjects, but in all cases studied the ratio was lower than the classically accepted value of 80 (Rush and Driscoll 1968), and it was in the range of 20–50. However, the r_{skull}/r_{brain} ratios of the individual subjects are readily reproducible. These results indicate that the r_{skull}/r_{brain} variations over subjects cannot be disregarded when solving the EEG inverse problem when a spherical model is used. In order to obtain an estimate of the sources of a given potential distribution over the scalp as precisely as possible, conductivities measured in the same subject should preferentially be used.

5
Localisation Methods Applied to Spontaneous Oscillatory Activities

A basic question in EEG/MEG studies is whether the main rhythmic activities—alpha and mu rhythms on the one hand and sleep spindles on the other—are generated in distinct or overlapping cortical areas. In order to solve this question, advanced spatiotemporal analysis methods are necessary. We should note that the estimation of equivalent dipole models is only meaningful if the scalp field has focal character and the number of possible active areas can be anticipated with reasonable accuracy. The recent development of a new algorithm (Manshanden et al. 2002) aimed at estimating sources of large data sets, as is the case for this kind of spontaneous EEG oscillation, allowed the issue of whether generators of spontaneous MEG/EEG alpha and mu rhythms and sleep spindles are distributed over distinct or over overlapping cortical areas to be addressed. The basic approach consisted of finding well-fitting dipoles using a dipole model applied to successive time samples of a burst of an oscillation. The equivalent dipoles encountered were plotted on the corresponding MRI slice of the brain, as shown in Fig. 2 (A for the EEG, and B for the MEG). It is important to consider what equivalent dipolar sources of spontaneous brain activity may represent. Sleep spindles, alpha rhythms and mu rhythms are spontaneously occurring brain rhythms that can be recorded from the scalp. This suggests that extended cortical areas are involved in the generation of these signals. The use of equivalent dipoles as source models for these distributed brain activities yields an oversimplified solution to the problem of determining the underlying sources of these signals. The equivalent dipoles should be viewed simply as descriptors of the "centre of gravity" that best describe, in a statistical sense, the spatial distribution of the corresponding active cortical area at a given time. The positions of the dipoles with respect to the cortical surface depend on the extent and geometry of the activated cortical area: superficially positioned dipoles (i.e. near to the cortical surface), such as those of the mu rhythm, correspond to more localised cortical activity, while deep-lying dipoles, like those of sleep spindles, instead represent the activity of extended cortical surfaces. Thus, dipole locations provide only an approximation of the localisation of the active brain area and the extension of the area. When comparing the results of the alpha rhythms and of the sleep spindles (Fig. 2), we should emphasise that there is no overlap of the centres of gravity of these two kinds of rhythms. This indicates that different regions of the cortex are involved in the generation of these brain rhythms. The same applies to the mu rhythm, which appeared to be generated in a different brain region compared to the alpha rhythm and sleep spindles. The superficial location of the mu rhythm dipoles (especially in MEG, Fig. 2b) suggests that the mu rhythm is generated in a relatively well-localised cortical area. Thus, the equivalent dipole model appears to be an adequate model for the estimation of mu sources. A comparison of the results obtained in the same subject based on EEG (Fig. 2a) or on MEG (Fig. 2b) data shows that the dipoles estimated using the latter occupy a more circumscribed number of voxels than those based on the former; this is particularly clear for the spatial distribution of the dipolar sources of sleep spindles and the mu rhythm. The close spatial relationship of the MEG mu rhythm dipoles to the dipoles of the N20 component of the medial nerve somatosensory evoked fields demonstrates that the mu rhythm arises from the cortex around the central sulcus.

5.1
EEG-Correlated fMRI

The advent of simultaneous EEG–fMRI acquisitions (Lemieux et al. 1997; Goldman et al. 2002; Krakow et al. 2000) has allowed the study of the haemodynamic correlates of spontaneous variations of alpha rhythm (Laufs et al. 2003; Moosmann et al. 2003), focussing on group results. In this kind of work it is important to study individual subjects, since there is a considerable variability with respect to these phenomena among normal subjects. Gonçalves et al. 2006; de Munck et al. 2007 found a negative correlation between the BOLD signal and the average power time series within the alpha band (8–12 Hz) in extensive areas of the occipital, parietal and frontal lobes, and a negative correlation was found between heartbeat intervals (reverse of heart rate) and alpha power (de Munck et al. 2007) although one subject only showed positive correlations, thus contradicting the negative BOLD alpha power cortical correlations that were found in most subjects. In small thalamic areas, the BOLD signal was positively correlated with the alpha power. Results suggest that the resting state varies among subjects, and sometimes even within one subject. As the resting state plays an important role in many fMRI experiments, the simultaneous recording of fMRI and EEG is advisable; see the chapters "Brain Rhythms", "Sleep", "EEG–fMRI in Adults with Focal Epilepsy", "EEG–fMRI in Idiopathic Generalised Epilepsy (Adults)" and "EEG–fMRI in Children with Epilepsy" for further discussions of this issue in the healthy and pathological brain.

6
Conclusions

Knowledge of the electrical and magnetic fields generated by local neuronal networks is of interest to the neuroscientist because these signals can yield relevant information about the activity modes of neuronal populations. This is particularly relevant when attempting to understand higher-order brain functions such as perception, action programming, and memory trace formation. It is becoming increasingly clear that these functions are mediated by dynamical assemblies of neurons. In this respect, knowledge of the properties of the individual neurons is not sufficient. It is necessary to understand how populations of neurons interact and undergo self-organisation processes to form dynamical assemblies. The latter constitute the functional substrate of complex brain functions. These neuronal assemblies generate patterns of dendritic currents and action potentials of course, but these patterns are usually difficult to evaluate experimentally due to the multitude of parameters and the complexity of the structures. Nevertheless, the concerted action of these assemblies can also be revealed in the LFPs that can be recorded at distance from the generators as EEG or MEG signals. However, extracting information from EEG or MEG signals about the functional state of a local neuronal network poses a number of nontrivial problems that must be solved by combining anatomical/physiological with biophysical/mathematical concepts and tools. Indeed, given a certain EEG or MEG signal, it is not possible to precisely reconstruct the behaviour of the underlying neuronal elements, since this inverse problem does not have a unique solution. Therefore, it is necessary to assume specific models of the neuronal elements and their interactions in dynamical assemblies in order to make sense of the LFPs. This implies that it is necessary to construct models that incorporate knowledge about cellular/membrane properties with those for the local circuits, their spatial organisation and organisation patterns. Furthermore, intracranial EEG studies (such as those in patients with epilepsy being evaluated for surgery) demonstrate that a significant amount of brain activity does not appear in the EEG or MEG. This consideration, along with the fundamental limitations of the EEG/MEG inverse problem and the difficulty involved in estimating large or complex networks of generators suggest that functional imaging combined with EEG can play a significant role in improving our understanding of brain activity.

References

Achermann P, Borbély AA (1997) Low-frequency (<1 Hz) oscillations in the human sleep electroencephalogram. Neuroscience 81(1):213–22

Adrian ED, Mathews BHC (1934) The interpretation of potential waves in the cortex. J Physiol 81:440–71

Amzica F, Steriade M (1997) The K-complex: its slow (<1-Hz) rhythmicity and relation to delta waves. Neurology 49(4):952–9

Baker SN, Kilner JM, Pinches EM, Lemon RN (1999) The role of synchrony and oscillations in the motor output. Exp Brain Res 128:109–17

Berger H (1929) Über des Elekrenkephalogramm des Menschen. Arch Psychiat Nervenkr 87: 527–70

Bouyer JJ, Montaron MF, Vahnée JM, Albert MP, Rougeul A (1987) Anatomical localization of cortical beta rhythms in cat. Neuroscience 22(3):863–9

Burghoff M, Sander TH, Schnabel A, Drung D, Trahms L, Curio G, Mackert BM (2004) DC-magnetoencephalography: direct measurements in a magnetically extremely-well-shielded room. Appl Phys Lett 85:6278–80

Buser P, Rougeul-Buser A (2005) Visual attention in behaving cats: attention shifts and sustained attention episodes are accompanied by distinct electrocortical activities. Behav Brain Res 164(1):42–51

Buxhoeveden DP, Casanova MF (2002) The minicolumn hypothesis in neuroscience. Brain 125: 935–51

Buzsáki G (2006) Rhythms of the brain. Oxford University Press, Oxford

Caton R (1875) The electric currents of the brain. Br Med J 2:278

Cram JR, Kohlenberg RJ, Singer M (1977) Operant control of alpha EEG and the effects of illumination and eye closure. Psychosom Med 39(1):11–8

de Munck JC, Gonçalves SI, Huijboom L, Kuijer JP, Pouwels PJ, Heethaar RM, Lopes da Silva FH (2007) The hemodynamic response of the alpha rhythm: an EEG/fMRI study. Neuroimage 35(3):1142–51

Eckhorn R, Bauer R, Jordan W, Brosch M, Kruse W, Munk M, Reitboeck HJ (1988) Coherent oscillations: a mechanism of feature linking in the visual cortex? Multiple electrode and correlation analyses in the cat. Biol Cybern 60(2):121–30

Favorov OV, Diamond ME (1990) Demonstration of discrete place-defined columns—segregates—in the cat SI. J Comp Neurol 298(1):97–112

Freeman WJ (2005) Origin, structure, and role of background EEG activity. Part 3. Neural frame classification. Clin Neurophysiol 116(5):1118–29

Freeman WJ, van Dijk BW (1987) Spatial patterns of visual cortical fast EEG during conditioned reflex in a rhesus monkey. Brain Res 422(2):267–76

Freiwald WA, Kreiter AK, Singer W (1995) Stimulus dependent inter-columnar synchronization of single unit responses in cat area 17. Neuroreport 6:2348–52

Fuchs M, Wagner M, Kastner J (2007) Development of volume conductor and source models to localize epileptic foci. J Clin Neurophysiol 24(2):101–19

Goldman RI, Stern JM, Engel J Jr, Cohen M (2002) Simultaneous EEG and fMRI of the alpha rhythm. NeuroReport 13(18):2487–92

Gonçalves SI, de Munck JC, Pouwels PJ, Schoonhoven R, Kuijer JP, Maurits NM, Hoogduin JM, Van Someren EJ, Heethaar RM, Lopes da Silva FH (2006) Correlating the alpha rhythm to BOLD using simultaneous EEG/fMRI: inter-subject variability. Neuroimage 30(1):203–13

Gonçalves SI, de Munck JC, Verbunt JP, Bijma F, Heethaar RM, Lopes da Silva F (2003) In vivo measurement of the brain and skull resistivities using an EIT-based method and realistic models for the head. IEEE Trans Biomed Eng 50(6):754–67

Gray CM, König P, Engel AK, Singer W (1989) Oscillatory responses in cat visual cortex exhibit inter-columnar synchronization which reflects global stimulus properties. Nature 338(6213): 334–7

Hämäläinen MS, Hari R, Ilmoniemi R, Knuutila J, Lounasmaa O (1993) Magnetoencephalography. Theory, instrumentation and applications to the noninvasive study of human brain function. Rev Mod Phys 65:413–97

Hari R, Salmelin R, Mäkelä JP, Salenius S, Helle M (1997) Magnetoencephalographic cortical rhythms. Int J Psychophysiol 26(1–3):51–62

Huang TY, Cherkas PS, Rosenthal DW, Hanani M (2005) Dye coupling among satellite glial cells in mammalian dorsal root ganglia. Brain Res 1036(1–2):42–9

Hughes SW, Crunelli V (2005) Thalamic mechanisms of EEG alpha rhythms and their pathological implications. Neuroscientist 11(4):357–72

Hughes SW, Lörincz M, Cope DW, Blethyn KL, Kékesi KA, Parri HR, Juhasz G, Crunelli V (2004) Synchronized oscillations at alpha and theta frequencies in the lateral geniculate nucleus. Neuron 42:253–68

Krakow K, Allen PJ, Symms MR, Lemieux L, Josephs O, Fish DR (2000) EEG recording during fMRI experiments: image quality. Hum Brain Mapp 10:10–15

Laufs H, Kleinschmidt A, Beyerle A, Eger E, Salek-Haddadi A, Preibisch C, Krakow K (2003) EEG-correlated fMRI of human alpha activity. Neuroimage 19:1463–76

Lehtelä L, Salmelin R, Hari R (1997) Evidence for reactive magnetic 10-Hz rhythm in the human auditory cortex. Neurosci Lett 222(2):111–4

Lemieux L, Allen PJ, Franconi F, Symms MR, Fish DR (1997) Recording of EEG during fMRI experiments: patient safety. Magn Reson Med 38:943–52

Lopes da Silva F (1991) Neural mechanisms underlying brain waves: from neural membranes to networks. Electroencephalogr Clin Neurophysiol 79(2):81–93

Lopes da Silva FH (2002) Electrical potentials. In: Ramachandran VS (ed) Encyclopedia of the human brain. Elsevier, New York, pp 147–67

Lopes da Silva FH, Storm van Leeuwen W (1977) The cortical source of the alpha rhythm. Neurosci Lett 6:237–41

Lopes da Silva FH, van Rotterdam A (2005) Biophysical aspects of EEG and magnetoencephalographic generation. In: Niedermeyer E, Lopes da Silva F (eds) Electroencephalography: basic principles, clinical applications and related fields, 5th edn. Lippincott, Williams & Wilkins, New York

Lopes da Silva FH, van Rotterdam A, Storm van Leeuwen W, Tielen AM (1970) Dynamic characteristics of visual evoked potentials in the dog. II. Beta frequency selectivity in evoked potentials and background activity. Electroencephalogr Clin Neurophysiol 29(3):260–8

Lorente de Nó R (1947) Action potential of the motoneurons of the hypoglossus nucleus. J Cell Comp Physiol 29:207–87

Mainen ZF, Sejnowski TJ (1996) Influence of dendritic structure on firing patterns in model neocortical neurons. Nature 382:363–6

Manshanden I, De Munck JC, Simon NR, Lopes da Silva FH (2002) Source localization of MEG sleep spindles and the relation to sources of alpha band rhythms. Clin Neurophysiol 113(12): 1937–47

Moosmann M, Ritter P, Krastel I, Brink A, Thees S, Blankenburg F, Taskin B, Obrig H, Villringer A (2003) Correlates of alpha rhythm in functional magnetic resonance imaging and near infrared spectroscopy. Neuroimage 20:145–58

Moruzzi G, Magoun HW (1949) Brain stem reticular formation and activation of the EEG. Electroencephalogr Clin Neurophysiol 1(4):455–73

Mountcastle VB (1997) The columnar organization of the neocortex. Brain 120:701–22

Munk MH, Roelfsema PR, König P, Engel AK, Singer W (1996) Role of reticular activation in the modulation of intracortical synchronization. Science 272(5259):271–4

Murakami S, Okada Y (2006) Contributions of principal neocortical neurons to magnetoencephalography and electroencephalography signals. J Physiol 575(3):925–36

Niedermeyer E (2005) The normal EEG in the waking adult. In: Niedermeyer E, Lopes da Silva FH (eds) Electroencephalography: basic principles, clinical applications and related fields, 5th edn. Lippincott, Williams & Wilkins, New York

Nunez PL (1995) Neocortical dynamics and human EEG rhythms. Oxford University Press, New York

Okada YC, Wu J, Kyuhou S (1997) Genesis of MEG signals in a mammalian CNS structure. Electroenceph Clin Neurophysiol 103:474–85

Paskewitz DA, Orne MT (1973) Visual effects on alpha feedback training. Science 181(97): 360–3

Pfurtscheller G, Lopes da Silva FH (1999) Event-related EEG/MEG synchronization and desynchronization: basic principles. Clin Neurophysiol 110(11):1842–57

Pfurtscheller G, Stancak A Jr, Neuper C (1996) Post-movement beta synchronization. A correlate of an idling motor area? Electroencephalogr Clin Neurophysiol 98:281–93

Roopun AK, Middleton SJ, Cunningham MO, LeBeau FE, Bibbig A, Whittington MA, Traub RD (2006) A beta2-frequency (20–30 Hz) oscillation in nonsynaptic networks of somatosensory cortex. Proc Natl Acad Sci USA 103(42):15646–50

Rougeul A, Bouyer JJ, Dedet L, Debray O (1979) Fast somato-parietal rhythms during combined focal attention and immobility in baboon and squirrel monkey. Electroencephalogr Clin Neurophysiol 46(3):310–9

Rougeul-Buser A, Buser P (1997) Rhythms in the alpha band in cats and their behavioural correlates. Int J Psychophysiol 26(1–3):191–203

Rush S, Driscoll DA (1968) Current distribution in the brain from surface electrodes. Anesth Analg 47:717–23

Simon NR, Manshanden I, Lopes da Silva FH (2000) A MEG study of sleep. Brain Res 860(1–2):64–76

Speckmann E-J, Elger CE (2005) Introduction to the neurophysiological basis of EEG and DC potentials. In: Niedermeyer E, Lopes da Silva FH (eds) Electroencephalography: basic principles, clinical applications and related fields, 5th edn. Lippincott, Williams & Wilkins, New York, pp 17–29

Stennett RG (1966) Alpha amplitude and arousal: a reply to Stennett. Psychophysiology 2(4): 372–76

Steriade M (2006) Grouping of brain rhythms in corticothalamic systems. Neuroscience 137(4): 1087–106

Steriade M, Contreras D, Amzica F, Timofeev I (1996) Synchronization of fast (30–40 Hz) spontaneous oscillations in intrathalamic and thalamocortical networks. J Neurosci 16(8): 2788–808

Stuart GJ, Sakman B (1994) Active propagation of somatic action potentials into neocortical pyramidal cell dendrites. Nature 367:68–72

Surwillo WW (1967) The inverted-U relationship: a reply to Stennett. Psychophysiology 3(3):321–2

Surwillo WW (1965) The relation of amplitude of alpha rhythm to heart rate. Psychophysiology 1(3):247–52

Traub RD, Jefferys JGR, Miles R, Whittington MA, Tóth K (1994) A branching dendritic model of a rodent CA3 pyramidal neurone. J Physiol 481:79–95

Traub RD, Miles R (1991) Neuronal networks of the hippocampus. Cambridge University Press, New York

Vanhatalo S, Voipio J, Kaila K (2005) Full-band EEG (FbEEG): an emerging standard in electroencephalography. Clin Neurophysiol 116(1):1–8

Von Helmholtz HLF (2004) Some laws concerning the distribution of electric currents in volume conductors with applications to experiments on animal electricity. Proc IEEE 92(5):868–70

The Basics of Functional Magnetic Resonance Imaging

3

Ralf Deichmann, Ulrike Nöth, and Nikolaus Weiskopf

1
The Basics of MR Imaging

1.1
Spins in an External Magnetic Field

In magnetic resonance imaging (MRI), the signal that is measured usually arises from the nuclei of the tissue's hydrogen atoms (i.e. *protons*). A proton possesses a physical property, its *spin*, which behaves roughly speaking like a compass needle: each spin has a small magnetic dipole moment and aligns in an external magnetic field. If tissue is brought into the strong magnetic field inside the magnetic resonance (MR) scanner bore, spins will align either antiparallel or parallel to the magnetic field B. At the field strengths relevant here, a tiny majority of the spins assume the latter alignment and their magnetic moments add up, giving rise to a net macroscopic magnetisation M which is parallel to B, representing a state of equilibrium (Fig. 1, left). Thus, the existence of this magnetisation inside the magnetic field is an indicator of the presence of protons, and the measurement of M with a certain spatial resolution can be used to construct a proton image.

Fig. 1 Spins align in an external magnetic field B, giving rise to a macroscopic *magnetisation M* which is parallel to B (*left*). If the protons inside the magnetic field B are exposed to an electromagnetic wave with the *Larmor frequency*, the magnetisation M is tilted (*right*)

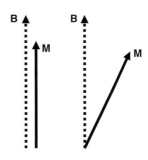

R. Deichmann (✉)
University Hospital, Brain Imaging Center, Haus 95H, Schleusenweg 2-16, 60528 Frankfurt-Main, Germany
e-mail: deichmann@med.uni-frankfurt.de

C. Mulert and L. Lemieux (eds.), *EEG- fMRI*
DOI: 10.1007/978-3-540-87919-0_3, © Springer Verlag Berlin Heidelberg 2010

Fig. 2 The tilted magnetisation rotates around the magnetic field vector, sending out an electromagnetic wave with the Larmor frequency

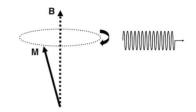

1.2
The Magnetic Resonance Effect

The measurement of M is possible due to the following physical effect: if the protons inside the magnetic field B are exposed to an electromagnetic wave with a specific frequency, the so-called *Larmor frequency*, the magnetisation M is tilted in proportion to the exposure duration (Fig. 1, right). The tilted magnetisation then rotates around the magnetic field vector (Fig. 2). This movement, called *precession*, is similar to the behaviour of an ordinary spinning top. During precession, the protons send out an electromagnetic wave that has the Larmor frequency (Fig. 2). The important point is that the Larmor frequency is proportional to the magnetic field B, with a value of 42.6 MHz/T. Thus, for a clinical 1.5 T scanner, the Larmor frequency amounts to about 64 MHz, which is close to the range of frequencies used for FM broadcasting. It should be noted that the tilted magnetisation gradually returns to its original state, or equilibrium. This effect, called *relaxation*, will be discussed below.

In summary, M (and thus the presence of protons) is detected in the following way: the sample is placed inside the MR scanner and thus exposed to a strong static magnetic field B. As a consequence, a macroscopic magnetisation M parallel to B builds up. An electromagnetic wave with the Larmor frequency and duration of a few milliseconds is transmitted using equipment similar to a small FM radio broadcasting station. This gives rise to a tilt and a subsequent precession of the magnetisation vector. After sending the initial electromagnetic pulse, a detector similar to an FM radio tuned to the Larmor frequency is switched on. If a signal is detected, there must be protons inside the sample under investigation. It is important to note that the initial step of tilting the magnetisation only works if the frequency of the transmitted electromagnetic signal is exactly the protons' Larmor frequency. Thus, we are dealing with a typical resonance effect, giving rise to the expression MRI. The MR effect was first described in 1946 (Bloch et al. 1946; Purcell et al. 1946).

1.3
Spatial Encoding in MR Imaging

As described so far, the MR effect only allows the detection of the presence of protons. The question of how spatial resolution of the protons throughout the sample can be achieved to produce an image now arises. This will be discussed step by step for three orthogonal directions that are defined relative to the brain as follows: x (left/right), y (anterior/posterior), and z (superior/inferior).

1.3.1
Frequency Encoding

Figure 3 (left) shows a so-called *pulse diagram*, a schematic description of an MR experiment. On the *RF (radiofrequency) axis*, there is the initial electromagnetic pulse that tilts the magnetisation, and the signal acquired subsequently. Below, there is the *gradient axis*, showing that during signal acquisition a *gradient* G_x is switched on. This means that during acquisition the magnetic field is modified in a way that it increases linearly in the x-direction. Thus, during acquisition, the protons' Larmor frequency depends on their position inside the brain, i.e. on their x-coordinate. Figure 3 (right) shows two small brain regions and the signal that protons inside these regions send out while the gradient is switched on: the protons in the region on the left-hand side are exposed to a slightly reduced magnetic field, so they send out an electromagnetic wave with a slightly lower frequency. The signal sent out by the protons in the region on the right hand side has a higher frequency. The "FM radio" detects the sum signal from all protons. This signal undergoes a *frequency analysis* (mathematically, this process is called a *Fourier transform*), resulting in the signal's frequency spectrum. The exact positions of the protons (or at least their x-coordinates) can then be deduced from the signal's frequency spectrum. Thus, this process is called *frequency encoding*. The gradient that is switched on during signal acquisition (or signal "readout") is called the *read gradient*. It should be noted that this gradient is on during acquisition only, not during the initial RF pulse. Otherwise, the spins would have different, position-dependent Larmor frequencies while the electromagnetic wave is being sent, so the magnetisation would be tilted for only some of the spins. The use of magnetic field gradients to achieve spatial resolution was first proposed by Lauterbur (1973).

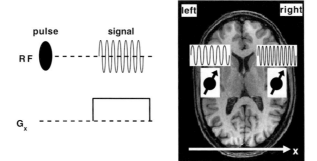

Fig. 3 The concept of frequency encoding: due to the *read gradient* (*x*-direction), the magnetic field increases linearly in the *x*-direction. Consequently, during acquisition, the protons' Larmor frequencies depend on their positions inside the brain. The exact positions of the protons (or at least their *x*-coordinates) can then be deduced from the frequency spectrum

1.3.2
Phase Encoding

The experiment described above allows for spatial resolution in one direction only. A 2D experiment is depicted in Fig. 4. This time, the pulse diagram comprises an RF axis and two gradient axes for gradients in the x- and y-directions. Parts of this experiment correspond to the one described above: the initial RF pulse tilts the magnetisation, and a signal is acquired while the read gradient G_x is switched on, so the protons' x-coordinates can be deduced from their signal frequencies. In addition, a gradient in the direction perpendicular to the read gradient, G_y, is switched on between the initial RF pulse and the acquisition process. The effect of this gradient is explained in Fig. 4 (right) for two brain regions with the same x-coordinates but different y-coordinates: while the gradient G_y is switched on, the protons in the anterior region have a higher Larmor frequency than the protons in the posterior one. The effect on the Larmor frequency only lasts as long as G_y is switched on. Once G_y is switched off and G_x is switched on, the signals from both regions have the same Larmor frequencies because they have the same x-coordinate. However, the starting points of the signals from the anterior and posterior regions are different: for the example shown in Fig. 4, the signal from the anterior region has a maximum value when acquisition starts, whereas the signal from the posterior region has a minimum value. Thus, the signals appear shifted in time—they have different *phases*. In summary, the x-coordinate can be deduced from the signal frequency and the y-coordinate from the signal phase. The gradient G_y is called the *phase encoding (PE) gradient*, and the process of switching an imaging gradient between spin excitation and signal acquisition is referred to as PE. It should be noted that an exact determination of the y-coordinate requires the repetition of the experiment depicted in Fig. 4 using different PE gradients. Thus, in Fig. 7, which shows a complete imaging experiment, the PE gradient (i.e. the gradient in the y-direction) is depicted as a "ladder" with an arrow, reflecting the different PE gradient amplitudes.

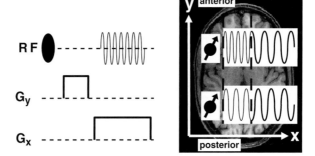

Fig. 4 The concept of phase encoding (PE): while the *phase gradient* (y-direction) is switched on, protons with different y-coordinates precess with different frequencies, leading to different starting points (*phases*) when the acquisition begins. Thus, the y-coordinate can be deduced from the phase and the x-coordinate from the frequency

Fig. 5 The concept of slice selection: due to the *slice gradient* (*z*-direction), protons with different *z*-coordinates have different Larmor frequencies. Thus, an RF pulse with a specific frequency can only excite protons within a certain slice

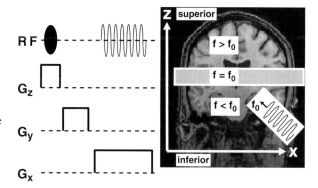

1.3.3
Slice Selection

Figure 5 shows an experiment with spatial resolution in three directions. Basically, this experiment corresponds to the one discussed above, comprising a phase gradient and a read gradient. However, this time a gradient G_z is switched on at the beginning of the experiment and remains on during the transmission of the RF pulse. Due to this gradient, the magnetic field strength and thus the protons' Larmor frequencies increase in this direction. Let us assume that within a certain axial slice the Larmor frequency has a value of f_0 (Fig. 5, *right*). If an RF pulse with this frequency is sent, it will tilt the magnetisation within this slice only. It cannot influence protons in the upper or lower parts of the brain, because their Larmor frequencies are higher or lower than f_0, so there is no resonance (in a certain way, this resembles a swing that can only be pushed effectively when using the correct rhythm/frequency). Thus, only protons inside the selected slice are tilted (or "excited") and can contribute to the signal. In summary, the combination of an RF pulse and a gradient causes a slice-selective excitation. The gradient G_z is also referred to as the *slice gradient* or *slice selective gradient*. The spatial encoding within the excited slice is then achieved with the help of the read gradient G_x and the phase gradient G_y, as described above. This process is repeated for different excitation frequencies in order to acquire multislice image datasets.

1.4
Relaxation Times T1 and T2

After an RF pulse has tilted the magnetisation vector, precession takes place, as shown in Fig. 2. However, as noted previously, precession has a limited duration: after a while, the magnetisation is once again parallel to the static magnetic field, i.e. at stable equilibrium. This process is called *relaxation*. Relaxation consists of two simultaneous processes, as follows.

The *longitudinal* component of the tilted magnetisation (i.e. the component parallel to the magnetic field) approaches a maximum value (the so-called *equilibrium value*) with the time constant T1, the *longitudinal relaxation time*. This process is also called *spin-lattice relaxation* because free water spins transfer energy to the surrounding environment, the *lattice*.

The *transverse* component of the tilted magnetisation (i.e. the component perpendicular to the magnetic field) vanishes with the time constant T2, the *transverse relaxation time*. This process is also called *spin-spin relaxation* because free water spins exchange small amounts of energy.

In the human brain, there are a wide variety of T1 values: at 3 T, approximate T1 values are 850 ms (white matter), 1,300 ms (grey matter), and 4,500 ms (CSF) (Wansapura et al. 1999). Thus, MRI acquisition sequences that exploit T1 contrast—so-called T1-weighted techniques such as T1-weighted spin echo sequences, T1-weighted fast gradient echo sequences like FLASH (Haase 1990), and magnetisation-prepared sequences such as MP-RAGE (Mugler III and Brookeman 1990) and MDEFT (Ugurbil et al. 1993)—are commonly used to visualise and quantify brain morphology.

For T2, there is less contrast between white matter and grey matter, with values amounting to about 80 and 110 ms, respectively, at 3 T (Wansapura et al. 1999). However, CSF has a very long T2 value (about 2,000 ms), providing a means of distinguishing between brain tissue and fluid compartments like oedema. Thus, T2-weighted acquisition techniques such as T2-weighted spin echo sequences are often used to detect lesions.

1.5
Gradient Echoes and the Relaxation Time T2*

The occurrence of *gradient echoes* is a striking phenomenon in MR techniques. Gradient echo methods are widely used, in particular for functional imaging. Figure 6 schematically describes a simple gradient echo experiment. An initial RF pulse tilts the magnetisation. A signal is acquired while a gradient is turned on in the *x*-direction. As described above, this means that during the duration of the gradient the magnetic field increases linearly in the *x*-direction. As a consequence, rapid signal decay is observed. However, after a reverse gradient (field magnitude increases in the *negative x*-direction) has been applied, the signal builds up again after a while. This effect is known as *gradient echo*. The first part of this experiment (the accelerated signal decay in the presence of a gradient) can be explained as follows: while the gradient is switched on, spins at different positions in space will be exposed to different field strengths, so they rotate with different Larmor frequencies. Figure 6 schematically shows the magnetisation vectors of two spin ensembles, the lower one having

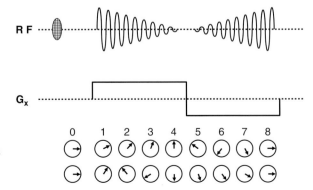

Fig. 6 Gradient echo: due to the magnetic field gradient, protons at different positions precess with different frequencies, resulting in signal losses due to destructive interference (*dephasing*). After inversion of the gradient, this process is reversed (*rephasing*) and the signal returns (*gradient echo*)

an increased Larmor frequency. Directly after the RF pulse (time point 0 in Fig. 6), the magnetisation vectors of the excited spins all point in the same direction. Thus, they add up to a strong net magnetisation, giving rise to a strong signal. While the gradient is on (time points 1–4), the spins *dephase*—i.e. their magnetisation vectors rotate at different speeds, thus pointing in different directions, so their contributions to the net magnetisation cancel each other, causing fast signal decay. In general, it can be said that any inhomogeneity of the static magnetic field will have a similar effect, resulting in accelerated signal decay. Thus, the signal decays with the *effective (apparent) transverse relaxation time* $T2^*$, which depends on the degree of field inhomogeneity and can be considerably shorter than T2. The second part of the experiment, which gives rise to the gradient echo, can be explained as follows. After gradient inversion, the distribution of field strengths changes. A spin that was initially exposed to an increased magnetic field now finds itself in an area of relatively low field strength and vice versa. Thus, a spin ensemble that initially rotated quickly now continues with a low frequency, and a spin ensemble that initially rotated slowly continues with a high frequency. This process continually reduces the phase difference between spins (time points 5–8), so that the spins are now *rephasing* and the resulting signal (the gradient echo) builds up, attaining maximum strength when the vectors are in phase again (time point 8).

Figure 7 shows a gradient echo imaging sequence. Before the acquisition, a negative gradient in the x-direction causes spin dephasing. When the positive read gradient is switched on, the spins rephase and a gradient echo occurs. In addition, a negative gradient is switched on after the slice gradient to compensate for dephasing effects due to this gradient that would otherwise reduce the signal strength. It should be noted that in gradient echo techniques, spin dephasing compensation only occurs for the gradients that are inverted. All other field inhomogeneities cause additional spin dephasing and thus reduce the $T2^*$ value. Thus, gradient echo images are $T2^*$ weighted, displaying lower image intensities in areas of reduced $T2^*$ due to local inhomogeneities of the static magnetic field.

The time difference between the initial RF pulse and the centre of the gradient echo is called the *echo time* TE (Fig. 7). It should be noted that the choice of TE determines the

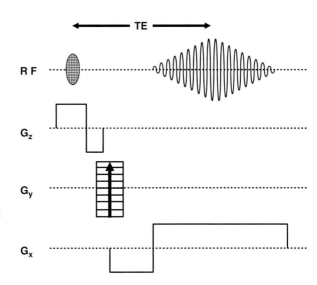

Fig. 7 A complete gradient echo imaging experiment. The *echo time TE* is defined as the time difference between the RF excitation and the centre of the gradient echo

T2* contrast: if TE is too short, the spins do not have sufficient time to dephase, so T2* weighting is poor. If on the other hand TE is considerably longer than T2*, the signal will have decayed by the time the acquisition starts, so the signal-to-noise ratio (SNR) of the image will be poor.

Gradient echo techniques are of major importance for functional imaging studies because neuronal activations lead to small changes of T2* in the surrounding brain tissue and thus to intensity variations in T2*-weighted gradient echo images. This effect, which is called the blood oxygenation level-dependent (BOLD) effect, will be discussed in a later section.

1.6
k-Space

The k-space is a mathematical concept that is extremely useful for describing MR acquisition sequences, in particular the echo-planar imaging sequence, which is the mainstay of functional magnetic resonance imaging (fMRI). This section will give a quick non-mathematical introduction to k-space.

Let us assume that a single data point is acquired, for example one of the data points forming a gradient echo. Between the acquisition of this data point and the preceding RF excitation pulse, a gradient G_x (in the read direction) and a gradient G_y (in the phase direction) are switched on for a certain duration. The data point's *k-values* k_x and k_y are then defined as the areas under the respective gradients (i.e. the product of gradient strength and gradient duration). For example, in Fig. 4 the k_y value of any data point constituting the signal is the area under the preceding PE gradient G_y, and the k_x value is the area under the read gradient G_x up to the time when the data point is acquired. This means that the data points constituting the signal in Fig. 4 have the same k_y value but different, increasing k_x values. Based on this definition, we can now analyse the k values of the data points in the various gradient echoes that are acquired according to Fig. 7. Please keep in mind that the experiment depicted in Fig. 7 is repeated several times using different values for the PE gradient G_y, i.e. several gradient echoes with different degrees of PE are acquired. Let us start with the k_x values: the first data point of each gradient echo is preceded by the negative gradient on the G_x axis only, so it has a negative k_x value. The other data points are preceded by the initial negative gradient plus the positive read gradient of increasing duration, so they have increasing k_x values. However, all data points belonging to the same echo are preceded by the same gradient G_y, so they have the same k_y value, which is negative for the first echo because G_y starts with a negative value. The different k values of the data points belonging to the gradient echo can be depicted in a 2D k-space diagram, as shown in Fig. 8 (left): obviously, the data points cover the bottom-most horizontal line in k-space. For the next echo, the PE gradient G_y has a higher value, so k_y is increased and the data points constituting this echo cover the next highest horizontal line in k-space (Fig. 8, left). In summary, one can say that for any particular MR imaging experiment, several data points with different combinations of k_x and k_y must be acquired, covering the complete 2D k-space, as shown in Fig. 8. For the experiment described in Fig. 7, k-space is covered in horizontal lines, filling each line successively from the left to the right.

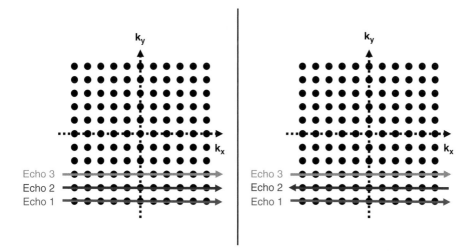

Fig. 8 *Left*: Schematic description of k-space coverage for the gradient echo experiment depicted in Fig. 7, filling *horizontal lines* successively from the *left* to the *right*. *Right*: schematic description of k-space coverage for the echo planar imaging (EPI) experiment depicted in Fig. 9, filling *odd horizontal lines* successively from the *left* to the *right* and even *horizontal lines* successively from the *right* to the *left*

1.7
Echo Planar Imaging (EPI)

The gradient echo sequence depicted in Fig. 7 is relatively time consuming, mainly because each repetition with a new PE gradient requires its own slice-selective excitation pulse. Special gradient echo techniques such as single-shot EPI have been developed to circumvent this limitation (Mansfield 1977). EPI is schematically described in Fig. 9. After slice-selective excitation, a series of gradient echoes are acquired by successive inversions of the read gradient. A short gradient pulse in the y-direction, the so-called blip, is switched on between successive acquisitions. Thus, the degree of PE for a specific echo is given by the initial negative gradient in the y-direction and the sum of the blips up to the echo acquisition time. In summary, this satisfies the conditions posed above for imaging (performance of a series of acquisitions while a read gradient in the x-direction is turned on, with each acquisition being preceded by phase gradients in the y-direction with different degrees of PE), so a full image can be constructed from the acquired data. There is only one excitation pulse, so the technique is very fast, with typical acquisition times of less than 100 ms per slice. Gradient echo EPI images are heavily T2* weighted, displaying reduced image intensity in areas affected by local magnetic field inhomogeneities, as explained above. As we will see below, T2*-weighting and speed of acquisition make this technique ideally suited for functional MRI.

The k-space analysis is relatively simple: for the first echo, the data points have increasing k_x values, ranging from a negative to a positive value, but the same negative k_y value due to the preceding PE gradient G_y. Thus, this echo covers the bottom-most horizontal line in k-space, as shown in Fig. 8 (right). For the second echo, k_y is increased due to the

Fig. 9 Schematic description of single-shot EPI: a series of gradient echoes is acquired by successive inversions of the read gradient. Due to short intermediate y-gradient pulses (*blips*), the echoes have different degrees of PE

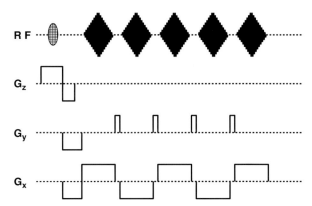

intermediate blip. The k_x values of this echo range from a positive to a negative value, so this echo covers the next horizontal line in k-space, but *in reverse order*. In summary, it can be said that k-space is covered in horizontal lines in EPI, with odd lines filled successively from the left to the right, and even lines from the right to the left. This k-space line-filling order reversal, which allows for fast data acquisition, can also give rise to artefacts (see the chapter on "Image Acquisition Artefacts").

1.8
Spin Echoes

For the sake of completeness, the occurrence of spin echoes will be briefly described in this section. The basic experiment is described in Fig. 10 (top). A 90° pulse tilts the magnetisation vector and a strong signal can be observed directly after the excitation (time point 1). This signal decays with the time constant T2*. After a short while, a 180° pulse is applied (between time points 2 and 3). As a consequence, the signal builds up again (time point 4). This effect is known as *spin echo* (Hahn 1950) and can be explained as follows (bottom part of Fig. 10). Directly after the excitation (time point 1), all of the spins are aligned, forming a strong signal. However, they start to rotate (black arrow), usually with different Larmor frequencies due to field inhomogeneities, as described above. For simplicity, let us assume there are three spin ensembles: a "fast" one (red), an "average" one (blue), and a "slow" one (green). After a while (time point 2), the "fast" spin is relatively advanced, whereas the "slow" spin is lagging behind. Consequently, the spins are dephased and the signal has decayed. The 180° pulse rotates the spins around the axis of initial alignment (green arrow). This leads to a fundamental change in constellation (time point 3): the "fast" spin is now lagging behind while the "slow" one is well advanced. However, the direction of precession remains unchanged (black arrow), so the "fast" spin catches up, and after a while (time point 4) the spins are realigned, once again forming a strong signal, the spin echo. This procedure compensates for the effects of all field inhomogeneities, so spin echoes are T2-weighted (in contrast to gradient echoes, which are T2*-weighted).

As described above, T2-weighted spin echo sequences are widely used in clinical practice for the detection of lesions. To shorten the experiment duration, a fast spin echo

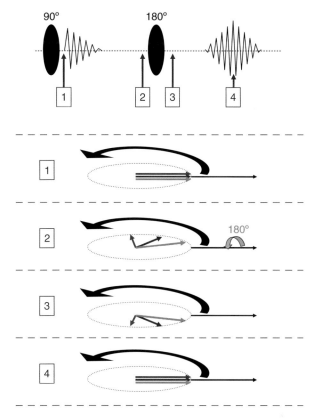

Fig. 10 Schematic description of the spin echo effect, indicating the magnetisation vectors of three spin ensembles with high (*red*), medium (*blue*), and low (*green*) Larmor frequencies. At time point 2, the signal is dephased because the *red* vector is advanced while the *green* one is lagging behind. After application of the 180° pulse, this constellation is inverted. As a consequence, the *red* vector "catches up", and at time point 4 the vectors are realigned, resulting in the spin echo signal

sequence dubbed RARE (Hennig et al. 1986) is frequently used (also known as the *turbo spin echo* sequence). This sequence is basically similar to the EPI technique described above; however, to achieve T2 weighting, a series of spin echoes (rather than gradient echoes) are acquired by applying 180° pulses between subsequent echoes.

1.9
The Specific Absorption Rate (SAR)

When RF pulses are applied in MRI experiments, energy is transferred to the spin system. The problem is that RF pulses also induce electrical currents in tissue, which lead to tissue heating. As a consequence, only a fraction of the transmitted RF energy is used for spin excitation and the remaining part causes unwanted heating effects. The SAR is the RF power absorbed by tissue, measured in watts per kilogram of body weight. For safety reasons, the SAR must not exceed certain limits. As an example, the maximum allowed SAR averaged over the head is 3.2 W/kg. The SAR depends strongly on the MRI technique in use. For example, EPI is a low-SAR technique because only a single RF pulse is required per imaging slice. In contrast, fast spin echo techniques like RARE (turbo spin echo) are high-SAR techniques because a series of 180° pulses is required to create a train of spin echoes. It should be noted that SAR values increase with the scanner's magnetic field strength. Due to the higher Larmor frequency and the fact that tissue conductivity increases with the frequency, a larger proportion of the energy is converted into heat. As a consequence, it may be difficult to run high-SAR sequences on high-field scanners.

The insertion of conductive material (such as EEG electrodes and leads) inside the scanner bore is problematic because induced currents can heat up the hardware, resulting in a risk of causing local RF burns where the hardware is in contact with the skin. Thus, high-SAR sequences should not be used in concurrent EEG–fMRI acquisitions. Additionally, in studies of this kind, the standard RF setup (whole-body coil for RF transmission and head coil for signal reception) should be avoided; a head transmit/receive coil should be used instead, to reduce the exposure of equipment to RF fields. The issue of safety in relation to EEG–fMRI is discussed in detail in the chapter "EEG Instrumentation and Safety".

2
The Cerebral Blood Flow (CBF)

2.1
Definition, Order of Magnitude, Measurement

Brain perfusion or CBF is a measure of the delivery of arterial blood, and thus of oxygen, to brain tissue. An increase in CBF is caused, for example, by brain activation due to a higher demand for oxygen during neuronal activity; this CBF increase results in a higher oxyhaemoglobin concentration at the site of activity, leading to the "BOLD effect" described in Sect. 4 of this chapter. Therefore, the site of brain activation can be determined by measuring CBF changes (Luh et al. 2000). On the other hand, a decrease in CBF will lead to low levels of oxygen (hypoxia), to which the brain is very vulnerable, and which can cause brain damage in severe cases, such as in cases of ischaemic stroke. In general, CBF is a crucial parameter for diagnosing, treating and understanding the mechanisms underlying various pathological conditions (Tofts 2003, pp. 465–471), in particular stroke (Chalela et al. 2000), epilepsy (Hamandi et al. 2008), and cancer (Barrett et al. 2007).

CBF can be quantified in terms of the rate of delivery of arterial blood $\Delta V_B/\Delta t$ (measured in ml per min) to the capillaries of a particular volume V or mass m of brain tissue (measured in units of 100 ml or 100 g, respectively; see also Fig. 11):

$$\mathrm{CBF} = \frac{1}{V} \cdot \frac{\Delta V_B}{\Delta t}.$$

Fig. 11 The cerebral blood flow (CBF) is the rate of delivery of arterial blood to the capillaries of a particular volume V or mass m of brain tissue. Only blood in the capillaries contributes to the CBF. Blood passing through tissue in arteries (or arterioles) and veins (or venules) does not contribute

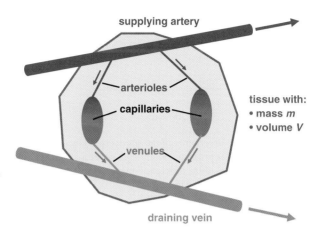

Approximate values for global CBF are 65 ml/100 ml/min in grey matter and 33 ml/ 100 ml/min in white matter (Yen et al. 2002).

It should be noted that only blood in the capillaries contributes to CBF, while blood passing through tissue in arteries (or arterioles) and veins (or venules) does not.

There are two major MR methods for measuring CBF, *dynamic susceptibility contrast (DSC) MRI* and *arterial spin labelling (ASL)*. DSC is also called *dynamic contrast enhanced (DCE)* MRI if imaging is based on T1 contrast.

DSC MRI uses a paramagnetic contrast agent (e.g. Gd-DTPA), which is injected intravenously as a tracer, so this method is invasive. The contrast agent locally reduces the relaxation times T1, T2 and T2*. The passage of the contrast agent bolus through the tissue of interest is usually monitored by acquiring a time series of T2- or T2*-weighted images (e.g. using the EPI sequence), because the respective imaging sequences have a higher temporal resolution than T1-weighted sequences. By analysing the signal time course of the bolus passage, which has a duration of typically a few seconds, information on the CBF, the cerebral blood volume (CBV), and the mean transit time (MTT) can be derived (Tofts 2003, pp. 365–390). Since the transverse relaxation rates 1/T2* and 1/T2 can be assumed to be proportional to the contrast agent concentration, the latter can be obtained from changes in signal intensity, from which concentration-time curves can be derived. The advantage of this method is a high SNR. However, CBF quantification is complicated (Buxton 2002, pp. 310–350), especially with intravascular contrast agents, and DSC MRI does not allow for repeated CBF measurements before complete washout of the contrast agent.

In contrast to the DSC method, ASL uses inverted blood spins as a tracer and is completely noninvasive. With a time resolution of 4–10 min (for quantitative high-resolution multislice CBF maps), it allows for serial determination of CBF. The disadvantage is the low SNR and the short lifetime of the tracer (which decays with T1). Therefore, ASL does profit from measurements at high magnetic field strengths that intrinsically provide increased SNR and longer T1 values. In the following paragraphs, only the noninvasive ASL method will be discussed because of its widespread use in human studies.

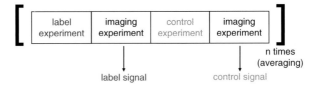

$$CBF \propto \Delta S = \text{control signal} - \text{label signal}$$

Fig. 12 Schematic description of the arterial spin labelling (ASL) method for CBF quantification: two types of images are acquired, through either a label experiment or a control experiment. The CBF is proportional to the difference image. To increase the signal-to-noise ratio, the acquisition is usually averaged several times

2.2
Arterial Spin Labelling Measurements

An ASL measurement consists of a label experiment, where a magnetisation preparation (inversion) of inflowing blood is performed before its entry into the imaging slice(s), and a control experiment, where no preparation of the inflowing blood is performed. Images are acquired after each experiment, giving the label and control signals (Fig. 12). The CBF is proportional to the difference in signal:

$$CBF \propto \Delta S = S_{\text{control}} - S_{\text{label}}$$

The fact that the signal difference only shows perfused areas can be explained as follows. The signal in the imaging slice arises from the static tissue spins and the moving blood spins. The static spins provide the same signal in the label and control scans, so they do not contribute to the difference image. The inflowing blood spins, however, are relaxed in the control scan and inverted in the label scan, which results in a positive signal in the difference image (Fig. 13).

It should be noted that ΔS is generally on the order of 1% of the average signal strength in the label and control images, so a small measurement error in S_{control} or S_{label} will result in a large error for CBF.

	control		label		difference
static spins	relaxed ↑		relaxed ↑		0
		⊖		⊜	
blood spins	relaxed ↑		inverted ↓		non-zero
net signal					non-zero

Fig. 13 Schematic description of the ASL method for CBF quantification: static spins are fully relaxed for both the control and the label experiment. In contrast, blood spins are inverted for the label experiment. Thus, the difference image shows the signal for blood spins only

2.3
Labelling Methods

ASL comes in two varieties: continuous (CASL) and pulsed (PASL) arterial spin labelling. CASL uses special long-duration RF pulses to continuously invert blood spins entering the brain inside a thin slice. This results in a continuous label of inverted blood, giving rise to a relatively high SNR. However, high RF power consumption, leading to tissue heating as well as eddy current effects due to strong gradients, can be a problem. A separate labelling coil is advantageous but technically more challenging because it requires an additional transmit channel. PASL uses short RF pulses to invert spins inside a broad slab, resulting in reduced power consumption and reduced eddy currents. However, instead of a continuous inflow of labelled blood there will be a bolus of inverted blood spins, the spatial extent of which is not usually well defined, leading to a reduced SNR. EPISTAR (Edelman et al. 1994), PICORE (Wong et al. 1997) and FAIR (Kim 1995; Schwarzbauer et al. 1996) are commonly used PASL implementations. Combined EEG-ASL acquisitions have been successfully performed in the field of epilepsy (Stefanovic et al. 2005; Hamandi et al. 2008; Carmichael et al. 2008); see the chapters "EEG–fMRI in Adults with Focal Epilepsy", "EEG–fMRI in Idiopathic Generalised Epilepsy (Adults)" and "EEG–fMRI in Children with Epilepsy".

2.4
Quantification Problems in ASL

There are several sources of systematic error in CBF quantification (Wong 2005) that are related to problems affecting static and blood spins. Static spins can be erroneously influenced by the label experiment via the magnetisation transfer effect (increasing with the duration of inversion pulses), eddy currents (increasing with decreasing inversion slice thickness) and imperfect slice profiles (increasing with slice thickness). Blood spins can lead to errors due to inflow from areas that are not affected by the label experiment (causing underestimation of the CBF), and intravascular signal from labelled blood designed to perfuse capillaries in more distal slices (causing overestimation of the CBF).

The following parameters influence the difference signal ΔS and need to be taken into account in CBF quantification: the transit delay δt (the time labelled blood needs to travel from the labelling site to the imaging slice), the natural time width τ of the bolus (depends on the thickness of the labelling slice and the velocity distribution of the spins inside), the T1 decay of labelled blood (leads to reduced SNR in the difference signal), and the exchange of water between labelled blood and the brain tissue which has a different T1.

Quantification can be simplified by using saturation pulses on the labelling slice that cut off the tail of the bolus, leading to a well-defined bolus length. This makes the method independent of (1) the natural time width of the bolus, as the bolus length is now defined by the time between the labelling pulse and saturation pulse, and (2) under certain conditions of the transit delay, too. The respective sequences are QUIPSS II (Wong et al. 1998), where a single broad saturation pulse is applied to the whole of the labelling slice (some quantification errors still remain due to imperfect slice profiles), and Q2TIPS (Luh et al.

1999), where a train of thin slice saturation pulses (with a much better slice profile) is applied at the distal end of the labelling slice (instead of one broad saturation pulse to the whole of the labelling slice), thus further improving quantification. Saturation of the imaging slice before the labelling/control experiment reduces errors for the static spins due to the imperfect slice profile of the broad labelling slice, and has the additional advantage that adding the label and control images yields an image showing the BOLD effect (Wong et al. 1997; Luh et al. 2000), as discussed later.

A more recent form of PASL is velocity-selective ASL (VS-ASL), where the labelling of blood is based on flow velocity and not on spatial location (Wu and Wong 2006). A detailed review of the issues discussed in this section can be found in Wong (2005).

3
The Cerebral Blood Volume (CBV)

3.1
Definition, Order of Magnitude, Measurement

The blood volume per tissue mass or volume (ml/100 g or ml/100 ml) is expressed as the CBV. In the human brain, typical values are approximately 5 ml/(100 ml) in grey matter and 2.5 ml/(100 ml) in white matter (Kuppusamy et al. 1996; Leenders et al. 1990). The CBV is an important parameter in normal brain physiology and pathophysiology. It is used as a measure of brain activity in fMRI (Belliveau et al. 1991; Lu et al. 2003; Vanduffel et al. 2001). In particular, direct measurements of CBV help to elucidate the complex interplay between CBF, CBV, and blood oxygenation underlying the BOLD effect used in the majority of current fMRI studies, and are important for the quantitative mapping of the cerebral metabolic rate of oxygen ($CMRO_2$; Kida et al. 2007). CBV is also used as a marker of disease; for example, in the assessment of brain vasculature diseases (Kader and Young 1996).

Various MR methods were developed to measure the CBV, and these fall into two main categories: methods using contrast agents (Belliveau et al. 1991; Ostergaard et al. 1998; Schwarzbauer et al. 1993; Vanduffel et al. 2001), and a more recently developed contrast agent-free method (vascular space occupancy; VASO) (Lu et al. 2003).

3.2
Contrast Agent-Based Methods

There are two main contrast agent-based methods: DSC imaging (which is also called DCE imaging) and steady-state imaging. In each case, a paramagnetic contrast agent (e.g. Gd-DTPA) is injected, reducing the intravascular relaxation times. In DSC imaging, the passage of a bolus of contrast agent after intravenous injection is traced by T2*/T2-weighted imaging. The signal time curve allows the CBV to be estimated based on a model of tracer kinetics (Tofts 2003, pp. 365–390). In steady-state imaging, changes in T1 are exploited by comparing images acquired before and after injection. A sufficient waiting time is employed to ensure that the contrast agent concentration in the blood has reached a steady state.

3.2.1
Dynamic Susceptibility Contrast Imaging

DSC (or DCE) imaging was described above: a paramagnetic contrast agent is injected as a bolus intravenously, and the signal time course is monitored with a T2 or T2*-weighted MR sequence. The area under the signal time curve is proportional to the CBV (Rosen et al. 1990). Since the proportionality constant is not generally known, the relative CBV (rCBV) can be calculated, where a value of 100% corresponds to pure blood. The rCBV can be obtained from the ratio of the signal in the region of interest to the signal from voxels that contain blood only (e.g. inside the superior sagittal sinus). Since DSC imaging requires a high temporal resolution of about a second to sample the signal time course adequately, the spatial resolution is limited. Thus, partial volume effects complicate the assessment of CBV and large vessels cannot be excluded (Lin et al. 1999). Moreover, the signal intensity may be too low in blood-only voxels during the bolus passage. Recirculation of the contrast agent after the first pass and an unknown arterial input function further complicate the assessment (Tofts 2003, pp. 365–390). Therefore, often only quotients of CBV values are reported, for example comparing two homologous brain areas in the left and right hemispheres or tissues of interest.

3.2.2
Steady-State Imaging

The CBV can also be estimated from steady-state imaging (Kuppusamy et al. 1996; Moseley et al. 1992; Schwarzbauer et al. 1993). For this method, it is assumed that two separate compartments contribute to the signal: an extravascular (brain parenchyma) and an intravascular (blood vessels) compartment. When a paramagnetic contrast agent is injected, it will selectively lower T1 in the intravascular compartment, leading to a signal increase in T1-weighted images. The increase in signal permits the size of the intravascular compartment, i.e. the CBV, to be calculated. Two acquisitions are performed, one before and one after the injection of the contrast agent, allowing for sufficient time to reach a steady-state distribution of the contrast agent. Since the data are acquired in the steady state, the imaging sequence does not need to be fast, allowing for higher spatial resolution and high SNR. Therefore, 3D gradient echo sequences are usually used for imaging.

In the original implementation, a quantitative T1 map was acquired before and after contrast agent injection (Schwarzbauer et al. 1993), using a spoiled, fast, low-angle shot (FLASH) technique (Haase 1990). The longitudinal relaxation rate $R1 = 1/T1$ is obtained for a voxel containing the tissue of interest and a control voxel containing blood only. The CBV can be computed as (Schwarzbauer et al. 1993):

$$CBV = \frac{R1_{post}(\text{tissue}) - R1_{pre}(\text{tissue})}{R1_{post}(\text{blood}) - R1_{pre}(\text{blood})}.$$

Since in spoiled FLASH the signal change $S_{post}-S_{pre}$ is roughly proportional to the underlying change in relaxation rate $R1_{post}-R1_{pre}$, the CBV can be directly estimated from the signals for the two voxels, bypassing $T1/R1$ quantification (Kuppusamy et al. 1996):

$$CBV = \frac{S_{post}(\text{tissue}) - S_{pre}(\text{tissue})}{S_{post}(\text{blood}) - S_{pre}(\text{blood})}.$$

Recently, the steady-state approach was modified to include an inversion of the longitudinal magnetisation prior to FLASH acquisition (Perles-Barbacaru and Lahrech 2007). The inversion time (TI) and the repetition time (TR) are chosen in a way that the signal from compartments with long T1 values is nulled, leading to complete suppression of the extravascular signal. In contrast, intravascular blood yields the maximum signal since the blood T1 is strongly reduced due to the contrast agent. Thus, the total signal S_{post} arises from intravascular blood only. A second measurement without T1 weighting is performed, choosing long TR and TI values, which yields a signal S_0 arising from all compartments. As a consequence, the CBV can be obtained from the quotient S_{post}/S_0. To exclude residual signal contributions, another T1-weighted measurement before contrast agent administration is performed, and the CBV is obtained from:

$$CBV = \frac{S_{post} - S_{pre}}{S_0}.$$

The steady-state methods assume that the intra- and extravascular compartments are separate. This assumption can be violated when, for example, the blood–brain barrier is damaged or if diffusion of water across the capillary walls is significant (Perles-Barbacaru and Lahrech 2007), thus resulting in a misestimation of the CBV.

3.3
Contrast Agent-Free Method: Vascular Space Occupancy Measurement

The VASO imaging technique measures CBV without an exogenous contrast agent. VASO imaging is primarily used qualitatively for fMRI, but quantitative CBV measurements are possible in combination with a contrast agent (Lu et al. 2005). Usually, a gradient echo EPI acquisition is preceded by a global inversion that nulls the blood signal. Thus, an increase in CBV results in a reduction of signal intensity. The original version of VASO-fMRI allowed for the acquisition of a single slice only (Lu et al. 2003), but was later extended to multislice acquisition (Lu et al. 2004).

Compared to contrast agent-based techniques, VASO-fMRI offers the advantage that it is noninvasive and can be repeated as often as necessary. Further, it is not sensitive to extravascular signal changes, since it uses the intravascular blood as an endogenous contrast agent. However, VASO-fMRI can systematically misestimate the changes in CBV due to brain activation (Donahue et al. 2006; Scouten and Constable 2007), which has been attributed to different factors. In particular, inflow effects, contributions of cerebrospinal fluid signal, and partial volume effects of white and grey matter affect the results and complicate their interpretation (Donahue et al. 2006; Scouten and Constable 2007).

4
The BOLD Effect and Functional MRI

Most functional MR imaging studies exploit the intrinsic BOLD contrast mechanism (Ogawa et al. 1990; Kwong et al. 1992). In the following discussion, we use the classic stimulus-induced activation model to explain the BOLD effect. However, it is important to keep in mind that numerous investigations such as EEG-correlated fMRI studies concern the resting state, in which one often seeks to reveal patterns of signal change that may not correspond to stimulus or task-driven effects, such as spontaneous fluctuations in brain activity: epilepsy, sleep, brain rhythms, etc. In general, it has been observed that in brain images based on gradient echo techniques with a suitable echo time TE, signal amplitudes are temporarily enhanced in regions of neuronal activation (increase in neuronal activity). This effect can be explained roughly as follows. During the resting state, local oxygen concentrations are relatively low, so blood contains a high concentration of *deoxyhaemoglobin*, which is *paramagnetic* (i.e. it locally increases the static magnetic field), whereas brain tissue is *diamagnetic* (i.e. it tends to slightly decrease the static magnetic field). This means that at the interfaces of vessels and brain tissue there are magnetic field inhomogeneities that shorten T2* and give rise to a signal reduction in T2*-weighted gradient echo images, as explained above. After neuronal activation, more oxygen is transported to the site of activation via an increased CBF, leading to a washout of deoxyhaemoglobin and an increased concentration of *oxyhaemoglobin*, which is diamagnetic. Thus, the magnetic properties of blood and brain tissue are more similar, field inhomogeneities are reduced, and the local image intensity increases.

In reality, matters are more complicated. Figure. 14 shows a typical signal time course following neuronal activation associated with an external stimulus (task) or spontaneous brain activity, the so-called *haemodynamic response*. Initially, there is a slight signal *decrease*. This *initial dip* is not always observed and has been reported for high field strengths (Buxton 2001). Afterwards, there is a *positive BOLD response* that persists for about 5–10 s. For the remaining time, up to 30 s after the onset of the stimulus, there is a signal *undershoot*. The physiology behind these effects is only partially understood. In particular, it is not clear how the coupling between neuronal activity and blood flow is mediated (Attwell and Iadecola 2002), and which aspect or aspects of neuronal activity it best reflects. This is one of the questions that studies combining electrophysiology/EEG with fMRI may help to elucidate (Logothetis et al. 2001; Shmuel et al. 2006; Laufs et al. 2003; Moosmann et al. 2003). Here, we focus on the vascular response itself, for which a thorough discussion of the various theories can be found in the literature (Buxton et al. 2004). In this section, one of the most commonly cited

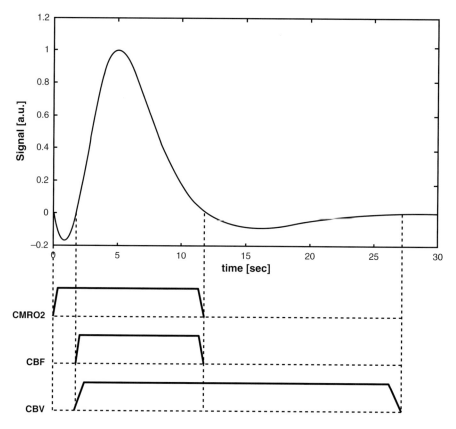

Fig. 14 A typical haemodynamic response function following a stimulus, showing a negative *initial dip*, a strong *positive BOLD response*, and a subsequent negative *undershoot*. These phenomena can be explained with the different time constants of the underlying physiological parameters: the metabolic rate of oxygen consumption (CMRO$_2$), the CBF, and the cerebral blood volume (CBV)

models will be presented. The important physiological parameters that influence the BOLD effect are the cerebral metabolic rate of oxygen consumption (CMRO$_2$), the CBF, and the CBV. The time courses of these parameters after activation are schematically sketched in Fig. 14.

Directly after the onset of neuronal activation, the CMRO$_2$ is increased. The consumption of oxygen leads to a higher concentration of deoxyhaemoglobin, which reduces the signal, resulting in the initial dip. However, after a very short while, the CBF and the CBV go up, with opposing effects: due to the increased CBF, oxygen is transported to the site of activation, giving rise to a decreased concentration of deoxyhaemoglobin and thus to a higher signal, as explained above. The increase in CBV is concomitant with a higher concentration of deoxyhaemoglobin, lowering the signal. However, the effect of the CBF increase outpaces the signal reduction caused by the higher CMRO$_2$ and CBV values, resulting in a positive BOLD response. After about 10 s, CMRO$_2$ and CBF return to their baseline levels. The relaxation of CBV is slower, so for a certain time there is an increased concentration of deoxyhaemoglobin due to the higher blood volume, which reduces the signal, resulting in the undershoot.

So far, we have focussed on the positive BOLD response for simplicity. However, it is important to note that the BOLD response curve may be inverted, in other words the large BOLD change that occurs after 5–10 s may be negative, as observed in various fMRI (Shmuel et al. 2006; Stefanovic et al. 2004) and EEG–fMRI studies (Hamandi et al. 2008; Laufs et al. 2003; Moosmann et al. 2003). Though the underlying mechanism is not completely understood, one important mechanism is a decrease in blood flow consistent with a decrease in neuronal activity in the cortex compared to the baseline (Hamandi et al. 2008; Carmichael et al. 2008). For example, it was shown that a decrease in global neuronal activity in primate visual cortex is accompanied by a negative BOLD response (Shmuel et al. 2006). Increased local field potential (LFP) activity, on the other hand, was shown to correlate well with the positive BOLD response (Logothetis et al. 2001). Although the majority of the studies exploited the main BOLD response after 5–10 s, some studies also targeted the initial dip for high-resolution fMRI (e.g. Kim et al. 2000). Moreover, the initial dip and the undershoot in the BOLD response were also studied in the context of models of the BOLD effect (see the review by Buxton et al. 2004).

The practical question of which echo time TE should be chosen for maximum BOLD contrast then arises. Figure 15 shows the theoretical BOLD signal depending on TE for a T2* value of 45 ms (which is the approximate T2* at a field strength of 3 T). The result corresponds to the discussion above (see the section on gradient echoes and T2*). For short TE, the spins do not have sufficient time to dephase, so the effect is small. For very long TE, there are signal losses due to relaxation effects. Optimum results can be obtained at 45 ms, i.e. when TE equals T2*. However, as described above, gradient echo sequences are susceptible to *all* field inhomogeneities, so there are signal losses in brain areas where the static magnetic field is typically distorted due to the vicinity of air-filled

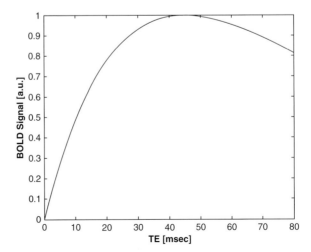

Fig. 15 Dependence of the theoretical BOLD sensitivity on the chosen echo time TE at 3 T

cavities (for example in the orbitofrontal and temporal areas). Thus, the TE chosen should be as short as possible. According to Fig. 15, there is still a strong BOLD signal for a TE of 30 ms, which is the recommended value for fMRI studies carried out on 3 T scanners. At 1.5 T, a TE of 50 ms should be chosen due to the prolonged T2* values at lower field strengths.

References

Attwell D, Iadecola C (2002) The neural basis of functional brain imaging signals. Trends Neurosci 25:621–625

Barrett T, Brechbiel M, Bernardo M, Choyke PL (2007) MRI of tumor angiogenesis. J Magn Reson Imaging 26:235–249

Belliveau JW, Kennedy DN Jr, McKinstry RC, Buchbinder BR, Weisskoff RM, Cohen MS, Vevea JM, Brady TJ, Rosen BR (1991) Functional mapping of the human visual cortex by magnetic resonance imaging. Science 254:716–719

Bloch F, Hansen WW, Packard M (1946) Nuclear induction. Phys Rev 69:127.

Buxton RB (2001) The elusive initial dip. Neuroimage 13:953–958

Buxton RB (2002) Introduction to functional magnetic resonance imaging: principles and techniques. Cambridge University Press, Cambridge

Buxton RB, Uludag K, Dubowitz DJ, Liu TT (2004) Modeling the hemodynamic response to brain activation. Neuroimage 23:S220–S233

Carmichael DW, Hamandi K, Laufs H, Duncan JS, Thomas DL, Lemieux L (2008) An investigation of the relationship between BOLD and perfusion signal changes during epileptic generalised spike wave activity. Magn Reson Imaging 26(7):870–873

Chalela JA, Alsop DC, Gonzalez-Atavales JB, Maldjian JA, Kasner SE, Detre JA (2000) Magnetic resonance perfusion imaging in acute ischemic stroke using continuous arterial spin labeling. Stroke 31:680–687

Donahue MJ, Lu H, Jones CK, Edden RA, Pekar JJ, van Zijl PC (2006) Theoretical and experimental investigation of the VASO contrast mechanism. Magn Reson Med 56:1261–1273

Edelman RR, Siewert B, Darby DG, Thangaraj V, Nobre AC, Mesulam MM, Warach S (1994) Qualitative mapping of cerebral blood flow and functional localization with echo-planar MR imaging and signal targeting with alternating radio frequency (STAR) sequences: applications to MR angiography. Radiology 192:513–520

Haase A (1990) Snapshot FLASH MRI: applications to T1, T2, and chemical-shift imaging. Magn Reson Med 13:77–89

Hahn EL (1950) Spin echoes. Phys Rev 80:580–594

Hamandi K, Laufs H, Nöth U, Carmichael DW, Duncan JS, Lemieux L (2008) BOLD and perfusion changes during epileptic generalised spike wave activity. Neuroimage 39:608–618

Hennig J, Nauerth A, Friedburg H (1986) RARE imaging: A fast imaging method for clinical MR. Magn Reson Med 3:823–833

Kader A, Young WL (1996) The effects of intracranial arteriovenous malformations on cerebral hemodynamics. Neurosurg Clin N Am 7:767–781

Kida I, Rothman DL, Hyder F (2007) Dynamics of changes in blood flow, volume, and oxygenation: Implications for dynamic functional magnetic resonance imaging calibration. J Cereb Blood Flow Metab 27:690–696

Kim DS, Duong TQ, Kim SG (2000) High-resolution mapping of iso-orientation columns by fMRI. Nat Neurosci 3:164–169

Kim SG (1995) Quantification of regional cerebral blood flow change by flow-sensitive alternating inversion recovery (FAIR) technique: Application to functional mapping. Magn Reson Med 34:293–301

Kuppusamy K, Lin W, Cizek GR, Haacke EM (1996) In vivo regional cerebral blood volume: quantitative assessment with 3D T1-weighted pre- and postcontrast MR imaging. Radiology 201:106–112

Kwong KK, Belliveau JW, Chesler DA, Goldberg IE, Weisskoff RM, Poncelet BP, Kennedy DN, Hoppel BE, Cohen MS, Turner R, Cheng HM, Brady TJ, Rosen BR (1992) Dynamic magnetic resonance imaging of human brain activity during primary sensory stimulation. Proc Natl Acad Sci USA 89:5675–5679

Laufs H, Kleinschmidt A, Beyerle A, Eger E, Salek-Haddadi A, Preibisch C, Krakow K (2003) EEG-correlated fMRI of human alpha activity. Neuroimage 19:1463–1476

Lauterbur PC (1973) Image formation by induced local interactions: Examples employing nuclear magnetic resonance. Nature 242:190–191

Leenders KL, Perani D, Lammertsma AA, Heather JD, Buckingham P, Healy MJ, Gibbs JM, Wise RJ, Hatazawa J, Herold S, Beany RP, Brooks DJ, Spinks T, Rhodes C, Frackowiak RSJ, Jones T (1990) Cerebral blood flow, blood volume and oxygen utilization. Normal values and effect of age. Brain 113(1):27–47

Lin W, Celik A, Paczynski RP (1999) Regional cerebral blood volume: A comparison of the dynamic imaging and the steady state methods. J Magn Reson Imaging 9(1):44–52

Logothetis NK, Pauls J, Augath M, Trinath T, Oeltermann A (2001) Neurophysiological investigation of the basis of the fMRI signal. Nature 412:150–157

Lu H, Golay X, Pekar JJ, van Zijl PC (2003) Functional magnetic resonance imaging based on changes in vascular space occupancy. Magn Reson Med 50:263–274

Lu H, Law M, Johnson G, Ge Y, van Zijl PC, Helpern JA (2005) Novel approach to the measurement of absolute cerebral blood volume using vascular-space-occupancy magnetic resonance imaging. Magn Reson Med 54:1403–1411

Lu H, van Zijl PC, Hendrikse J, Golay X (2004) Multiple acquisitions with global inversion cycling (MAGIC): A multislice technique for vascular-space-occupancy dependent fMRI. Magn Reson Med 51:9–15

Luh WM, Wong EC, Bandettini PA, Hyde JS (1999) QUIPSS II with thin-slice TI1 periodic saturation: a method for improving accuracy of quantitative perfusion imaging using pulsed arterial spin labeling. Magn Reson Med 41:1246–1254

Luh WM, Wong EC, Bandettini PA, Ward BD, Hyde JS (2000) Comparison of simultaneously measured perfusion and BOLD signal increases during brain activation with T_1-based tissue identification. Magn Reson Med 44:137–143

Mansfield P (1977) Multiplanar image formation using NMR spin echoes. J Phys C Solid State Phys 10:L55–L58

Moosmann M, Ritter P, Krastel I, Brink A, Thees S, Blankenburg F, Taskin B, Obrig H, Villringer A (2003) Correlates of alpha rhythm in functional magnetic resonance imaging and near infrared spectroscopy. Neuroimage 20:145–158

Moseley ME, Chew WM, White DL, Kucharczyk J, Litt L, Derugin N, Dupon J, Brasch RC, Norman D (1992) Hypercarbia-induced changes in cerebral blood volume in the cat: a 1H MRI and intravascular contrast agent study. Magn Reson Med 23:21–30

Mugler III JP, Brookeman JR (1990) Three-dimensional magnetization-prepared rapid gradient-echo imaging (3D MP RAGE). Magn Reson Med 15:152–157

Ogawa S, Lee TM, Nayak AS, Glynn P (1990) Oxygenation-sensitive contrast in magnetic resonance image of rodent brain at high magnetic fields. Magn Reson Med 14:68–78

Ostergaard L, Smith DF, Vestergaard-Poulsen P, Hansen SB, Gee AD, Gjedde A, Gyldensted C (1998) Absolute cerebral blood flow and blood volume measured by magnetic resonance imaging bolus tracking: Comparison with positron emission tomography values. J Cereb Blood Flow Metab 18:425–432

Perles-Barbacaru AT, Lahrech H (2007) A new magnetic resonance imaging method for mapping the cerebral blood volume fraction: the rapid steady-state T1 method. J Cereb Blood Flow Metab 27:618–631

Purcell EM, Torrey HC, Pound RV (1946) Resonance absorption by nuclear magnetic moments in a solid. Phys Rev 69:37–38

Rosen BR, Belliveau JW, Vevea JM, Brady TJ (1990) Perfusion imaging with NMR contrast agents. Magn Reson Med 14:249–265

Schwarzbauer C, Syha J, Haase A (1993) Quantification of regional blood volumes by rapid T1 mapping. Magn Reson Med 29:709–712

Schwarzbauer C, Morrissey SP, Haase A (1996) Quantitative magnetic resonance imaging of perfusion using magnetic labeling of water proton spins within the detection slice. Magn Reson Med 35:540–546

Scouten A, Constable RT (2007) Applications and limitations of whole-brain MAGIC VASO functional imaging. Magn Reson Med 58:306–315

Shmuel A, Augath M, Oeltermann A, Logothetis NK (2006) Negative functional MRI response correlates with decreases in neuronal activity in monkey visual area V1. Nat Neurosci 9:569–577

Stefanovic B, Warnking JM, Kobayashi E, Bagshaw AP, Hawco C, Dubeau F, Gotman J, Pike GB (2005) Hemodynamic and metabolic responses to activation, deactivation and epileptic discharges. Neuroimage 28:205–215

Stefanovic B, Warnking JM, Pike GB (2004) Hemodynamic and metabolic responses to neuronal inhibition. Neuroimage 22:771–778.

Tofts P (2003) Quantitative MRI of the brain: measuring changes caused by disease. Wiley, Chichester

Ugurbil K, Garwood M, Ellermann J, Hendrich K, Hinke R, Hu X, Kim SG, Menon R, Merkle H, Ogawa S, Salmi R (1993) Imaging at high magnetic fields: Initial experiences at 4 T. Magn Reson Quart 9:259–277

Vanduffel W, Fize D, Mandeville JB, Nelissen K, Van Hecke P, Rosen BR, Tootell RB, Orban GA (2001) Visual motion processing investigated using contrast agent-enhanced fMRI in awake behaving monkeys. Neuron 32:565–577

Wansapura JP, Holland SK, Dunn RS, Ball WS (1999) NMR relaxation times in the human brain at 3.0 Tesla. J Magn Reson Imaging 9:531–538

Wong EC (2005) Quantifying CBF with pulsed ASL: technical and pulse sequence factors. J Magn Reson Imaging 22:727–731

Wong EC, Buxton RB, Frank LR (1997) Implementation of quantitative perfusion imaging techniques for functional brain mapping using pulsed arterial spin labeling. NMR Biomed 10:237–249

Wong EC, Buxton RB, Frank LR (1998) Quantitative imaging of perfusion using a single subtraction (QUIPPS and QUIPSS II). Magn Reson Med 39:702–708

Wu WC, Wong EC (2006) Intravascular effect in velocity-selective arterial spin labeling: The choice of inflow time and cutoff velocity. Neuroimage 32:122–128

Yen YF, Field AS, Martin EM, Ari N, Burdette JH, Moody DM, Takahashi AM (2002) Test-retest reproducibility of quantitative CBF measurements using FAIR perfusion MRI and acetazolamide challenge. Magn Reson Med 47:921–928

Locally Measured Neuronal Correlates of Functional MRI Signals

4

Amir Shmuel

Functional MRI (fMRI) utilizes changes in metabolic and hemodynamic signals in order to infer the underlying local changes in neuronal activity. fMRI signals are therefore an indirect measure of neuronal activity, with the involvement of intermediary processes of neurovascular coupling and MRI measurements. This chapter summarizes the current concepts surrounding the neuronal correlates of fMRI signals measured locally and the mechanisms by which neurovascular coupling is achieved.

1
Blood Oxygenation Level Dependent Functional MRI Signals

The majority of functional brain imaging studies in humans rely on functional MRI (fMRI; Bandettini et al. 1992; Kwong et al. 1992; Ogawa et al. 1992). fMRI utilises task-invoked metabolic and haemodynamic responses in order to infer the underlying local changes in neuronal activity. fMRI signals may therefore be considered to constitute only an indirect measure of neuronal activity, with the intermediary processes of neurovascular coupling and MRI measurements also being involved. Understanding how metabolic and haemodynamic signals are derived from the underlying neuronal activity is therefore essential to the utilisation of fMRI as an effective method of studying brain function.

The most commonly used fMRI contrast is the blood oxygenation level dependent signal (BOLD; Ogawa et al. 1990; see Chapter 3 "The Basics of Functional Magnetic Resonance Imaging"). The BOLD signal is inversely proportional to the local content of deoxyhaemoglobin (deoxyHb) (Ogawa et al. 1990). Following increases in neuronal activity, local arterial cerebral blood flow (CBF) increases are larger than the increases in oxygen consumption (Fox and Raichle 1986; Hoge et al. 1999), resulting in lower deoxyHb content in the local capillaries, venules and draining veins, and an increased BOLD signal (Buxton et al. 2004).

A. Shmuel
Montreal Neurological Institute, McGill University, Montreal, QC, Canada
e-mail: amir.shmuel@mcgill.ca

C. Mulert and L. Lemieux (Eds.), *EEG-fMRI*
DOI: 10.1007/978-3-540-87919-0_4, © Springer Verlag Berlin Heidelberg 2010

2
Synaptic Activity and Local Field Potentials; Spiking and Multiunit Activity

Excitable neurons receive input signals via their synapses. Excitatory and inhibitory inputs take the form of excitatory and inhibitory postsynaptic potentials (EPSPs and IPSPs), respectively. These potentials can be measured using intracellular or patch clamp neurophysiological recordings, which are more commonly used in studies with brain slices than in in-vivo studies. Postsynaptic *input* excitatory and inhibitory potentials propagate along the dendrites towards the soma. Depending on the ratio between excitatory and inhibitory inputs, as well as on the synchronization between excitatory inputs, action potentials may then be initiated at the axon hillock. Action potentials propagate along the axons towards the cell's presynaptic axonal terminals. Here they transmit the *output* of the neuron to recipients via neurotransmitters released from vesicles into the synaptic cleft.

Most intracortical neurophysiological recordings are extracellular. This type of recording does not measure membrane potential; instead it measures signals within the extracellular space that reflect synaptic and spiking activity. When the membrane potentials between two separate regions of a neuron are different, a flow of current is triggered within that neuron. This current is matched by a return current flowing through the extracellular space. Active regions of the membrane together form a current sink, while inactive regions act collectively as a current source. The current sink is localized at the site of synaptic excitation, where there is a net influx of positive ions. Net effluxes of positive ions from other parts of the same neuron form the current source, thus establishing a current loop between the source and sink (Nicholson 1973). The broadband extracellularly recorded signal reflects the summation of extracellular currents that are secondary to ionic fluxes produced by synaptic and spiking activity across the nerve cell membrane. Local field potential (LFP) refers to currents established by activity in a number of surrounding neurons and measured together in vivo.

LFPs are not perfect indicators of neuronal activity. The amplitudes of LFPs depend not only on the strength of the synaptic input and on the transmembrane currents, but also on the spatial distribution of the current sources and sinks, as well as on the synchrony of the currents. The functional anatomy, positions and orientations of activated cells also influence the measured LFPs. For example, the appropriate stimulation of Purkinje cells in the cerebellum gives rise to large LFPs. This is also true of pyramidal cells in the cerebral cortex. These cells have large LFPs because their dendrites are predominantly parallel to each other. By contrast, interneurons do not contribute to LFPs, as their dendrites are distributed in a radial, star-shaped pattern (Lauritzen 2005). Fields generated by two or more neurons may add up or cancel out, depending upon the relative timing of their action potentials and their relative geometrical arrangement. The synchronous activation of many neurons lying in parallel within the brain will result in a large field potential (for reviews on field potentials, see Freeman 1975 and Logothetis 2002).

In extracellular neurophysiological recordings, the broadband recorded signal is composed of scattered action potentials superimposed on relatively slow-varying field potentials. Practically, LFPs and multiunit activity (MUA) are extracted from the broadband signal by temporal filtering: content with a frequency above ~300 Hz is taken to be the MUA, while content with a frequency below ~150 Hz is considered the LFP. This band separation has been justified theoretically (Logothetis 2002). EPSPs and IPSPs are both relatively slow events (10–100 ms long) compared to action potentials (0.4–2 ms long). This difference in duration is reflected in the difference between the power spectra of a single synaptic event and that of a single spike. The difference is again apparent when comparing the frequency spectrum caused by a series of scattered synaptic events to the spectrum caused by spiking events. The average spectrum of a spike is within the band used to compute MUA (i.e. above 300 Hz). The average spectrum of simulated EPSPs shows substantially higher energy in the low-frequency range (below 150 Hz) than in the MUA range. Experimental evidence linking LFPs to synaptic activity comes from experiments in which intra- and extracellular recordings were combined (e.g. Pedemonte et al. 1998). These experiments indicated that LFPs have a synaptic–dendritic origin. Further support for the synaptic origin of LFPs comes from current-source density analysis. This analysis indicates that LFPs reflect a weighted average of synchronized dendrosomatic components of synaptic signals. These signals originate from the neural population within 0.5–3 mm of the electrode tip (Mitzdorf 1987; Juergens et al. 1999). Given this evidence, it is reasonable to assert that LFPs predominantly reflect synaptic events, including synchronized afferent inputs and synaptic inputs originating from local neurons. LFPs represent a summation of synaptic activity from neurons within ~2–3 mm of the recording electrode tip. In contrast, the MUA represents a weighted sum of the extracellular signatures of action potentials occurring within a ~200–300 µm radius of the electrode tip (Logothetis 2002). The MUA is thought to be dominated by the action potentials of pyramidal cells, though action potentials from axons of passage, from dendritic spikes and from spikes originating in local interneurons also play a role.

3
Neurophysiological Activity and fMRI Signals: Time and Space

In the temporal domain, the BOLD response appears as a delayed, low-pass-filtered version of the neurophysiological response. This is because changes in blood flow occur over a much slower timescale than changes in electrophysiological activity. Changes in electrophysiological activity may happen within milliseconds or tens of milliseconds, whereas changes in blood flow or BOLD response take anywhere from hundreds of milliseconds to seconds. Consider the specific example of neurons in the primary visual cortex (V1). Subsequent to the onset of a visual stimulus, the response of V1 neurons begins within 20–50 ms, while a peak response is achieved within 30–70 ms (Maunsell and Gibson 1992). The onset of the subsequent vascular response becomes apparent only after 1.5–2.5 s. How quickly the corresponding positive BOLD response can be measured depends on the paradigm, the signal-to-noise ratio (SNR), the amplitude of the response and the analytical parameters. Typically, peak blood flow and BOLD response are not achieved until 5–6 s after the onset of the stimulus. As a result, a vascular response to a synaptic input is still developing when a second stimulus arrives at the active region. Complicating matters, the vascular response to subsequent stimuli is influenced by the preceding stimulus because of the temporal overlap between responses (Lauritzen 2005).

　　In the spatial domain, the resolution of the fMRI signal depends on the choice of fMRI contrast and the strength of the magnetic field. It also depends on which component of the vasculature is being probed (e.g. capillaries, venules, or veins). The point spread function of T2* BOLD response in the human visual area V1 has been estimated as ~3.5 mm at 1.5 T (Engel et al. 1997), and as less than 2 mm at 7 T (Shmuel et al. 2007).

4
Neurophysiological Activity and fMRI Signals: Amplitude and Reliability

The vast majority of studies analysing the relationship between neuronal, metabolic and haemodynamic responses have reported that a monotonic increase in metabolic and haemodynamic responses occurs subsequent to increases in neuronal activity. Many studies have indicated not only an increasing monotonous relationship between the different physiological responses, but even an approximately linear relationship. An example of such a study is one showing that relative changes in blood oxygenation in cat area 18 are proportional to increases in neuronal activity during the initial phase ("initial dip") of the associated haemodynamic response (Shmuel and Grinvald 1996) (Fig. 1a). Similarly, a study in rat somatosensory cortex showed that the rate of oxygen consumption is proportional to increases in neuronal activity during the late phase of the haemodynamic response (Smith et al. 2002) (Fig. 1b). It has also been shown that the CBF response to the stimulation of climbing fibres in the rat cerebellum is proportional to the integrated neuronal responses induced by that stimulation (Mathiesen et al. 1998) (Fig. 2a).

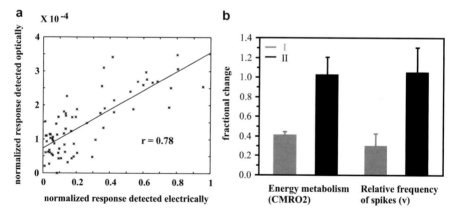

Fig. 1a–b Relationship between oxygen consumption and spiking activity. **a** Relationship between changes in blood oxygenation obtained optically and the underlying spike activity. These data were obtained during the initial phase ("initial dip") of the response. The line is the best linear fit to the data obtained by linear regression. A high degree of linearity is demonstrated. Modified from Fig. 7 of Shmuel and Grinvald (1996) with permission. **b** Relative changes in oxygen consumption and spiking activity evoked by rat forepaw stimulation. Responses obtained from baseline conditions I and II are shown in *grey* and *black*, respectively. The baseline condition II was lowered by ~30% from baseline condition I because of a higher dosage of α-chloralose; however, the incremental response from condition II was larger. In each modality, energy metabolism and spiking activity, approximately the same levels of activation are reached on stimulation from both starting baseline levels. Modified from Fig. 3 of Smith et al. (2002) with permission

Somatosensory evoked potential amplitudes were linearly correlated to the BOLD responses in rat sensory cortex when activated by forepaw stimulation across a range of stimulus frequencies (Brinker et al. 1999). A similar result was found in humans in response to stimulation of the median nerve using different stimulus intensities (Arthurs and Boniface 2003). Finally, the utilisation of visual stimuli with different luminance contrasts elicited BOLD responses that were proportional to the corresponding increases in neuronal activity (Logothetis et al. 2001).

Though a number of studies found linear relationships between electrophysiological and vascular responses, nonlinear relationships have also been observed. In the cerebellum, the CBF response to the stimulation of the parallel fibres shows a sigmoidal relation to the summated increases in neuronal activity (Mathiesen et al. 1998) (Fig. 2b). Using optical measurements of haemodynamic signals and simultaneous recordings of neural activity, Devor et al. (2003) demonstrated a nonlinear relationship between neuronal and haemodynamic responses in an event-related paradigm. Specifically, the haemodynamic response continues to grow beyond the saturation of electrical activity. Similar results were reported by Jones et al. (2004) and Sheth et al. (2004). The neurovascular coupling relationship within rat somatosensory cortex in the latter study was consistently better described by the nonlinear power law or threshold models. Hoffmeyer et al. (2007) examined neurovascular coupling in rat sensory cortices in response to direct stimulation of transcallosal pathways. They showed that an exponential relation exists between CBF responses and the summed amplitudes of increases in neuronal activity. Yet another type of nonlinearity that has been observed suggests that a certain minimum threshold of coordinated synaptic activity must be reached in order to trigger a haemodynamic response (Nielsen and Lauritzen 2001). This relationship implies that small changes in neuronal activity may be undetectable by

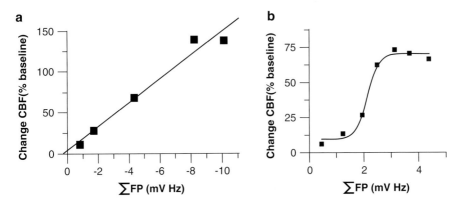

Fig. 2a–b Relationship between neuronal and haemodynamic responses in rat cerebellum. **a** Frequency-dependent CBF increases in response to climbing fibre stimulation are correlated with the sum of active and passive postsynaptic activity. The figure presents the scatter plot of CBF increases vs. summed field potentials, i.e. the product of field potential amplitudes and stimulation frequency. The *line* demonstrates the linear regression ($r = -0.985$, $P = 0.0022$). **b** CBF responses increase with increasing summed field potentials in response to parallel fibre stimulation at increasing frequency. The figure presents CBF increases (ordinate) vs. summed field potentials (abscissa) from one rat, showing a sigmoidal relationship. Both panels were modified from Mathiesen et al. (1998) (Figs 4d and 5d) with permission

perfusion-based imaging techniques. Synaptic activity needs to surpass a minimum threshold in order to cause an increase in CBF.

Overall it appears that, within a limited dynamic range of stimulus conditions, haemodynamic signals couple linearly to neuronal activity. In some networks, the haemodynamic responses become saturated, so that an increase in neuronal activity above a maximum level induces no further increase in the haemodynamic response. In other networks, the electrophysiological responses saturate, whereas the haemodynamic responses do not. Therefore, simply subtracting fMRI data obtained using two different stimuli might not properly indicate the difference in overall neuronal activity between the two neural states in a proportional manner (Lauritzen 2005).

The interpretation of fMRI signals is complicated by not only the partially nonlinear relation between haemodynamics and neural activity, but also by differences in the SNRs of these signals. The SNR of the neurophysiological signal associated with induced neuronal activity is about two orders of magnitude greater than that of BOLD (Logothetis et al. 2001). Such a difference can, in principle, result in the statistical rejection of valid activity during mapping experiments, despite the fact that the underlying neural response is significant. These findings are consistent with the demonstration that extensive averaging of fMRI data allows more brain regions to be correctly classified as activated regions (Saad et al. 2003).

5
The Driving Force of the Haemodynamic Response: Synaptic or Spiking Activity?

To correctly interpret the results of fMRI experiments, it is imperative to know whether fMRI signals primarily reflect the input to a specific region in the form of synaptic activity, or the output from a specific region in the form of spiking activity.

Several studies have reported an approximately linear relationship between metabolic and haemodynamic responses and spiking activity. Shmuel and Grinvald (1996) used optical imaging of intrinsic signals in conjunction with extracellular recordings in cat area 18. They compared the optically measured decrease in blood oxygenation ("initial dip") in grey matter regions to the action potential response to visual stimuli of drifting gratings, and reported an approximately linear relationship (Fig. 1a). Thus, the oxygen consumption during the initial phase of the BOLD response, before the increases in CBF, is correlated with spiking activity. Smith et al. (2002) reported a similar correlation between oxygen consumption and spiking activity for the subsequent phase of the BOLD response, after the increase in CBF. They measured changes in the spiking activities of neuronal ensembles during forepaw stimulation of anaesthetized rats. In addition, they derived the localised changes in oxygen consumption under the same conditions from BOLD fMRI data in conjunction with measured changes in CBF and cerebral blood volume (CBV). The changes in oxygen consumption were found to be proportional to the associated changes in spiking activity.

Rees et al. (2000) compared visual motion stimuli induced fMRI responses in human MT+ to spike rates obtained from single neurons in monkey MT using identical stimuli. Responses in human MT+ showed a strong and highly linear dependence on increasing coherence of motion signal, similar to action potential responses obtained from monkeys. Their results support the notion that fMRI responses are directly proportional to average neuronal firing rates. A comparison of BOLD responses in human V1 and action potential responses in monkey V1 to stimuli of varying luminance contrast resulted in similar conclusions (Heeger et al. 2000).

Under physiological conditions, synaptic activity is highly correlated with the firing rates of the presynaptic neurons. Synaptic activity is also coupled to the firing rate of the neuron to which the synapses under consideration belong. Therefore, if spiking activity is correlated with haemodynamic responses, synaptic activity is expected to be correlated too. This is especially true in the cerebral cortex, in which the majority of synapses (both excitatory and inhibitory) can be traced to a local network of connections originating in the nearby cortical neighbourhood, leaving only a small minority of inputs from more remote cortical and subcortical structures (Braitenberg and Schuz 1991; Peters and Payne 1993; Peters and Sethares 1991). An increase in the average firing rate causes a proportional increase in local synaptic activity. This in turn causes a proportional increase in metabolic demand and a proportional change in the vascular response.

Therefore, it is not surprising that in many cases the BOLD signal correlates equally well with LFPs and spiking activity. For example, Mukamel et al. (2005) recorded single unit activity and LFPs in the auditory cortices of two neurosurgical patients, and compared them with the fMRI signals of healthy subjects during the presentation of an identical movie segment. The predicted fMRI signals derived from single units and the measured fMRI signals from auditory cortex showed a highly significant correlation. The results showed a high linear correlation between spiking activity, high-frequency LFP, and fMRI BOLD signal measured in human auditory cortex during natural stimulation. As the spiking activity in the stimulation paradigm used by Mukamel et al. (2005) was highly correlated with the high-frequency LFP, the results could not identify one or the other as the driving force behind the BOLD signal. However, regardless of the mechanism underlying the BOLD signal, at least under natural stimulus conditions, BOLD fMRI signals can be a faithful measure of the average firing rate of the underlying neuronal population.

The local connectivity in the cortex is dense, resulting in high correlation between synaptic activity and firing rates of the pre- and postsynaptic neurons. These anatomical and functional features imply that the correlation of action potential rates to metabolic or haemodynamic response does not necessarily mean that action potentials consume most of the energy or are the cause of the CBF response. To indicate a type of neuronal activity that could be reflected in the fMRI signal under most conditions, one needs to dissociate the types of neuronal activities under consideration.

Strong evidence of the larger energy consumption of synaptic activity compared to spiking activity comes from Schwartz et al. (1979), who managed to spatially dissociate these types of activity. These authors measured regional brain-glucose metabolism in rats using 2-deoxyglucose tissue autoradiography (Sokoloff et al. 1977). They subjected rats to an osmotic load that was sufficient to stimulate cell bodies in the supraoptic and paraventricular nuclei of the hypothalamus. Importantly, the axon terminals of these cells reside in the posterior pituitary gland, at a significant distance from the cell bodies. This made it possible to unequivocally compare the metabolic activities in the two locations. The metabolism increased significantly in the area of the axon terminals in the posterior pituitary gland, and not measurably in the cell bodies residing in the hypothalamus. This result is consistent with the known correlation between the cost of maintaining ionic gradients and the surface-to-volume ratio of the involved cellular elements (Cohen and DeWeer

1977; Ritchie 1967; Raichle and Mintum 2006). Overall, the data support the concept that the mechanisms that drive CBF must be found at the synaptic–dendritic level, higher than the axosomatic level (see Lauritzen 2005 for additional evidence).

A dissociation between synaptic and spiking activity was also achieved by Mathiesen et al. (1998), who used laser Doppler flow measurements and extracellular neurophysiological recordings to examine the mechanisms of activity-dependent increases in CBF in the rat cerebellum. Stimulation of the monosynaptic climbing fibre system evoked extracellular field potentials and complex spikes in Purkinje cells with concomitant increases in CBF, indicating that both synaptic and spiking activities may contribute to the increased CBF. Stimulation of the disynaptic parallel fibre system inhibited the spiking activity in Purkinje cells, while the postsynaptic activity probed by the simultaneously recorded field potential increased. In spite of the decreases in spiking activity, CBF increased (Fig. 3a). This finding demonstrated that activity-dependent CBF increases in the cerebellum depend on synaptic excitation, including excitation of inhibitory interneurons, whereas the net activity of Purkinje cells, the principal neurons of the cerebellar cortex, is unimportant for the vascular response.

More recently, evidence from the same laboratory (Thomsen et al. 2004) demonstrated that spiking activity of Purkinje cells in the cerebellum is insufficient to cause increases in CBF. This study examined the effect of enhanced spike activity per se on CBF in rat cerebellum under conditions of disinhibition, achieved by blocking GABA(A) receptors using either bicuculline or picrotoxin. Disinhibition increased Purkinje cell spiking rate to 200–300% of control activity without incurring any increase in basal CBF. This demonstrates that increased spike activity per se is not sufficient to affect basal CBF. The neurovascular coupling between excitatory synaptic activity and CBF responses evoked by inferior olive (climbing fibre) stimulation was preserved during disinhibition. Thus, the unchanged basal CBF in the presence of the dramatic rise in Purkinje cell spiking rate could not be explained by impaired synaptic activity–CBF coupling. Therefore, increased spiking activity of principal neurons is neither sufficient nor necessary to elicit CBF responses, and activation-dependent vascular signals primarily reflect excitatory synaptic activity.

The complex connectivity of the cortex makes it difficult to dissociate synaptic and spiking activity. Nevertheless, such dissociation can be achieved in some cases. Logothetis et al. (2001) introduced simultaneous intracortical recordings of neural signals and fMRI responses, and used this technique to study the relationship of the BOLD signal to LFPs and spiking activity in the monkey visual cortex. In response to visual stimulation, the largest increases in power were observed within the gamma range of the LFPs. At recording sites characterized by transient responses of MUA and spiking activity, LFPs were the only signal that significantly correlated with the haemodynamic response (Fig. 3b). At such sites, the spiking activity and MUA showed strong adaptation, returning to the baseline before the LFPs. The latter remained elevated in some cases for the duration of the visual stimulus, better reflecting the duration of the BOLD response. In contrast, there were no sites found in which transient LFP responses and sustained MUA and BOLD responses could be observed. Linear systems analysis on a trial-by-trial basis showed that LFPs yield a better estimate of BOLD responses than the multiunit responses. A similar study in alert monkeys showed that although both LFP and MUA make significant contributions to the BOLD response, LFPs are better and more reliable predictors of the BOLD signal (Goense and Logothetis 2008).

Similar results were reported by Niessing et al. (2005). These authors recorded neurophysiological and optically measured haemodynamic responses simultaneously in the cat

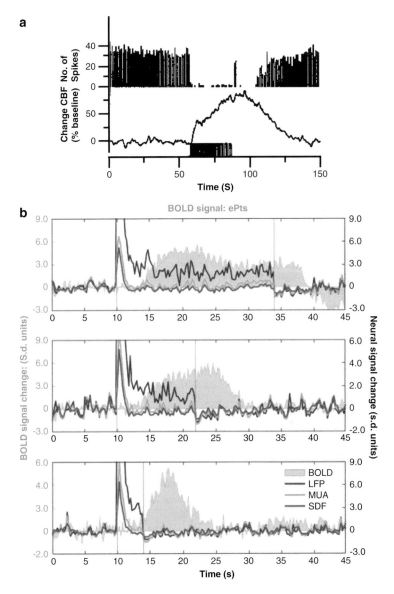

Fig. 3a–b CBF and BOLD responses correlate with LFPs. **a** Activity-dependent CBF increases and spike activity in response to parallel fibre stimulation in the cerebellum. Purkinje cell spike firing activity almost vanished after 1–3 s of stimulation, and spontaneous firing did not return to basal levels until 19–25 s after the end of stimulation (*upper plot*). CBF increased during stimulation, continued to increase for 5–10 s after the end of stimulation, and returned to baseline after 40–50 s (*lower plot*). Modified from Fig. 3a of Mathiesen et al. (1998) with permission. **b** Simultaneous neural and BOLD recordings from a cortical site showing a transient neural response. Responses to a pulse stimulus of 24, 12 and 4 s are shown in the *top*, *middle* and *bottom* plots, respectively. Both single- and multiunit responses adapt a couple of seconds after stimulus onset, with LFP remaining the only signal correlated with the BOLD response. *SDF*, spike-density function; *ePts*, BOLD time series from an ROI around the electrode. Modified from Fig. 3 of Logothetis et al. (2001) with permission

visual cortex. Increasing stimulus strength enhanced spiking activity, high-frequency LFP oscillations, and haemodynamic responses. With constant stimulus intensity, the haemodynamic response fluctuated; these fluctuations were only loosely related to the rate of action potentials, but were tightly correlated to the power of LFP oscillations in the gamma range. When sorting all trials according to the amplitude of the haemodynamic response, clear differences were observed with respect to the frequency distribution of the respective oscillatory responses in the LFPs. In trials with the weakest optically measured response, low-frequency oscillations in the delta, theta and alpha frequency bands were most prominent, while the high-frequency oscillations were weak. With increasing haemodynamic response strength, oscillation frequency shifted from the theta and alpha bands to the beta and lower gamma frequency bands. The strongest haemodynamic responses were associated with the most prominent oscillations in the lower and upper gamma frequency bands. Quantifying the relationships between the strength of haemodynamic responses and the oscillation power in different LFP frequency bands showed that low frequency activity in the delta band was negatively correlated with haemodynamic signal strength. Theta, alpha and beta activities were not significantly correlated with this signal. Weak and strong positive correlations existed for activity of oscillations in the lower and upper gamma bands, respectively. These oscillations increase with the synchrony of synaptic events, which suggests a close correlation between haemodynamic responses and neuronal synchronization.

Yet another dissociation of synaptic and spiking activity was demonstrated by Viswanathan and Freeman (2007) in cat primary visual cortex. During colocalised recordings of neural and tissue oxygen, they presented visual stimuli composed of gratings drifting at different temporal frequencies. With increasing temporal frequency, the spiking activity decreased while the LFPs in the lower gamma band prevailed. During stimulation at 20 Hz, spiking and low-gamma responses were ~15 and 85% of their respective maximal responses obtained at 4 Hz. Responses in the delta, theta, alpha, beta and high-gamma bands dropped to ~40% of their respective maximal responses. The tissue oxygen, a measure related to BOLD signal, dropped to ~60% of its maximal response at 4 Hz, suggesting coupling of these measures to the LFPs. Comparing responses to temporal frequencies of 4 Hz and 30 Hz, Viswanathan and colleagues observed strong coupling between LFPs and changes in tissue oxygen concentration in the absence of spikes, implying that the BOLD signal is more closely coupled to synaptic activity.

In a recent report, Rauch et al. (2008) induced a dissociation of MUA from LFP activity with injections of the neuromodulator BP554 into the primary visual cortex of anaesthetized monkeys. BP554 is a 5-HT$_{1A}$ agonist acting primarily on the membrane of efferent neurons by potassium-induced hyperpolarisation. Its infusion in visual cortex reliably reduced MUA responses without significantly affecting either LFP or BOLD activity. This finding suggests that the efferents of a neuronal network represent relatively little metabolic burden compared with the overall presynaptic and postsynaptic processing of incoming afferents. These findings suggest that the BOLD contrast mechanism mainly reflects the presynaptic and postsynaptic processing of incoming afferents to a region, and only to a lesser extent the activity of its output efferents.

Thus far, we have mentioned both instances of coupling and of dissociation between spiking activity and the BOLD signal. What determines whether the BOLD signal reflects the spiking output of neurons in any specific paradigm? Nir et al. (2007) have recorded isolated unit activity and LFP using multiple electrodes in the human auditory cortex. They found a wide range of coupling levels between the activities of individual neurons and gamma LFPs. However, this large variability could be explained predominantly ($r = 0.66$) by the degree of firing-rate correlations between neighbouring neurons. Gamma LFP was well coupled to BOLD measured across different individuals ($r = 0.62$). By contrast, the coupling of single units to BOLD was highly variable but tightly related to interneuronal firing-rate correlations ($r = 0.70$). Therefore, whether the BOLD signal reflects output spiking activity seems to depend on whether the paradigm evokes a high-degree interneuronal correlation.

6
Neuronal Correlates of Negative Bold Responses

In addition to increases in CBF and BOLD signals, sustained negative responses are pervasive in functional imaging. Some studies have hypothesized a purely vascular origin (for example, "vascular blood steal") for this phenomenon, suggesting that the negative BOLD response (NBR) bears little direct relation to underlying neuronal activity (Harel et al. 2002; Kannurpatti and Biswal 2004). Shmuel et al. (2002) measured BOLD and CBF, and demonstrated a robust, sustained NBR in the human occipital cortex, triggered by stimulating part of the visual field. The NBR was associated with reductions in CBF and with decreases in oxygen consumption. The findings from this study support the contribution to the NBR of a significant component of a reduction in neuronal activity. Similar associations of NBRs with decreases in CBF and oxygen consumption have been reported recently in the visual cortex (Uludag et al. 2004; Pasley et al. 2007) and in the motor cortex (Stefanovic et al. 2004, 2005). Using a similar stimulation paradigm to the one they used in humans, Shmuel et al. (2006) demonstrated a NBR beyond the stimulated regions of the monkey primary visual cortex. Through simultaneous fMRI and electrophysiological recordings, these authors showed that the NBR was associated with local decreases in neuronal activity below spontaneous activity. Trial-by-trial amplitude fluctuations revealed tight coupling between the NBR and decreases in neuronal activity. The NBR was associated with comparable decreases of LFPs and MUA. These findings indicate that a significant component of the NBR originates from decreases in neuronal activity (Fig. 4).

More recently, Devor et al. (2007) used optical imaging techniques in the rat primary somatosensory cortex to study the neuronal and vascular mechanisms underlying NBRs. Stimulation of the rat forepaw evoked a central region of net neuronal depolarisation surrounded by net hyperpolarisation. Haemodynamic measurements revealed that predominant depolarisation corresponded to an increase in oxygenation, whereas predominant hyperpolarisation corresponded to a decrease in oxygenation. At the microscopic level of single surface arterioles, the response was composed of a combination of dilatory and constrictive phases. The relative strength of vasoconstriction covaried with the relative strength of neuronal hyperpolarisation and the corresponding oxygenation decrease. These results suggest that neuronal inhibition and concurrent arteriolar vasoconstriction correspond to a decrease in blood oxygenation, which would be consistent with a negative BOLD fMRI response.

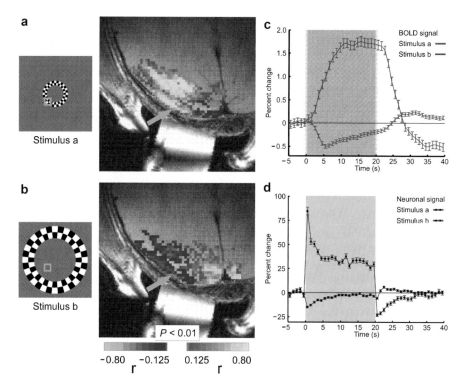

Fig. 4a–d Neuronal correlates of negative BOLD response (NBR). **a, b** Patterns of response to a central and a peripheral visual field stimulus. One oblique anatomical slice is shown, with the fMRI response superimposed. *Green arrows*, location of the recording electrode within visual area V1. *Green squares*, aggregate receptive field of the neurons in the vicinity of the electrode. The stimulus in **a** overlapped with the receptive field and induced a positive BOLD response in the vicinity of the electrode. The stimulus in **b** did not overlap with the receptive field and induced a NBR in that same vicinity. **c** Time course (mean ± s.e.m.) of the BOLD response sampled from the ROI around the electrode. **d** Neuronal responses to the stimuli presented in **a** and **b**. Time courses (mean ± s.e.m.) of the fractional change in the comprehensive neuronal signal in response to stimuli that overlapped (*red*) or did not overlap (*blue*) with the receptive field are shown. The data in **c** and **d** were averaged over all trials from 15 sessions. All panels were modified from Shmuel et al. (2006) (Figs. 1a, b, d and 2a) with permission

7
Neuronal Correlates of Spontaneous Fluctuations in fMRI Signals

The relationship between BOLD and neural events during the resting state is of particular current interest. While early human fMRI studies considered large spontaneous signal fluctuations typically seen during rest to be uninteresting "noise", a great deal of recent work has focussed on measuring and interpreting these signals (Biswal et al. 1995; Fox and Raichle 2007). These spontaneous fluctuations in fMRI signals are reminiscent of previously demonstrated spontaneous fluctuations in cortical neuronal signals obtained from cats (Arieli et al. 1996) and monkeys (Leopold et al. 2003). Importantly, fluctuations in fMRI signals at rest are correlated over large parts of the human brain (Biswal et al. 1995), a phenomenon termed functional connectivity.

Previous studies identified contributions of non-neuronal origin to spontaneous fluctuations in fMRI signals. These contributions include vascular vasomotion (Mayhew et al. 1996) and respiration (Birn et al. 2006; Wise et al. 2004). In contrast, until recently the link between spontaneous fluctuations in fMRI signals and the underlying neural activity remained tenuous.

Through simultaneous fMRI and intracortical neurophysiological recording, Shmuel and Leopold (2008) demonstrated a correlation between slow fluctuations in BOLD signals and concurrent fluctuations in the underlying locally measured neuronal activity. This correlation varied with the time lag of BOLD relative to neuronal activity, resembling a traditional haemodynamic response function with peaks at 6 s lag of the BOLD signal. The correlations were reliably detected when the neuronal signal consisted of either relative power changes in the LFP gamma band (see also Logothetis et al. 2001, Fig. 4a), the MUA band, or the spiking rate of a small group of neurons. Analysis of the correlation between the voxel-by-voxel fMRI time series and the neuronal activity measured within one cortical site showed that widespread areas of visual cortex in both hemispheres were significantly correlated with neuronal activity from a single recording site in V1. These results were obtained in anaesthetized, paralysed monkeys that were either staring at a uniform grey field or were in complete darkness. These findings generalised over sessions with grey images or in darkness. To the extent that Shmuel and Leopold's (2008) V1 findings can be generalised to other cortical areas, fMRI-based functional connectivity between remote regions in the resting state can be linked to the synchronisation of slow fluctuations in the underlying neuronal signals.

8
Neurovascular Coupling

Thus far we described how fMRI signals relate to the underlying neuronal activity. The last section describes the mechanisms that control this relationship, by initiating and maintaining the hemodynamic response.

Arterial blood is delivered to the cerebral cortex via arteries and arterioles located within the pia mater, the innermost layer of the meninges adjacent to the surface of the cortex. Pial arteries and arterioles penetrate the cortex or give rise to branches that penetrate the cortex in a direction orthogonal to the cortical sheet (Duvernoy et al. 1981). These arteries and arterioles consist of an endothelial cell layer, a smooth muscle layer with contractile properties, and an outer layer known as the adventitia. The arterioles give rise to capillaries, which consist of endothelial cells and pericytes with contractile properties. Within the cortex, both the arterioles and capillaries are in direct contact with the end-feet of astrocytic glial cells.

At the baseline level of neuronal activity, cerebrovascular autoregulation takes place: cerebral arteries relax when arterial pressure decreases, and constrict when arterial pressure increases. This autoregulation counteracts the effects of fluctuations in arterial pressure, assuring stable cerebral blood pressure and perfusion (Heistad and Kontos 1983). When a change in neuronal activity is induced, perturbing the activation rate away from baseline, this activity is coupled with local increases in CBF (Roy and Sherrington 1890). This phenomenon is termed "functional hyperaemia". "Neurovascular coupling" refers to the complex mechanism underlying functional hyperaemia.

Recent findings have led to the emergence of the concept of an integrated "neurovascular unit", which comprises neurons, glia and cerebral blood vessels (Fig. 5). This "neurovascular unit" is responsible for triggering and controlling functional hyperaemia (Iadecola 2004; Girouard and Iadecola 2006). At first, the mechanism controlling functional hyperaemia was thought to rely solely on feedback processes, where a deficit in energy following increased neuronal activity triggers an increase in CBF. A specific example of this mechanism is the catabolism of ATP molecules, which results in the production of the vasodilator adenosine. In contrast, the hypoxia and hypoglycaemia that follow stimulation are transient and of low magnitude. This suggests that the feedback mechanisms triggered by the hypoxia and hypoglycaemia are unlikely to be the exclusive driving forces underlying functional hyperaemia.

It has recently been suggested that a feedforward mechanism exists. In this mechanism, increases in neuronal activity initiate functional hyperaemia through neurotransmitter-related signalling; this happens even before hypoxia and hypoglycemia take place (Attwell and Iadecola 2002). This hypothesis came about due to a comparison between the timing and magnitude of CBF responses and the timing and magnitude of the release of vasoactive cations (Lou et al. 1987; Lassen 1991). There are a number of possible components of this feedforward mechanism. These include the release of ions, the release of metabolic by-products, and the release of vasoactive neurotransmitters, as well as the production of vasoactive substances triggered by neurotransmitters. Vasoactive mediators that are by-products of, or that play an integral role in, increases in neuronal activity include ions (e.g. K^+ and H^+), neurotransmitters (e.g. γ-aminobutyric acid (GABA)), and neuromodulators (e.g. acetylcholine; Edvinsson and Krause 2002; Hamel 2004). Glutamate, a common neurotransmitter in the cerebral cortex, stimulates the production of vasodilators such as nitric oxide (NO) (Faraci and Breese 1993). Suppressing the actions of any of these mediators reduces the CBF response without abolishing it completely. Therefore, functional hyperaemia seems to be triggered by several vasoactive mediators, but does not depend entirely on any of them (Iadecola 2004).

The release of vasoactive materials appears to be necessary (but not sufficient) for functional hyperaemia to occur. If diffusion of vasoactive metabolites was the only mechanism that controlled functional hyperaemia, then one would not expect increases in CBF to be as rapid and spatially specific as they are. Neurons (specifically interneurons) with processes impinging on blood vessels seem to release vasoactive factors at the onset of an increase in neuronal activity (Cauli et al. 2004). This theory is supported by experiments in mice lacking stellate neurons in the molecular layers of their cerebella. Mice lacking these stellate neurons show reduced CBF response to somatosensory stimulation (Yang et al. 2000). In addition to interneurons, astrocytes also play a role in controlling functional hyperaemia. Astrocytes, glial cells located in proximity to arterioles and capillaries, are involved in energy metabolism. Increases in intracellular Ca^{2+} concentrations in astrocyte end-feet

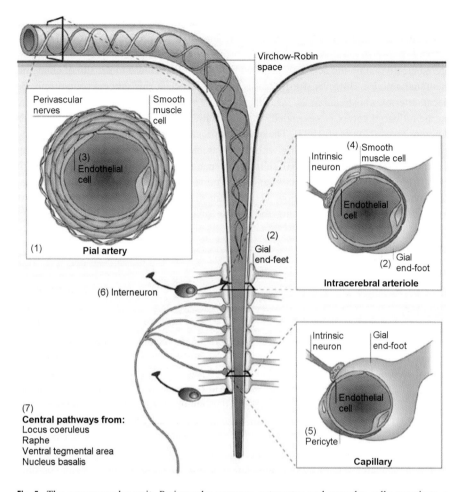

Fig. 5 The neurovascular unit. Perivascular neurons, astrocytes and vascular cells constitute a functional unit. Neurons and astrocytes are in close proximity and are functionally coupled to smooth muscle cells and endothelial cells (*1*). As the arterioles penetrate deep into the brain, the vascular basement membrane comes into direct contact with the glia-astrocytic end-feet (*2*). Endothelial cells (*3*) produce powerful vasodilators such as nitric oxide (NO), prostacyclin and carbon monoxide, and vasoconstrictors such as endothelin. Endothelial vasoactive substances are released by agonists that activate specific receptors, or by changes in shear stress at the cell surface produced by changes in the rate of blood flow. Gap junctions permit intracellular responses to be transmitted to adjacent endothelial cells. Smooth muscle cells (*4*) and pericytes (*5*) convert the chemical signals that originate from endothelial cells, neurons and astrocytes into changes in vascular diameter. These signals constrict or relax smooth muscle cells by inducing changes in the concentration of intracellular Ca^{2+} and altering the phosphorylation state of light-chain myosin. Astrocytic end-feet almost completely surround intraparenchymal blood vessels (*2*). They are involved in gliovascular signalling, the regulation of brain water permeability, neuronal energy metabolism, and synaptic function. Glutamate and GABA (γ-aminobutyric acid) released from neurons initiate calcium waves in astrocytes that induce perivascular release of vasoactive agents that participate in neurovascular signalling. Intracerebral arterioles and capillaries are contacted by neural processes that originate from local interneurons (*6*) or from central pathways (*7*; intrinsic neurons). These processes contain many neurotransmitters. Modified from Box 2 of Iadecola (2004) with permission

constrict the diameters of small arterioles (Mulligan and MacVicar 2004). Astrocytes release vasoactive mediators, including NO, K^+, adenosine and arachidonic acid metabolites.

Thus far we have introduced the mechanisms by which functional hyperaemia is triggered locally within the cerebral cortex and the cerebellum, close to the site of changing neuronal activity. However, for increases in CBF to occur, this process cannot only be local: arterioles upstream in the vascular tree must also dilate. Indeed, increased activity in the rat barrel cortex is associated with the dilation of pial arterioles several hundreds microns away (Cox et al. 1993). The upstream propagation of vasodilation appears to be mediated by retrograde signalling within the vascular wall; this may take place via gap junctions that couple endothelial cells and, separately, smooth muscle cells (Dietrich et al. 1996). Another proposed mechanism suggests that intracortical, downstream vasodilation can cause increased flow in upstream vessels, thereby increasing the shear stresses on these vessels, causing the release of endothelium-dependent vasodilators (Iadecola 1998).

9
Summary

Functional MRI (fMRI) utilizes metabolic and hemodynamic responses to stimuli or actions in order to infer the underlying local changes in neuronal activity. fMRI signals may therefore be considered only an indirect measure of neuronal activity, with the involvement of intermediary processes of neurovascular coupling and MRI measurements. This chapter summarizes the current concepts surrounding the neuronal correlates of fMRI signals measured locally and the mechanisms by which neurovascular coupling is achieved.

The majority of studies on the neuronal correlates of fMRI signals have reported a monotonous increase in metabolic and hemodynamic responses to increases in neuronal activity. Many of these measurements have indicated not only a monotonous relationship, but even an approximate linear relationship. The signal-to-noise ratio of increases in neuronal activity compared with fluctuations in baseline is substantially higher than that of BOLD. Under most conditions, the cortical BOLD response appears to be similarly related to both the synaptic input to a region and to its spiking output. Studies in which dissociations between synaptic and spiking activity were achieved indicate that the BOLD response reflects the former more than the latter. Negative BOLD responses have been shown to be associated with decreases in neuronal activity. Spontaneous fluctuations in fMRI signals reflect fluctuations in the locally measured neuronal activity mixed with a significant component of non-neuronal origin, e.g. respiration.

An integrated "neurovascular unit", comprised of neurons, glia and cerebral blood vessels, seems to be responsible for triggering and controlling changes in cerebral blood flow coupled to neuronal activity. Increases in neuronal activity cause the release of various vasoactive agents, such as ions, metabolic by-products and neurotransmitters. The propagation of vasodilation upstream is thought to be mediated by retrograde signalling within the vascular wall.

References

Arieli A, Sterkin A, Grinvald A, Aertsen A (1996) Dynamics of ongoing activity: Explanation of the large variability in evoked cortical responses. Science 273:1868–1871

Arthurs OJ, Boniface SJ (2003) What aspect of the fMRI BOLD signal best reflects the underlying electrophysiology in human somatosensory cortex? Clin Neurophysiol 114:1203–1209

Attwell D, Iadecola C (2002) The neural basis of functional brain imaging signals. Trends Neurosci 25:621–625

Bandettini PA, Wong EC, Hinks RS, Tikofsky RS, Hyde JS (1992) Time course EPI of human brain function during task activation. Magn Reson Med 25:390–397

Birn RM, Diamond JB, Smith MA, Bandettini PA (2006) Separating respiratory-variation-related fluctuations from neuronal-activity-related fluctuations in fMRI. Neuroimage 31:1536–1548

Biswal B, Yetkin FZ, Haughton VM, Hyde JS (1995) Functional connectivity in the motor cortex of resting human brain using echo-planar MRI. Magn Reson Med 34:537–541

Braitenberg V, Schuz A (1991) Anatomy of the cortex. Springer, Berlin

Brinker G, Bock C, Busch E, Krep H, Hossmann KA, Hoehn-Berlage M (1999) Simultaneous recording of evoked potentials and T2*-weighted MR images during somatosensory stimulation of rat. Magn Reson Med 41:469–473

Buxton RB, Uludag K, Dubowitz DJ, Liu TT (2004) Modeling the hemodynamic response to brain activation. Neuroimage 23:S220–S233

Cauli B, Tong XK, Rancillac A, Serluca N, Lambolez B, Rossier J, Hamel E (2004) Cortical GABA interneurons in neurovascular coupling: relays for subcortical vasoactive pathways. J Neurosci 24:8940–8949

Cohen LB, De Weer P (1977) Structural and metabolic processes directly related to action potential propagation. In: Brookhart JM, Mountcastle VB (eds) Handbook of physiology: the nervous system. American Physiological Society, Bethesda, pp 137–159

Cox SB, Woolsey TA, Rovainen CM (1993) Localized dynamic changes in cortical blood flow with whisker stimulation corresponds to matched vascular and neuronal architecture of rat barrels. J Cereb Blood Flow Metab 13:899–913

Devor A, Dunn AK, Andermann ML, Ulbert I, Boas DA, Dale AM (2003) Coupling of total hemoglobin concentration, oxygenation, and neural activity in rat somatosensory cortex. Neuron 39:353–359

Devor A, Tian P, Nishimura N, Teng IC, Hillman EMC, Narayanan SN, Ulbert I, Boas DA, Kleinfeld D, Dale AM (2007) Suppressed neuronal activity and concurrent arteriolar vasoconstriction may explain negative blood oxygenation level-dependent signal. J Neurosci 27:4452–4459

Dietrich HH, Kajita T, Dacey RG (1996) Local and conducted vasomotor responses in isolated rat cerebral arterioles. Am J Physiol Heart Circ Physiol 271:H1109–H1116

Duvernoy HM, Delon S, Vannson JL (1981) Cortical blood vessels of the human brain. Brain Res Bull 7:519–579

Edvinsson L, Krause DN (eds) (2002) Cerebral blood flow and metabolism. Lippincott Williams and Wilkins, Philadelphia, pp 191–211

Engel SA, Glover GH, Wandell BA (1997) Retinotopic organization in human visual cortex and the spatial precision of functional MRI. Cereb Cortex 7:181–192

Faraci FM, Breese KR (1993) Nitric oxide mediates vasodilation in response to activation of N-methyl-D-aspartate receptors in brain. Circ Res 72:476–480

Fox MD, Raichle ME (2007) Spontaneous fluctuations in brain activity observed with functional magnetic resonance imaging. Nat Rev Neurosci 8(9):700–711

Fox PT, Raichle ME (1986) Focal physiological uncoupling of cerebral blood-flow and oxidative-metabolism during somatosensory stimulation in human-subjects. Proc Natl Acad Sci USA 83:1140–1144

Freeman WJ (1975) Mass action in the nervous system. Academic, New York

Girouard H, Iadecola C (2006) Neurovascular coupling in the normal brain and in hypertension, stroke, and Alzheimer disease. J Appl Physiol 100:328–335

Goense JBM, Logothetis NK (2008) Neurophysiology of the BOLD fMRI signal in awake monkeys. Curr Biol 18:631–640

Hamel E (2004) Cholinergic modulation of the cortical microvascular bed. Prog Brain Res 145: 171–178

Harel N, Lee SP, Nagaoka T, Kim DS, Kim SG (2002) Origin of negative blood oxygenation level-dependent fMRI signals. J Cereb Blood Flow Metab 22:908–917

Heeger DJ, Huk AC, Geisler WS, Albrecht DG (2000) Spikes versus BOLD: what does neuroimaging tell us about neuronal activity? Nat Neurosci 3:631–633

Heistad DD, Kontos HA (1983) Cerebral circulation. In: Shepherd JT, Abboud FM, Geiger SR (eds) Handbook of physiology, Sect 2, Vol III, Pt 1. The cardiovascular system. Circulation and organ blood flow (Chap 5). American Physiological Society, Bethesda, pp 137–182

Hoffmeyer HW, Enager P, Thomsen KJ, Lauritzen MJ (2007) Nonlinear neurovascular coupling in rat sensory cortex by activation of transcallosal fibers. J Cereb Blood Flow Metab 27: 575–587

Hoge RD, Atkinson J, Gill B, Crelier GR, Marrett S, Pike GB (1999) Linear coupling between cerebral blood flow and oxygen consumption in activated human cortex. Proc Natl Acad Sci USA 96:9403–9408

Iadecola C (1998) Cerebral circulatory dysregulation in ischemia. In: Ginsberg MD, Bogousslavsky J (eds) Cerebrovascular diseases. Blackwell Science, Cambridge, pp 319–332

Iadecola C (2004) Neurovascular regulation in the normal brain and in Alzheimer's disease. Nat Rev Neurosci 5:347–360

Jones M, Hewson-Stoate N, Martindale J, Redgrave P, Mayhew J (2004) Nonlinear coupling of neural activity and CBF in rodent barrel cortex. Neuroimage 22:956–965

Juergens E, Guettler A, Eckhorn R (1999) Visual stimulation elicits locked and induced gamma oscillations in monkey intracortical- and EEG-potentials, but not in human EEG. Exp Brain Res 129:247–259

Kannurpatti SS, Biswal BB (2004) Negative functional response to sensory stimulation and its origins. J Cereb Blood Flow Metab 24:703–712

Kwong KK, Belliveau JW, Chesler DA, Goldberg IE, Weisskoff RM, Poncelet BP, Kennedy DN, Hoppel BE, Cohen MS, Turner R, Cheng HM, Brady TJ, Rosen BR (1992) Dynamic magnetic resonance imaging of human brain activity during primary sensory stimulation. Proc Natl Acad Sci USA 89:5675–5679

Lassen NA (1991) Cations as mediators of functional hyperemia in the brain. In: Lassen NA, Ingvar DH, Raichle ME, Friberg L (eds) Brain work and mental activity. Munksgaard, Copenhagen, pp 68–79

Lauritzen M (2005) Reading vascular changes in brain imaging: is dendritic calcium the key? Nat Rev Neurosci 6:77–85

Leopold DA, Murayama Y, Logothetis NK (2003) Very slow activity fluctuations in monkey visual cortex: implications for functional brain imaging. Cereb Cortex 13:423–433

Logothetis NK (2002) The neural basis of the blood-oxygen-level-dependent functional magnetic resonance imaging signal. Philos Trans R Soc Lond B Biol Sci 357:1003–1037

Logothetis NK, Pauls J, Augath M, Trinath T, Oeltermann A (2001) Neurophysiological investigation of the basis of the fMRI signal. Nature 412:150–157

Lou HC, Edvinsson L, MacKenzie ET (1987) The concept of coupling blood flow to brain function: revision required? Ann Neurol 22:289–297

Mathiesen C, Caesar K, Akgoren N, Lauritzen M (1998) Modification of activity dependent increases of cerebral blood flow by excitatory synaptic activity and spikes in rat cerebellar cortex. J Physiol 512:555–566

Maunsell JH, Gibson JR (1992) Visual response latencies in striate cortex of the macaque monkey. J Neurophysiol 68:1332–1344

Mayhew JE, Askew S, Zheng Y, Porrill J, Westby GW, Redgrave P, Rector DM, Harper RM (1996) Cerebral vasomotion: a 0.1-Hz oscillation in reflected light imaging of neural activity. Neuroimage 4:183–193

Mitzdorf U (1987) Properties of the evoked potential generators: current source-density analysis of visually evoked potentials in the cat cortex. Int J Neurosci 33:33–59

Mukamel R, Gelbard H, Arieli A, Hasson U, Fried I, Malach R (2005) Coupling between neuronal firing, field potentials, and fMRI in human auditory cortex. Science 309:951–954

Mulligan SJ, MacVicar BA (2004) Calcium transients in astrocyte endfeet cause cerebrovascular constrictions. Nature 431:195–199

Nicholson C (1973) Theoretical analysis of field potentials in anisotropic ensembles of neuronal elements. IEEE Trans Biomed Eng 20:278–288

Nielsen A, Lauritzen M (2001) Coupling and uncoupling of activity-dependent increases of neuronal activity and blood flow in rat somatosensory cortex. J Physiol 533:773–785

Niessing J, Ebisch B, Schmidt KE, Niessing M, Singer W, Galuske RA (2005) Hemodynamic signals correlate tightly with synchronized gamma oscillations. Science 309:948–951

Nir Y, Fisch L, Mukamel R, Gelbard-Sagiv H, Arieli A, Fried I, Malach R (2007) Coupling between neuronal firing rate, gamma LFP, and BOLD fMRI is related to interneuronal correlations. Curr Biol 17:1275–1285

Ogawa S, Lee TM, Kay AR, Tank DW (1990) Brain magnetic resonance imaging with contrast dependent on blood oxygenation. Proc Natl Acad Sci USA 87:9868–9872

Ogawa S, Tank DW, Menon R, Ellermann JM, Kim SG, Merkle H, Ugurbil K (1992) Intrinsic signal changes accompanying sensory stimulation: Functional brain mapping with magnetic-resonance-imaging. Proc Natl Acad Sci USA 89:5951–5955

Pasley BN, Inglis BA, Freeman RD (2007) Analysis of oxygen metabolism implies a neural origin for the negative BOLD response in human visual cortex. Neuroimage 36:269–276

Pedemonte M, Barrenechea C, Nunez A, Gambini JP, Garcia-Austt E (1998) Membrane and circuit properties of lateral septum neurons: relationships with hippocampal rhythms. Brain Res 800:145–153

Peters A, Payne BR (1993) Numerical relationships between geniculocortical afferents and pyramidal cell modules in cat primary visual cortex. Cereb Cortex 3:69–78

Peters A, Sethares CJ (1991) Organization of pyramidal neurons in area 17 of monkey visual cortex. J Comp Neurol 306:1–23

Raichle ME, Mintum MA (2006) Brain work and brain imaging. Annu Rev Neurosci 29:449–476

Rauch A, Rainer G, Logothetis NK (2008) The effect of a serotonin-induced dissociation between spiking and perisynaptic activity on BOLD functional MRI. Proc Natl Acad Sci USA 105:6759–6764

Rees G, Friston K, Koch C (2000) A direct quantitative relationship between the functional properties of human and macaque V5. Nat Neurosci 3:716–723

Ritchie JM (1967) The oxygen consumption of mammalian non-myelinated nerve fibers at rest and during activity. J Physiol 188:309–329

Roy C, Sherrington C (1890) On the regulation of the blood supply of the brain. J Physiol 11:85–108

Saad ZS, Ropella KM, DeYoe EA, Bandettini PA (2003) The spatial extent of the BOLD response. Neuroimage 19:132–144

Schwartz WJ, Smith CB, Davidsen L, Savaki H, Sokoloff L, et al. (1979) Metabolic mapping of functional activity in the hypothalamo-neurohypophysial system of the rat. Science 205:723–725

Sheth SA, Nemoto M, Guiou M, Walker M, Pouratian N, Toga AW (2004) Linear and nonlinear relationships between neuronal activity, oxygen metabolism, and hemodynamic responses. Neuron 42:347–355

Shmuel A, Augath M, Oeltermann A, Logothetis NK (2006) Negative functional MRI response correlates with decreases in neuronal activity in monkey visual area V1. Nat Neurosci 9:569–577

Shmuel A, Grinvald A (1996) Functional organization for direction of motion and its relationship to orientation maps in cat area 18. J Neurosci 16:6945–6964; and cover illustration

Shmuel A, Leopold DA (2008) Neuronal correlates of spontaneous fluctuations in fMRI signals in monkey visual cortex: Implications for functional connectivity at rest. Human Brain Mapp 29:751–761

Shmuel A, Yacoub E, Chaimow D, Logothetis NK, Ugurbil K (2007) Spatio-temporal point-spread function of fMRI signal in human gray matter at 7 Tesla. Neuroimage 35:539–552

Shmuel A, Yacoub E, Pfeuffer J, Van de Moortele PF, Adriany G, Hu XP, Ugurbil K (2002) Sustained negative BOLD, blood flow and oxygen consumption response and its coupling to the positive response in the human brain. Neuron 36:1195–1210

Smith AJ, Blumenfeld H, Behar KL, Rothman DL, Shulman RG, Hyder F (2002) Cerebral energetics and spiking frequency: the neurophysiological basis of fMRI. Proc Natl Acad Sci USA 99:10765–10770

Sokoloff L, Reivich M, Kennedy C, Des Rosiers MH, Patlak CS, Pettigrew KD, Sakurada O, Shinohara M (1977) The [^{14}C] deoxyglucose method for the measurement of local glucose utilization: Theory, procedure and normal values in the conscious and anesthetized albino rat. J Neurochem 28:897–916

Stefanovic B, Warnking JM, Kobayashi E, Bagshaw AP, Hawco C, Dubeau F, Gotman J, Pike GB (2005) Hemodynamic and metabolic responses to activation, deactivation and epileptic discharges. Neuroimage 28:205–215

Stefanovic B, Warnking JM, Pike GB (2004) Hemodynamic and metabolic responses to neuronal inhibition. Neuroimage 22:771–778

Thomsen K, Offenhauser N, Lauritzen M (2004) Principle neuron spiking: neither necessary nor sufficient for cerebral blood flow at rest or during activation in rat cerebellum. J Physiol 560:181–189

Uludağ K, Dubowitz DJ, Yoder EJ, Restom K, Liu TT, Buxton RB (2004) Coupling of cerebral blood flow and oxygen consumption during physiological activation and deactivation measured with fMRI. Neuroimage 23:148–155

Viswanathan A, Freeman RD (2007) Neurometabolic coupling in cerebral cortex reflects synaptic more than spiking activity. Nat Neurosci 10:1308–1312

Wise RJS, Ide K, Poulin MJ, Tracey I (2004) Resting state fluctuations in arterial carbon dioxide induce significant low frequency variations in BOLD signal. Neuroimage 21:1652–1664

Yang G, Huard JM, Beitz AJ, Ross ME, Iadecola C (2000) Stellate neurons mediate functional hyperemia in the cerebellar molecular layer. J Neurosci 20:6968–6973

What Can fMRI Add to the ERP Story?

5

Christoph Mulert

1
Introduction

ERPs are unique measurements of brain activity offering information about the reactivity of the brain with a high temporal resolution. ERPs can be used to investigate cognition, somatosensory processing and pain, auditory and visual processing, to mention but a few of the most important applications. A high degree of specialisation has emerged, so for example researchers interested in language processing can use the N400 potential (Kutas and Hillyard 1980; Friederici et al. 1993; Kiang et al. 2008), scientists looking at auditory attention can use the N1 potential (Hillyard et al. 1973; Naatanen and Picton 1987; Mulert et al. 2001), and groups interested in face processing may focus on the N170 (Sagiv and Bentin 2001; Taylor et al. 2004; Itier et al. 2006). While it is almost impossible to identify a single starting point of the ERP story since the early steps in evoked potential research started in the 1930s (Davis 1939), the discovery of the P300 in 1965 was an important milestone (Sutton et al. 1965). Researchers then started "to consider that we are involved in a breakthrough—evoked potentials are not just another physiological measure like the galvanic skin response, or pupillography, or heart rate, but something much more exciting—a direct reflection of time-locked activity of the brain associated with specific conscious processes in awake human subjects" (Sutton 1969). Even at that time, the authors described the influence of stimulus probability on the amplitude of the P300 potential (see Fig. 1).

This study provided evidence that is it not only the character of the stimulus that influences the evoked potential, but that there is also an endogenous influence of the reaction or attitude to the potential waveform.

Similar milestones were, for instance, the identification of the contingent negative variation (CNV) (Walter et al. 1964) and the detection of an influence of selective attention on the N1 potential (Hillyard et al. 1973).

C. Mulert
Functional Brain Imaging Branch, Department of Psychiatry and Psychotherapy, LMU Munich, Nussbaumstrasse 7, 80336 Munich, Germany
e-mail: christoph.mulert@med.uni-muenchen.de

C. Mulert and L. Lemieux (eds.), *EEG–fMRI*
DOI: 10.1007/978-3-540-87919-0_5, © Springer Verlag Berlin Heidelberg 2010

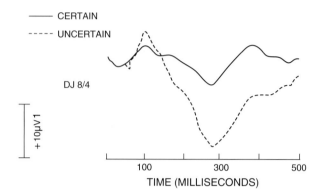

Fig. 1 This is part of the original figure from the first publication describing the P300 potential (Sutton et al. 1965; Fig. 1, pp 1187). The P300 was evoked with a stimulus uncertainty paradigm using paired stimuli (cue and test stimuli, $P = 0.33$ occurrence of uncertain test stimuli) and not with the "oddball paradigm", which is commonly used today. Reprinted with the permission of AAAS

ERPs have been used extensively in investigations of patients with neuropsychiatric diseases (for a review, see Pogarell et al. 2007). For example, reduced P300 amplitudes are a common finding in patients with schizophrenia (Salisbury et al. 1998; Mathalon et al. 2000; Jeon and Polich 2003). This reduction seems to be especially pronounced in patients with poor premorbid adjustment, early and insidious onset, a chronic and deteriorating course of disease, negative symptoms, and a tendency to develop tardive dyskinesia (Hegerl et al. 1995). A small P300 has been found to predict nonresponse to neuroleptics concerning positive symptoms (Ford et al. 1994). In addition, patients with a "cycloid psychosis" (according to the classification by Leonhard), which is characterised by a favourable therapeutic response and long-term prognosis, do not show any reduction in P300 amplitude, or even an increase in amplitude in comparison to healthy controls (Strik and Dierks 1993a, b; Strik et al. 1997).

Recent interest in ERP research has emerged due to the fact that ERPs often show a high heritability, in the range from 0.6 to 0.8 (Katsanis et al. 1997; Wright et al. 2001). Several ERP components (e.g. P300, P50) are now seen as intermediate phenotypes or endophenotypes and meet the criteria suggested by Gotesman (Gottesman and Gould 2003). ERPs have recently been introduced in the drug development process for psychiatric disorders such as schizophrenia. Since they can be modelled in preclinical studies, they offer opportunities for use as translational biomarkers (Javitt et al. 2008).

Apart from the enormous and ongoing success of ERPs in several different research areas, the localisation aspect of ERPs remains an area of investigation. In particular, it is obvious that all ERP analyses suffer more or less from the difficulty in determining precisely which parts of the brain are involved in the generation of a specific event-related potential. As described in the chapter "EEG: Origin and Measurement", this difficulty is fundamental: it is called the "inverse problem" and was described more than 150 years ago (Helmholtz 1853). It means that different combinations of intracerebral sources can result in the same potential distribution on the scalp, and therefore that the inverse problem has no unique solution. Thus, attempts at EEG-based localisations are merely reasonable estimates. A starting assumption is that the combination of fMRI and ERPs may help in resolving this problem.

Fig. 2 Summary of intracranial findings concerning the generation of different aspects of the P300 potential (P3a and P3b). Reprinted from Halgren et al. (1998) with the permission of Elsevier

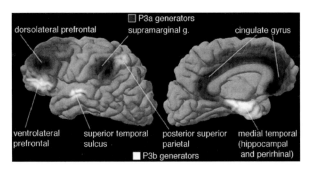

2
ERP Generator Localisation

One traditional approach to learning about the localisation of brain function as well as the generation of ERP has been to look at subjects with brain lesions. For example, an investigation of patients with bilateral damage to the hippocampus complex but undisturbed scalp P300 potentials suggested that the hippocampus does not contribute to the scalp P300 (Polich and Squire 1993), although the hippocampus is typically found to be responsive to targets but not to irrelevant stimuli using intracranial recordings (McCarthy et al. 1989). Intracranial recordings are another very interesting source of knowledge concerning the localisation of ERP generators (Halgren et al. 1994, 1995a, b; Brazdil et al. 2005; Rosburg et al. 2005, 2007); see Fig. 2.

However, both approaches (lesion studies, intracranial recordings) are limited, although they may offer general information about ERP generation. Since both lesions and intracranial recordings can only be investigated in specifically selected groups, these strategies are not directly applicable for research questions concerning healthy controls or even the vast majority of neuropsychiatric patients.

3
The Inverse Problem of EEG

In the authoritative textbook entitled *Electroencephalogaphy*, Fernando Lopes da Silva writes: "The ultimate aim of electroencephalography is to find the intracranial sources of the potentials recorded at the scalp" (Lopes da Silva 1993). However, this is a difficult task because of the Non-Unicity of the solution to the inverse problem of EEG. Focusing on this issue, several suggestions have been made during the last few decades for specific assumptions that may enable us to obtain plausible estimates of the underlying neural generators.

Apart from specific assumptions concerning the method of solving the inverse problem, additional assumptions have to be made concerning the (physical, geometric, anatomical)

properties of the generator, conductive media and recording electrodes. Early head models were simple spheres (typically four concentric spheres representing the brain tissue, the cerebrospinal fluid, the skull and the scalp), but in the last few years more realistic head models using MRI information have been developed (Schneider 1974; Sencaj and Aunon 1982; Meijs et al. 1988; Hamalainen and Sarvas 1989).

Concerning the choice of generator model, one option to solve the inverse problem is the strategy of calculating a (equivalent) dipole (Schneider 1972; Henderson et al. 1975; Cuffin 1985; Scherg and von Cramon 1985, 1986; Scherg and Berg 1991). Such a dipole is a mathematical abstraction that is assumed to generate a potential on the scalp. By changing the parameters of the dipole (position, orientation), "forward solutions" can be calculated in order to get a possible scalp potential distribution. If the difference between a forward solution and the original scalp potential is small, the solution is generally sound. However, this does not mean that the solution is correct in terms of the real generators of brain activity—it only means that the solution is basically possible. This kind of solution is generally nonlinear. Since the correct estimation of the number of dipoles used in a model is an essential issue when attempting to find a valid localisation, dipole source analyses have been used successfully in situations with a small number of active sources, such as localisation of epileptic spikes (Scherg et al. 1999) or simple evoked potentials with activity mainly in the early sensory areas (Hegerl et al. 1994). In general, this strategy has some advantages if the number of active brain regions is small and additional information about the possible positions of the sources is available.

Another strategy for solving the inverse problem can be used with minimal prior information about the nature of the generators apart from anatomical contraints, which usually limit the solution space to the grey matter. The latter may be obtained from subject-specific or generic MRI scans. This kind of strategy has been introduced as minimum-norm estimation (MNE) by Hämäläinen and Ilmoniemi (Hamalainen and Ilmoniemi 1984, 1994; Wang et al. 1992; Ilmoniemi 1993). This method has developed further over the last few years, including into "weighted" minimum-norm solutions (WMN). For example, using MNE, separate time behaviours of the temporal and frontal mismatch negativity sources were found (Rinne et al. 2000).

The next important development was LORETA, which incorporates the "smoothness assumption" (Pascual-Marqui et al. 1994, 1999). Based on neurophysiological findings in a number of animal studies that neighbouring neurons are most likely to be active synchronously and simultaneously (Llinas 1988; Gray et al. 1989), Pascual-Marqui proposed to assume that grid points in a current source model are more likely to be synchronised than grid points that are far from each other. This method has become quite popular during the last few years because comparisons of localisation results with imaging methods such as fMRI or PET have often revealed a considerable overlap (see Fig. 3) (Pizzagalli et al. 2003; Mulert et al. 2004, 2005).

Recent developments such as sLORETA (Pascual-Marqui 2002) and eLORETA have demonstrated even better localisation accuracy (Wagner et al. 2004). Linear methods like LORETA seem to be advantageous if there is likely to be a large number of active sources, and if no information is available about the positions of the electrical generators. LORETA has been used in numerous studies over the last few years, including investigations of

Fig. 3 Localisation of
brain activation evoked by
an oddball paradigm:
activations in the fMRI
analysis (*left*), and
simultaneously acquired
ERP activity localised
independently with
LORETA (*right*).
Reprinted from Mulert
et al. (2004) with the
permission of Elsevier

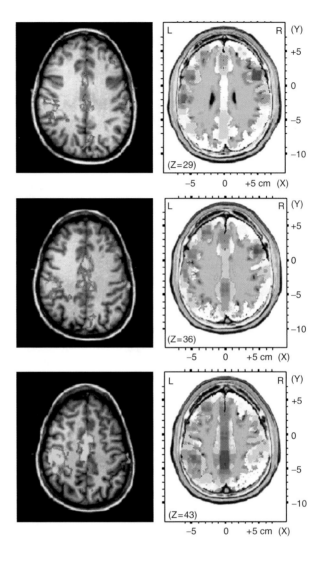

ERP (Anderer et al. 2003), resting EEG activity (Gianotti et al. 2007), sleep spindles (Ventouras et al. 2007), and patients with depression (Pizzagalli et al. 2001), schizophrenia (Mulert et al. 2001) and epilepsy (Bela et al. 2007).

The development of methods for EEG-based localisation is a very active field with numerous propositions during the last few years, including hierarchical and empirical Bayesian approaches (Phillips et al. 2005; Friston et al. 2008; Trujillo-Barreto et al. 2008).

Obviously, the ongoing process of developing solutions for the inverse problem proves two points. Firstly, there is enormous interest in obtaining information about the neural generators of ERPs. Secondly, there is currently no method that is able to solve all of the complex "real-world" questions concerning ERP localisation. However, today, we do have strategies to solve the inverse EEG problem with reasonable localisation accuracy that can be used reliably for a number of experimental questions.

4
Does fMRI Help to Solve the Inverse Problem?

There are practical issues with combining ERP and fMRI information that are discussed in more detail in other chapters of this book, as well as theoretical aspects that are concerned with understanding the workings of the brain. Generally, different methods are sensitive to different aspects of brain function; while EEG/ERP emphasises the aspect of the synchronisation of neural ensembles, fMRI tends to point to regional specialisation. Therefore, theoretically, a combination of EEG and fMRI is likely to significantly enhance our understanding of brain function.

From an ERP research point of view, the ability to correctly localise brain activity within millimetres, as offered by fMRI, is very attractive in terms of the additional information afforded to almost every aspect of ERP research. This perspective was apparently the starting point for studies that used a typical ERP paradigm for a fMRI study to identify the neural generators of the ERP components. Examples of this kind of study are provided by Menon et al. (1997); McCarthy et al. (1997); Linden et al. (1999). In these studies, the "oddball" paradigm was used, where frequent and infrequent stimuli are presented and attention must be paid to the infrequent stimulus (controlled by button pressing or counting). This paradigm is a classical ERP one that evokes the P300 component after a rare and relevant event.

The authors have described activity in the supramarginal gyrus and other inferior parietal regions and frontal midline areas. Since these regions were already found using intracranial recordings, lesion studies or ERP-based inverse solutions, the idea of combining ERP with fMRI to get spatial information was supported (McCarthy et al. 1997; Menon et al. 1997; Linden et al. 1999).

At this point, it should be mentioned that there are, of course, several constellations in which a one-to-one relationship between scalp EEG/ERP information and BOLD signal changes cannot be expected. For example, neural activity may be related to BOLD signal changes but not to scalp EEG changes if—due to the spatial orientations of the electrical generators (e.g. self-cancelling sources in sulci or neuronal assemblies without a strictly parallel orientation)—the electrical signals are not measurable on the scalp. In addition, nonpyramidal neuron activity will not lead to measurable electrical activity on the scalp (Nunez and Silberstein 2000).

On the other hand, the highly synchronous activities of a small number of neurons or phase shifts/changes in phase synchrony could result in a detectable EEG signal, but the associated haemodynamic changes may be small and not sufficiently above baseline values to survive statistical testing.

This issue of limited overlap between EEG measures and fMRI results has been addressed using different strategies. Obviously, it is especially relevant for any fMRI-constrained source analysis. Generally, when using fMRI activations as "seeding points" for dipoles, a close relationship between fMRI activation and electrical activity is assumed.

However, if dipoles are seeded in a BOLD cluster that does not contribute to scalp potential, the whole dipole model and all resulting information (e.g. about the time courses of dipoles) could be inaccurate. Several validation strategies to deal with this problem have been suggested, such as scanning the whole brain with "probe sources" that suggest additional electrical generators not seen in the fMRI analysis (Bledowski et al. 2007).

Another very promising approach with respect to the relationship of EEG and fMRI is to use single-trial variations of the EEG as regressors for an fMRI analysis (Nagai et al. 2004; Hinterberger et al. 2005; Debener et al. 2005; Eichele et al. 2005; Mulert et al. 2008). The full potential of this approach has been shown in a study by Eichele and colleagues, who separated different aspects of the BOLD signal with regard to their relationships with single EEG single-trial variations of different ERP components. One example of EEG–fMRI single-trial coupling is demonstrated in Fig. 4 (own data). Here, single-trial variations of the P300 potential were used to estimate the corresponding BOLD signal.

Single-trial coupling of EEG and fMRI is necessary if the focus of interest is the haemodynamic correlate of a specific ERP component. However, the results provided by this technique could also include brain regions that are not the actual electrical generators of the respective ERP component. This kind of strategy could also include BOLD activations of regions that are functionally very closely connected to the electrical generators of the respective ERP components, but are not the actual electrical generators themselves. Keeping this in mind, this kind of EEG-informed fMRI analysis is even more interesting considering the possibility of providing the functional neural networks engaged in a task.

At this point, it can be stated that fMRI has the potential to push forward our knowledge regarding the electrical generators of ERPs, but also that oversimplifications must be avoided since no general one-to-one relationship between EEG/ERP signal and fMRI signal can be premised.

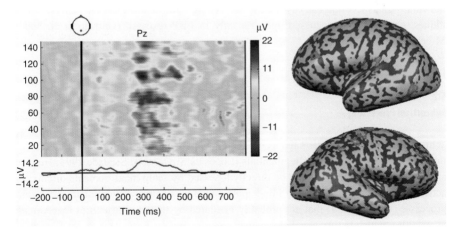

Fig. 4 *Left side*: single-trial variations of the P300 potential at Pz. *Right side*: specific P300-related fMRI activations based on single-trial coupling of the P300 amplitude variation and the corresponding BOLD signal (own data)

5
Further Aspects

While most chapters of this book deal with the direct combination of EEG and fMRI, it may also be worth posing the question of whether there could be an indirect influence of the fast-growing use of fMRI for many different research questions that have traditionally been investigated with ERPs. While such an assessment tends to be fragmentary and speculative, there may be at least two interesting aspects of it.

5.1
Serial Processing vs. Parallel and Reciprocal Network Activity

ERPs are usually defined in the time domain. Therefore, ERP components are obtained and described in sequence. For example, in auditory processing, early (brainstem) potentials can be numbered and distinguished from mid-latency potentials and late potentials. Accordingly, a sequence of information processing can be assumed. This assumption of serial information processing has influenced strategies to describe "mental chronometry" (Posner 2005), for instance the separation of evoked responses in stimulus evaluation processes and response-selection processes with separately measurable latencies (Falkenstein et al. 1994), or even four sequential steps (stimulus registration, stimulus selection, stimulus identification, stimulus categorisation) (Dien et al. 2004). Since fMRI does not offer comparable time resolution, fMRI-based mental chronometry analyses are rare (Formisano et al. 2002; Formisano and Goebel 2003). However, functional connectivity analyses, initially developed for fMRI data, have stressed the issue of reciprocal relationships between brain regions in a common neural network—an aspect that can easily be missed using traditional EEG/ERP analysis techniques, and was only focussed upon recently in ERP research (Garrido et al. 2007; Mulert et al. 2007).

5.2
Subcortical Processing

While subcortical structures such as the thalamus play an important role in the generation of brain rhythms and brain potentials (Lopes da Silva 1991; Steriade 1994; Hughes and Crunelli 2005), they cannot be directly assessed by scalp measurements of cortical activity. Accordingly, there is a "blind spot" and (for example) "attentional searchlight processes" (Crick 1984) that are probably mediated by thalamic structures (McAlonan et al. 2006), which in turn may have an enormous impact on cortical (electrical) processing and cannot be assessed with scalp EEG/ERP alone. Since (high-field) fMRI can be used to gather information about thalamic activity, EEG/ERP research may also be stimulated here.

6
Conclusions

ERP research has been performed successfully for decades and will continue to be a major tool for brain research due to its unique properties (e.g. concerning temporal resolution). However, localisation has always been a problematic but key issue in ERP research. Obviously, fMRI, with its ability to correctly localise to within millimetres, is capable of providing valuable information in relation to almost every research question that has already been addressed with just ERPs. While, in general, it cannot be expected that there is a one-to-one relationship between ERPs and the fMRI signal, it is still interesting that both signals are related directly or indirectly to synaptic activity. In the future, combining EEG and fMRI may prove to be crucial to obtaining a deeper understanding of brain activity. At the moment, practical issues (e.g. artefact correction) and basic questions (e.g. the precise relationship between EEG and fMRI signals) remain the source of debate. Nevertheless, several studies have already shown the enormous impact of combination strategies, and further improvements in technical aspects are expected to turn simultaneous EEG–fMRI into a routine method for the investigation of human brain function.

References

Anderer P, Saletu B, et al. (2003) Non-invasive localization of P300 sources in normal aging and age-associated memory impairment. Neurobiol Aging 24(3):463–479

Bela C, Monika B, et al. (2007) Valproate selectively reduces EEG activity in anterior parts of the cortex in patients with idiopathic generalized epilepsy. A low resolution electromagnetic tomography (LORETA) study. Epilepsy Res 75(2 & 3):186–191

Bledowski C, Linden DE, et al. (2007) Combining electrophysiology and functional imaging— different methods for different questions. Trends Cogn Sci 11(12):500–502

Brazdil M, Dobsik M, et al. (2005) Combined event-related fMRI and intracerebral ERP study of an auditory oddball task. Neuroimage 26(1):285–293

Crick F (1984) Function of the thalamic reticular complex: the searchlight hypothesis. Proc Natl Acad Sci USA 81(14):4586–4590

Cuffin BN (1985) A comparison of moving dipole inverse solutions using EEG's and MEG's. IEEE Trans Biomed Eng 32(11):905–910

Davis PA (1939) Effects of accoustic stimuli on the waking human brain. J Neurophysiol 2: 494–499

Debener S, Ullsperger M, et al. (2005) Trial-by-trial coupling of concurrent electroencephalogram and functional magnetic resonance imaging identifies the dynamics of performance monitoring. J Neurosci 25(50):11730–11737

Dien J, Spencer KM, et al. (2004) Parsing the late positive complex: mental chronometry and the ERP components that inhabit the neighborhood of the P300. Psychophysiology 41(5):665–678

Eichele T, Specht K, et al. (2005) Assessing the spatiotemporal evolution of neuronal activation with single-trial event-related potentials and functional MRI. Proc Natl Acad Sci USA 102(49):17798–17803

Falkenstein M, Hohnsbein J, et al. (1994) Effects of choice complexity on different subcomponents of the late positive complex of the event-related potential. Electroencephalogr Clin Neurophysiol 92(2):148–160

Ford JM, White P, et al. (1994) Schizophrenics have fewer and smaller P300s: a single-trial analysis. Biol Psychiatry 35(2):96–103

Formisano E, Linden DE, et al. (2002) Tracking the mind's image in the brain I: time-resolved fMRI during visuospatial mental imagery. Neuron 35(1):185–194

Formisano E, Goebel R (2003) Tracking cognitive processes with functional MRI mental chronometry. Curr Opin Neurobiol 13(2):174–181

Friederici AD, Pfeifer E, et al. (1993) Event-related brain potentials during natural speech processing: effects of semantic, morphological and syntactic violations. Brain Res Cogn Brain Res 1(3):183–192

Friston K, Harrison L, et al. (2008) Multiple sparse priors for the M/EEG inverse problem. Neuroimage 39(3):1104–1120

Garrido MI, Kilner JM, et al. (2007) Evoked brain responses are generated by feedback loops. Proc Natl Acad Sci U S A 104(52):20961–20966

Gianotti LR, Kunig G, et al. (2007) Correlation between disease severity and brain electric LORETA tomography in Alzheimer's disease. Clin Neurophysiol 118(1):186–196

Gottesman II, Gould TD (2003) The endophenotype concept in psychiatry: etymology and strategic intentions. Am J Psychiatry 160(4):636–645

Gray CM, Konig P, et al. (1989) Oscillatory responses in cat visual cortex exhibit inter-columnar synchronization which reflects global stimulus properties. Nature 338(6213):334–337

Halgren E, Baudena P, et al. (1995a) Intracerebral potentials to rare target and distractor auditory and visual stimuli. I. Superior temporal plane and parietal lobe. Electroencephalogr Clin Neurophysiol 94(3):191–220

Halgren E, Baudena P, et al. (1994) Spatio-temporal stages in face and word processing. 2. Depth-recorded potentials in the human frontal and Rolandic cortices [published erratum appears in J Physiol Paris 1994;88(2):following 151]. J Physiol Paris 88(1):51–80

Halgren E, Baudena P, et al. (1995b) Intracerebral potentials to rare target and distractor auditory and visual stimuli. II. Medial, lateral and posterior temporal lobe. Electroencephalogr Clin Neurophysiol 94(4):229–250

Halgren E, Marinkovic K, Chauvel P (1998) Generators of the late cognitive potentials in auditory and visual oddball tasks. Electroencephalogr Clin Neurophysiol 106:159–164

Hamalainen M, Ilmoniemi RJ (1984) Interpreting measured magnetic fields of the brain: estimates of current distributions (Technical Report TKK-F-A559). Helsinki University of Technology, Finland

Hamalainen MS, Ilmoniemi RJ (1994) Interpreting magnetic fields of the brain: minimum norm estimates. Med Biol Eng Comput 32(1):35–42

Hamalainen MS, Sarvas J (1989) Realistic conductivity geometry model of the human head for interpretation of neuromagnetic data. IEEE Trans Biomed Eng 36(2):165–171

Hegerl U, Gallinat J, et al. (1994) Intensity dependence of auditory evoked dipole source activity. Int J Psychophysiol 17(1):1–13

Hegerl U, Juckel G, et al. (1995) Schizophrenics with small P300: a subgroup with a neurodevelopmental disturbance and a high risk for tardive dyskinesia? Acta Psychiatr Scand 91(2): 120–125

Helmholtz H (1853) Über einige Gesetze der Vertheilung elektrischer Ströme in körperlichen Leitern mit der Anwendung auf die thierisch-elektrischen Versuche. Annalen der Physik und Chemie 89:211–233; 353–377

Henderson CJ, Butler SR, et al. (1975) The localization of equivalent dipoles of EEG sources by the application of electrical field theory. Electroencephalogr Clin Neurophysiol 39(2):117–130

Hillyard SA, Hink RF, et al. (1973) Electrical signs of selective attention in the human brain. Science 182(108):177–180

Hinterberger T, Veit R, et al. (2005) Neuronal mechanisms underlying control of a brain-computer interface. Eur J Neurosci 21(11):3169–3181

Hughes SW, Crunelli V (2005) Thalamic mechanisms of EEG alpha rhythms and their pathological implications. Neuroscientist 11(4):357–372

Ilmoniemi RJ (1993) Models of source currents in the brain. Brain Topogr 5(4):331–336

Itier RJ, Latinus M, et al. (2006) Face, eye and object early processing: what is the face specificity?
Neuroimage 29(2):667–676

Javitt DC, Spencer KM, et al. (2008) Neurophysiological biomarkers for drug development in
schizophrenia. Nat Rev Drug Discov 7(1):68–83

Jeon YW, Polich J (2003) Meta-analysis of P300 and schizophrenia: patients, paradigms, and
practical implications. Psychophysiology 40(5):684–701

Katsanis J, Iacono WG, et al. (1997) P300 event-related potential heritability in monozygotic and
dizygotic twins. Psychophysiology 34(1):47–58

Kiang M, Kutas M, et al. (2008) An event-related brain potential study of direct and indirect
semantic priming in schizophrenia. Am J Psychiatry 165(1):74–81

Kutas M, Hillyard SA (1980) Event-related brain potentials to semantically inappropriate and
surprisingly large words. Biol Psychol 11(2):99–116

Linden DE, Prvulovic D, et al. (1999) The functional neuroanatomy of target detection: an fMRI
study of visual and auditory oddball tasks. Cereb Cortex 9(8):815–823

Llinas RR (1988) The intrinsic electrophysiological properties of mammalian neurons: insights
into central nervous system function. Science 242(4886):1654–1664

Lopes da Silva F (1991) Neural mechanisms underlying brain waves: from neural membranes to
networks. Electroencephalogr Clin Neurophysiol 79(2):81–93

Lopes da Silva F (1993) EEG analysis: theory and practice. In: Niedermeyer E, Lopes DS (eds)
Electroencephalography. Williams and Wilkins, Baltimore, p 1117

Mathalon DH, Ford JM, et al. (2000) Trait and state aspects of p300 amplitude reduction in schizophrenia: a retrospective longitudinal study. Biol Psychiatry 47(5):434–449

McAlonan K, Cavanaugh J, et al. (2006) Attentional modulation of thalamic reticular neurons.
J Neurosci 26(16):4444–4450

McCarthy G, Luby M, et al. (1997) Infrequent events transiently activate human prefrontal and
parietal cortex as measured by functional MRI. J Neurophysiol 77(3):1630–1634

McCarthy G, Wood CC, et al. (1989) Task-dependent field potentials in human hippocampal formation. J Neurosci 9(12):4253–4268

Meijs JW, Peters MJ, et al. (1988) Relative influence of model assumptions and measurement
procedures in the analysis of the MEG. Med Biol Eng Comput 26(2):136–142

Menon V, Ford JM, et al. (1997) Combined event-related fMRI and EEG evidence for temporal-
parietal cortex activation during target detection. Neuroreport 8(14):3029–3037

Mulert C, Jager L, et al. (2005) Sound level dependence of the primary auditory cortex:
Simultaneous measurement with 61-channel EEG and fMRI. Neuroimage 28(1):49–58

Mulert C, Gallinat J, et al. (2001) Reduced event-related current density in the anterior cingulate
cortex in schizophrenia. Neuroimage 13(4):589–600

Mulert C, Leicht G, et al. (2007) Auditory cortex and anterior cingulate cortex sources of the early
evoked gamma-band response: relationship to task difficulty and mental effort. Neuropsychologia
45(10):2294–2306

Mulert C, Jager L, et al. (2004) Integration of fMRI and simultaneous EEG: towards a comprehensive understanding of localization and time-course of brain activity in target detection.
Neuroimage 22(1):83–94

Mulert C, Seifert C, et al. (2008) Single-trial coupling of EEG and fMRI reveals the involvement of
anterior cingulate cortex activation in effortful decision making. Neuroimage 42(1):158–168

Naatanen R, Picton T (1987) The N1 wave of the human electric and magnetic response to sound:
a review and an analysis of the component structure. Psychophysiology 24(4):375–425

Nagai Y, Critchley HD, et al. (2004) Brain activity relating to the contingent negative variation: an
fMRI investigation. Neuroimage 21(4):1232–1241

Nunez PL, Silberstein RB (2000) On the relationship of synaptic activity to macroscopic measurements: does co-registration of EEG with fMRI make sense? Brain Topogr 13(2):79–96

Pascual-Marqui RD (2002) Standardized low-resolution brain electromagnetic tomography (sLORETA): technical details. Methods Find Exp Clin Pharmacol 24(Suppl D):5–12

Pascual-Marqui RD, Lehmann D, et al. (1999) Low resolution brain electromagnetic tomography (LORETA) functional imaging in acute, neuroleptic-naive, first-episode, productive schizophrenia. Psychiatry Res 90(3):169–179

Pascual-Marqui RD, Michel CM, et al. (1994) Low resolution electromagnetic tomography: a new method for localizing electrical activity in the brain. Int J Psychophysiol 18(1):49–65

Phillips C, Mattout J, et al. (2005) An empirical Bayesian solution to the source reconstruction problem in EEG. Neuroimage 24(4):997–1011

Pizzagalli DA, Oakes TR, et al. (2003) Coupling of theta activity and glucose metabolism in the human rostral anterior cingulate cortex: an EEG/PET study of normal and depressed subjects. Psychophysiology 40(6):939–949

Pizzagalli D, Pascual-Marqui RD, et al. (2001) Anterior cingulate activity as a predictor of degree of treatment response in major depression: evidence from brain electrical tomography analysis. Am J Psychiatry 158(3):405–415

Pogarell O, Mulert C, et al. (2007) Event-related potentials in psychiatry. Clin EEG Neurosci 38(1):25–34

Polich J, Squire LR (1993) P300 from amnesic patients with bilateral hippocampal lesions. Electroencephalogr Clin Neurophysiol 86(6):408–417

Posner MI (2005) Timing the brain: mental chronometry as a tool in neuroscience. PLoS Biol 3(2):e51

Rinne T, Alho K, et al. (2000) Separate time behaviors of the temporal and frontal mismatch negativity sources. Neuroimage 12(1):14–19

Rosburg T, Trautner P, et al. (2007) Hippocampal event-related potentials to tone duration deviance in a passive oddball paradigm in humans. Neuroimage 37(1):274–281

Rosburg T, Trautner P, et al. (2005) Subdural recordings of the mismatch negativity (MMN) in patients with focal epilepsy. Brain 128(pt 4):819–828

Sagiv N, Bentin S (2001) Structural encoding of human and schematic faces: holistic and part-based processes. J Cogn Neurosci 13(7):937–951

Salisbury DF, Shenton ME, et al. (1998) First-episode schizophrenic psychosis differs from first-episode affective psychosis and controls in P300 amplitude over left temporal lobe [published erratum appears in Arch Gen Psychiatry 1998;55(5):413]. Arch Gen Psychiatry 55(2):173–180

Scherg M, Bast T, et al. (1999) Multiple source analysis of interictal spikes: goals, requirements, and clinical value. J Clin Neurophysiol 16(3):214–224

Scherg M, Berg P (1991) Use of prior knowledge in brain electromagnetic source analysis. Brain Topogr 4(2):143–150

Scherg M, von Cramon D (1986) Evoked dipole source potentials of the human auditory cortex. Electroencephalogr Clin Neurophysiol 65(5):344–360

Scherg M, von Cramon D (1985) Two bilateral sources of the late AEP as identified by a spatio-temporal dipole model. Electroencephalogr Clin Neurophysiol 62(1):32–44

Schneider M (1974) Effect of inhomogeneities on surface signals coming from a cerebral current-dipole source. IEEE Trans Biomed Eng 21(1):52–54

Schneider MR (1972) A multistage process for computing virtual dipolar sources of EEG discharges from surface information. IEEE Trans Biomed Eng 19(1):1–12

Sencaj RW, Aunon JI (1982) Dipole localization of average and single visual evoked potentials. IEEE Trans Biomed Eng 29(1):26–33

Steriade M (1994) Sleep oscillations and their blockage by activating systems. J Psychiatry Neurosci 19(5):354–358

Strik WK, Dierks T, et al. (1993a) Differences in P300 amplitudes and topography between cycloid psychosis and schizophrenia in Leonhard's classification. Acta Psychiatr Scand 87(3):179–183

Strik WK, Fallgatter AJ, et al. (1997) Specific P300 features in patients with cycloid psychosis. Acta Psychiatr Scand 95(1):67–72

Strik WK, Dierks T, et al. (1993b) Amplitudes of auditory P300 in remitted and residual schizophrenics: correlations with clinical features. Neuropsychobiology 27(1):54–60

Sutton S (1969) The specification of psychological variables in an average evoked potential experiment. In: Donchin E, Lindsley DB (eds) Average evoked potentials. Methods, results and evaluations (NASA SP-191). Columbia University Press, New York, pp 237–262

Sutton S, Braren M, et al. (1965) Evoked-potential correlates of stimulus uncertainty. Science 150(700):1187–1188

Taylor MJ, Batty M, et al. (2004) The faces of development: a review of early face processing over childhood. J Cogn Neurosci 16(8):1426–1442

Trujillo-Barreto NJ, Aubert-Vazquez E, et al. (2008) Bayesian M/EEG source reconstruction with spatio-temporal priors. Neuroimage 39(1):318–335

Ventouras EM, Alevizos I, et al. (2007) Independent components of sleep spindles. Conf Proc IEEE Eng Med Biol Soc 1:4002–4005

Wagner M, Fuchs M, et al. (2004) Evaluation of sLORETA in the presence of noise and multiple sources. Brain Topogr 16(4):277–280

Walter WG, Cooper R, et al. (1964) Contingent negative variation: an electric sign of sensorimotor association and expectancy in the human brain. Nature 203:380–384

Wang JZ, Williamson SJ, et al. (1992) Magnetic source images determined by a lead-field analysis: the unique minimum-norm least-squares estimation. IEEE Trans Biomed Eng 39(7):665–675

Wright MJ, Hansell NK, et al. (2001) Genetic influence on the variance in P3 amplitude and latency. Behav Genet 31(6):555–565

The Added Value of EEG–fMRI in Imaging Neuroscience

6

Rainer Goebel and Fabrizio Esposito

1
Introduction

The main objective of functional neuroimaging is to detect and characterise (in space and time) relevant changes in brain states and their relation to neuronal activity. Functional MRI (fMRI), electroencephalography (EEG) and magnetoencephalography (MEG) are the most widespread noninvasive techniques that are available to experimental and clinical neuroscientists to achieve this objective starting from in vivo measures of brain electrical activity. Both fMRI and EEG assume that a given brain state can be decoded from the precise anatomical localisation and the detailed temporal evolution of neuroelectrical brain activation signals, respectively. Starting from these common assumptions, fMRI neuroscientists have developed many different approaches for mapping brain states at a spatial resolution of a few millimetres and testing many different neurophysiological and neuropathological hypotheses in normal and clinical populations, despite the limited temporal resolution of the available signals (see previous chapters). On the other hand, EEG neuroscientists have posed analogous questions and addressed similar problems by developing different approaches for the detailed temporal analysis of EEG recordings, despite the limited spatial detail in their findings.

The previous chapter illustrated how fMRI can be used by EEG neuroscientists to improve the quality of EEG results and to help with the problem of source localisation.

The purpose of this chapter is to illustrate how the fMRI neuroscientist can integrate detailed temporal information by incorporating simultaneously recorded EEG signals into standard as well as sophisticated fMRI spatiotemporal modelling. We discuss how this can be achieved in such a way that new effects become detectable in the fMRI domain even when the original event or state change causing possible fMRI effects can only be characterised at very rapid temporal scales (e.g. milliseconds) or frequency bands (above 1 Hz). Our discussion occurs at a conceptual level, and we refer the reader to other chapters in Part 2 for more details regarding problems such as EEG preprocessing.

F. Esposito (✉)
Department of Cognitive Neuroscience, University of Maastricht, 6200 MD Maastricht, The Netherlands
e-mail: fabrizio.esposito@maastrichtuniversity.nl

C. Mulert and L. Lemieux (eds.), *EEG–fMRI*
DOI: 10.1007/978-3-540-87919-0_6, © Springer Verlag Berlin Heidelberg 2010

We start from the problem of optimising a common source space for fMRI and EEG signal projection through the use of anatomical and functional MRI models and EEG distributed inverse models. Then we explore different frameworks for the integrated analysis of simultaneously acquired EEG–fMRI data sets in the same space.

The basic limitation of both fMRI and EEG is the indirect nature of measured brain signals, which always implies that substantial interpretational efforts are required, and means that neuroscientists should be cautious before drawing any general conclusions about the location and the electrical nature of the neural sources related to the investigated phenomena. Nonetheless, this general limitation can be elegantly counterbalanced by multimodal simultaneous acquisition and comparative analysis approaches, which emphasise the diversity of the physical origins of fMRI and EEG signals with respect to the same neural generators. Nowadays, one of the most important goals of fMRI and EEG developers is to provide analysis tools that optimally orient the neuroscientist towards the real-time comparative evaluation and interpretation of fMRI and EEG data.

Historically, fMRI and EEG methodologies have followed asynchronous and independent paths of research and development with rather a limited degree of interaction until the end of the twentieth century, mostly due to technological reasons. Starting from the beginning of the twenty-first century, however, the advent of new systems equipped for the simultaneous acquisition of EEG and fMRI data from the same subject has boosted research into integrated data modelling and analysis.

The combination of EEG and fMRI data sets into one unique data model is still the focus of intensive research, and enormous effort is required to integrate independent fields of knowledge such as physics, computer science and neuroscience. In fact, besides the classical problems of head modelling in EEG and haemodynamic modelling in fMRI, there is the added difficulty of needing to understand and model the ongoing correlations of EEG and fMRI data.

In this chapter, we discuss different strategies that are available to the neuroimaging researcher for combining and integrating EEG data into the standard framework of fMRI image analysis. Specifically, we discuss how the fMRI analyst can fruitfully incorporate the rich content of temporal information associated with a simultaneously acquired EEG time series into a standard fMRI analysis. We emphasise the potential and the importance of anatomically and functionally informing distributed EEG solutions in the context of the classical EEG inverse problem when attempting to link the spatial information extracted from fMRI data to the temporal information from EEG data in a common shared anatomical space.

2
The EEG–fMRI Integrated Source Space

Functional MRI data sets are normally acquired over the whole brain, with voxel sizes ranging from 2 to 4 mm. Starting from high-resolution coregistered T1-weighted MRI scans with 1 mm isotropic resolution, fMRI signals can be interpolated up to 1- or 2-mm voxels. Moreover, the precise segmentation of the white matter volumes from the T1-weighted

MRI images allows the white matter/grey matter boundary to be identified. From this inner cortical boundary, dense cortex meshes can be reconstructed with vertices located along the modelled surface (Dale et al. 1999). In many cognitive studies, voxel-based functional MRI time-series and spatial patterns can be projected onto the cortical meshes by sampling the activity within grey matter along the normal vector of each vertex. This results in mesh time series for typically 100,000–200,000 vertices per hemisphere. EEG signals are acquired from scalp channels that may range in number from 20 to 300, although MRI-compatible devices rarely allow more than 100 channels. In order to aid the creation of a common source space for fMRI and EEG signal projection, cortex meshes obtained from MRI data are usually simplified by geometry-preserving mesh decimation algorithms, resulting in meshes with a few thousand vertices (Fig. 1). As an alternative, regular 3D rectangular grids made up of 3–10 mm voxels can be defined directly in the MRI volume space and used for fMRI resampling and EEG projection. In order to constrain the analysis on the cortical voxels, these grids are usually applied to segmentation-derived cortical masks.

BOLD–fMRI temporal resolution is in the range of a few hundreds of milliseconds, and is physically limited by the sluggishness of the haemodynamic response, which imposes time constants on the order of seconds (Boynton et al. 1996). EEG temporal resolution is on the order of 1 ms or less, but, even for high-density channel configurations, the effective spatial resolution of any detectable neural effects is physically limited by the distance of the neural sources from the electrodes and the inhomogeneous volume conductivity of the head, which influences the propagation of electric currents from the source to the electrodes through the different compartments of the cranium. In order to be detectable at distant electrodes, sufficiently large neuronal populations must be synchronously active, and the dendritic compartments of participating neurons must be oriented in parallel.

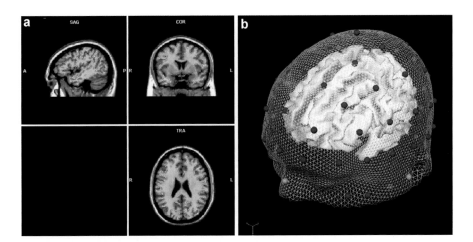

Fig. 1 a–b Example of the definition of the EEG–fMRI source space for the MNI template brain and the standard MNI 81-electrode EEG configuration. Source points are visible in the volume space (**a**) and correspond to the vertices of the cortical mesh (**b**) automatically registered to the EEG configuration. In the *right* panel (**b**), *red* spheres represent electrode positions, *pink* spheres represent fiducials, and *yellow* and *white* meshes represent reconstructed head and cortex surfaces, respectively

In the last few decades, important fMRI and EEG/MEG studies have been reported that support the notion that the preparation of anatomically informed source spaces for time-series projection and neural activity representation significantly enhances the spatiotemporal patterns yielded by fMRI and EEG/MEG measurements with respect to neural source localisation and dynamic brain state analysis (see e.g. Kiebel et al. 2000; Dale and Sereno 1993; Dale et al. 2000).

In EEG–fMRI studies, voxel-level fMRI time series are acquired simultaneously with EEG channel time series. EEG configurations are normally digitised on the head of the subject prior to the MRI scanning session in such a way that automatic 2D–3D MRI image registration and surface-based reconstruction of the head and brain allow EEG and fMRI signals to be spatially referred to the same 3D coordinate system. Based on this coregistration prerequisite, various approaches have been suggested for modelling EEG source signals, including placing current dipoles in fMRI hot spots (Scherg 1990) and distributed source modelling (Hamalainen and Ilmoniemi 1984), which will be described in more detail below.

As described above, fMRI voxel-level BOLD time courses can be projected from the voxel space to the cortex source space by sampling along the normal of a vertex from the inner (white matter/grey matter) to the outer (grey matter/CSF) boundary, and the corresponding time courses are averaged to yield one unique time course at that vertex. As a result, fMRI data modelling and analysis can be performed directly in the cortex source space.

EEG channel time series can be projected from the channel space to the cortex source space by placing a single current dipole at each vertex of the mesh and estimating the distributed solution for the EEG inverse problem constrained to the vertex positions (Dale and Sereno 1993; Dale et al. 2000).

More generally, assuming a mesh of N vertices and a linear (discrete) equivalent current dipole (ECD) model as a data model (see e.g. Mosher and Leahy 1998; Mosher et al. 1999; Baillet et al. 2001), M channel time series can be expressed as linear combinations of N dipolar source time series:

$$\mathbf{y}(t) = \begin{pmatrix} y_1(t) \\ \dots \\ y_M(t) \end{pmatrix} = \mathbf{A} \cdot \begin{pmatrix} \mathbf{s}_1(t) \\ \dots \\ \mathbf{s}_N(t) \end{pmatrix} + \mathbf{n}(t) = \mathbf{A} \cdot \mathbf{s}(t) + \mathbf{n}(t). \tag{1}$$

In Eq. 1, the columns of matrix $\mathbf{A}$ ($M \times 3N$) contain the lead fields of the dipolar sources for the given M-channel EEG configuration, while $\mathbf{s}_i(t) = [s_x(t), s_y(t), s_z(t)]^t$ represents the source activity time series of the dipole placed at the ith vertex of the mesh and $\mathbf{n}(t)$ represents the channel noise.

The lead fields for the EEG configurations are normally extracted from a precomputed volume conductor model applied to the head of the subject (Sarvas 1985; Berg and Scherg 1994, Mosher et al. 1999). Optionally, the dimensionality of the linear problem (Eq. 1) is reduced by a factor of three by constraining not only the number and the locations of the dipoles but also their orientations, for example using the unit normal vectors of the reconstructed cortical surface mesh (see e.g. Dale et al. 2000; Lin et al. 2004, 2006).

All linear ECD-based inverse solutions can be expressed as a collection of spatial filters (one per source dipole component) that can be directly applied to channel data to generate the estimated source time series at all vertices of the mesh:

$$\mathbf{x}(t) = \mathbf{W} \cdot \mathbf{y}(t). \tag{2}$$

Matrix $\mathbf{W}$ ($3N \times M$) contains the spatial filter weights (one collection per source dipole component), and $\mathbf{x}(t)$ is the estimated source time series for all components and locations. Once the filter weights have been estimated (see below), Eq. 2 can be used to generate a "point" source time series at each vertex of the mesh (virtual electrode; see e.g. Brookes et al. 2005), or, as an alternative, subsets of adjacent vertices in one or more prespecified regions (regional sources) can be jointly summarised in terms of their orientations and temporal (or spectrotemporal) variance via (for example) principal component analysis (PCA) (Kayser and Tenke 2003). Solution (2) for one or more sources can be visualised in the channel space in the form of 2D or 3D EEG channel topographies. For regional sources and free-orientation EEG solutions, one possible way to reduce Eq. 2 to a single set of channel weights is to first average WMN coefficients across all regional vertices separately for each orientation (X, Y and Z), and then project the weights along the orientation explaining the maximum variance of the projected data by means of a singular value decomposition (SVD). For orientation-constrained solutions, the maximum variance projection is not necessary.

The estimation of the inverse solution $\mathbf{W}$ can proceed by filling either one, two or three rows of $\mathbf{W}$ at each source location ("scanning" approach), or by attempting a total inversion of the distributed ECD model across the entire source space ("imaging" approach) (see e.g. Darvas et al. 2004). For instance, dipole fitting methods (Scherg 1990), linearly constrained minimum variance (LCMV) beamformers (van Veen et al. 1997), and multiple signal classification (MUSIC, Mosher and Leahy 1998) are commonly used "scanning" approaches. Imaging approaches always require some form of regularisation due to the ill-posed nature of the problem of inverting the linear model in Eq. 1 for $N > M$. A commonly adopted "imaging" approach is the weighted minimum norm (WMN) solution (Hamalainen and Ilmoniemi 1984; Hamalainen et al. 1993; Leahy et al. 1996) expressed by the formula:

$$\mathbf{W} = \mathbf{RA^t} \left(\mathbf{ARA^t} + \lambda^2 \mathbf{C_N} \right)^{-1}, \tag{3}$$

where matrix $\mathbf{R}$ represents the a priori source covariance, and is used to "inform" the source activities, $\mathbf{C_N}$ is the covariance matrix of the channel noise, and λ is a regularisation parameter (Tikhonov and Arsenin 1977). A typical weighting scheme (depth weighting, Lawson and Hanson 1974; Jeffs et al. 1987) specifies $\mathbf{R}$ as a diagonal matrix with nonzero entries that are inversely proportional to the γth power of lead field norms (γ being the depth-weighting parameter; see also Lin et al. 2004, 2006).

Other common imaging approaches, such as the Laplacian-weighted minimum norm (LORETA, Pascual-Marqui et al. 1994) and the local autoregressive average (LAURA, Grave de Peralta et al. 2004) (see also previous chapter and Michel et al. 2004 for review), are analogous to WMN but allow for additional constraints on the source covariance in a nondiagonal matrix $\mathbf{R}$. Finally, some form of normalisation (e.g. dynamic SPM, Dale et al. 2000) or standardisation (s-LORETA, Pascual-Marqui 2002) with respect to the source noise and signals can be applied to the filter weights in matrix $\mathbf{W}$ before application to the channel time series. Finally, the WMN scheme has been also used for fMRI-constrained distributed inverse modelling by "modulating" the diagonal entries with local fMRI activity (e.g. via BOLD percent signal change estimates), and the off-diagonal entries with some functional connectivity measure such as inter-regional BOLD signal correlations (see e.g. Liu et al. 1998; Dale et al. 2000; Babiloni et al. 2003).

3
Integration Strategies for EEG–fMRI Studies

The major motivation for the development of EEG–fMRI systems stems from the need to link the precise and detailed spatial characterisation of neural phenomena achievable with modern high-field fMRI to the precise and detailed temporal characterisation of neuronal phenomena achievable with modern high-density EEG. Despite the important problem of dealing with the presence of fMRI-specific artefacts in the collected EEG traces, the simultaneous acquisition of EEG and fMRI signals provides a strong neurophysiological and neuropsychological basis for establishing this link, by making sure that the same brain is studied at the same time while performing a cognitive task. Nonetheless, new issues—physical and physiological—have arisen about the intrinsic nature and the validity of EEG–fMRI signal correlations. The former refer to a lack of knowledge about the real extent of temporal and spatial effect coupling between the two modalities. The latter refer to the different perspectives and expectations of neuroscientists from the fMRI and EEG fields. Based on these observations, we propose to consider two different symmetric approaches to the comparative analysis of simultaneously acquired EEG–fMRI data.

In one approach, EEG data are first analysed in the channel or source space, and one or more sources are characterised in the (time or frequency) temporal domain. A temporal model for fMRI responses, e.g. a general linear model (GLM, Friston et al. 1995), is thus derived by extracting the trial-by-trial variation (modulation) or the spectrotemporal evolution of one or more predetected EEG sources (integration of fMRI and EEG in the temporal domain, Fig. 2). The effective integration of EEG data into the fMRI temporal model requires the application of a correction for fMRI haemodynamics, e.g. via linear convolution with a model haemodynamic response function (Boynton et al. 1996), and, with the sole exception of resting-state fMRI studies (Laufs et al. 2003), the orthogonalisation of the EEG measures to the standard fMRI response (Feige et al. 2005; Eichele et al. 2005). The GLM results will then reveal brain regions related to an EEG-derived temporal reference.

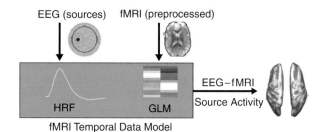

Fig. 2 Integration of fMRI and EEG in the temporal domain

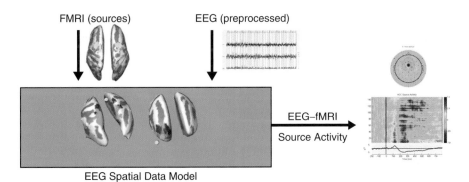

Fig. 3 Integration of fMRI and EEG in the spatial domain

In a second approach (integration of fMRI and EEG in the spatial domain; see Fig. 3), fMRI spatial patterns are first extracted in the cortex source space and then used in combination with forward and inverse solutions to generate fMRI-derived channel topographies (inverse filters) in the context of EEG spatial modelling. A detailed time or time–frequency characterisation is then associated with the fMRI spatial pattern. The fMRI spatial information can either be incorporated into the estimation of the distributed inverse solution (see e.g. Liu et al. 1998; Babiloni et al. 2003) or it can simply be used to select the regions of activity in the cortex source space in order to create the corresponding channel topography (regional source).

4
Illustration of the Integration of fMRI and EEG in the Temporal Domain

EEG-relevant neural processes can be characterised in the time or the frequency domain. Short-lasting (a few milliseconds) and broadband EEG processes are usually evaluated in the time domain and detected as amplitude peaks in the response at a specific latency, with positive or negative polarity (see previous chapter). Long-lasting and narrow-band EEG processes are usually evaluated in the frequency domain in terms of their spectral power and phase distribution in certain frequency ranges (Engel et al. 2001). Although it is possible to observe these processes in single or multiple channels, many studies have shown the importance of projecting EEG time series from the channel space to a different space where specific subcomponents are well separated and better studied. For instance, temporal independent component analysis (ICA) (Hyvarinen et al. 2001) is a statistical technique that decomposes channel time series into independent components by removing statistical redundancy between channel observations, and it has been proposed as a powerful tool for separating and rejecting EEG artefacts and for generating new hypotheses about the underlying source dynamics and origins (Makeig et al. 2002). As an alternative, and especially when the principal aim of the study is to produce a local validation of the EEG source and a local interpretation of EEG–MRI effect coupling, the preprocessed

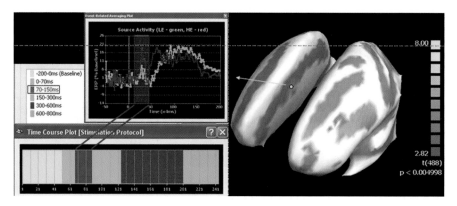

Fig. 4 Results from the EEG distributed source analysis in the cortical space

EEG channel time series can be first projected into an anatomically informed source space (e.g. a cortex source space) and then analysed for the main or differential effects of a specific temporal feature.

Examples of this integration strategy are depicted in Figs. 4–6. Figure 4 shows the results of a cortically constrained distributed source analysis performed on a 5,000-vertex source space after estimation and application of a WMN filter to the preprocessed EEG time series from a single-subject EEG–fMRI experiment where a simple auditory-guided choice task was performed under two levels of decision effort (LE: low effort, HE: high effort); for a detailed description of the experimental paradigm, see Mulert et al. (2005). Figure 5 shows the source ERP images for the two conditions (upper panels), and the equivalent dipoles estimated from the local peaks of the ERPs (lower panels). Figure 6 shows the FMRI (volume) map obtained from the incorporation of the trial-by-trial amplitude modulation of the ERP source in the anterior cingulate cortex (ACC) during the HE session.

5
Illustration of the Integration of fMRI and EEG in the Spatial Domain

In the example in the previous section, the high temporal resolution of simultaneously acquired EEG data was used to augment the fMRI temporal model and to study neural events whose actual occurrence or effective characterisation would otherwise be impossible at the fMRI temporal scale.

An alternative approach is to assume that standard fMRI temporal models are sufficient to map the BOLD effects of the stimulus-evoked brain activity, thus producing a detailed spatial picture of the temporally evolving cognitive states as a standalone modality. In such cases, it could be extremely interesting for the fMRI cognitive scientist to enrich the meaning and the interpretation of fMRI spatiotemporal patterns with spatially selective EEG features using the simultaneous EEG data available.

Using the cortex source space as a common space for both fMRI and EEG data projection, it is possible to establish a spatial link between the ongoing fMRI activity in one or

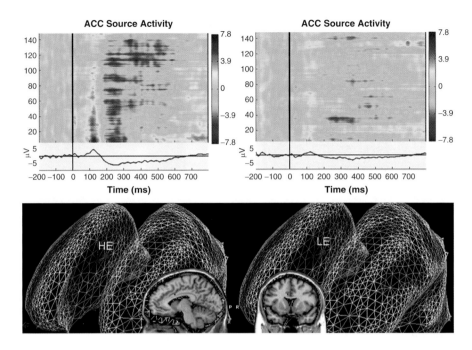

Fig. 5 Results from the EEG distributed source analysis in the cortical space and projection in the volume. *Upper panels*: source ERP images (single-trial and trial-averaged responses) for the HE (*left*) and LE (*right*) conditions. *Lower panels*: equivalent current dipole sources for the HE (*left*) and LE (*right*) conditions. The source location is displayed in the volume space (*left*: sagittal view; *right*: coronal view) as a *red* point

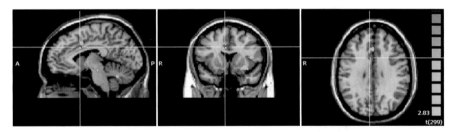

Fig. 6 FMRI (volume) GLM map obtained from the incorporation of the trial-by-trial amplitude modulation of the ERP source in the anterior cingulated cortex (ACC) during the HE session (triplanar view centred on the EEG source location)

more (functionally connected) regions and the temporal or spectrotemporal variance of simultaneously acquired EEG data. Figures 7–9 refer to the application of just such an integration strategy (schematically illustrated in Fig. 3) to an EEG–fMRI block-design experiment (own data) based on a typical working-memory task, the *N*-back task (see e.g. Esposito et al. 2006). According to this strategy, an fMRI spatial pattern is first obtained from mesh time series by performing standard GLM mapping of the linear differential contrasts among

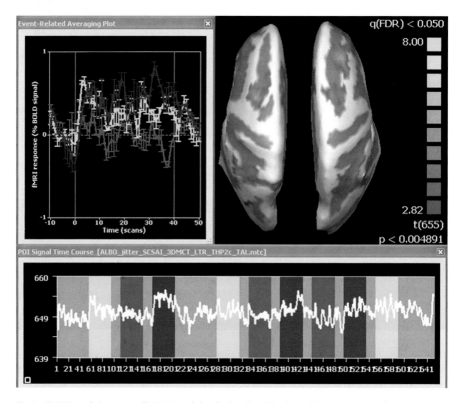

Fig. 7 FMRI spatial pattern of BOLD activity during the *N*-back working-memory task. Statistically significant (conjunction test, $P < 0.05$, FDR-corrected) parametric BOLD responses are projected onto the cortex source space

memory conditions in the cortex source space (Fig. 7 shows the conjunction map for the contrasts "2-back vs. 1-back" and "1-back vs. 0-back"). The set of regions exhibiting statistically significant BOLD responses is then used to generate a corresponding set of EEG regional sources (Fig. 8) using a cortically constrained distributed inverse solution (WMN) estimated on the same source space (Fig. 8). The WMN channel weightings for each regional source are visualised in the channel space as EEG topographies. In this way, the active fMRI network "selects" a network of EEG regional sources that can be jointly analysed for their spectrotemporal features using PCA for example. For instance, the normalised distribution of the source power spectral density across all sources in different frequency bands can be analysed and the variances of fundamental EEG rhythms during the fMRI experiment can be visualised (Fig. 8). Based on this strategy, the fMRI network parametrically activated during the *N*-back task of Fig. 7 exhibited prevalent peaks in the theta band (mainly in the lateral frontal and superior lateral parietal sources) and, in more composite spectra, in the alpha and gamma bands (anterior and posterior midline sources). The time–frequency plots, the theta power traces and the temporal correlations of the theta power traces with the experimental conditions are shown in Fig. 9. A positive parametric trend in the EEG theta signal with the cognitive load of the working-memory condition is evident.

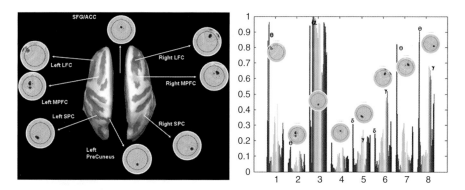

Fig. 8   FMRI regions of activity are converted to EEG topographies via the application of a WMN filter in the cortex source space (*left*). FMRI-derived regional sources are jointly analysed in the temporal evolution of their frequency spectral distribution in the range between 0 and 50 Hz for the entire fMRI run (*right*). In this plot the normalised spectrotemporal variance contribution in different bands from each source is emphasised via colour coding from the lowest (*blue-cyan*) to the highest (*yellow-red*) frequencies. Peaks of temporal variance in the delta, theta, alpha, beta and gamma bands are marked on the plot

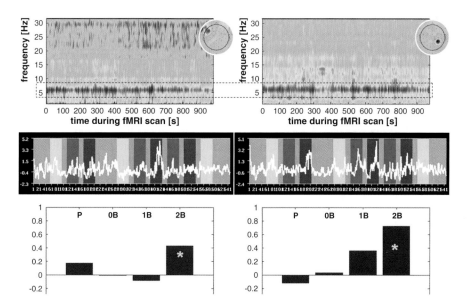

Fig. 9   Time–frequency plots (*upper panels*), theta power traces (*central panels*) and temporal correlations of the theta traces with the experimental conditions (*lower panels*) for the "principal" theta sources, associated with the left lateral frontal cortex (*left panels*) and right superior parietal cortex (*right panels*)

6
Discussion

In this chapter, we have presented two alternative strategies that are available to the fMRI researcher for combining simultaneously acquired EEG and fMRI data sets into one integrated conceptual framework. We briefly illustrated the two approaches on two real-world single-subject EEG–fMRI data sets. Although these illustrations made use of specific data models and statistical techniques, the described frameworks should be considered general with respect to the implementation of other fMRI or EEG data models. The proposed analysis pathways of Figs. 2 and 3 conceptually represent the general motivations and expectations of imaging neuroscientists with regard to the practical applications of EEG–fMRI from two opposite but symmetric views.

When integrating fMRI and EEG in the temporal domain (Fig. 2), the high temporal resolution of simultaneously acquired EEG data is used to augment the fMRI temporal model and study neural events whose actual occurrence or effective characterisation would not otherwise be possible at the fMRI temporal scale. As a result, we gain the ability to map the fMRI correlates of new events that cannot be characterised using a single experimental design. From the fMRI modelling and analysis viewpoint, this approach turns out to be very similar to the integration of on-line external or behavioural measures, such as reaction times, ratings, etc., which is common practice in fMRI research. Nonetheless, two critical aspects are implicit to this approach. First, not only must an EEG source exist with a given observed feature (e.g. an ERP component within a given interval of latencies), but also substantial trial-by-trial modulation must exist during the entire experiment in order to produce a relatively noise-free fMRI predictor for a statistically powerful GLM. Normally the variance of EEG-derived predictors after orthogonalisation to the standard stimulus-coding predictors can be very low, thus impairing the single-subject and group-level random-effects GLM statistics. Orthogonalisation is necessary to distinguish the variance already explained by the stimulus function and isolate the real added value of embedding EEG features into the GLM. The use of large cohorts may result in additional variability caused by the different EEG reactivities of the subjects (Meltzer et al. 2007a, b). Second, significant effects are mapped for the EEG–fMRI correlations on a purely temporal basis. Therefore, additional difficulties can arise in the interpretation of fMRI hot spots that are not well co-localised with the EEG source or are even far from it. In fact, while a full understanding of local EEG–fMRI correlations ultimately requires more sophisticated physical and empirical models for effect coupling, both types of findings require that interpretations should be approached with extreme caution. The known limitations of EEG inverse models may sometimes produce "ghost" sources (see e.g. Michel et al. 2004), thereby making the source projection itself of limited validity or even biasing the integration of EEG features in the fMRI temporal model. In relation to this point, the use of an intermediate nonanatomically informed source projection such as ICA may provide better results due to the temporal decorrelation of the signals. Although the co-localisation of EEG and fMRI sources is sometimes presented and invoked as a source cross-validation scheme (see e.g. Wibral et al. 2008), it may well also be the case that some of the EEG generators are spatially masked by volume conductor effects but pop out nicely anyway due to the fMRI functional connectivity. This is especially true for subcortical and thalamic effects, which have been shown to be visible with EEG–fMRI (Feige et al. 2005) but are also very difficult to isolate via EEG spatial modelling alone (Nunez and Srinivasan 2006). In such cases, the added value of the simultaneous EEG measure cannot be restricted to a pure cross-validation tool.

When integrating fMRI and EEG in the spatial domain (Fig. 3), the high spatial resolution and the local physical origin of the fMRI signals are used to inform an EEG spatial model and to characterise brain activity and cognitive states at typical EEG time and frequency scales. As a result, it becomes possible to enrich detailed pictures of fMRI-derived spatiotemporal patterns with high temporal resolution EEG-derived information.

The use of EEG distributed inverse models and a typical "imaging" approach (such as WMN) in a common anatomically informed (cortex) source space has been highlighted in this chapter. This solution presents a number of attractive properties in the context of EEG–fMRI experiments where single or a few isolated regions are not selected but instead distributed networks are involved in controlling the information flow, processing and execution of complex cognitive functions. In fact, although theoretically and technically possible, the use of ECD dipole-fitting procedures would require that at least one single dipole is placed in each region of activity, whereas scanning approaches such as beamforming implicitly pose theoretical constraints on remote source correlations (van Veen et al. 1997). One more attractive property of imaging solutions for EEG–fMRI studies is the possibility of adding distributed fMRI constraints directly to the WMN estimation (see e.g. Liu et al. 1998; Dale et al. 2000; Babiloni et al. 2003). Nonetheless, for the purpose of the case illustrated here, we did not want to bias the contribution of the EEG sources with condition-specific fMRI effects.

We have shown how it is possible in practice to spatially select a set of regional EEG sources from fMRI patterns and to jointly analyse their spectrotemporal contribution to the measured EEG variance in a simultaneous EEG–fMRI experiment. This is the first step before correlating any EEG spectrotemporal feature (e.g. band-specific power traces) to the experimental conditions of the EEG–fMRI experiments.

There are, however, several caveats for this approach too, which also requires caution during interpretation. First, according to this scheme, significant effects are mapped while assuming that EEG–fMRI correlation occurs on a purely spatial basis. Similar to combination in the temporal domain, combination in the spatial domain also requires the development of more sophisticated physical and empirical models for EEG–fMRI effect coupling. Second, the known limitations of EEG inverse models do not allow conclusions to be drawn about the presence of one or more single EEG generators in each fMRI region (Liu et al. 2006). It may well be that global effects or strong local effects from "close" regions contribute substantially to the spectral and temporal features of a given regional source. In this sense, a joint PCA of multiple remote regional sources can be a more robust approach for identifying the presence of global effects (i.e. common to all regional sources) and differentially evaluating the relative contribution of each single region within the network.

Due to volume conduction effects, scalp recordings are known to be biased towards global activity (Nunez and Srinivasan 2006), and the purpose of the inverse spatial filters estimated via EEG spatial modelling is to remove this bias as much as possible and to enhance local activity. It must be also stated, however, that the presence of global activity throughout the selected EEG sources is not necessarily an artefact, whereas the excessive dominance of one source over all of the others (especially if this happens over an extended time–frequency range) is likely due to residual artefacts in the EEG data.

Several conjectures about fMRI and EEG brain dynamics have agreed that "high values of complexity necessarily correspond to an optimal synthesis of functional specialisation and functional integration within a system" (Edelman and Tononi 2000; Nunez and Srinivasan 2006). Following up this conceptual framework, the technical search for the optimal integration of EEG and fMRI data will likely evolve towards a search for the optimal balance between global and local effect coupling.

In summary, fMRI researchers can enrich topographically accurate fMRI data with precise timing information when performing simultaneous EEG–fMRI experiments. The approaches outlined in this chapter may lead to new insights into the neuronal basis of cognitive processes, but they require sophisticated combined data analysis, preferentially in a common cortex space, as well as careful interpretation of the spatiotemporal results obtained.

References

Babiloni F, Babiloni C, Carducci F, Romani GL, Rossini PM, Angelone LM, Cincotti F (2003) Multimodal integration of high-resolution EEG and functional magnetic resonance imaging data: A simulation study. Neuroimage 19(1):1–15

Baillet S, Mosher JC, Leahy RM (2001) Electromagnetic brain mapping. IEEE Signal Process Mag 18(6):14–30

Berg P, Scherg M (1994) A fast method for forward computation of multiple-shell spherical head models. Electroencephalogr Clin Neurophysiol 90:58–64

Boynton GM, Engel SA, Glover GH, Heeger DJ (1996) Linear systems analysis of functional magnetic resonance imaging in human V1. J Neurosci 16(13):4207–4221

Brookes MJ, Gibson AM, Hall SD, Furlong PL, Barnes GR, Hillebrand A, Singh KD, Holliday E, Francis ST, Morris PG (2005) GLM-beamformer method demonstrates stationary field, alpha ERD and gamma ERS co-localisation with fMRI BOLD response in visual cortex. Neuroimage 26:302–308

Dale AM, Fischl B, Sereno MI (1999) Cortical surface-based analysis: I. Segmentation and surface reconstruction. Neuroimage 9:179–194

Dale AM, Liu AK, Fischl BR, Buckner RL, Belliveau JW, Lewine JD, Halgren E (2000) Dynamic statistical parametric mapping: combining fMRI and MEG for high-resolution imaging of cortical activity. Neuron 26:55–67

Dale AM, Sereno MI (1993) Improved localization of cortical activity by combining EEG and MEG with MRI cortical surface reconstruction: A linear approach. J Cogn Neurosci 5:162–176

Darvas F, Pantazis D, Kucukaltun-Yildirim E, Leahy RM (2004) Mapping human brain function with MEG and EEG: Methods and validation. Neuroimage 23:S289–S299

Edelman GM, Tononi G (2000) A universe of consciousness. Basic Books, New York

Eichele T, Specht K, Moosmann M, Jongsma ML, Quiroga RQ, Nordby H, Hugdahl K (2005) Assessing the spatiotemporal evolution of neuronal activation with single-trial event-related potentials and functional MRI. Proc Natl Acad Sci USA 102(49):17798–17803

Engel AK, Fries P, Singer W (2001) Dynamic predictions: oscillations and synchrony in top-down processing. Nat Rev Neurosci 2(10):704–716

Esposito F, Bertolino A, Scarabino T, Latorre V, Blasi G, Popolizio T, Tedeschi G, Cirillo S, Goebel R, Di Salle F (2006) Independent component model of the default-mode brain function: assessing the impact of active thinking. Brain Res Bull 70(4–6):263–269

Friston KJ, Holmes AP, Poline JB, Grasby PJ, Williams SC, Frackowiak RS, Turner R (1995) Analysis of fMRI time-series revisited. Neuroimage 2(1):45–53

Feige B, Scheffler K, Esposito F, Di Salle F, Hennig J, Seifritz E (2005) Cortical and subcortical correlates of electroencephalographic alpha rhythm modulation. J Neurophysiol 93(5):2864–2872

Grave de Peralta R, Murray MM, Michel CM, Martuzzi R, Gonzalez Andino S (2004) Electrical neuroimaging based on biophysical constraints. Neuroimage 21:527–539

Jeffs B, Leahy R, Singh M (1987) An evaluation of methods for neuromagnetic image reconstruction. IEEE Trans Biomed Eng 34:713–723

Hamalainen M, Hari R, Ilmoniemi R, Knuutila J, Lounasmaa O (1993) Magnetoencephalography: theory, instrumentation, and application to non-invasive studies of the working human brain. Rev Mod Phys 65:413–497

Hamalainen M, Ilmoniemi RJ (1984) Interpreting measured magnetic fields of the brain: estimates of current distributions (Technical Report TKK-F-A559). Helsinki University of Technology, Finland

Hyvarinen A, Karhunen J, Oja E (2001) Independent component analysis. Wiley, New York

Kayser J, Tenke CE (2003) Optimizing PCA methodology for ERP component identification and measurement: theoretical rationale and empirical evaluation. Clin Neurophysiol 114(12): 2307–2325

Kiebel SJ, Goebel R, Friston KJ (2000) Anatomically informed basis functions. Neuroimage 11(6):656–667

Laufs H, Krakow K, Sterzer P, Eger E, Beyerle A, Salek-Haddadi A, Kleinschmidt A (2003) Electroencephalographic signatures of attentional and cognitive default modes in spontaneous brain activity fluctuations at rest. Proc Natl Acad Sci USA 100(19):11053–11058

Lawson CL, Hanson RJ (1974) Solving least squares problems. Prentice Hall, Englewood Cliffs

Leahy RM, Mosher JC, Philips JW (1996) A comparative study of minimum norm inverse methods for MEG imaging. In: Proceedings of the Tenth International Conference of Biomagnetism, BIOMAG'96, Santa Fe, NM, USA, 16–21 Feb 1996, pp 274–275

Lin FH, Witzel T, Ahlfors SP, Stufflebeam SM, Belliveau JW, Hämäläinen MS (2006) Assessing and improving the spatial accuracy in MEG source localization by depth-weighted minimum-norm estimates. Neuroimage 31:160–171

Lin FH, Witzel T, Hämäläinen MS, Dale AM, Belliveau JW, Stufflebeam SM (2004) Spectral spatiotemporal imaging of cortical oscillations and interactions in the human brain. Neuroimage 23:582–595

Liu AK, Belliveau JW, Dale AM (1998) Spatiotemporal imaging of human brain activity using functional MRI constrained magnetoencephalography data: Monte Carlo simulations. Proc Natl Acad Sci USA 95(15):8945–8950

Liu Z, Kecman F, He B (2006) Effects of fMRI–EEG mismatches in cortical current density estimation integrating fMRI and EEG: a simulation study. Clin Neurophysiol 117(7):1610–1622

Makeig S, Westerfield M, Jung TP, Enghoff S, Townsend J, Courchesne E, Sejnowski TJ (2002) Dynamic brain sources of visual evoked responses. Science 295(5555):690–694

Meltzer JA, Negishi M, Mayes LC, Constable RT (2007a) Individual differences in EEG theta and alpha dynamics during working memory correlate with fMRI responses across subjects. Clin Neurophysiol 118(11):2419–2436

Meltzer JA, Zaveri HP, Goncharova II, Distasio MM, Papademetris X, Spencer SS, Spencer DD, Constable RT (2007b) Effects of working memory load on oscillatory power in human intracranial EEG. Cereb Cortex 18(8):1843–1855

Michel CM, Murray MM, Lantz G, Gonzalez S, Spinelli L, Grave de Peralta R (2004) EEG source imaging. Clin Neurophysiol 115(10):2195–2222

Mosher JC, Leahy RM (1998) Recursive MUSIC: a framework for EEG and MEG source localization. IEEE Trans Biomed Eng 45(11):1342–1355

Mosher JC, Leahy R, Lewis P (1999) EEG and MEG: forward solutions for inverse methods. IEEE Trans Biomed Eng 46(3):245–259

Mulert C, Menzinger E, Leicht G, Pogarell O, Hegerl U (2005) Evidence for a close relationship between conscious effort and anterior cingulate cortex activity. Int J Psychophysiol 56:65–80

Nunez PL, Srinivasan R (2006) Electric fields of the brain. The neurophysics of EEG, 2nd edn. Oxford University Press, New York

Pascual-Marqui R (2002) Standardized low resolution brain electromagnetic tomography (sLORETA): technical details. Methods Find Exp Clin Pharmacol 24D:5–12

Pascual-Marqui R, Michel C, Lehman D (1994) Low resolution electromagnetic tomography: a new method for localizing electrical activity in the brain. Int J Psychophysiol 18:49–65

Sarvas J (1985) Basic mathematical and electromagnetic concepts of the biomagnetic inverse problem. Phys Med Biol 32:11–22

Scherg M (1990) Fundamentals of dipole source potential analysis. Adv Audiol 6:40 69

Tikhonov A, Arsenin V (1977) Solutions to ill-posed problems. Wiley, New York

van Veen B, van Drongelen W, Yuchtman M, Suzuki A (1997) Localization of brain electrical activity via linearly constrained minimum variance spatial filtering. IEEE Trans Biomed Eng 44(9):867–880

Wibral M, Turi G, Linden DE, Kaiser J, Bledowski C (2008) Decomposition of working memory-related scalp ERPs: crossvalidation of fMRI-constrained source analysis and ICA. Int J Psychophysiol 67(3):200–211

Part II

Technical and Methodological Aspects of Combined EEG–fMRI Experiments

EEG Instrumentation and Safety

7

Philip J. Allen

Abbreviations

AC	Alternating current
DC	Direct current
ECG	Electrocardiogram
EEG	Electroencephalography
emf	Electromotive force
EMG	Electromyography
EPI	Echo planar imaging
fMRI	Functional magnetic resonance imaging
MR	Magnetic resonance
MRI	Magnetic resonance imaging
RF	Radiofrequency
rms	Root mean square
SAR	Specific absorption rate

1
Introduction

The successful combination of electroencephalography (EEG) and fMRI demands careful consideration of three important issues: patient safety, EEG quality and image quality. In this chapter we first consider the implications these factors have on the design of EEG instrumentation, and then examine the precautions that must be taken in order that these recordings can be performed safely.

P. J. Allen
Department of Clinical Neurophysiology, The National Hospital for Neurology and Neurosurgery, Queen Square, London, WC1N 3BG, UK
e-mail: Philip.allen@uclh.nhs.uk

C. Mulert and L. Lemieux (eds.), *EEG– fMRI*
DOI: 10.1007/978-3-540-87919-0_7, © Springer Verlag Berlin Heidelberg 2010

2
EEG Instrumentation

EEG instrumentation comprises electrodes, an acquisition system to amplify and digitise the EEG signals, and review facilities for the display and analysis of the recorded waveforms. The design of EEG instrumentation appropriate for use in the magnetic resonance (MR) scanner must take into account a number of factors that are not applicable to conventional EEG equipment: the presence of static and time-varying magnetic fields and their associated EEG artefacts; the need to limit radiofrequency (RF) emissions to preserve image quality; and finally the obvious requirement to avoid the introduction of ferrous materials into the scanner environment. These considerations dictate that EEG monitoring equipment used for diagnostic recordings in a clinical setting are not suitable for optimal EEG–fMRI monitoring. In this section, we examine the influence the above factors exert on the design of EEG instrumentation. We start at the beginning of the EEG signal chain with a consideration of the electrodes. EEG artefact post-processing correction methods are discussed in detail in the chapters "EEG Quality: Origin and Reduction of the EEG Cardiac-Related Artefact" and "EEG Quality: The Image Acquisition Artefact".

2.1
Electrodes

The term EEG electrode is used here to describe the combination of the electrode head and connecting lead. In addition to the EEG and image quality issues discussed in this section, EEG electrodes also raise safety issues when used in the MR scanner; these will be discussed in Sect. 3 of this chapter.

2.1.1
Electrode Lead Arrangement

The electromotive force (emf) induced in a conductive loop is proportional to the rate of change of magnetic flux cutting the loop and the loop area:

$$V_{induced} = A \times \frac{dB}{dt},$$
(1)

where
 $V_{induced}$ = emf induced in the loop,
 A = loop area perpendicular to the field,
 $\frac{dB}{dt}$ = rate of change of magnetic flux cutting the loop.

Hence, it is important to minimise the area of any loop formed by the electrode leads in order to reduce signal artefacts induced by the changing magnetic fields. A number of methods to achieve this have been reported (Goldman et al. 2000; Anami et al. 2003;

Hoffmann et al. 2000; Negishi et al. 2004; Vasios et al. 2006); in essence, these involve bunching electrode leads together at a single point on the head and then further minimising the loop area, typically by twisting the wires together as far as possible along their entire path from the subject's head to the amplifier inputs. This not only keeps the leads in close proximity to each other but also results in the cancellation of the induced emfs in adjacent twists. Nevertheless, EEG is recorded between separate points on the head, and hence some loop area is inevitable. Goldman et al. proposed minimising this by recording from a chain of linked bipolar pairs connected to individual differential amplifiers (Goldman et al. 2000). Although this can present a smaller loop than encountered in common reference recordings, it is more restrictive in terms of electrode placement, particularly when the number of channels is large. More common is the use of electrode caps, which combine the advantage of multichannel referential recordings with relatively low loop areas (Baumann and Noll 1999; Bonmassar et al. 1999; Srivastava et al. 2005; Laufs et al. 2003; Iannetti et al. 2002) (Fig. 1).

Although some groups have advocated shielding of the electrode leads (Hoffmann et al. 2000) and electrodes (Anami et al. 2003), presumably to reduce artefacts caused by electrostatic coupling to electric field sources in the scanner, a quantitative assessment of the benefit of this technique has not yet been reported. Minimisation of loop area is also important to ensure patient safety; this will be addressed in Sect. 3 of this chapter.

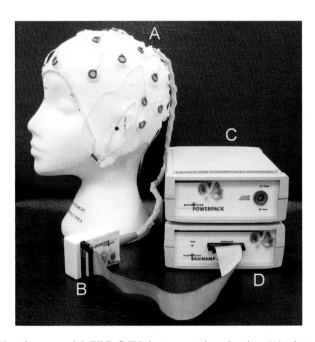

Fig. 1 Example of commercial EEG–fMRI instrumentation showing (**A**) electrode cap, (**B**) connector box containing current-limiting resistors, (**C**) battery power pack and (**D**) 32 channel EEG amplifier/digitiser. This instrumentation is sited adjacent to the scanner bore and transmits data to a receiver outside the Faraday shield via fibre optic links

2.1.2
Electrode Lead Movement

EEG artefacts are induced not only by changing magnetic fields cutting a static loop but also by variation in loop area in the static field. Such variation can result from the movement of the electrode leads caused by a ballistocardiogram (Debener et al. 2007; Allen et al. 1998), small head movements (Hill et al. 1995) and scanner vibration (Garreffa et al. 2004). A variety of methods have been used to minimise these artefacts, such as weighing down the electrode leads where they pass out of the scanner using sand bags (Benar et al. 2003), placing padding under the leads and amplifier (Hoffmann et al. 2000), placing a tight bandage over the patient's head to secure individual electrode leads (Benar et al. 2003), or the use of an electrode cap (Kruggel et al. 2000). There is general agreement that such fixation methods can reduce artefacts significantly.

Another important factor in reducing electrode lead movements (although not strictly part of the EEG instrumentation) is the reduction of patient head movement. Such immobilisation has been achieved using a vacuum cushion filled with polystyrene spheres (Benar et al. 2003; Anami et al. 2003). This method has been reported to be effective and well tolerated, the latter being an important factor in prolonged EEG–fMRI experiments, since any patient discomfort is likely to provoke gross movement, with its associated artefacts in both the EEG and magnetic resonance imaging (MRI) data.

In a comparison of three different methods for reducing lead and head movement (weighing down the leads, electrodes secured by a tight bandage, head fixed by vacuum cushion), Benar et al. found that the former was the most important and the vacuum cushion the least (Benar et al. 2003). It is interesting to note, however, that whereas artefact in the range 30–50 μV were observed for the subjects in this study, Kruggel et al. observed artefact of up to 500 μV using a broadly comparable arrangement (stretchable cap, twisted leads weighed down with rice bags, head restrained by cushions) (Kruggel et al. 2000). This tenfold difference (which cannot be attributed entirely to the different scanner fields in these studies, of 1.5 and 3 T respectively) suggests that these artefact minimisation techniques are very sensitive, and hence local experimentation may be necessary to find the optimal arrangement.

2.2
EEG Recording System

The EEG recorded in the MR scanner is contaminated by two different sources of interference that do not afflict clinical EEG recordings. The first is often referred to as pulse (or sometimes ballistocardiogram) artefact, and is caused by cardiac-related movement of the electrodes or blood flow in the static field. It is typically 10–100 μV in amplitude and overlaps the EEG frequency range (Allen et al. 1998). A variety of techniques have been developed to reduce these artefacts (Allen et al. 1998; Goldman et al. 2000; Bonmassar et al. 2002; Benar et al. 2003); these make no additional demands on the EEG instrumentation above those required for conventional clinical EEG.

The second source of interference is often referred to as imaging (or sometimes gradient) artefact, and represents the emfs induced in the electrode lead loops by the changing magnetic fields applied during imaging. It has two distinct components, attributable to the gradient and RF fields respectively. The former range in frequency from the slice repetition interval (typically 10–20 Hz) up to the kHz range. The RF fields have a fundamental component at the Larmor frequency of the scanner, ranging from 63 MHz for 1.5 T up to 300 MHz for 7 T, but also lower-frequency components reflecting the rate at which the RF is pulsed (Hoffmann et al. 2000) and the pulse shape. In contrast to pulse artefact, imaging artefact is normally significantly larger in amplitude than the EEG, often obscuring the waveforms completely (Allen et al. 2000). In the early days of this technique, the EEG and fMRI were interleaved. In studies of epilepsy, this was typically achieved by triggering fMRI acquisition immediately after observing an epileptiform spike in the EEG (Warach et al. 1996; Seeck et al. 1998). It was accepted that the EEG recording during the image acquisition would be obscured. Subsequent developments in artefact subtraction methods have now made truly simultaneous EEG and fMRI recording routine. Although this makes greater demands on the EEG instrumentation, particularly with regard to filtering, sampling rate and dynamic range, it offers much greater freedom in experimental design and is now accepted as an essential requirement.

2.2.1
Filters

As RF artefacts occur at a frequency many orders of magnitude higher than those of EEG, they can be reduced to an acceptable level by low-pass filtering with a -3 dB cut-off point that is substantially higher than the EEG bandwidth. For example, Anami et al. demonstrated that a 3,000 Hz cut-off low-pass filter reduced the RF artefact to below 100 µV, substantially less than that of the gradient artefact (Anami et al. 2003) (Fig. 2). This filtering should, however, be implemented at the front end of the instrumentation to avoid possible demodulation of the RF into the EEG frequency range due to nonlinearities in subsequent active amplifier stages. Gradient artefacts, in contrast, overlap the EEG spectrum and hence cannot be removed by low-pass filtering alone. Nevertheless, analogue low-pass filtering prior to the main gain stage in the EEG amplifier is normally essential to prevent saturation by the high-amplitude gradient artefact. In order to maximise the attenuation of these artefacts, the cut-off frequency of this filter should be set as low as possible consistent with the recommended EEG bandwidth, typically 70 Hz (Deuschl and Eisen 1999). Attenuation of gradient artefact can be improved by using a higher-order (three or greater) analogue low-pass filter with a steeper roll-off. However, this comes at the expense of poorer phase-frequency linearity, which may result in distortion of EEG transients (Janssen et al. 1986) and hence should be avoided.

2.2.2
Sampling Rate

Given that low-pass filtering alone cannot remove all of the imaging artefact, a variety of post-processing artefact subtraction methods have been developed. The artefact removal method most commonly used to date is based on the subtraction of an artefact template

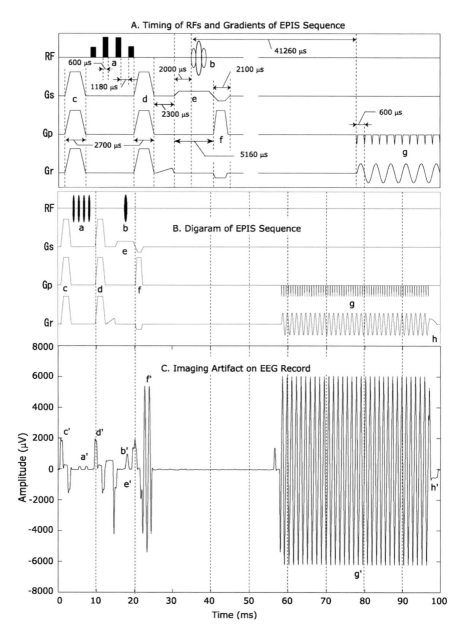

Fig. 2 **A** Timings of RF emission and gradient pulses in an fMRI sequence (EPIS, Siemens: ep2d_fid_60b2080_62_64.ekc). *RF*, radiofrequency wave; *Gs*, slice selection gradient; *Gp*, phase encoding gradient; *Gr*, readout gradient. *a*, Fat suppression pulses (1–3–3–1 pulses); *b*, slice selection RF; *c*, *d*, *h*, spoilers; *e*, slice selection gradient; *f*, dephasing and rephrasing gradient; *g*, readout gradient. **B** Schematic diagram of whole EPIS sequence. **C** Imaging artefact waveform for one slice scan on a dummy EEG record with a phantom using the EPIS sequence. The artefact corresponding to each gradient component described above in (**A**) can be identified, and is denoted by the same alphabet as that denoting the original gradient but with a prime. From Anami et al. (2003)

derived from averaging the artefact over a number of scan repetitions (Allen et al. 2000). Successful artefact subtraction by this method (and many of its subsequent enhancements; see for example Negishi et al. 2004; Benar et al. 2003) is dependent on accurate calculation of the artefact template. As the imaging artefact contains rapidly changing components, a fast sampling rate (typically 5 kHz) is required in order to capture these signals adequately (Allen et al. 2000). This is ten times higher than the rate used in conventional EEG equipment. Even at this high sampling rate, temporal jitter in the EEG sampling can lead to inaccuracies in the artefact template estimation that limit the effectiveness of this method (Cohen et al. 2001). Although technically feasible, increasing the sampling rate further results in very large data-sets, especially for prolonged recordings using a large number of channels. Hence, an alternative approach has been proposed whereby the EEG sampling is synchronised to the MR scanner clock (Cohen et al. 2001). Mandelkow et al. demonstrated that this method can reduce the residual artefact, particularly the higher-frequency EEG components, and achieves good artefact reduction even when using a conventional EEG sampling rate of 500 Hz (Mandelkow et al. 2006). It is worth noting, however, that the EEG in this study was originally sampled at 5 kHz then down-sampled to 500 Hz after the application of a seventh-order digital filter, an important step for preventing aliasing. As the authors comment, the application of such a high-order filter implemented in hardware prior to digitising at 500 Hz would inevitably distort the EEG due its nonlinear phase response. Nevertheless, the method holds great promise for improving artefact suppression, particularly when there is a requirement to analyse higher-frequency EEG components such as the gamma bands. It therefore follows that the facility to synchronise the EEG sampling rate precisely to an external clock is a useful addition to the EEG instrumentation specification. This synchronisation also requires hardware to reduce the scanner clock to the EEG sampling rate (10 MHz to 5 kHz in the report by Mandelkow), but this can be achieved independently of the EEG instrumentation, for example by phase-locked loop circuitry (Mandelkow et al. 2006) or a clock divider.

2.2.3
Signal Range

The amplitude of gradient imaging artefact in the EEG is proportional to the loop area and the rate of change of magnetic flux cutting the loop, as described in Eq. 1. Allen et al. calculated that for a relatively high slew rate of 125 T m^{-1} s^{-1} and a worst case EEG lead loop area of 100 cm^2 located 0.2 m from the scanner isocentre, the induced artefact due to gradient fields is ±250 mV (Allen et al. 2000), more than two orders of magnitude greater than the recommended range (±1 mV) for conventional EEG equipment (Nuwer et al. 1999). In practice, careful alignment of electrode leads can help reduce the artefact amplitude substantially. Anami et al. recorded imaging artefact from electrodes on a phantom in a 1.5 T scanner using a typical blipped echo planar imaging (EPI) sequence (see the chapter "EEG Quality: Origin and Reduction of the EEG Cardiac-Related Artefact"), wide bandwidth [direct current (DC) to 3,000 Hz] and 20 kHz sampling (Anami et al. 2003). This revealed a substantially lower maximum gradient artefact of 40 mV (Fig. 2). However, the use of faster slew rates or the acquisition of different physiological parameters such as electrocardiogram (ECG) and electromyography (EMG), which may necessarily involve larger loop areas, would result in proportionally larger artefact. It is therefore still important that the EEG instrumentation has sufficient range throughout the entire signal path to record these signals without saturating—if the artefact saturates then the underlying physiological signal will be lost. It is important to note that saturation is not always obvious by inspection of the recorded EEG signal, due to the effect on the waveform of subsequent circuit stages such as alternating current (AC) coupling and additional high- and low-pass filters. The following factors need consideration when assessing whether EEG instrumentation has sufficient range: the amplitude and spectral distribution of the imaging artefact, the frequency response and location in the overall system of the analogue low-pass filters, and the signal range at each stage of the EEG instrumentation. For example, Allen et al. described an EEG amplifier with an overall dynamic range in the passband of 33.3 mV, which, through the judicious use of gain and filter stages, could handle artefact of ±250 mV pk–pk at source without saturating (Allen et al. 2000).

2.2.4
Signal Resolution

In addition to providing sufficient signal range, the EEG instrumentation must also have adequate resolution. The minimum recommended resolution for conventional EEG equipment is 0.5 µV (Nuwer et al. 1999). Given the need for a large signal range of the order 20–30 mV as described above, this resolution would require 16 bits, which in practice requires a digitiser with more than 16 bits. However, given that the residual artefact from current pulse- and imaging-artefact subtraction methods is at least 5 µV (Allen et al. 2000), and that this error occurs independent of digitisation errors, 16-bit digitisation yielding 14–15 effective bits and hence a resolution of 1–2 µV is adequate. As artefact subtraction methods improve, greater bit depth may be justified, especially when recording lower-amplitude EEG activity such as event-related potentials (ERPs). The dynamic range can, however, be increased for these by averaging, albeit at the expense of longer recording time.

2.3
RF Emissions

The MRI scanner contains an extremely sensitive RF detector. Any RF emissions from the EEG instrumentation may lead to artefacts in the MR images if they fall in the frequency range detected by the scanner. Potential sources of these emissions are active circuitry in EEG instrumentation located in the scanner room or the ingress of RF signals via conductors that breach the scanner's Faraday shield. For the former, careful design is required to minimise RF emissions, as even relatively low-frequency digital circuitry can generate signals in the RF range due to the presence of harmonics. These may pass into the head coil by conduction along the electrode leads or by radiation through space. A number of techniques can be used to minimise this interference: RF signals should be minimised at source by using low-power digital components, thereby minimising switching currents; all active circuitry should be enclosed in a conductive enclosure (Allen et al. 2000; Gualniera et al. 2004; Garreffa et al. 2004); and all conductive signal paths (for example connections to EEG electrodes and external battery packs) breaching this enclosure should do so via in-line RF filters (Fig. 3). Where active EEG instrumentation is located in the scanner room,

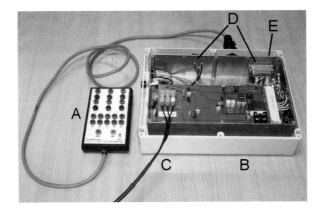

Fig. 3 Example of early in-house MRI-compatible EEG instrumentation developed in 2000 by our group. *A*, Nonferrous electrode connector box suitable for mounting in the bore of the magnet. *B*, EEG amplifier and digitiser; *C*, fibre optic cables transmitting digitised EEG data to a receiver unit outside the scanner room; *D*, in-line RF filters fitted to all signal lines breaching the shielded enclosure; *E*, shielded enclosure limiting RF emissions

EEG data is normally transmitted to a receiver in the console room via fibre optic cables, thereby eliminating the ingress of RF from outside the scanner (Figs. 1 and 2). This approach has been implemented in a number of commercial products.

Alternatively, the EEG instrumentation can be sited in the console room, with connection to the subject made via long electrode leads which pass through the Faraday shield (Huang-Hellinger et al. 1995; Anami et al. 2003). If the impedance of these leads is low, RF filtering must be applied at the point where the electrode leads breach the Faraday shield (Huang-Hellinger et al. 1995). Careful consideration must also be given to the safety implications of using such long cable runs with direct electrical connection to the patient, especially with regard to the accidental application of external voltage sources to these cables.

As stated previously, RF emissions will only cause image artefacts if they fall in the frequency range detected by the scanner receive coil and within the receiver bandwidth used for the imaging experiment, which occupies a narrow range either side of the Larmor frequency. Hence, it is perfectly possible that EEG instrumentation that does not generate image artefact when used with one scanner may cause interference in another. Hence, an empirical test of image artefact should be undertaken prior to introducing new EEG instrumentation.

2.4
Miscellaneous Factors

In addition to the essential characteristics described above for high-quality EEG recording in the MR scanner, EEG equipment should broadly meet the requirements for conventional EEG. The key parameters are as follows: maximum noise at input of 1.5 μV pk–pk; bandwidth 0.16–70 Hz, input impedance $\geq$100 MΩ; common mode rejection $\geq$110 dB (Nuwer et al. 1999). A DC input range of ±300 mV is sufficient to handle the likely range of electrode potentials (Kamp and Lopes Da Silva 1998). Built-in electrode impedance checking and a 50/60 Hz notch filter are desirable. Finally, the EEG review facilities should not be overlooked. Although the conventional requirements such as remontaging flexible sensitivity and time base must obviously be provided, one specific additional requirement for EEG–fMRI instrumentation is the facility to correlate (e.g. mark and export) specific EEG events the corresponding fMRI data simply and accurately.

2.5
Summary

The 15 years that have passed since the first reported recording of EEG during fMRI (Ives et al. 1993) have seen a burgeoning of interest in this technique. This has prompted the commercial development of EEG instrumentation designed specifically to meet many of the technical requirements described above, further extending the availability of the technique. Although further improvements in artefact minimisation would be desirable to record lower-amplitude activity such as ERPs or fast gamma activity, an EEG quality appropriate for studies of epilepsy and basic EEG rhythms can readily be achieved. However, it remains essential to pay careful attention to the entire recording setup comprising the subject, electrodes and EEG recording system in order to achieve optimal EEG signal quality. This will become even more important as higher-field scanners and studies of more subtle EEG activity become increasingly common.

3
Safety

Recording EEG in the MR scanner raises important safety issues. First, there is the hazard associated with the introduction of ferromagnetic materials into the scanner. Secondly, currents induced in the electrodes and attached wires by the changing fields applied during imaging can present a hazard due to the following mechanisms: eddy current heating of the electrode heads; currents induced in loops formed between the electrode leads; and currents induced along electrode leads. The safety implications of induced currents are determined by the field frequency, with different biological mechanisms for damage for the gradient- and RF-related fields. We begin by considering the relevant safety limits before moving on to a more detailed examination of each specific hazard.

3.1
Safety Limits

In the absence of a safety standard specifically addressing combined EEG–fMRI, the onus has been on users of this technique to demonstrate compliance with the standards applicable individually to MR and EEG equipment. Hence, the following safety limits derived from these standards apply: (1) maximum permissible cerebral temperature of 38°C, implying a maximum temperature increase due to scanner induced heating of 1°C (IEC 2002a); (2) maximum permissible temperature of an applied part in skin contact (such as an electrode) of 43°C (IEC 2005); and (3) maximum permissible tissue contact currents ranging from 0.5 mA rms (≈1 kHz) to 10 mA rms > 100 kHz (IEC 2005).

In addition, EEG instrumentation must meet the safety requirements for general medical electrical equipment (IEC 2005) and the particular standard for EEG equipment (IEC 2002b).

3.2
Static Field

The principal safety issue associated with the static field is the force it exerts on ferromagnetic material. Fortunately, this is not a significant limitation since there are a range of nonferromagnetic materials that meet the requirements for high-quality EEG. These include combinations of silver, silver chloride, gold, carbon and conductive plastic for scalp recordings, and iridium/platinum for intracerebral recordings. However, care should be taken to exclude the presence of ferromagnetic material in ancillary items, such as securing springs in electrode caps or amplifier connectors. Stainless steel sphenoidal electrodes are clearly unacceptable.

Any new EEG instrumentation introduced into the scanner must also be tested for displacement force and torque (Baumann and Noll 1999; Woods 2007). In addition, it should be noted that any electronic components dependent on ferromagnetic behaviour (such as some switching DC-DC converters, ferrites) may not function when placed in close proximity to the static field.

One further potential hazard is the current induced in an electrode lead loop moved through the nonuniform region of the static field, for example when the patient is introduced into the scanner. This current will flow between electrodes and hence through the patient. Lemieux et al. investigated this at 1.5 T and identified that the effect was very small and hence no additional safety measures were required (Lemieux et al. 1997), although this may require reassessment with the development of higher-field shielded magnets.

3.3
Gradient Fields

The emf induced in an electrode lead loop by the gradient fields is proportional to the rate of change of magnetic flux cutting the loop and the loop area, as defined in Eq. 1. As the frequency of these fields typically does not extend much higher than 1 kHz, the dominant physiological effect is neuromuscular stimulation. Lemieux et al. calculated that for a relatively high slew rate of 120 T m^{-1} s^{-1} and a worst case loop area of 400 cm^2, loop resistance must be at least 3.3 kΩ in order to meet the safe limit of 0.5 mA rms under a single fault condition, namely the electrode leads accidentally shorting together (Lemieux et al. 1997). As a much higher value of current limiting resistor is normally required to limit heating due to RF-induced currents, this does not present an additional constraint. Indeed, the inevitable tissue contact impedance presented at each electrode (of the order of 1 kΩ), combined with careful electrode lead arrangement to reduce the loop area below the pessimistic 400 cm^2, means that the current limit requirements can feasibly be met even if a current limiting resistor is omitted. However, this would need further consideration if substantially higher slew rates were used or loop area was increased, for example by recording from very widely spaced possibly noncephalic electrodes.

3.4
Eddy Currents

The RF fields applied during scanning induce eddy currents in the electrodes (Lemieux et al. 1997). These currents are much greater than those induced in human tissue, due to the relatively higher electrical conductivity of the electrode material, and may result in Joule heating of the electrode (Roth et al. 1992). Lemieux et al. investigated eddy current heating of a silver/silver chloride electrode in a 1.5 T scanner [averaged specific absorption rate (SAR) 0.06 W/kg] and found a maximum temperature increase of <1°C, comfortably within the permitted limit (Lemieux et al. 1997). Similar results have been found at higher field strengths: Mirsattari et al. found no temperature rise in a gold-plated pure silver electrode in a 1.5 T scanner (averaged SAR up to 1.6 W/Kg) (Mirsattari et al. 2004); Stevens et al. found no significant heat increase in the same electrode or in a silver/silver chloride in carbon embedded plastic electrode at 4 T with a high-power pulse sequence (8 W average per TR) (Stevens et al. 2007).

There is, however, evidence that eddy current heating may prove more significant at 7 T: Vasios et al. recorded a 2.2°C rise in a full-ring electrode following 22 min of high-power turbo spin echo (TSE) with a maximum local SAR of 11 W/Kg (Vasios et al. 2006), a power level just above the maximum SAR limit (IEC 2002a). Although this heating may not be due entirely to eddy currents (the temperature increase was recorded from a 32 electrode configuration and hence would include heating effects from currents induced in the associated conducting loops and elongated conductors), these clearly made a significant contribution since the temperature rise for the same configuration was reduced to 0.8°C when the full-ring electrodes were replaced with half rings designed specifically to reduce eddy currents.

In summary, these experimental investigations indicate that at field strengths of 4 T or less, electrode heating due to eddy currents does not appear to pose a risk to patients. Above 4 T, more specialised electrode design and/or SAR limits may be required. See the chapter "Specific Issues Related to EEG–fMRI at $B_0 > 3$ T" for further discussion.

3.5
RF Fields

The dominant physiological effect of induced high-frequency currents (>100 kHz) is tissue heating. The interaction between the scanner's RF (B_1) field and electrode leads can result in heating via two related mechanisms. Firstly, the magnetic component of the B_1 field will induce an emf in any conductive loop formed by the electrode leads. This emf is proportional to the loop area cut by the field and the rate of change of the field (1). If tissue forms part of the loop, the induced emf will drive a current through this, causing heating. It is worth noting that in contrast to gradient field induced currents, the capacitance between bundled electrode leads presents relatively low-impedance conductive loops at RF frequencies, even if the leads are not accidentally shorted together, i.e. the non-fault condition (Lemieux et al. 1997). Secondly, the electric component of the B_1 field can induce a current along the extended conductor formed by an electrode lead (the antenna effect). The magnitude of this current is influenced by a wide range of factors, including the proximity of the wires to the source of electric field in the MR transmitter coil (Hofman et al. 1996) and the resonant length of the electrode leads in relation to the RF wavelength, with a theoretical maximum induced current for multiples of half wavelength (Pictet et al. 2000). As a broad guide, the resonant length of a straight wire in air is 2.35 m at 1.5 T and 1.17 m at 3 T (Dempsey et al. 2001), but this varies significantly according to the wire diameter, shape, insulation thickness and permittivity, and tissue conductivity and permittivity (Yeung et al. 2002). Although it is known that the maximum temperature increase associated with these currents occurs in tissue adjacent to the tip of a conductor, where the electric field is maximum (Yeung et al. 2002), accurate prediction of the associated temperature rise for a given scenario remains problematical. Both mechanisms for interaction of the electrodes and leads with the scanner RF fields are exacerbated by resonant conditions where the induction of much larger currents occurs (Dempsey et al. 2001); it is thus necessary to avoid these conditions.

In the first systematic study of safety due to RF heating of EEG electrodes in the MR scanner, Lemieux et al. investigated induced currents due to the electric and magnetic fields separately and concluded that the latter dominated and that a current-limiting resistor (12 kΩ) was required in the scalp electrode leads in order to limit contact currents to acceptable levels for a worst case electrode lead loop (400 cm²) and high SAR for a 1.5 T scanner (Lemieux et al. 1997). This additional resistance is small relative to the typical input impedance of an EEG amplifier (at least 10 MΩ) and hence does not degrade EEG signal quality significantly. This study was undertaken using a head RF transmit coil—the safety of EEG–fMRI for body RF coils has not yet received a thorough investigation. The authors stressed the importance of performing a local risk assessment of the specific electrode and scanner setup using the methodology presented. Data supplied by the manufacturer on the relationship between B_1 and SAR for the quadrature transmit and receive head coil used in the GE Signa Excite 3 T scanner demonstrates that the RMS value of B_1 for a given SAR value (and body weight) is less than 50% of the value at 1.5 T, and therefore so will be the current induced in the EEG system-patient circuit, suggesting that the proposed safety measure is also adequate for this instrument, even taking into account the effect of the higher RF frequency.[1]

Our group has performed over 300 EEG–fMRI recordings at both 1.5 and 3 T using electrodes with current limiting resistors without incident. Current limiting resistors are included in a number of commercial electrodes and electrode caps designed for

---

[1]This corresponds to the fact that more heating is induced per unit B_1 at 3 T than at 1.5 T. The lower expected induced currents reflect the fact that the regulatory SAR limits are independent of field strength.

EEG–fMRI. Such studies have been performed at multiple centres worldwide over the last ten years; as far as the author is aware there have been no reports of adverse incidents resulting from these recordings. It has been proposed, on the basis of in vivo temperature measurements in a small number of subjects for a particular experimental setup, that additional resistors are not in fact necessary (Lazeyras et al. 2001). However, their use does provide reassurance that even under worst-case conditions (including a single fault), the subject will not be harmed, with only a minimal associated increase in EEG noise.

An alternative approach to establishing the safety of RF/EEG electrode interactions is the measurement of temperature changes during the scanning of electrodes attached to a head phantom. This method has been used extensively in the safety assessment of implants in the MR scanner (Carmichael et al. 2007a; Baker et al. 2004; Yeung et al. 2002; Gray et al. 2005) and more recently for EEG electrodes (Vasios et al 2006; Angelone 2006). The reliability of the temperature changes recorded using this approach is of course strongly influenced by the accuracy of the physical model. In particular, the head phantom must have realistic geometric, thermal and electrical properties (Angelone et al. 2006; Rezai et al. 2002; Park et al. 2003). Although the absence of thermoregulation from the head models used to date is clearly an inaccuracy, this merely leads to a conservative estimate of the temperature increases expected in human studies (Akca et al. 2007). The electrode lead length is also important: Yeung et al. observed substantial differences in heating at the tip of a length of wire in response to small changes in its length (of the order of a few centimetres) (Yeung et al. 2002). Similarly, the proximity of conducting leads to the transmit coil (where the electric component of the RF field is maximal) can affect heating significantly (Dempsey et al. 2001; Georgi et al. 2004). It is also important to use electrode gel in order to accurately replicate the electrical contact between the phantom and electrode (Vasios et al. 2006). The precise location of a temperature probe in the electrode gel can also introduce significant measurement variability (Angelone et al. 2006). In summary, careful experimental technique combined with a knowledge of the wide range of factors that influence MR-induced heating is an essential prerequisite for a reliable safety assessment based on this methodology (Shellock 2007). Finally, it is important to note once again that measurements performed on one scanner are not transferable to other scanners, and hence a local assessment combined with strict adherence to an experimental protocol is essential (Kainz 2007; Carmichael et al. 2007a).

One limitation of this empirical approach is the restricted spatial sampling that can be achieved with current MR compatible thermometry (typically four sites). This requires assumptions to be made regarding the location of the greatest temperature rise, which may be difficult to predict with certainty for a particular arrangement of electrode and leads in the scanner. One potential solution is to calculate temperature changes from a computational simulation of the electric field distribution resulting from the application of RF fields to a realistic head/electrode model. This approach allows the direct visualisation of the local SAR (and hence by application of the heat equation, the associated temperature changes; Collins et al. 2004) throughout the entire head volume, rather than just at selected sites.

Angelone et al. have used this method to investigate RF heating of EEG electrodes at 7 T (Angelone et al. 2006). Electric field and SAR values were calculated using the finite difference time domain method applied to numerical models of the electrodes, leads, RF coil and anatomically accurate homogeneous head model. The simulated temperature changes were validated by comparison with those measured for an equivalent electrode/phantom head arrangement in the scanner, the two methods showing broad agreement in spatiotemporal distribution of temperature change. A maximum temperature rise inside the head of 3.4°C (i.e. above the 1°C safe limit) was identified for a high-power TSE sequence, indicating the need to limit SAR below the normal maximum permissible level (IEC 2002a). Interestingly, the authors found minimal difference between the simulated SAR distributions for electrodes with and without a modelled current limiting resistor. It is possible that at such high frequencies (300 MHz for 7 T), parasitic capacitance in the resistor reduces its impedance, thereby limiting its current limiting capability. This suggests that discrete current reducing resistors may not provide effective protection against SAR increases inside the head at 7 T, although their effect on contact currents, which might be expected to be maximal immediately adjacent to the electrodes (i.e. on the surface of the phantom), was less clear. Lower-temperature increases were recorded when using carbon leads, suggesting that distributed resistance in the electrode leads may be advantageous. See the chapter "Specific Issues Related to EEG–fMRI at $B_0 > 3$ T" for further discussion of the specific issues related to high-field EEG–fMRI.

Carbon leads may also reduce magnetic susceptibility artefacts in the images (Van Genderingen et al. 1989; Van Audekerke et al. 2000). Although promising, the use of computational simulation to assess the safety of RF/EEG electrode interactions is relatively new: further validation is required before this technique can be used on its own to establish patient safety. Combining this computational method with temperature measurement in a comparable physical model may prove advantageous, with the former being used to identify the site of maximum heating and the latter to verify the temperature changes at the equivalent position in the physical model.

Finally, although many studies have recommended the use of SAR limits to ensure the safety of EEG–fMRI experiments (Angelone et al. 2004; Lemieux et al. 1997), such limits are both scanner- and RF coil-specific. Indeed, Baker et al. have demonstrated that the relationship between scanner-reported SAR and the associated heating of an implanted electrode can be highly variable, even between scanners of identical field strength from the same manufacturer (Baker et al. 2004). It is likely that this is also the case for scalp EEG electrodes, and hence it is important to recognise that a universal SAR limit calculated for a specific electrode set, although attractive in its simplicity, may not be reliable.

3.6
Implanted Electrodes

The above discussion of safety issues has only addressed scalp electrodes. Imaging for post-surgical localisation of intracranial electrodes is currently performed in a number of centres. Retrospective examination of patients with implanted electrodes who underwent MR imaging indicate that the risks are generally low (Davies et al. 1999; Brooks et al. 1992). In addition, a small number of studies have investigated the safety of imaging implanted electrodes and found no evidence of displacement force and RF heating beyond safe limits (Boucousis et al. 2005; Kanal et al. 1999). However, these studies only investigated single electrodes, whereas in practice these recordings involve multiple electrodes, thereby introducing inter-electrode lead loops. More recently, Carmichael et al. measured RF heating for a combination of subdural strips and depth electrodes at 1.5 and 3 T (Carmichael et al. 2007b). This

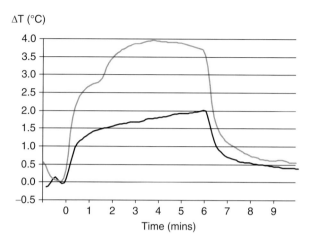

Fig. 4 Temperature increase with time for a subdural grid electrode contact, high SAR (2.4–2.5 W/kg). The *grey line* shows the temperature rise when all the electrode tails were in electrical contact, the *blue line* when they were all separated

showed that, for high SAR (≈2.5 W/kg), the worst case temperature increase only exceeded the 1°C limit at 1.5 T when the electrode tails were shorted together (contrary to the manufacturer's recommendations); at 3 T the limit was exceeded even when the tails were isolated (Fig. 4). Clearly, a local investigation of temperature increases for a given specific electrode arrangement, scanner and pulse sequence is essential in order to identify the safe SAR limit.

This study (Carmichael et al. 2007b) only investigated the safety of electrode/RF interactions for MR-based electrode *localisation*. Recording from intracranial electrodes may be important in the application of EEG–fMRI to epilepsy. However, recording EEG from these electrodes during MR requires additional cabling to link the electrodes (which typically have tails of only 30 cm in length) to the EEG amplifier. Such conductors are likely to alter the resonant length of the overall EEG electrode assembly, potentially modifying the associated temperature changes. Further studies of RF heating are required to establish the safety of EEG–fMRI for implanted electrodes.

3.7
Summary

RF heating of electrodes or brain tissue is the principal safety issue in EEG–fMRI. The degree of heating is dependent on a wide range of factors, including: the number of electrodes and their shape; lead arrangement, length and proximity to the scanner transmit coil; scanner hardware, software and scanning sequence. EEG–fMRI recordings using scalp electrodes with current limiting resistors and minimised electrode lead loops have been shown to be safe at 1.5 T. Such studies have been performed at multiple centres with scanners up to 3 T for many years with no adverse incidents reported. However, extending these findings to body RF coils and higher field scanners requires further investigation. In particular, the effectiveness of current limiting resistors at higher RF frequencies is unclear. In view of the range and sensitivity of the factors influencing RF heating, a local risk assessment and adherence to a strict experimental protocol is essential.

Acknowledgements   I am grateful to Dr D.W. Carmichael for helpful comments regarding this chapter.

References

Akca IB, Oner Ferhanoglu MS, Yeung CJ, et al. (2007) Measuring local RF heating in MRI: simulating perfusion in a perfusionless phantom. J Magn Reson Imaging 26:1228–1235

Allen PJ, Josephs O, Turner R (2000) A method for removing imaging artefact from continuous EEG recorded during functional MRI. Neuroimage 12:230–239

Allen PJ, Polizzi G, Krakow K, et al. (1998) Identification of EEG events in the MR scanner: the problem of pulse artefact and a method for its subtraction. Neuroimage 8:229–239

Anami K, Mori T, Tanaka F, et al. (2003) Stepping stone sampling for retrieving artefact-free electroencephalogram during functional magnetic resonance imaging. Neuroimage 19:281–295

Angelone LM, Potthast A, Segonne F, et al. (2004) Metallic electrodes and leads in simultaneous EEG-MRI: specific absorption rate (SAR) simulation studies. Bioelectromagnetics 25:285–295

Angelone LM, Vasios CE, Wiggins G, et al. (2006) On the effect of resistive EEG electrodes and leads during 7T MRI: simulation and temperature measurement studies. Neuroimage 24:801–812

Baker KB, Tkach JA, Nyenhuis JA, et al. (2004) Evaluation of specific absorption rate as a dosimeter of MRI-related implant heating. J Magn Reson Imaging 20:315–320

Baumann SB, Noll DC (1999) A modified electrode cap for EEG recordings in MRI scanners. Clin Neurophysiol 110:2189–2193

Benar CG, Aghakhani Y, Wang, et al. (2003) Quality of EEG in simultaneous EEG–fMRI for epilepsy. Clin Neurophysiol 114:569–580

Bonmassar G, Anami K, Ives J, et al. (1999) Visual evoked potential (VEP) measured by simultaneous 64-channel EEG and 3T fMRI. Neuroreport 10:1893–1897

Bonmassar G, Purdon PL, Jaaslelainen IP, et al. (2002) Motion and ballistocardiogram artefact removal for interleaved recording of EEG and EPs during MRI. Neuroimage 16:1127–1141

Boucousis S, Edwards J, Goodyear BG, et al. (2005) Safety and feasibility of intracranial EEG–fMRI at 3 Tesla. Epilepsia 46 S8:37 (abstract 1.071)

Brooks ML, O'Connor MJ, Sperling MR, et al. (1992) Magnetic resonance imaging in localization of EEG depth electrodes for seizure monitoring. Epilepsia 33:888–891

Carmichael DW, Pinto S, Limousin-Dowsey P, et al. (2007a) Functional MRI with active, fully implanted, deep brain stimulation systems: safety and experimental confounds. Neuroimage 37:508–517

Carmichael DW, Thorton JS, Allen PJ, et al. (2007b) Safety of localizing intracranial EEG electrodes using MRI. Proc Intl Soc Magn Reson Med 15:1073

Cohen MS, Goldman RI, Jerome E Jr (2001) Simultaneous EEG and fMRI made easy. Proc Annual Meeting of the Organization for Human Brain Mapping, Brighton, UK, 10–14 June 2001, p. 6

Collins CM, Liu W, Wang J, et al. (2004) Temperature and SAR calculations for a human head within volume and surface coils at 64 and 300 MHz. J Magn Reson Imaging 19:650–656

Davies LM, Spencer DD, Spencer SS, et al. (1999) MR imaging of implanted depth and subdural electrodes: is it safe? Epilepsy Res 35:95–98

Debener S, Mullinger KJ, Niazy RK, et al. (2007) Properties of the ballistocardiogram artefact as revealed by EEG recordings at 1.5, 3 and 7 T static magnetic field strength. Int J Pyschophysiol 67:188–199; doi:10.1016/j.ijpsycho.2007.05.015

Dempsey MF, Condon B, Hadley DM (2001) Investigation of the factors responsible for burns during MRI. J Magn Reson Imaging 13(4):627–631

Deuschl G, Eisen A (1999) Recommendations for the practice of clinical neurophysiology: guidelines of the International Federation of Clinical Neurophysiology, 2nd edn. Elsevier, Amsterdam

Garreffa G, Bianciardi M, Hagberg GE, et al. (2004) Simultaneous EEG–fMRI acquisition: how far is it from being a standardized technique? Magn Reson Imaging 22:1445–1455

Georgi JC, Lawrence AD, Mehta MA, et al. (2004) Active deep brain stimulation during MRI: a feasibility study. Magn Reson Med 51:380–388

Goldman RI, Stern JM, Engel J Jr, et al. (2000) Acquiring simultaneous EEG and functional MRI. Clin Neurophysiol 111:1974–1980

Gray RW, Bibens WT, Shellock FG (2005) Simple design changes to wires to substantially reduce MRI-induced heating at 1.5T: implications for implanted leads. Magn Reson Imaging 23: 887–891

Gualniera G, Garreffa G, Morasso P, et al. (2004) A method for real-time artefact filtering during simultaneous EEG–fMRI acquisition: preliminary results. Neurocomputing 58–60:1171–1179

Hill RA, Chiappa KH, Huang-Hellinger F, et al. (1995) EEG during MR imaging: differentiation of movement artefact from paroxysmal cortical activity. Neurology 45:1942–1943

Hoffmann A, Jager L, Werhahn KJ, et al. (2000) Electroencephalography during functional echo-planar imaging: detection of epileptic spikes using post-processing methods. Magn Reson Med 44:791–798

Hofman MBM, De Cock CC, van der Linden JC, et al. (1996) Transesophageal cardiac pacing during magnetic resonance imaging: feasibility and safety considerations. Magn Reson Med 35:413–422

Huang-Hellinger FR, Breiter HC, McCormak G, et al. (1995) Simultaneous functional magnetic resonance imaging and electrophysiological recording. Hum Brain Mapp 3:13–23

Iannetti GD, Bonaventura CD, Pantano P, et al. (2002) fMRI/EEG in paroxysmal activity elicited by elimination of central vision and fixation. Neurology 58:976–979

IEC (2002a) International standard, medical equipment, part 2–33: particular requirements for the safety of magnetic resonance equipment for medical diagnosis. International Electrotechnical Commission 60601-2-33, Geneva

IEC (2002b) International standard, medical electrical equipment, part 2–26: particular requirements for the safety of electroencephalographs. International Electrotechnical Commission 60601-2-26, Geneva

IEC (2005) International standard, medical equipment, part 1: general requirements for basic safety and essential performance. International Electrotechnical Commission 60601-1:2005, Geneva

Ives JR, Warach S, Schmitt F, et al. (1993) Monitoring the patient's EEG during echo planar MRI. Electroenceph Clin Neurophysiol 87:417–420

Janssen R, Benignus VA, Grimes LM, et al. (1986) Unrecognized errors due to analog filtering of the brain-stem auditory evoked response. Electroenceph Clin Neurophysiol 65:203–211

Kainz W (2007) MR heating tests of MR critical implants. J Magn Reson Imaging 26:450–451

Kamp A, Lopes Da Silva F (1998) Technological aspects of EEG recording. In: Niedermeyer E, Lopes Da Silva F (eds) Electroencephalography. Basic principles, clinical applications and related fields, 4th edn. Williams and Wilkins, Baltimore

Kanal E, Cida Meltzer C, Adelson PD, et al. (1999) Platinum subdural grid: MR imaging compatibility testing. Radiology 211:886–888

Kruggel F, Wiggins CJ, Herrmann CS, et al. (2000) Recording of the event related potentials during functional MRI at 3.0 Tesla field strength. Magn Reson Med 44:277–282

Laufs H, Kleinschmidt A, Beyerle A, et al. (2003) EEG-correlated fMRI of human activity. Neuroimage 19:1463–1476

Lazeyras F, Zimine I, Blanke O, et al. (2001) Functional MRI with simultaneous EEG recording: feasibility and application to motor and visual activation. J Magn Reson Imaging 13:943–948

Lemieux L, Allen PJ, Franconi F, et al. (1997) Recording of EEG during fMRI experiments: patient safety. Magn Reson Med 38:943–952

Mandelkow H, Halder P, Boesiger P, et al. (2006) Synchronisation facilitates removal of MRI artefacts from concurrent EEG recordings and increases usable bandwidth. Neuroimage 32:1120–1126

Mirsattari SM, Lee DH, Jones D, et al. (2004) MRI compatible EEG electrode system for routine use in the epilepsy monitoring unit and intensive care unit. Clin Neurophysiol 115:2175–2180

Negishi M, Abildgaard M, Nixon T, et al. (2004) Removal of time varying gradient artefacts from EEG data acquired during continuous fMRI. Clin Neurophysiol 115:2181–2192

Nuwer MR, Comi G, Emerson R et al (1999) IFCN standards for digital recording of clinical EEG. In: Deuschl G, Eisen A (eds) Recommendations for the practice of clinical neurophysiology: guidelines of the International Federation of Clinical Neurophysiology, 2nd edn. Elsevier, Amsterdam

Park SM, Nyenhuis JA, Smith CD, et al. (2003) Gelled versus nongelled phantom material for measurement of MRI-induced temperature increases with bioimplants. IEEE Trans Magn 39:3367–3371

Pictet J, Meuli R, Wicky S, et al. (2000) Radiofrequency heating effects around resonant lengths of wire in MRI. Phys Med Biol 47:2973–2985

Rezai AR, Finelli D, Nyenhuis JA, et al. (2002) Neurostimulation systems for deep brain stimulation: in vitro evaluation of magnetic resonance imaging-related heating at 1.5T. J Magn Reson Imaging 15:241–250

Roth BJ, Pascual-Leone A, Cohen LG, et al. (1992) The heating of metal electrodes during rapid-rate magnetic stimulation: a possible safety hazard. Electroenceph Clin Neurophysiol 85:116–123

Seeck M, Lazeyras F, Michel CM, et al. (1998) Non-invasive epileptic focus localization using EEG-triggered functional MRI and electromagnetic tomography. Electroenceph Clin Neurophysiol 106:508–512

Shellock FG (2007) Comments on MR heating tests for critical implants. J Magn Reson Imaging 26:1182–1185

Srivastava G, Crottaz-Herbette S, Lau KM, et al. (2005) ICA-based procedures for removing ballistocardiogram artefacts from EEG data acquired in the MRI scanner. Neuroimage 24:50–60

Stevens TK, Ives JR, Martyn Klassen L, et al. (2007) MR compatibility of EEG electrodes at 4 Tesla. J Magn Reson Imaging 25:872–877

Van Audekerke J, Peeters R, Verhoye M, et al. (2000) Special designed RF-antenna with integrated non-invasive carbon electrodes for simultaneous magnetic resonance imaging and electroencephalography acquisition at 7T. Magn Reson Imaging 18:887–891

Van Genderingen HR, Sprenger M, de Ridder JW, et al. (1989) Carbon-fiber electrodes and leads for electrocardiography during MR imaging. Radiology 171:872

Vasios CE, Angelone LM, Purdon PL, et al. (2006) EEG/(f)MRI measurements at 7 Tesla using a new EEG cap ("Inkcap"). Neuroimage 33:1082–1092

Warach S, Ives JR, Schlaug G, et al. (1996) EEG-triggered echo-planar functional MRI in epilepsy. Neurology 47:89–93

Woods TO (2007) Standards for medical devices in MRI: present and future. J Magn Reson Imaging 26:1186–1189

Yeung CJ, Susil RC, Atalar E (2002) RF safety index of wires in interventional MRI: using a safety index. Magn Reson Med 47:187–193

EEG Quality: Origin and Reduction of the EEG Cardiac-Related Artefact

8

Stefan Debener, Cornelia Kranczioch, and Ingmar Gutberlet

1
Introduction

With the advent of purpose-built "MR-compatible" EEG recording hardware, the simulta-neous acquisition of EEG and fMRI has recently become more widespread (for reviews, see Herrmann and Debener 2007; Laufs et al. 2008). Nevertheless, the MRI scanner remains a hostile environment for EEG recordings, and ensuring good EEG signal quality can be a challenging task (e.g. Parkes et al. 2006). The level of EEG data quality that can be achieved from simultaneous recordings is a matter of ongoing investigation, but a com-mon view is that a certain loss of quality is unavoidable and must be tolerated (Debener et al. 2007b). Nonetheless, combined EEG and fMRI data acquisitions in a single session are an attractive alternative to separate acquisitions in some circumstances, as discussed throughout this book (Babiloni et al. 2004; Debener et al. 2006; Horwitz and Poeppel 2002). The reduction of artefacts that contaminate the EEG signal as much as possible is necessary to make full use of the potential of EEG–fMRI.

The MRI environment is known to introduce several different types of EEG artefact, among them the gradient artefact and the cardiac pulse-related (often referred to as balli-stocardiogram or BCG) artefact.[1] This chapter focuses on the pulse artefact: its origin, characteristics of it, and methods of reducing or eliminating it. After introducing the con-ceptual and statistical characteristics that define the pulse artefact, we discuss the mecha-nisms that give rise to the pulse artefact and present a two-factor pulse artefact model. We will review and compare different ways of removing it. We will focus on several recording

---

[1]In this work we use the term "pulse-related artefact" or "pulse artefact" to designate what many authors call the BCG. This choice reflects the editors' wish to use a term that can encompass all possible (not just ballistic) mechanisms that give rise to the EEG artefact (see Sect. 3).

Prof. Dr. Stefan Debener (✉)
Biomagnetic Center, Dept. of Neurology, University Hospital Jena, Erlanger Allee 101, D-07747 Jena, Germany
e-mail: stefan@debener.de

C. Mulert and L. Lemieux (eds.), *EEG–fMRI*
DOI: 10.1007/978-3-540-87919-0_8, © Springer Verlag Berlin Heidelberg 2010

and analysis details that have been barely acknowledged in the literature and can have a significant impact on the quality of the pulse artefact correction step, and thus on the final EEG data quality.

With amplitudes that can be several orders of magnitudes larger than the neuronal EEG signal, the MR image acquisition artefact is more prominent than the pulse artefact. However, the imaging artefact's perfect predictability and relative reproducibility (its amplitude and shape can be affected by subject motion) mean that it can be removed relatively easily from the EEG by postprocessing. Moreover, the impact of the gradient artefact could, in principle, be reduced by employing interleaved recording designs (see the chapter "Experimental Design and Data Analysis Strategies").

2
Characteristics of the Pulse Artefact

The pulse artefact is clearly visible on EEGs recorded inside the MR scanner even in the absence of scanning, and contributes amplitudes and frequencies that are close to the range of the usual EEG signal, with an amplitude that is on the order 50 µV (at 1.5 T) and has a resemblance to epileptic spikes. As will be discussed in the next section, the pulse artefact is a typical example of a mesogenous artefact, since it results from the interaction between the active cardiovascular system (endogenous contribution) and the main static (B_0) field inside the MRI scanner (exogenous contribution).[2]

Figure 1 shows a typical example of the pulse artefact and how it interferes with ongoing EEG signals recorded inside a 1.5 T MRI scanner. Its defining feature is synchrony with the cardiac rhythm captured on simultaneously recorded ECG. Careful comparison of the pulse artefact and ECG reveals a delay of approximately 200 ms between the R peak and the peak artefact in the EEG traces (Allen et al. 1998), indicating that the artefact is not simply a volume-conducted electrical ECG artefact, with fluctuations in the interartefact interval reflecting fluctuations in the subject's heart rate (and likely in other cardiovascular parameters). As can be seen, the artefact amplitude can be substantially larger than occipital EEG alpha oscillations. The peak amplitude can vary markedly across individuals, channels and MRI scanners. As a rule of thumb, EEG electrodes far from the EEG reference electrode express larger amplitudes, and a high-field MRI scanner causes larger amplitudes than a scanner with a lower field (Debener et al., 2008). In addition, the artefact's morphology can vary between EEG channels, and these channel-by-channel differences do not seem to be completely accounted for by scaling differences. The interchannel variability in artefact latency and morphology as well as in morphology over time (e.g. channel P7 in Fig. 1) is a key consideration for artefact reduction methods.

It is noteworthy that the spatial features of the pulse artefact have rarely (Allen et al. 1998; Nakamura et al. 2006) been investigated in detail (Debener et al., 2007). Figure 2

---

[2]The pulse artefact was originally described in clinical EEGs recorded outside the MRI and in the supine position, which can cause a pulsatile, rocking head rotation. Here we limit the pulse artefact to intra-MRI EEG recordings.

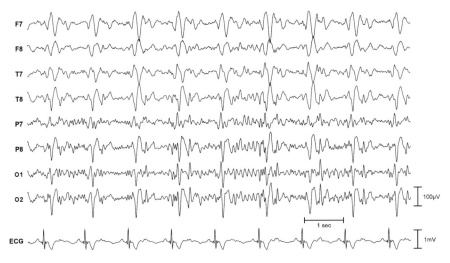

Fig. 1 Example of the pulse artefact in ongoing EEG data recorded in a 1.5 T MRI scanner without MRI scanning. EEG traces at lateral sites over the left and right hemispheres, where the artefact is usually most pronounced, are shown. Note the temporal pattern, which corresponds to the cardiac cycle and is delayed in relation to the R peak of the ECG (*bottom trace*) by about 200 ms. Also apparent are the different morphologies of the artefact at different scalp sites, and, across electrodes, the asymmetric and asynchronous patterns of activity. The ECG was recorded simultaneously from an electrode attached to the lower back and referenced to the EEG recording reference (Cz), a favourable ECG recording scheme. Exposure to a strong magnetic field distorts the ECG signal most during the ST interval, whereas the QRS interval is unchanged compared to outside MRI scanner recordings

illustrates the main spatial features of the pulse artefact, showing the time-domain averaged signal (the *evoked pulse artefact*) and topographies at some peak latencies. In order to obtain the evoked pulse artefact, the onset of each cardiac cycle was determined and used as a time-locking event (in this example, this was the Q wave in the ECG recording). The upper part of the figure shows the evoked artefact traces at all EEG electrodes together with the mean global field power (GFP). The GFP summarizes activity irrespective of the polarity of the potentials and corresponds to the spatial standard deviation across all recorded channels (Skrandies 1990). It can be seen that the pulse artefact starts approximately 150 ms after the Q peak and has two peaks at approximately 230 and 330 ms. Also, the pulse artefact lasts until at least ~500 ms after the ECG Q wave. Corresponding voltage maps at selected GFP peak latencies reveal some interesting features. First, in most cases the artefact topography can be characterised by a low spatial frequency. Therefore, the pulse artefact can be best characterised by more complete spatial coverage of the head sphere. Poor spatial coverage, for instance due to a focus on a few electrodes around the vertex (Nakamura et al. 2006) may miss important features of the artefact. Second, the topography changes substantially over time. Repeating patterns can be observed (for example, compare the maps at 176 and 464 ms in Fig. 2), although they are slightly rotated relative to each other. We have consistently observed this moving topographical pulse artefact pattern, irrespective of the number of EEG channels (30–62), the MRI scanner manufacturer (Siemens, Philips), the MRI

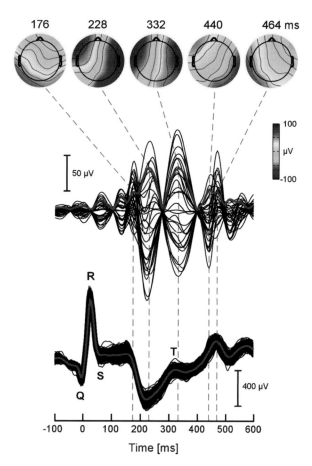

Fig. 2 Temporal characteristics of the pulse artefact, based on a typical 30-channel EEG recording in a 1.5 T MRI scanner. The *upper traces* show the evoked pulse artefact at all EEG channels. Overlaid in *red* is the mean global field power (GFP), which corresponds to the spatial standard deviation. Voltage maps are shown for selected GFP peak latencies. Note that, while some maps (176 and 464 ms; 228 and 440 ms) look similar, they are rotated differently, illustrating the temporal dynamics and spatial nonstationarity of the artefact. The distorted ECG is shown in the *bottom* part of the figure (see Fig. 1 for ECG recording details). Here, *black* traces refer to single cardiac cycles, with the Q wave used as the time-locking event and the *red* trace representing the average ECG. The T wave can be identified at about 300 ms, on top of the field-induced deflection at approximately 150-450 ms. The polarity of the ECG deflection depends on the orientation of the MRI B_0 field, and so it can be different at different MRI scanner sites

scanner type (head scanner, whole-body scanner), and the MRI B_0 field strength (1.5, 3 and 7 T). Therefore, the pulse artefact contributes a very dynamic - moving, rotating and polarity inverting - signal to the EEG, thus adding a range of topographies and signatures.

The lower part of Fig. 2 shows individual pulse artefacts and the averaged ECG, which shows that the ECG waveform is distorted by the influence of the magnetic field. Whereas the QRS complex appears to be relatively unaffected, an additional deflection during the ejection phase of the cardiac cycle can be seen. An additional deflection can be observed between the onset of the S wave and the offset of the T wave (not present at 0 T). The latency range of this deflection roughly corresponds to the maximum artefact in the EEG, and can be substantially larger than the R wave (Debener et al. 2008). It is important to note, though, that the sign of this deflection depends on the polarity of the scanner's B_0 field, which varies between manufacturers.

Figures 1 and 2 illustrate the artefact in a case that is representative of commonly observed features: ECG-artefact delay and general topography, with its dynamic, rotational and polarity-inverting aspects.[3] The factors that can lead to differences in the artefact are linked to the subject and experimental setup. First of all, the theories for both of the postulated generative mechanisms, namely BCG and the Hall effect, predict that the artefact scales approximately proportionally with B_0 (Tenforde et al. 1983). This has been confirmed; the pulse artefact is much smaller at 1.5 T than at 3 and 7 T, with important consequences for the choice of artefact removal technique (Debener et al. 2008). Second, there are interindividual differences in patterns of cardiac activity, such as changes in heart rate, in peak latencies and morphology (Debener et al. 2008). Therefore, for those individuals with a higher heart rate (shorter interbeat interval), the pulse artefact activities between adjacent cardiac cycles may overlap to some extent, which could further complicate artefact removal (Vincent et al. 2007). Thirdly, the quality of the ECG recording may vary across subjects and/or sites, and it may not always be possible to identify the onset of every single cardiac cycle precisely. This can impair the performance of the pulse artefact removal procedures that rely on the detection of each cardiac cycle's onset. We conclude that the pulse artefact represents a rather complicated, dynamic contribution to the EEG. Thus, the development, application and comparison of pulse artefact removal procedures represents a real challenge.

3
Origin of the Pulse Artefact, Simulations and Modelling

The physical principles of electromagnetism state that any movement of electrically conductive material in a static magnetic field results in electromagnetic induction, and this is the fundamental cause of the pulse artefact. Therefore, motion related to cardiac activity can give rise to induced electromotive forces in the circuit formed by the EEG recording leads and subject, and be picked up by the EEG amplifier (see Fig. 3). However, the type of motion that is relevant to the pulse artefact is a matter of discussion. Some authors have suggested that axial head rotation is the primary cause (e.g. Nakamura et al. 2006), while others point to the possible local effect of pulsatile movements of scalp vessels on adjacent electrodes. In addition to ballistic effects, motion of the blood (i.e. abrupt changes in blood velocity) can lead to the Hall effect (a voltage difference is created on opposite sides of a

---

[3]For a movie illustration of the BCG time course and topography, the interested reader may wish to visit http://www.debener.de.

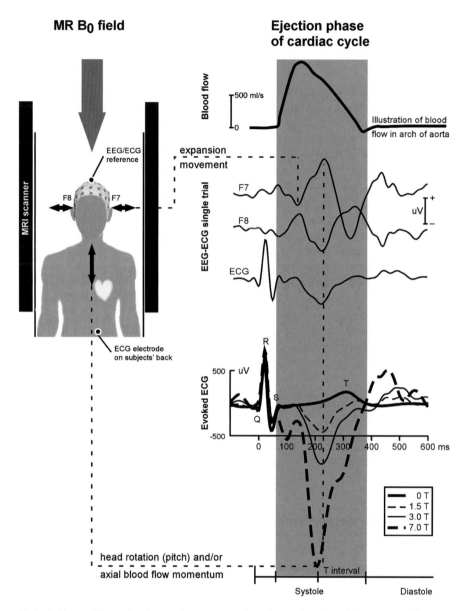

Fig. 3 A diagram illustrating factors that can cause the pulse artefact. Two different types of movement are indicated, axial nodding rotation of the head and expansion at lateral and temporal scalp sites. The *left* part of the figure illustrates a subject in the supine position inside an MRI scanner. The locations of the EEG electrodes, the EEG/ECG reference site and the ECG recording site on the lower back are indicated. The *lower right* part of the figure shows evoked ECG traces from one individual, recorded outside the MRI (0 T) and inside three different MRI scanners (1.5, 3.0, 7.0 T). A typical single trial of ECG and EEG activity is shown above the evoked ECG traces, and at the *top* , the time course of the blood fl ow in the arch of the aorta (as adapted from cardiac physiology textbooks) is shown. As highlighted by the *grey* background, the artefact mostly occurs during the ejection phase of the cardiac cycle. This figure is reprinted from Debener et al. 2008, with kind permission from Elsevier Publishers

moving conductor through which an electric current is flowing when placed in a strong magnetic field), which may also contribute to the pulse artefact.

In order to simulate the topographies of nodding head rotation and lateral electrode expansion, we recorded EEG data from a spherical phantom covered with a layer of conductive gel placed in a 1.5 T MRI scanner (see Fig. 4).[4] Lateral electrode expansion was simulated by inflating two balloons underneath the lateral electrodes, and axial head rotation was simulated by slightly rocking the whole phantom in the axial direction (i.e. in the direction of the B_0 field). Lateral electrode expansion lead to spatially circumscribed contributions, which could comprise positive, negative or biphasic deflections. The topographies resulting from axial and nodding head rotation closely resembled those observed in real subjects. Both basic, spatially unspecific map and polarity differences between the left and right hemisphere electrodes and polarity reversal (probably related to forwards–backwards motion) were evident in this simulation. Thus, this result clearly supports the role of nodding head rotation as a generator of the pulse artefact (Nakamura et al. 2006). However, the simulations did not reveal the rotational, moving aspect that is clearly present in real recordings. Accordingly, we conclude that rocking axial head rotation is the major, but not the only motion-related contribution to the pulse artefact.

Figure 3 summarizes multiple possible contributions to pulse artefact generation. The left hand part of the figure illustrates a subject in the supine position in the MRI scanner, along with the EEG and ECG electrode configuration usually used in our lab. The right hand part illustrates the typical time course of a cardiac cycle, with the blood flow illustration adapted from cardiac physiology textbooks. It can be seen that the onset of the pulse artefact roughly corresponds to the onset of the systole; that is, the onset of the blood ejection phase. During this period, the major pulse artefact deflections in both the EEG and ECG channels seem to occur. Note also the single-trial activities in channels F7 and F8 that are characterised by different polarities and also show the polarity reversal pattern over time. We speculate that the rotational aspect of the dynamic pulse artefact topography points towards a mixing of lateral electrode expansion and axial nodding head rotation. Unfortunately, at present, not enough is known about the temporal behaviour of these two processes, and the simulation study we reported above does not provide any insight into this matter. However, this type of information would be necessary in order to model topographies that could result from the interplay of lateral electrode expansion and axial nodding head rotation. Clearly, more studies are needed in order to isolate these potential pulse artefact contributions. This type of research could help to further our understanding of the pulse artefact, and thus help to achieve better EEG data quality from inside MRI scanner recordings.

Some authors recommended that an attempt should be made to reduce pulse artefacts prior to amplification by carefully laying out and immobilising the leads, twisting the leads, and using a bipolar electrode chain arrangement and a head vacuum cushion (Goldman et al 2000; Benar et al 2003). It is noteworthy that in EEG–fMRI studies in epilepsy, some investigators have found these measures to be sufficient, at least at 1.5 T, to analyse the EEG of epileptic patients. However, it is more common to combine these efforts with postprocessing artefact methods.

---

[4]These recordings were made at the Sir Peter Mansfield MRI Centre in Nottingham, UK. We are very grateful to Richard Bowtell and Karen Mullinger for sharing their ideas and our enthusiasm about EEG–fMRI and the pulse-related artefact.

Fig. 4 Results of a motion simulation study. A spherical phantom was covered with a layer of electrode gel, fitted with an EEG cap, and positioned in the centre of an MRI scanner (**a**). Different types of motion were induced while EEG was recorded, among them bilateral expansion motion (**b**), as caused by the inflation of balloons positioned underneath temporal electrodes, and axial, nodding head motion (**c**). Recordings and the respective voltage topographies shown in (**b**) and (**c**) are based on averages over a few repetitions. Lateral expansion motion caused rather locally circumscribed voltages, which may resemble tangential (*left*) or radial (*right*) features. Axial nodding head rotation, on the other hand, contributed a low spatial frequency map, which was characterized by a polarity change over time, and by different polarities between left and right hemisphere electrodes

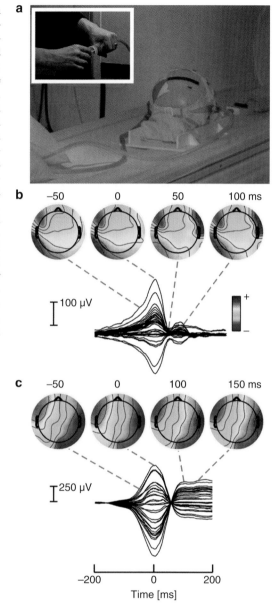

4
Reducing the Pulse Artefact Using Waveform Removal Approaches

In 1998, a seminal study on removing the pulse artefact was published (Allen et al. 1998). In this paper, Allen et al. introduced the average artefact subtraction (AAS) algorithm, which has become one of the most influential and frequently used methods. The algorithm is predicated on the assumption that the EEG signals of interest (neuronal activity) and the ECG are not correlated, and that the artefact is relatively stable across a number of successive heartbeats. Therefore, in the ideal situation of a perfectly stable heartbeat, subtraction of the EEG averaged over a number of preceding heartbeats from the ongoing EEG will result in the removal of the artefact. While different implementations and developments of the AAS exist (Laufs et al. 2008), the basic principle of the AAS is common to all variants (see Fig. 5).

Figure 5 illustrates and highlights the main steps of the AAS method. First, the AAS approach requires knowledge of the precise onset of each cardiac cycle, which is usually obtained by simultaneously recording the ECG and detecting the onset of each cardiac cycle (e.g. all R peaks in the ECG). After this has been achieved, the next step is to define an artefact template. Importantly, this is done for each EEG channel separately and achieved by averaging the EEG over a predefined epoch preceding and time-locked to each cardiac cycle onset. The resulting artefact template represents the evoked pulse artefact with the ongoing EEG activity averaged out. The result is a moving average and subtraction procedure where the resulting template is subtracted from the current EEG epoch and thereby reduces the artefact. The procedure is repeated for every EEG channel and can be implemented in real time. In theory, the quality of the template increases with the number of epochs used. However, averaging more epochs reduces the sensitivity of the template to capture temporal fluctuations of the artefact. In spite of this limitation, many groups have found that the AAS procedure, which has been implemented in commercially

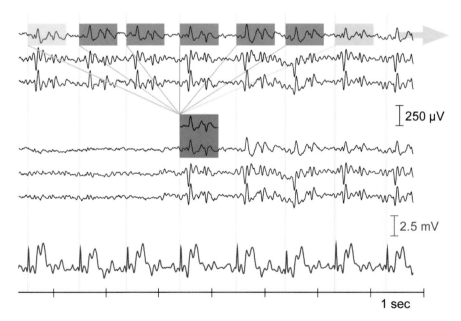

250 μV

2.5 mV

1 sec

Fig. 5 Schematic of the average artefact subtraction procedure. For each channel, a waveform template is generated by averaging EEG epochs over adjacent cardiac cycles, with the time- locking event being derived from the ECG. The template generation is combined with a moving average procedure, and new templates are generated for each cardiac cycle. The procedure is repeated for each EEG channel

available and open source software packages, can give satisfactory EEG data quality (e.g. Hamandi et al. 2008; Sammer et al. 2005).

The limitations of the AAS algorithm result from deviations from the basic assumptions: a lack of correlation between stimulus (and response) and cardiac activity; temporal stability of the artefact; reliable and precise detection of the onset of each cardiac cycle. Any degree of correlation between cardiac activity and neuronal activity can be problematic from the point of view of EEG data quality, but the effects can be reduced by proper experimental design in evoked response studies (e.g. interstimulus interval jitter). Deviations from the stability assumption result in inaccurate artefact estimation and therefore lead to greater residual artefact after subtraction. Shortening the moving average window size cannot fully redress this problem, since a smaller moving average window would leave more residual EEG activity in the template.

The choice of template length is also potentially problematic due to variations in the R–R interval. Mismatch between template window length and artefact duration will lead to greater residual artefact. This has led to the introduction of alternative template generation schemes that either scale the pulse artefact template with a percentage of the mean R-R period in the moving average window (Ellingson et al. 2004) or that build a template which incorporates the pulse artefact data for all R-R period lengths present in the current moving average window (BrainVision Analyzer software). In the latter case, this template is then adaptively applied to each QRS period based on its R-R period, thus ensuring that no portion of the pulse artefact remains uncorrected due to a suboptimal template length.

Alternative template constructions that are based on weighted averages (Goldman et al. 2000) or median instead of mean values (Sijbers et al. 2000) have been devised. Also, some implementations allow for the selection of trials contributing to the template generation depending on whether they correlate sufficiently with other trials or not. This option helps to ensure that trials containing other EEG artefacts are excluded, thus improving the quality of the template used for subtraction. While all of these features may improve pulse artefact correction, they are not able to fully account for interartefact variability.

The cardiac cycle onset can be difficult to identify due to ECG channel contamination resulting from gradient switching and the effect of B_0 leading to missed cycles or inaccurate template estimation window alignment, and consequently degraded template estimates and residual artefacts. Accurate marker position improves the quality of the pulse artefact correction, in particular with regard to residual noise in the high-frequency range of the EEG signal. In our experience, efforts to ensure good ECG recording quality with a focus on a clear R wave through careful consideration of the positioning of electrodes are worthwhile. We usually derive the ECG from a single electrode attached to the lower back and referenced against the EEG reference (vertex or nearby) (e.g. Debener et al. 2005b, 2007, 2008). This scheme ensures large R peaks while avoiding respiratory and other movement-related artefacts on the ECG channel. While derivation schemes such as the classical Einthoven II ECG can yield clear R waves, they cannot easily be implemented inside the scanner, as they require long electrode leads that could also potentially pose a safety risk to the subjects. As a result, automatic R-wave detection algorithms developed for normal recording conditions may fail for intrascanner recordings and may provide inaccurate positioning of the event markers. One way to explore this further is to compute the standard deviation of the delays between the actual marker positions (e.g. Q wave) and the following R wave latencies (Debener et al. 2008). Some implementations of the AAS algorithm, such as the BrainVision Analyzer (Brain Products GmbH, Munich, Germany), already take jitter information into account, and automatically align markers statistically such that the overall jitter is minimised before correction.

The problems inherent in the AAS approach have been investigated further by Niazy and colleagues (Niazy et al. 2005), and similarly by Negishi et al. (2004), who proposed a new way of constructing a pulse artefact template. These authors suggested generating pulse artefact templates based on a channel-wise temporal principal components analysis (PCA), thereby relaxing the stability requirement. Niazy and colleagues named this approach the optimal basis set (OBS) method, which refers to the first few principal components as representations of several distinct pulse artefact templates. These templates explain most of the artefact variance in any given EEG channel and are jointly used to regress the pulse artefact from the EEG data. The OBS approach therefore tries to account for greater temporal variation in the artefact shape. The resulting software tool is a freely available Matlab plug-in that interacts with the open-source EEGLAB environment (Delorme and Makeig 2004). A potential limitation of this approach is that the number of necessary artefact templates are not indicated by the software and need to be determined by the user.

Other channel-by-channel correction approaches exist that account for the template duration problem. For instance, Bonmassar et al. utilized an adaptive Kalman filter approach (Bonmassar et al. 2002), which requires an extra motion sensor signal to be recorded as a reference signal. However, it might be feasible to use electrooculogram (EOG) signals instead (In et al. 2006). A novel method for recording motion has been proposed by Masterton et al. (2007), who attached three loops as motion sensors on an electrode cap. This group reported a more complete model of head movements and, when employing a linear adaptive filter technique, good correction of the pulse-related artefact and (other) head movement artefacts. While apparently producing good corrections, the Kalman filter approach appears to be computationally demanding, and is based on the questionable assumption that the EEG signal has a white noise characteristic (In et al. 2006). Other methods such as a wavelet-based nonlinear reduction of the pulse artefact (Wan et al. 2006) are also computationally demanding and are therefore unlikely to supplant AAS in the near future. Recently, Vincent and colleagues (Vincent et al. 2007) proposed a moving general linear model approach (mGLM), along with evidence of improved performance compared to the AAS. These authors address the specific issue of pulse artefact that lasts longer than a cardiac cycle. It remains to be determined whether this is indeed a significant problem, and whether the mGLM approach provides a major improvement over the AAS.

5
Removing the Pulse Artefact Using Spatial Pattern Removal Approaches

The abovementioned AAS, OBS and mGLM approaches all aim to model the pulse artefact waveform. This is usually done for each EEG channel separately, taking into account the fact that different channels show different artefact morphologies. However, as already shown in Fig. 2, the pulse artefact can be also characterised by a number of typical topographies, which may be sufficiently different from topographies of neuronal origin to be identifiable. The potential virtue of spatial approaches, which aim to remove those topographies, is that exact knowledge of the onset of each cardiac cycle is not necessarily required. Thus, in principle, a spatial approach can avoid problems that are inherent to AAS and OBS, as discussed above.

Motivated by the success of spatial approaches for the removal of EEG eye blink and eye movement artefacts, two spatial pulse artefact correction approaches have been proposed (Benar et al. 2003): PCA and independent component analysis (ICA). The assumption behind these is that the pulse artefact contribution is physiologically independent from, or in the case of PCA orthogonal to, ongoing EEG activity. Therefore, pulse artefact activity is presumed to be contained in a small number of components, whereas all other EEG activity should be represented by the remaining components. In the original work by Benar and colleagues, pulse artefact components were visually identified by exploring the similarity of all component time courses to the simultaneously recorded ECG signal (Benar et al. 2003). Back-projection of remaining components resulted in reconstructed EEG traces with reduced artefact. Benar and colleagues found that both ICA and PCA were well suited for this task, as they eliminated pulse artefact activity while preserving the relative amplitudes of epileptic spikes.

However, the subjective selection of components is a limitation of this approach, since it makes its performance user dependent and requires training. Indeed, it can be rather difficult to visually identify and select the components that represent pulse artefact activity beyond the first few strongest and most obvious ones. Srivastava et al. (2005) proposed the identification of independent components based on their degree of correlation with the ECG. A comparison of a fully automatic implementation of ICA, OBS and OBS-ICA methods found that the latter two provided superior performance (Debener et al. 2007). Possible explanations for the difference are as follows. First, the selection-by-correlation approach does not identify the correct components (that is, those reflecting the pulse artefact) because the independent components represent a linear decomposition of the EEG artefact rather than the electrical ECG signal. Second, it may be that ICA is not able to disentangle ongoing and event-related EEG activity from pulse artefact activity due to violations of the spatial stationarity assumption that underlies temporal ICA. With regard to the first concern, an alternative approach for component identification can be used, as shown in Fig. 6. Here, the components were identified by the amount of variance they contributed to the evoked pulse artefact, rather than based on the degree of correlation with the ECG. As illustrated, five components explained nearly all of the pulse artefact variance in this particular dataset (30-channel EEG recorded at 1.5 T). When compared to the identification-by-correlation criterion, we found evidence that this latter approach gives better results (Debener et al. 2008).

While several groups have reported success in using ICA for pulse artefact removal (e.g. Benar et al. 2003; Briselli et al. 2006; Eichele et al. 2005; Huiskamp 2005; Mantini et al. 2007; Nakamura et al. 2006), some results have been less positive (Debener et al.2007, 2008). A possible reason for this discrepancy is the field strength of the scanners used in these studies. A study using resting-state EEG data from the one individual was performed at 1.5, 3 and 7 T and the results were compared to recordings made at 0 T.

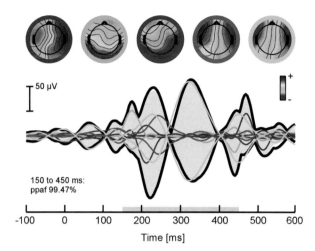

Fig. 6 Typical example of the use of ICA to remove the pulse artefact. Using the EEGLAB function "envtopo", the independent components that explain most of the variance of an evoked signal in a specified time range (here 150–450 ms) can be identified. In this case, five components were selected and accounted for >99% of the variance of the evoked signal. Shown are the envelope of the sensor data (*black*), which reflects the minima and maxima across all channels, and the envelope of the joint back-projection of the five independent components (*grey shaded area*). For each component, the map (i.e. inverse weights) and the envelope of the back-projection (coloured traces) are shown. *ppaf*, percentage of power accounted for

At 1.5 T, the ICA decomposition was found to be comparable to that obtained from data recorded outside the MRI, while the decompositions for data recorded at 3 and 7 T were markedly different. These findings are consistent with field-strength-dependent violations of the ICA assumptions. For example, the spatial stationarity assumption may be violated by the pulse artefact amplitude and spatial variability, which increases at higher fields, possibly reflecting the moving, rotating patterns previously described. As a result, ICA requires more components to model the pulse artefact at higher field strengths, and may be incompatible with the assumption of one (or a few) fixed sources (Nakamura et al. 2006). Further analyses of EEG and ECG are consistent with the notion that two different processes give rise to the BCG: blood movement or axial head rotation and electrode movement on the sides of the head. A BCG model has been proposed which may help to explain some of the observed inconsistencies in the usefulness of ICA for BCG removal (Debener et al. 2008).

In summary, the available evidence suggests that the spatial filtering approaches such as ICA and PCA may not be as efficient when used as template methods, particularly at fields of 3 T and higher. The application of ICA in combination with ECG-triggered template subtraction methods such as AAS and OBS offers a possible way forward.

Kim and coworkers combined a wavelet-based denoising approach with recursive adaptive filtering as postprocessing only in cases where AAS failed (Kim et al. 2004). Likewise, Niazy et al. (2005) suggest the use of adaptive noise cancellation following OBS to increase performance. A comparison of ICA with the identification-by-correlation approach (Srivastava et al. 2005), OBS (Niazy et al. 2005), and a combination of both (Debener et al. 2005b) showed that ICA, when used on its own, while reducing the pulse artefact substantially, also reduced the signal-to-noise ratios (SNRs) of ERPs. This suggests that artefact and signal could not be disentangled very well by ICA. However, when used after OBS, infomax ICA improved the ERP SNR and the ERP topography. Moreover, this combination can be used to remove eye blinks, and to identify brain-related signals (Debener et al. 2005a, b, 2006).

6
Evaluation of Pulse Artefact Removal Approaches

There is a lack of consistency in the evaluation of EEG artefact removal methods. There is a tendency to focus on the reduction of the pulse artefact removed from the signal. However, this approach does not necessarily address the issue of signal preservation. In the extreme case, all of the signal could be suppressed, including the undesirable artefact. Depending on the application, it may be best to avoid the use of a particular artefact correction method. Therefore, performance evaluation schemes must also address the correction algorithm's specificity—its capacity to preserve genuine neuronal signals. It is therefore a better strategy to quantify the amount of pulse artefact correction *and* the preservation of the aspect of the EEG that is of interest (epileptic spike, ERP, brain rhythm, spectrogram). If possible, the signal measured inside the scanner should be compared to an equivalent dataset recorded outside the scanner (≈ 0 T). For example, in studies designed to evaluate the performance of a correction method to be applied to event-related potential recordings, it is important to measure the SNR of the ERP component of interest and its topography (Handy 2005). The topographic quality of the corrected ERPs could be quantified by calculating the deviation to a reference recording topography or source reconstruction (Debener et al. 2007, 2008). Also, measures of the recovery of the EEG spectrum can be included, particularly if the EEG variable of interest is in the frequency or time-frequency domain (e.g. Allen et al. 1998). Moreover, hybrid simulation studies may be very informative when evaluating EEG signal quality. In any case, a better understanding of the mechanisms that give rise to the cardiac-related artefacts should lead to improved artefact reduction and expand the scope for the application of EEG–fMRI.

7
Conclusions

The pulse artefact is readily visible in EEGs recorded inside MR scanners and is generally larger at higher field strengths. It can interfere with the identification of events of interest, from large spikes in the recordings from epileptic patients to EEG oscillations and low-amplitude ERPs. While it is possible to reduce its magnitude at the source, this is unlikely to be sufficient for most applications, and particularly in the field of ERP. Different methods have been proposed for removing the pulse artefact, and an increasing number of publications that aim to tackle this issue are being published, which is encouraging and will help to further improve the EEG signal quality that can be achieved. Further progress in this field could be achieved with a more detailed knowledge of the precise origin of the pulse artefact. Nevertheless, when used correctly, existing methods such as AAS and OBS can, depending on the application, provide EEG data of sufficient quality. We have highlighted divergent views on the virtues of spatial filter tools such as ICA for pulse artefact removal. Data-driven methods such as ICA, when used in combination with AAS or OBS, appear capable of further reducing residual artefacts, and may play an increasingly important role in the integration of EEG and fMRI beyond mere artefact removal. Finally, the field would benefit from standardised artefact reduction evaluation procedures and methods that are capable of providing absolute performance measures and therefore facilitate comparisons.

References

Allen PJ, Polizzi G, Krakow K, Fish DR, Lemieux L (1998) Identification of EEG events in the MR scanner: the problem of pulse artefact and a method for its subtraction. Neuroimage 8(3): 229–239

Babiloni F, Mattia D, Babiloni C, Astolfi L, Salinari S, Basilisco A, Rossini PM, Marciani MG, Cincotti F (2004) Multimodal integration of EEG, MEG and fMRI data for the solution of the neuroimage puzzle. Magn Reson Imaging 22(10):1471–1476

Benar CG, Aghakhani Y, Wang YH, Izenberg A, Al-Asmi A, Dubeau F, Gotman J (2003) Quality of EEG in simultaneous EEG–fMRI for epilepsy. Clin Neurophysiol 114(3):569–580

Bonmassar G, Purdon PL, Jaaskelainen IP, Chiappa K, Solo V, Brown EN, Belliveau JW (2002) Motion and ballistocardiogram artefact removal for interleaved recording of EEG and EPs during MRI. Neuroimage 16(4):1127–1141

Briselli E, Garreffa G, Bianchi L, Bianciardi M, Macaluso E, Abbafati M, Grazia Marciani M, Maraviglia B (2006) An independent component analysis-based approach on ballistocardiogram artefact removing. Magn Reson Imaging 24(4):393–400

Debener S, Makeig S, Delorme A, Engel AK (2005a) What is novel in the novelty oddball paradigm? Functional significance of the novelty P3 event-related potential as revealed by independent component analysis. Cogn Brain Res 22(3):309–321

Debener S, Mullinger KJ, Niazy RK, Bowtell RW (2008) Properties of the ballistocardiogram artefact as revealed by EEG recordings at 1.5, 3 and 7 T static magnetic field strength. Int J Psychophysiol 67(3):189–199

Debener S, Strobel A, Sorger B, Peters J, Kranczioch C, Engel AK, Goebel R (2007) Improved quality of auditory event-related potentials recorded simultaneously with 3-T fMRI: Removal of the ballistocardiogram artefact. Neuroimage 34(2):590–600

Debener S, Ullsperger M, Siegel M, Engel AK (2006) Single-trial EEG/fMRI reveals the dynamics of cognitive function. Trends Cogn Sci 10(12):558–563

Debener S, Ullsperger M, Siegel M, Fiehler K, von Cramon DY, Engel AK (2005b) Trial-by-trial coupling of concurrent electroencephalogram and functional magnetic resonance imaging identifies the dynamics of performance monitoring. J Neurosci 25(50):11730–11737

Delorme A, Makeig S (2004) EEGLAB: An open source toolbox for analysis of single-trial EEG dynamics including independent component analysis. J Neurosci Methods 134(1):9–21

Eichele T, Specht K, Moosmann M, Jongsma ML, Quiroga RQ, Nordby Hand Hugdahl K (2005) Assessing the spatiotemporal evolution of neuronal activation with single-trial event-related potentials and functional MRI. Proc Natl Acad Sci USA 102(49):17798–17803

Ellingson ML, Liebenthal E, Spanaki MV, Prieto TE, Binder JR, Ropella KM (2004) Ballisto-cardiogram artefact reduction in the simultaneous acquisition of auditory ERPS and fMRI. Neuroimage 22(4):1534–1542

Goldman RI, Stern JM, Engel J, Cohen MS (2000) Acquiring simultaneous EEG and functional MRI. Clin Neurophysiol 111(11):1974–1980

Hamandi K, Laufs H, Nöth U, Carmichael DW, Duncan JS, Lemieux L (2008) BOLD and perfusion changes during epileptic generalised spike wave activity. Neuroimage 39(2):608–618

Handy TC (2005) Event-related potentials: a methods handbook. The MIT Press, Cambridge

Herrmann CS, Debener S (2007) Simultaneous recording of EEG and BOLD responses: a historical perspective. Int J Psychophysiol 67(3):161–168

Horwitz B, Poeppel D (2002) How can EEG/MEG and fMRI/PET data be combined? Hum Brain Mapp 17(1):1–3

Huiskamp, G.J. (2005). Reduction of the Ballistocardiogram Artifact in Simultaneous EEG-fMRI using ICA. Conf Proc IEEE Eng Med Biol Soc, 4, 3691–3694

In, M.H., Lee, S.Y., Park, T.S., Kim, T.S., Cho, M.H., & Ahn, Y.B. (2006). Ballistocardiogram artifact removal from EEG signals using adaptive filtering of EOG signals. Physiological Measurement, 27, 1227–1240

Kim KH, Yoon HW, Park HW (2004) Improved ballistocardiac artefact removal from the electro-encephalogram recorded in fMRI. J Neurosci Methods 135(1–2):193–203

Laufs H, Daunizeau J, Carmichael DW, Kleinschmidt A (2008) Recent advances in recording electrophysiological data simultaneously with magnetic resonance imaging. Neuroimage 40(2): 515–528

Mantini D, Perrucci MG, Cugini S, Ferretti A, Romani GL, Del Gratta C (2007) Complete artefact removal for EEG recorded during continuous fMRI using independent component analysis. Neuroimage 34(2):598–607

Masterton, R.A., Abbott, D.F., Fleming, S.W., & Jackson, G.D. (2007). Measurement and reduction of motion and ballistocardiogram artefacts from simultaneous EEG and fMRI recordings. Neuroimage, 37, 202–211

Nakamura W, Anami K, Mori T, Saitoh O, Cichocki A, Amari S (2006) Removal of ballistocardiogram artefacts from simultaneously recorded EEG and fMRI data using independent component analysis. IEEE Trans Biomed Eng 53(7):1294–1308

Negishi M, Abildgaard M, Nixon T, Constable RT (2004) Removal of time-varying gradient artefacts from EEG data acquired during continuous fMRI. Clin Neurophysiol 115(9):2181–2192

Niazy RK, Beckmann CF, Iannetti GD, Brady JM, Smith SM (2005) Removal of FMRI environment artefacts from EEG data using optimal basis sets. Neuroimage 28(3):720–737

Parkes LM, Bastiaansen MC, Norris DG (2006) Combining EEG and fMRI to investigate the post-movement beta rebound. Neuroimage 29(3):685–696

Sammer G, Blecker C, Gebhardt H, Kirsch P, Stark R, Vaitl D (2005) Acquisition of typical EEG waveforms during fMRI: SSVEP, LRP, and frontal theta. Neuroimage 24(4):1012–1024

Sijbers J, Van Audekerke J, Verhoye M, Van der Linden A, Van Dyck D (2000) Reduction of ECG and gradient related artefacts in simultaneously recorded human EEG/MRI data. Magn Reson Imaging 18(7):881–886

Skrandies W (1990) Global field power and topographic similarity. Brain Topogr 3(1):137–141

Srivastava G, Crottaz-Herbette S, Lau KM, Glover GH, Menon V (2005) ICA-based procedures for removing ballistocardiogram artefacts from EEG data acquired in the MRI scanner. Neuroimage 24(1):50–60

Tenforde TS, Gaffey CT, Moyer BR, Budinger TF (1983) Cardiovascular alterations in *Macaca* monkeys exposed to stationary magnetic fields: experimental observations and theoretical analysis. Bioelectromagnetics 4(1):1–9

Vincent JL, Larson-Prior LJ, Zempel JM, Snyder AZ (2007) Moving GLM ballistocardiogram artefact reduction for EEG acquired simultaneously with fMRI. Clin Neurophysiol 118(5): 981–998

Wan X, Iwata K, Riera J, Ozaki T, Kitamura M, Kawashima R (2006) Artefact reduction for EEG/fMRI recording: Nonlinear reduction of ballistocardiogram artefacts. Clin Neurophysiol 117(3):668–680

EEG Quality: The Image Acquisition Artefact

9

Petra Ritter, Robert Becker, Frank Freyer, and Arno Villringer

Abbreviations

ANC	Adaptive noise cancellation
FASTR	FMRI artefact slice template removal
FT	Fourier transform
IAR	Imaging artefact reduction
ICA	Independent component analysis
ITAS	Interpolation–template–alignment–subtraction
LPF	Low-pass filter
PCA	Principal component analysis
RF	Radiofrequency
SNR	Signal-to-noise ratio
TDC	Template drift compensation
TDD	Template drift detection

1
Origin of the Image Acquisition Artefact

In this chapter, we focus on the artefacts that arise in the EEG during the fMRI acquisition process. Functional MRI using echo planar imaging (EPI) sequences involves the application of rapidly varying magnetic field gradients for spatial encoding of the MR signal and radiofrequency (RF) pulses for spin excitation (see the chapter "The Basics of Functional Magnetic Resonance Imaging"). Early in the implementation of EEG–fMRI, it was observed that the acquisition of an MR image results in complete obscuration of

P. Ritter (✉)
Department of Neurology, Charité Universitätsmedizin Berlin, Chariteplatz 1, 10117 Berlin, Germany
e-mail: Petra.ritter@charite.de

C. Mulert and L. Lemieux (eds.), *EEG– fMRI*
DOI: 10.1007/978-3-540-87919-0_9, © Springer Verlag Berlin Heidelberg 2010

the physiological EEG (Ives et al. 1993; Allen et al. 2000). Electromagnetic induction in the circuit formed by the electrodes, leads, patient and amplifier exposed to a time-varying magnetic field causes an electromotive force. Artefacts induced in the EEG by the scanning process have a strong deterministic component, due to the preprogrammed nature of the RF and gradient switching sequence, and therefore artefact correction is generally considered a lesser problem than pulse-related artefacts (see the chapter "EEG Quality: Origin and Reduction of the EEG Cardiac-Related Artefact"). According to Faraday's law of induction, the induced electromotive force is proportional to the time derivative of the magnetic flux (summation of the magnetic field perpendicular to the circuit plane over the area circuit), $d\Phi/dt$, and can therefore reflect changes in the field (gradient switching, RF) or in the circuit geometry or position relative to the field due to body motion (Lemieux et al. 1997). Therefore, the combination of body motion with image acquisition artefacts can lead to random variations that represent a real challenge for artefact correction.

2
Characteristics of the Image Acquisition Artefact

In a typical EPI BOLD acquisition, the amplitude of the image acquisition artefact can be more than two orders of magnitude higher than the physiological EEG signal (Allen et al. 2000; Felblinger et al. 1999). The largest rate of change of the magnetic field occurs during the application of the RF pulses (about 30,000 T/s) (Huang-Hellinger et al. 1995). However, the frequency of the RF pulses (e.g. 64 MHz at 1.5T), lies well outside the frequency range of conventional EEG amplifiers resulting in greatly attenuated artefacts (Anami et al. 2003). For example, fMRI in a 1.5 T Siemens Magnetom Vision Scanner (Siemens Erlangen, Germany) produced image acquisition artefacts with amplitudes of up to 12 mV (Figs. 1 and 2). At 1.5 and 3 T, artefacts induced by gradient switching (10^3–10^4 μV) are generally much larger than those arising from RF pulses (up to 10^2 μV) (Anami et al. 2003).

The recorded artefact from one gradient pulse has the approximate differential waveform of the corresponding gradient pulse (Anami et al. 2003). The relative polarity and amplitude of the artefact varies across channels, but the timing of the rising and falling edges is the same across all channels. The frequency range of the image acquisition artefact exceeds that of standard clinical EEG equipment. The frequency of the readout gradient typically lies in the range of 500–900 Hz. Figures 1 and 2 illustrate typical time courses of the slice acquisition artefact. During periodic EPI BOLD scanning, the EEG is dominated by harmonics of the slice repetition frequency, typically in the range of 10–25 Hz (Fig. 3), convolved with harmonics of the volume repetition frequency of about 0.2–2 Hz (Mandelkow et al. 2006; Ritter et al. 2008a). The power spectrum of the image acquisition artefact thus overlaps that of the EEG.

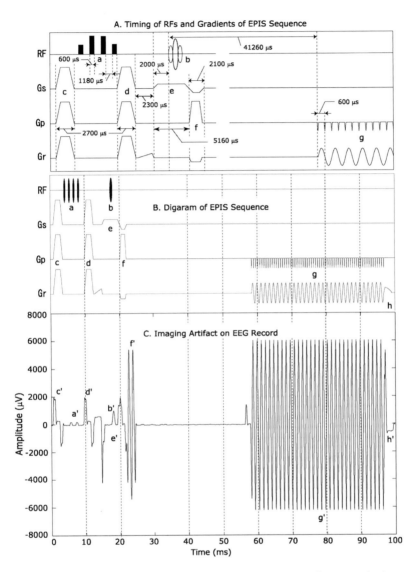

Fig. 1A–C The waveform of the image acquisition artefact can be accurately measured using a sufficiently high digitisation rate and a band-pass filter—here 20kHz/3kHz. This is a representative artefact waveform from a EPI BOLD fMRI (EPI) sequence. **A** Timings of RF and gradients in an fMRI sequence (EPIS, Siemens: ep2d_fid_60b2080_62_64.ekc). *RF*, radiofrequency wave; *Gs*, slice selection gradient; *Gp*, phase encoding gradient; *Gr*, readout gradient. *a*, Fat suppression pulses (1-3-3-1 pulses); *b*, slice selection RF; *c, d, h*, spoilers; *e*, slice selection gradient; *f*, dephasing and rephasing gradient; *g*, readout gradient. **B** Schematic diagram of whole EPIS sequence. **C** Image acquisition artefact waveform for one slice scan on a dummy EEG record with a phantom using the EPIS sequence. The artefact corresponding to each gradient component described above in **A** can be identified and is denoted by the same alphabet as that denoting the original gradient but with a prime (Anami et al. 2003)

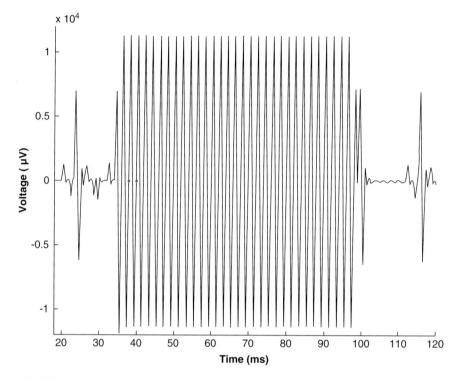

Fig. 2 The waveform of an image acquisition artefact during a single-slice acquisition (stepping stone sequence) using a 1.5 T scanner (Siemens Vision). The artefact was recorded at a sampling rate of 5 kHz and using a 1 kHz hardware low-pass filter. Here the readout gradient has a frequency of 500 Hz (the *two red dots* indicate one gradient period of length 2 ms).

3
Avoiding Image Acquisition Artefacts: Interleaved EEG–fMRI Protocols

Depending on the type of brain activity one is interested in studying, interruptions in scanning can reduce the impact of image acquisition artefacts. In EEG-triggered fMRI, short series of fMRI images are acquired following the (random) occurrence of predefined EEG events such as epileptic discharges (Baudewig et al. 2001; Krakow et al. 1999; Lemieux et al. 2001; Seeck et al. 1998; Symms et al. 1999; Warach et al. 1996). Assuming that the peak of the BOLD changes associated with the neural activity of interest occurs with the same time delay as those of normal stimuli (typically 3–8 s), the delayed onset of fMRI acquisition relative to the neural response does not pose a problem. However, this approach requires that the T1 saturation effects are modelled explicitly (Krakow et al. 2002), and fMRI signal changes that occur over long time scales cannot be easily accounted for, given the irregular sampling.

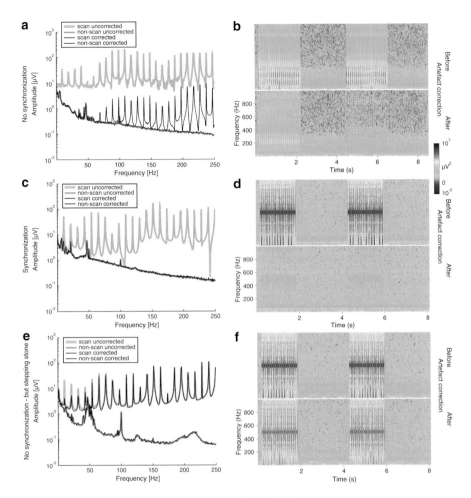

Fig. 3a–f Fourier spectrum and time–frequency plots of EEG data from synchronised and unsynchronised EEG and fMRI data acquisitions before and after image acquisition artefact correction using a slightly modified interpolation–template–alignment–subtraction (ITAS) algorithm (Ritter et al. 2007). Fourier spectra were calculated for scan periods and for non-scan periods. The Fourier spectrum of the imaging artefact afflicted EEG is dominated by harmonics of the slice repetition frequency (10 Hz in this study). **a** Unsynchronised EEG–fMRI (1.5 T Siemens Sonata) with an unstable MR sequence. The application of a correction algorithm comprising interpolation, timing error correction and artefact template subtraction (using a slightly modified ITAS algorithm as described in Ritter et al. 2007) yields good results in the frequency spectrum below 70 Hz. In **b**, for the same EEG data, time–frequency plots *before* and *after* image artefact correction are depicted. **c** Synchronised EEG–fMRI (1.5 T Siemens Vision) with a temporally stable *stepping-stone* MR sequence; simple artefact template subtraction can yield good results across the entire frequency spectrum. **d** Here the time-frequency plot of the imaging artefact corrected EEG data shows only mild residual artefacts in the 500 Hz range, reflecting the switching rate of the readout gradient. **e** Interestingly, the same algorithm used in **a** and **b** is much less efficient when applied to an EEG obtained from an unsynchronised EEG–fMRI setup with a stepping-stone sequence. Strong image acquisition artefacts are visible after imaging artefact correction, even in the lower frequency bands. This failure of the algorithm can be attributed to the oscillatory amplitude fluctuations of the image acquisition artefacts seen in Fig. 4a. **f** Here, the time–frequency plot of the imaging artefact corrected EEG is severely contaminated with residual artefacts.

In the periodic interleaved approach, MR acquisition is suspended at regular intervals, resulting in periods free of image acquisition artefacts on the EEG (Goldman et al. 2000, 2002; Ives et al. 1993; Kruggel et al. 2000; Sommer et al. 2003; Ritter et al. 2008a). Although interleaved protocols are generally less flexible and experimentally efficient than continuous measurements, they are suitable for certain forms of brain activity such as slowly varying rhythms and evoked responses. With longer acquisition times, unintentional fluctuations in attention and vigilance gain more relevance.

In multimodal studies of average evoked potentials/BOLD responses, a simultaneous EEG–fMRI setup is not always necessary (Horovitz et al. 2002, 2004; Opitz et al. 1999). In such cases separate EEG and fMRI measurements offer a reasonable alternative. There are, however, a number of questions that can only be addressed by truly simultaneous EEG–fMRI acquisition, such as studies on single trials and spontaneous non-task-related activity; see the chapters "Principles of Multimodal Functional Imaging and Data Integration" and "Experimental Design and Data Analysis Strategies".

4
Reduction of Image Acquisition Artefacts

4.1
Reduction at the Source

Minimising conductor loop area and avoiding conductor motion should help to reduce image acquisition artefacts in concurrent EEG–fMRI. Movement can be reduced by stabilising the subject's or patient's head with a vacuum cushion and fixing the EEG electronic devices and wires using sandbags, for example (Anami et al. 2003; Benar et al. 2003). Electrodes should be made of nonferromagnetic materials such as silver, silver/silver chloride, gold-coated silver and carbon (Van Audekerkea et al. 2000) in order to prevent motion relative to the scalp resulting from the strong static magnetic field. Artefact-reducing materials for the leads connecting electrode rings and amplifier are, for example, carbon fibres (Goldman et al. 2000) or very thin copper leads (Easy Cap, FMS, Munich). Twisted dual leads have the advantage that currents induced by motion and gradient switching cancel out since the currents induced in consecutive twists flow in opposing directions (Goldman et al. 2000). When possible, switching off the scanner's helium pump and patient monitoring devices can help to reduce vibration- and RF-related artefacts in the EEG (Fig. 4).

4.1.1
Stepping-Stone Sampling

Due to the short durations of image acquisition artefacts, a special MR sequence has been developed that allows EEG sampling at a digitisation rate of 1 kHz exclusively in the period in which the artefact resides around baseline level (Anami et al. 2003). This "stepping stone" sampling of EEG data is only possible in combination with synchronisation of the EEG digitisation and scanner clock. Artefact amplitude is strongly attenuated (Fig. 5d), for example

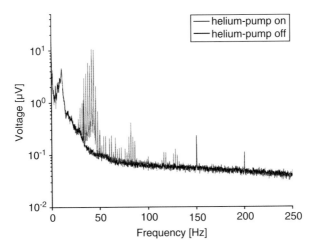

Fig. 4 Effects of the helium pump of the MR tomograph on the frequency spectrum of the EEG. These data (of 5 minutes duration for each condition) were obtained in a 1.5 Tesla Siemens Sonata scanner during non-MR-acquisition periods. Similar artefacts have been found in other MR-systems, such as the 1.5 Tesla Siemens Vision and 3 T Siemens Trio scanners. Helium-pump associated artefacts are not related to MR-image acquisition. They occur continuously, i.e. also in non-MR-acquisition periods. These artefacts are caused by the piston of the helium cooling head, which strikes the aluminium tube that functions as a cold shield. This causes vibrations of the tube at its resonance frequency of typically around 40 Hz. Vibrations of the tube induce eddy currents that generate magnetic field changes leading to the observed artefacts. The spectral peak visible in the Fourier spectrum at 50 Hz and its higher harmonics can be assigned to line noise.

to less than 5% in the study by Anami et al. (2003). Consequently, a greater dynamic range is available for the physiological EEG, allowing resolutions of 0.1 µV and below (Ritter et al. 2006; Freyer et al. 2009).

Non-MR signals such as EEG have been recorded using surplus RF receive bandwidth (Hanson et al. 2007). To this end, EEG signals amplified and digitised within the scanner are transmitted as radio waves that are detectable by the MR system and subsequently reconstructed to fill the periphery of the MRI field of view. Gradient artefacts can be greatly reduced when sampled in periods free of gradient switching using a variant of the stepping-stone technique based on a gradient field detection and gating mechanism that does not require modification of the MR sequence, in contrast to the method by Anami et al. 2003.

4.2
Synchronisation of EEG and fMRI Data Acquisitions

The EEG and fMRI acquisition systems can run independently of each other or in synchrony, with important implications for data quality (see the chapter "EEG Instrumentation and Safety" for a discussion of EEG instrumentation). While simpler to implement than synchronised acquisitions, free-running independent EEG and fMRI data acquisitions can result in a great degree of variability in the shape of the artefact (Fig. 5a and 6a), which may be more difficult to remove using post-processing methods (discussed in the next section

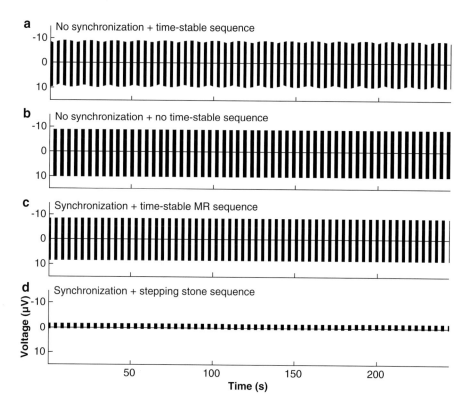

Fig. 5a–d Comparison of imaging artefact waveforms obtained from three different interleaved EEG–fMRI acquisitions: 4 min of EEG data acquired simultaneously with fMRI. Sixty MR volumes were acquired in the 4-min recording time. Due to the high amplitudes of the artefacts, physiological EEG traces in-between the image acquisition artefacts are only visible as a *flat line*. **a** Unsynchronised EEG and fMRI with a stable MR sequence and a TR that is an integer multiple of the EEG sampling rate yields EEG data containing image acquisition artefacts of high amplitudes and periodically varying shapes. **b** Unsynchronised EEG and fMRI with unstable MR sequence yields EEG data containing image acquisition artefacts of high amplitude and aperiodically varying shapes (see Fig. 5 for a zoomed-in depiction). **c** Synchronised EEG and fMRI in combination with a stable MR sequence yields image acquisition artefacts of high amplitude but constant shape (see Fig. 5). **d** Application of the *stepping-stone* sequence and synchronised EEG–fMRI yields image acquisition artefacts of lower amplitudes with constant shapes.

of this chapter). Synchronised acquisitions can be advantageous if the MR scan repetition time is chosen to be an integer multiple of the EEG sampling interval, resulting in stationary image acquisition artefacts (Fig. 5c, d and 6b), assuming that the artefact shape and amplitude do not change due to electrode movement and that the timing of the MR sequence is precise (Anami et al. 2003). In these circumstances it is possible to reduce the EEG sampling rate down to 500 Hz with satisfactory results following post-processing artefact correction (Mandelkow et al. 2006).

It should be noted that for multislice EPI sequences, the type of slice acquisition must be considered, since it influences the precision of the TR (Mandelkow et al. 2006). When slice acquisitions are equidistant in time, the actual TR can deviate from the prescribed TR by the product of the scanner clock precision and the number of slices. A stationary image acquisition artefact will be obtained if the actual TR matches a common multiple of the EEG sample time (0.2 ms for 5 kHz) and of the product of scanner clock precision (0.1 μs for 10 MHz) and number of slices. For nonequidistant slice acquisitions with pauses between successive volume acquisitions, the TR is rounded to the full precision of the scanner clock, and stationary artefacts will be obtained if TR is a multiple of the EEG sample time. Such rounding differences have been reported for the Philips 3 T Achieva system running software release 1.2.2 (Mandelkow et al. 2006) and have been found by our group for the Siemens 1.5 T Sonata system running NUMARIS/4, version syngo MR 2004A.

In a phantom measurement, Mandelkow et al. (2006) demonstrated that residual artefact power dominates the post-processed EEG spectra above roughly 80 Hz for recordings without synchronisation. This is also visible in Fig. 3a, b, which show data from a healthy subject at 1.5 T. With synchronisation, however, spectral power up to 200 Hz remains largely within 10 dB of the spectrum obtained without simultaneous fMRI (Mandelkow et al. 2006). Figure 3c, d demonstrates the superior quality of the synchronised EEG of a subject at 1.5 T.

Synchronised EEG and fMRI digitisation has been used to study high-frequency (600 Hz) and very low amplitude (few 100 nV) components of the somatosensory evoked potential (Ritter et al. 2008a ; Freyer et al. 2009) and spontaneous variations in the theta (3–6 Hz) and gamma (28–40 Hz) ranges (Giraud et al. 2007).

5
Correction of the Image Acquisition Artefact Using EEG Post-Processing

5.1
Artefact Template Subtraction

A widely applied processing method based on artefact template subtraction was demonstrated by Allen et al. (2000). This approach assumes that the shape of the gradient artefact does not change rapidly and that it is not correlated with the physiological signal (Hill et al. 1995). Channel-specific artefact templates are computed by averaging the EEG over a prespecified number of TR-related epochs and subtracted from the EEG traces in the current epoch. The epochs can be identified by recording a signal generated by the scanner that marks each image acquisition. The technique can be implemented in real time (Allen et al. 2000).

The averaging procedures implemented in different algorithms differ with respect to the number and selection of averaging epochs and their weighting. In the original implementation, the template consisted of a weighted sliding average of artefact epochs to account for possible changes of the artefact waveform over time and to account for a level of timing error, and used adaptive noise cancellation (ANC) to further reduce residual image acquisition artefacts (Allen et al. 2000). A least mean square (LMS) algorithm could be used to adjust the weights of the ANC filter. This approach, however, needed a high sampling frequency, and some unsatisfactory results were obtained, even at sampling rates of 10 kHz (Niazy et al. 2005).

The Vision Analyzer algorithm (V.1.05.0002, BrainProducts, Munich, Germany) offers three different methods of template estimation: (1) all epochs, (2) a sliding average of a certain number of epochs, or (3) a predefined number of initial scan epochs plus subsequent epochs exceeding a predefined cross-correlation with the initial template. Instead of a specific scanner-generated signal, epochs can be identified by searching for steep gradients or high amplitudes in the EEG exceeding a defined threshold. Recently we have introduced a modified approach for dynamic template estimation where artifact epochs in the template are weighted according to a Fourier spectrum-based similarity measure. This approach allowed the recovery of ultrahigh-frequency EEG signatures with amplitudes in the nanovolt range even during image acquisition periods (Freyer et al. 2009).

Image acquisition artefact template subtraction has been successfully adopted for the reconstruction of spontaneous EEG signatures such as alpha rhythm (Goncalves et al. 2005; Laufs et al. 2003; Moosmann et al. 2003), rolandic rhythms (Ritter et al. 2008b) and epileptic activity (Benar et al. 2003; Salek-Haddadi et al. 2002, 2003) and evoked potentials in the visual (Becker et al. 2005) and somatosensory system (Schubert et al. 2008).

As noted in the previous section (on synchronisation), the quality of artefact removal by template subtraction depends on the assumption of a stationary artefact, which is best satisfied when using synchronised systems (Fig. 3c) and when the exact TR of the MR sequence is a multiple of the sampling rate of the EEG. Jitter between EEG sampling and MR acquisition results in greater residual artefacts following imaging-artefact reduction (IAR), which are particularly prominent in the frequency spectrum approximately above 50 Hz (Figs. 3c, d and 5c). Low-pass filtering (cut-off around 50 and 80 Hz) can reduce residual artefacts. Although physiological signals above the cut-off frequency are removed by this procedure too, it can still be useful for the visual evaluation of the low-frequency EEG.

An alternative to the IAR method based on the frame-by-frame identification of the artefact uses an adaptive finite impulse response (FIR) filter (Wan et al. 2006). This method also assumes that the image acquisition artefacts are temporally stationary, except for a small frame-by-frame time shift. Using a Taylor expansion based on the average artefact waveform, the time-shifted image acquisition artefact of each frame was estimated using the average artefact waveform and its derivatives by LMS fitting. The algorithm outperformed simple average artefact template subtraction, which equals a zeroth-order FIR filter, but was not compared to artefact template subtraction combined with timing error correction.

An alternative to average artefact template subtraction, but one that is closely related to it, is based on online subtraction of a model of the image acquisition artefact that is estimated prior to EEG recording and subsequently fitted to the ongoing EEG for subtraction (Garreffa et al. 2003). A commercial software solution is also available for real-time imaging-artefact correction based on gradient template subtraction and template drift compensation (TDC) (Vision RecView, MRI correction module, Brainproducts, Munich, Germany). In this case, synchronised EEG–fMRI is highly beneficial.

5.2
Computing and Correcting Timing Errors

Since image acquisition artefacts contain higher frequencies than the EEG sampling rate, timing errors can lead to considerable changes of the image acquisition artefact waveform in unsynchronised acquisitions. Therefore, timing errors must be considered in the calculation of the average artefact template and in subsequent template subtraction to achieve adequate artefact reduction.

One method is to divide data into epochs, each containing an MRI volume or scan acquisition period. The epochs are then interpolated (usually by a sinc function with a factor of 10–15) and subsequently aligned by maximising the cross-correlation to a reference period. After adjusting, epochs are downsampled to the original sampling frequency and subsequently averaged to calculate an artefact template (Allen et al. 2000; Negishi et al. 2004).

Another method relies on the calculation of multiple image acquisition artefact templates, each representing another waveform of the artefact (Benar et al. 2003). This algorithm is implemented in Vision Analyzer (V.1.05.0004), providing so-called template drift detection (TDD) and subsequent TDC. Using the drift information provided by TDD, different average-artefact templates are calculated. Each individual artefact is assigned to one template. Artefact correction is then obtained by subtracting the corresponding template from the respective artefact epoch.

Figure 5 shows two cases of unsynchronised EEG–fMRI acquisitions that require different strategies for optimal artefact correction. Figure 5a shows an EEG recorded during fMRI with a temporally stable sequence and with a TR that is an integer multiple of the EEG sampling time. In this case of periodically changing artefact waveforms, an efficient correction would be to bin the observed types of artefact waveforms and then perform selective template calculation and subtraction. Interpolation of artefact periods would not eliminate the systematic differences between successive periods. Figure 5b depicts unsynchronised EEG acquisition during an fMRI sequence that was neither temporally stable nor an integer multiple of the EEG sampling interval. This case would benefit from the interpolation of artefact epochs rather than from binning, due to the large inter-artefact waveform variability.

5.3
Temporal Principal Component Analysis

Violations of the stationarity assumption can occur independent of the degree of EEG and fMRI acquisition due to electrode movement in relation to the gradient coil and RF antenna, leading to a degradation in artefact template subtraction performance.

Negishi and colleagues proposed the application of temporal principal component analysis (PCA) to each EEG channel independently in order to remove residual artefacts (Negishi et al. 2004). Temporal PCA utilises the differential statistical characteristics of the variance of EEG epochs during and in-between scan acquisitions, yielding results similar to those obtained using IAR + ANC (Negishi et al. 2004).

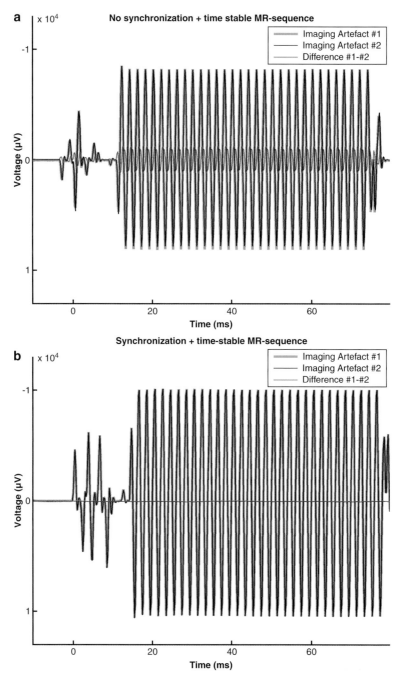

Fig. 6a–b Stability of image acquisition artefacts: single-slice artefacts of two consecutive imaging volume artefacts are superimposed for comparison (black and grey line). Red indicates the difference wave for the two artefacts. **a** In the unsynchronised EEG–fMRI approach, consecutive image acquisition artefacts differ considerably, resulting in a distinct difference wave. **b** In the synchronised EEG–fMRI approach, consecutive image acquisition artefacts are identical, resulting in a difference wave that is almost zero and zero (i.e. only the physiological EEG signal is present).

The method called fMRI artefact slice template removal (FASTR) employs both arte-fact template subtraction and temporal PCA (Niazy et al. 2005). Again, slice-specific arte-fact templates are constructed as the local moving average plus a linear combination of basis functions describing the variation of residuals. The basis functions are derived by performing temporal PCA on the artefact residuals and selecting the dominant components to serve as a basis set. Finally, imaging artefact residuals are removed by an ANC filter (see below). This algorithm has been successfully applied in a continuous EEG–fMRI study of laser-evoked responses at 3 T (Iannetti et al. 2005) When the EEG signature of interest is of very high frequency, the beneficial outcome of a PCA-based postprocessing can be further enhanced by employing a band-specific PCA in the high-frequency band in addi-tion to the PCA on the broad-band EEG. This cascaded PCA postprocessing enables the recovery of ultrafast EEG signatures, which were otherwise obscured by imaging artifact residuals (Freyer et al. 2009).

5.4
Independent Component Analysis

Another approach to imaging artefact correction is independent component analysis (ICA) in addition to artefact template subtraction (Mantini et al. 2007). ICA is a signal processing technique that recovers independent sources from a set of simultaneously recorded signals that result from a linear mixing of the source signals (Hyvarinen 1999; Mantini et al. 2007). Since EEG and image acquisition artefacts are generated by different independent pro-cesses and are therefore uncorrelated, ICA seems to be an appropriate approach. Mantini and colleagues categorised the ICA sources into two signal categories: brain signals and artefacts. This was done by visual inspection or in an automated approach by correlation to reference signals. Only sources classified as nonartificial were back-projected and used for further analysis. This approach proved to be capable of not only removing residual image acquisition artefacts but also ballistocardiogram and ocular artefacts.

Grouiller et al. (2007) compared an ICA-based imaging artefact removal approach to three other fundamental approaches to imaging artefact correction: IAR (Allen et al. 2000), FMRIB (Niazy et al. 2005) and Fourier transform (FT) filtering (Hoffmann et al. 2000). They used the implementation of the Infomax ICA algorithm in the EEGLAB toolbox (Computational Neurobiology Laboratory, Salk Institute, La Jolla, CA, USA: http://www.sccn.ucsd.edu/eeglab/) (Bell and Sejnowski 1995). The authors selected the components that were correlated with the imaging artefact template. Selected components had a norma-lised cross-correlation coefficient higher than the average plus one standard deviation of that coefficient computed for all the components. The components representing image acquisition artefacts were excluded from the EEG reconstruction. Results for the perfor-mance of ICA, however, differed between simulations and real data (for details, see Sect. 6). Results obtained by Grouiller et al. (2007) indicate that ICA may not be applicable for efficiently estimating independent components in long time series of EEG data. A theoreti-cal reason for this may be the spatial nonstationarity of the EEG and (especially) of the imaging artefact signal.

5.5
Filtering in the Frequency Domain

Image acquisition artefacts are periodic and distributed over a limited range of frequencies, suggesting that correction may be performed satisfactorily on the frequency domain. One such method is based on the comparison of the spectral content of EEG data acquired with and without simultaneous MR acquisition. The Fourier components of the signal corresponding to the MR-specific frequencies are set to zero for subsequent reprojection in signal space (Hoffmann et al. 2000). This algorithm was implemented in the FEMR program provided by Schwarzer (Munich, Germany). The disadvantage of this method is that, due to a spectral overlap between the physiological EEG and image acquisition artefacts, some of the physiological EEG signal is removed as well. The method is characterised by ringing artefact (Benar et al. 2003), which results from discontinuities (e.g. gaps between scan acquisitions in interleaved EEG–fMRI) in the signals to be corrected. A similar approach relies on channel-wise subtraction of an average gradient artefact power spectrum—adapted by a scaling factor to the spectrum of the individual artefact—from the power spectrum of the artefact-distorted EEG (Sijbers et al. 1999). To filter image acquisition artefacts in the frequency domain, one group (Grouiller et al. 2007) first calculated the FT of the imaging artefact template. Then, weights were applied to the spectral components of the FT of the EEG. For spectral components of the artefact afflicted EEG corresponding to strong spectral components in the artefact template, spectral filtering weights were set to the inverse. Thus, coefficients corresponding to the image acquisition artefact were attenuated. To obtain the corrected EEG, the inverse FT was applied. Grouiller et al. (2007) reported weighting coefficients to be inversely proportional to FT coefficients of the artefacts instead of zeroing them (Hoffmann et al. 2000) improved signal preservation and reduced ringing.

6
Evaluation of Correction Methods

To date, artefact correction performance evaluation has not been performed consistently. In many EEG–fMRI studies, a single algorithm is chosen without proper justification, and often the quality of gradient artefact correction is assessed by visual inspection only. However, a more systematic approach to the choice of correction method may be advised for certain applications, such as the analysis of single events and nonaveraged EEG data, when residual artefacts do not cancel out, or those that rely on the quantitation of EEG power in certain spectral bands. The task of selecting a suitable correction algorithm would be greatly facilitated by standardising their evaluation and carefully considering the experimental requirements in terms of the EEG–fMRI protocol and features of the signal of interest (spectral signature, amplitude). In the following we describe the main evaluation strategies employed to date.

Knowledge of the true signal is highly advantageous for the evaluation of signal filtering methods. This can be obtained in tests on phantoms and using signals generated by instruments offering the opportunity to assess both signal preservation and artefact reduction (Negishi et al. 2004; Schmid et al. 2006). Simulations have also been employed in which artificially generated signals (e.g. those extracted from recordings made under the control condition or simulated mathematically) are added to true artefacts (Allen et al. 2000; Groullier et al. 2007). The main disadvantage of this approach is a lack of realism, in terms of the complexity of true physiological signals, noise, subject movement and intersubject and inter-recording variability.

For tests based on real EEG, EEG recorded outside the MR environment should constitute the best gold standard. However, the specific evaluation of image acquisition artefact reduction methods can be performed adequately from signals recorded inside the scanner to compare signals captured without scanning (reference) and with scanning (and correction). For example, Allen et al. compared the signal's spectral content using this approach (Allen et al. 2000). In theory, a drawback of this approach is a lack of knowledge of the true EEG signal, in part due to the additional effects of the pulse artefact but also the sequential nature of the samples used for comparison. On the other hand, image acquisition artefact correction method performance evaluations based on signals recorded exclusively inside the scanner have the advantage that the pulse artefact is a common factor. Nonetheless, sequential measurements under the two experimental conditions may be particularly problematic for signals of interest with a high intrinsic variability, such as brain rhythms or epileptic discharges, but are possibly less so for evoked responses, where reproducible neuronal signals are more likely, although this bias can be reduced through adequate sampling.

Benar et al. (2003) compared Fourier filtering and template subtraction using EEGs obtained from patients with epilepsy, which were inspected by a trained observer after the application of both artefact correction methods. Visual subtraction was found to result in higher EEG quality than Fourier filtering.

Different gradient artefact correction algorithms based on the approach of template artefact subtraction were evaluated on data recorded with an unsynchronised EEG–fMRI setup using a visual stimulus presented to subjects at rest (Ritter et al. 2007). In this study, a combination of the following analyses was employed for performance estimation: (1) the degree of artefact reduction was evaluated by comparing the spectral content of the corrected data to that of gradient artefact free EEG epochs for six predefined frequency bands ranging from theta to omega (1–250 Hz); (2) the preservation of non-gradient artefact components of the EEG after correction was evaluated twofold—by comparing the spectral content of non-acquisition EEG epochs before and after gradient artefact correction for the six predefined frequency bands, and by exploring the impact of artefact correction on artificially generated signals added to the EEG. The study demonstrated that the amount of artefact reduction and the degree of physiological signal preservation are important complementary performance measures.

Another approach to the comparison of different artefact correction algorithms was based on the generation of artificial EEG and artificial image acquisition artefacts by a simple forward model (Grouiller et al. 2007). Modulations of the imaging artefact amplitude caused by subject motion and MRI and EEG clock asynchrony—which are typical of unsynchronised EEG-MRI setups—in combination with different EEG sampling rates were implemented in the model. The advantages of this approach include: it allows the effects of

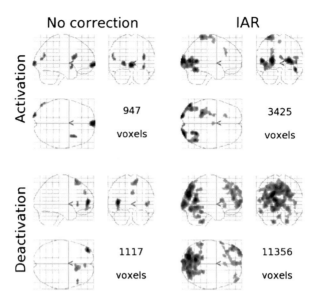

Fig. 7 Dependence of FMRI correlates of the alpha rhythm on the quality of image acquisition arte-fact correction. Glass brains were obtained using the power in the alpha band as a regressor con-volved with the HRF (p = 0.005, uncorrected). Left: Without any artefact correction. Right: Using IAR image acquisition artefact removal. (Modified from Grouiller et al. 2007).

different experimental or empirical parameters to be tested; knowledge of ground truth. The same group also evaluated artefact correction in real EEG data. To this end, after arte-fact correction, they calculated correlation coefficients between the alpha power modu-lated by an eyes-open/eyes-closed paradigm and the task function and also correlation coefficients between interictal spikes acquired inside and outside the scanner. For the sim-ulated data, the authors found that the ICA algorithm was the method that presented by far the best average results, although with a high performance variability, indicating that this approach might be unstable. FASTR and IAR were approximately equivalent and FT per-formed significantly less well. For the real data, the IAR and FASTR algorithms obtained the best results. There was considerable discrepancy between the results obtained from simulations and from experimental data for the ICA approach, indicating a possible weak-ness of the modelling.

The authors assessed the effect of artefact correction on the fMRI results by comparing statistical parametric maps obtained from models based on alpha power with and without imaging artefact correction (Fig. 7). "Summarized, the discussed repertoire of available hardware and software solutions enables satisfying imaging-artefact correction. However, individual results can vary and therefore a continuous critical re-evaluation of results is necessary to ensure reasonable data quality."

Acknowledgements We would like to thank Daniel Margulies and Matthias Reinacher for proofreading the manuscript. This work was supported by the German Federal Ministry of Edu-cation and Research BMBF (Berlin Neuroimaging Center; Bernstein Center for Computational Neuroscience) and the German Research Foundation DFG (Berlin School of Mind and Brain).

References

Allen PJ, Josephs O, Turner R (2000) A method for removing imaging artifact from continuous EEG recorded during functional MRI. Neuroimage 12(2):230–239

Anami K, Mori T, Tanaka F, Kawagoe Y, Okamoto J, Yarita M, Ohnishi T, Yumoto M, Matsuda H, Saitoh O (2003) Stepping stone sampling for retrieving artifact-free electroencephalogram during functional magnetic resonance imaging. Neuroimage 19(2 Pt 1):281–295

Baudewig J, Bittermann HJ, Paulus W, Frahm J (2001) Simultaneous EEG and functional MRI of epileptic activity: a case report. Clin Neurophysiol, 112: 1196–200

Becker R, Ritter P, Moosmann M, Villringer A (2005) Visual evoked potentials recovered from fMRI scan periods. Hum Brain Mapp 26(3):221–230

Bell AJ, Sejnowski TJ (1995) An information-maximization approach to blind separation and blind deconvolution. Neural Comput 7(6):1129–1159

Benar C, Aghakhani Y, Wang Y, Izenberg A, Al Asmi A, Dubeau F, Gotman J (2003) Quality of EEG in simultaneous EEG–fMRI for epilepsy. Clin Neurophysiol 114(3):569–580

Felblinger J, Slotboom J, Kreis R, Jung B, Boesch C (1999) Restoration of electrophysiological signals distorted by inductive effects of magnetic field gradients during MR sequences. Magn Reson Med 41(4):715–721

Freyer F, Becker R, Anami K, Curio G, Villringer A, Ritter P. Ultrahigh-frequency EEG during fMRI: Pushing the limits of imaging-artifact correction. Neuroimage, 2009

Garreffa G, Carni M, Gualniera G, Ricci GB, Bozzao L, De Carli D, Morasso P, Pantano P, Colonnese C, Roma V, et al. (2003) Real-time MR artifacts filtering during continuous EEG/fMRI acquisition. Magn Reson Imaging 21(10):1175–1189

Giraud AL, Kleinschmidt A, Poeppel D, Lund TE, Frackowiak RS, Laufs H (2007) Endogenous cortical rhythms determine cerebral specialization for speech perception and production. Neuron 56(6):1127–1134

Goldman RI, Stern JM, Engel J Jr., Cohen MS (2000) Acquiring simultaneous EEG and functional MRI. Clin Neurophysiol 111(11):1974–1980

Goldman RI, Stern JM, Engel J, Jr., Cohen MS (2002) Simultaneous EEG and fMRI of the alpha rhythm. Neuroreport, 13: 2487–92

Goncalves SI, de Munck JC, Pouwels PJ, Schoonhoven R, Kuijer JP, Maurits NM, Hoogduin JM, Van Someren EJ, Heethaar RM, Lopes da Silva FH. (2005) Correlating the alpha rhythm to BOLD using simultaneous EEG/fMRI: Inter-subject variability. Neuroimage

Grouiller F, Vercueil L, Krainik A, Segebarth C, Kahane P, David O (2007) A comparative study of different artefactartefact removal algorithms for EEG signals acquired during functional MRI. Neuroimage 38(1):124–137

Hanson LG, Lund TE, Hanson CG (2007) Encoding of electrophysiology and other signals in MR images. J Magn Reson Imaging 25(5):1059–1066

Hill RA, Chiappa KH, Huang-Hellinger F, Jenkins BG (1995) EEG during MR imaging: differentiation of movement artifact from paroxysmal cortical activity. Neurology, 45: 1942–3

Hoffmann A, Jager L, Werhahn KJ, Jaschke M, Noachtar S, Reiser M (2000) Electroencephalography during functional echo-planar imagingecho-planar imaging: detection of epileptic spikes using post-processing methods. Magn Reson Med 44(5):791–798

Horovitz SG, Rossion B, Skudlarski P, Gore JC (2004) Parametric design and correlational analyses help integrating fMRI and electrophysiological data during face processing. Neuroimage., 22: 1587–95

Horovitz SG, Skudlarski P, Gore JC (2002) Correlations and dissociations between BOLD signal and P300 amplitude in an auditory oddball task: a parametric approach to combining fMRI and ERP. Magn Reson.Imaging, 20: 319–25

Huang-Hellinger FR, Breiter HC, McCormack GM, Cohen MS, Kwong KK, Savoy RL, Weisskoff RM, Davis TL, Baker JR, Belliveau JW, et al. (1995) Simultaneous functional magnetic resonance imaging and electrophysiological recording. Human Brain Mapp 3:13–23

Hyvarinen A (1999) Fast and robust fixed-point algorithms for independent component analysis. IEEE Trans Neural Netw, 10: 626–34

Iannetti GD, Niazy RK, Wise RG, Jezzard P, Brooks JC, Zambreanu L, Vennart W, Matthews PM, Tracey I (2005) Simultaneous recording of laser-evoked brain potentials and continuous, high-field functional magnetic resonance imaging in humans. Neuroimage 28(3):708–719

Ives JR, Warach S, Schmitt F, Edelman RR, Schomer DL (1993) Monitoring the patient's EEG during echo planar MRI. Electroencephalogr. Clin. Neurophysiol 87: 417–20

Krakow K, Woermann FG, Symms MR, Allen PJ, Lemieux L, Barker GJ, Duncan JS, Fish DR (1999) EEG-triggered functional MRI of interictal epileptiform activity in patients with partial seizures. Brain, 122: 1679–88

Kruggel F, Wiggins CJ, Herrmann CS, von Cramon DY (2000) Recording of the event-related potentials during functional MRI at 3.0 Tesla field strength. Magn Reson.Med., 44: 277–82

Laufs H, Kleinschmidt A, Beyerle A, Eger E, Salek-Haddadi A, Preibisch C, Krakow K (2003) EEG-correlated fMRI of human alpha activity. Neuroimage., 19: 1463–76

Lemieux L, Allen PJ, Franconi F, Symms MR, Fish DR (1997) Recording of EEG during fMRI experiments: patient safety. Magn Reson Med 38(6):943–952

Lemieux L, Krakow K, Fish DR (2001) Comparison of spike-triggered functional MRI BOLD activation and EEG dipole model localization. Neuroimage 14: 1097–104

Mandelkow H, Halder P, Boesiger P, Brandeis D (2006) Synchronization facilitates removal of MRI artefacts from concurrent EEG recordings and increases usable bandwidth. Neuroimage 32(3):1120–1126

Mantini D, Perrucci MG, Cugini S, Ferretti A, Romani GL, Del Gratta C (2007) Complete artifact removal for EEG recorded during continuous fMRI using independent component analysis. Neuroimage 34(2):598–607

Moosmann M, Ritter P, Krastel I, Brink A, Thees S, Blankenburg F, Taskin B, Obrig H, Villringer A (2003) Correlates of alpha rhythm in functional magnetic resonance imaging and near infra-red spectroscopy. Neuroimage, 20: 145–58

Negishi M, Abildgaard M, Nixon T, Constable RT (2004) Removal of time-varying gradient artifacts from EEG data acquired during continuous fMRI. Clin Neurophysiol 115(9): 2181–2192

Niazy RK, Beckmann CF, Iannetti GD, Brady JM, Smith SM (2005) Removal of FMRI environment artifacts from EEG data using optimal basis sets. Neuroimage 28(3):720–737

Opitz B, Mecklinger A, Von Cramon DY, Kruggel F (1999) Combining electrophysiological and hemodynamic measures of the auditory oddball. Psychophysiology, 36: 142–7

Ritter P, Becker R, Graefe C, Villringer A (2007) Evaluating gradientgradient artifact correction of EEG data acquired simultaneously with fMRI. Magn Reson Imaging 25(6):923–932

Ritter P, Freyer F, Becker R, Anami K, Curio G, Villringer A (2006) Recording of ultrafast (600 Hz) EEG oscillations with amplitudes in the nanovolt range during fMRI-acquisition periods. 14th Scientific Meeting ISMRM, Seattle, WA, USA, 6–12 May 2006

Ritter P, Freyer F, Curio G, Villringer A (2008a) High frequency (600 Hz) population spikes in human EEG delineate thalamic and cortical fMRI activation sites. Neuroimage 42(2): 483–490

Ritter P, Moosmann M, Villringer A (2008b) Rolandic alpha and beta EEG rhythms' strengths are inversely related to fMRI-BOLD signal in primary somatosensory and motor cortex. Hum Brain Mapp 30(4):1168–1187

Salek-Haddadi A, Lemieux L, Merschhemke M, Friston KJ, Duncan JS, Fish DR (2003) Functional magnetic resonance imaging of human absence seizures. Ann.Neurol, 53: 663-7

Salek-Haddadi A, Merschhemke M, Lemieux L, Fish DR (2002) Simultaneous EEG-Correlated Ictal fMRI. Neuroimage, 16: 32–40

Schmid MC, Oeltermann A, Juchem C, Logothetis NK, Smirnakis SM (2006) Simultaneous EEG and fMRI in the macaque monkey at 4.7 Tesla. Magn Reson.Imaging., 24: 335–42

Schubert R, Ritter P, Wustenberg T, Preuschhof C, Curio G, Sommer W, Villringer A (2008) Spatial attention related SEP amplitude modulations covary with BOLD signal in S1–a simultaneous EEG–fMRI study. Cereb Cortex, 18: 2686–700

Seeck M, Lazeyras F, Michel CM, Blanke O, Gericke CA, Ives J, Delavelle J, Golay X, Haenggeli CA, de Tribolet N, Landis T (1998) Non-invasive epileptic focus localization using EEG-triggered functional MRI and electromagnetic tomography. Electroencephalogr.Clin. Neurophysiol 106: 508–12

Sijbers J, Michiels I, Verhoye M, Van Audekerke J, Van der LA, Van Dyck D (1999) Restoration of MR-induced artifacts in simultaneously recorded MR/EEG data. Magn Reson Imaging 17(9):1383–1391

Symms MR, Allen PJ, Woermann FG, Polizzi G, Krakow K, Barker GJ, Fish DR, Duncan JS (1999) Reproducible localization of interictal epileptiform discharges using EEG-triggered fMRI. Phys.Med.Biol., 44: N161–N8

Sommer M, Meinhardt J, Volz HP (2003) Combined measurement of event-related potentials (ERPs) and fMRI. Acta Neurobiol.Exp.(Wars.), 63: 49–53

Van Audekerkea J, Peeters R, Verhoye M, Sijbers J, Van der LA (2000) Special designed RF-antenna with integrated non-invasive carbon electrodes for simultaneous magnetic resonance imaging and electroencephalography acquisition at 7T. Magn Reson Imaging 18(7):887–891

Warach S, Ives JR, Schlaug G, Patel MR, Darby DG, Thangaraj V, Edelman RR, Schomer DL (1996) EEG-triggered echo-planar functional MRI in epilepsy. Neurology, 47: 89–93

Wan X, Iwata K, Riera J, Kitamura M, Kawashima R (2006) Artifact reduction for simultaneous EEG/fMRI recording: adaptive FIR reduction of imaging artifacts. Clin Neurophysiol 117(3):681–692

Image Quality Issues

10

David Carmichael

1
fMRI Pulse Sequences

The requirement of a fMRI pulse sequence is BOLD sensitivity, which means predominantly T2*-weighted[1] sequences such as GE-EPI, although spin echo sequences such as spin echo EPI (SE-EPI) can also be used (Bandettini et al. 1994; Norris et al. 2002; Schmidt et al. 2005).

SE-EPI suffers from reduced volume coverage relative to GE-EPI due to the longer echo times required, and generally shows smaller signal changes (Bandettini et al. 1994; Schmidt et al. 2005). However, spin echo sequences do not suffer from signal dropout and therefore perform much better in areas of large through-plane susceptibility gradients (Norris et al. 2002). There is mixed opinion as to whether, or in which parts of the brain, spin echo sequences may be advantageous (Parkes et al. 2005; Schmidt et al. 2005), but they are likely to be most usefully employed at field strengths of >3 T (Duong et al. 2002; Nair and Duong 2004). Some considerable research has recently been devoted to using steady-state free-precession sequences for fMRI (Miller et al. 2003, 2004, 2006; Zhong et al. 2007). While these sequences have shown promise, they are generally employed for niche applications (Miller et al. 2006). It is also worth noting that hybrid approaches using spin and gradient echoes such as GRASE (Feinberg et al. 1995; Fernandez-Seara et al. 2005) are also capable of being used to obtain high-quality fMRI data.

---

[1]The transverse relaxation time including a contribution from slowly changing or constant background magnetic fields.

D. Carmichael
Institute of Neurology, University College London, Queen Square, London WC1N 3BG, UK
e-mail: d.carmichael@ion.ucl.ac.uk

C. Mulert and L. Lemieux (eds.), *EEG- fMRI*
DOI: 10.1007/978-3-540-87919-0_10, © Springer Verlag Berlin Heidelberg 2010

2
GE-EPI

The sequence of choice for most fMRI applications is GE-EPI, due to its high speed and a high signal-to-noise ratio (SNR) per unit time. An image can typically be obtained in 20–50 ms using modern hardware, giving whole brain coverage in 2–4 s (Schmitt et al. 1998; Mansfield 1977; Ordidge 1999; Turner and Ordidge 2000).

In the following section, we will restrict our discussion to Cartesian k-space trajectory EPI because it is the most frequently used and generally offers highly competitive performance in terms of speed and artefact level. Other k-space trajectories commonly used for EPI include spirals where both read and phase-encoding gradients are equivalent in pulse shape and amplitude, but offset in phase and oscillate in a sinusoidal manner (Ahn et al. 1986; Glover and Law 2001; Preston et al. 2004; Sangill et al. 2006). This can reduce image distortion, for example, due to faster traversal of k-space (especially compared to the phase-encoding direction of Cartesian EPI), but may not necessarily yield an overall increase in performance over the whole brain (Block and Frahm 2005).

An EPI sequence diagram is shown in Fig. 1. A gradient echo is formed when the transverse magnetisation is dephased and then rephased by linear magnetic field gradients alone (unlike a spin echo). The EPI experiment involves a single RF excitation pulse followed by a train of these echoes that are read out by applying a series of gradients with equal areas and opposite magnitude. Each echo has a different net phase-encoding gradient due to the extra gradients (blips) applied between the readout gradient reversals (Wielopolski et al. 1998). In EPI, all of the PE steps are acquired in one TR, making it a fast technique. This implementation of EPI is termed "single shot" because it requires only one RF excitation of the magnetisation to obtain an entire image dataset.

The echo time (TE) is centred on the middle PE step, where the net phase-encoding gradient is zero. It is clear that as each echo is at a different position in time, the magnetisation will have experienced different amounts of dephasing from any local magnetic field differences. These are caused by interfaces between materials of different magnetic susceptibility, such as the head and air. Any inconsistency between successive echoes, obtained at different times, has associated problems that will be discussed at greater length later. EPI can suffer from a number of other problems that are directly related to its strategy of full k-space coverage in a single shot. EPI readouts are naturally longer than for other pulse sequences, because a greater distance through k-space must be travelled in one go (see Fig. 1). Additional problems are associated with having reversed the direction travelled through k-space in alternate lines (see Schmitt et al. 1998 for an additional description of EPI artefacts and their causes). Here, we first look to explain the most common sources of EPI artefact in a qualitative manner, and we describe the range of methods available to moderate their effects before going on to determine how the addition of EEG equipment may exacerbate these image quality issues.

2.1
Image Blurring

Blurring of image detail occurs because of T2*/T2-related signal decay over the length of the acquisition (i.e. not all points in k-space are sampled at the same effective TE). For EPI,

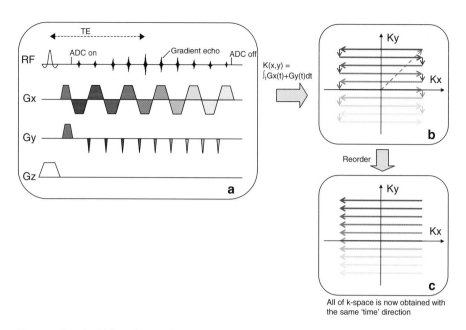

All of k-space is now obtained with
the same 'time' direction

Fig. 1a–c Standard blipped Cartesian EPI pulse sequence and corresponding k-space trajectory. The blipped EPI pulse sequence is shown (**a**). On the *top line* is the RF showing the slice-selective excitation pulse followed by a series of gradient echoes. Each of the gradient echoes is formed by a readout gradient of opposite polarity. Additionally, for each gradient reversal a different phase encode line is readout by the application of a phase-encoding gradient during the read gradient reversal. ADC is the analogue-to-digital converter that is switched on to record the signal. **b** The k-space trajectory is shown; the position in k-space is determined by the gradient area. The colour of the gradient corresponds to the k-space trajectory. Initially, the *grey* gradients take us to the k-space corner, and then the readout gradient alternately traverses from *right* to *left* while the phase-encoding blips make the jumps from *top* to *bottom* at the end of each readout gradient. It is worth noting that the order that k-space is acquired in the phase-encoding direction can be reversed (here the blips are negative), and this will alter the distortion (see Fig. 3 and consider the effect on the k-space trajectory of opposite-sign phase-encoding blips). **c** Alternate lines of data are reversed in direction prior to reconstruction. This effectively means that each line of k-space data should look as if it has been obtained under the same polarity of gradient (otherwise each line appears as if time was reversed). Any mismatch between positive and negative gradients creates a mismatch along the Ky direction in alternate lines and causes an N/2 ghost

the large time difference between adjacent k-space data points, particularly in the phase-encoding direction, causes greater signal decay and thus increased blurring. This can be thought of as the effective application of a filter in k-space described by the signal decay during the readout with the blurring caused in the image described by the Fourier transform of this filter, which is called the point spread function (PSF) (see Fig. 2). In tissue with a shorter T2*, due to stronger local susceptibility-related magnetic fields that are increased by utilising higher main magnetic field strengths, this problem is increased. Blurring will thus also be increased where stronger local susceptibility-related magnetic fields are produced by EEG equipment. Reduced blurring is achieved by shorter readout lengths or higher resolution images without increased readout duration. Methods to shorten readouts include multishot segmented EPI (Menon et al. 1997; Wielopolski et al. 1998), related

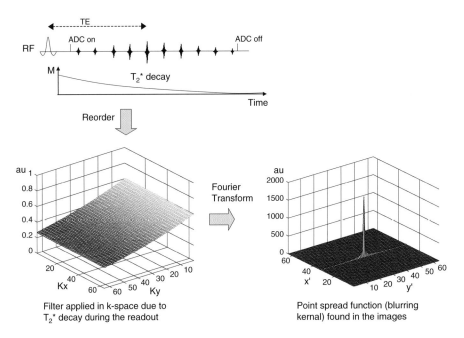

Fig. 2 Blurring in EPI images. Due to the properties of the Fourier transform we can separately consider each of the different components that modulate the underlying k-space signal produced by an object (that are all multiplied together in actual data). Each of these components can be thought of as a filter. The effect seen in the image is blurring from a convolution of the object by the Fourier transform of each k-space filter. There is a large amount of signal decay during the long EPI read out (*top*), which can thus be considered independently of other signal modulations (e.g. those imposed by imaging gradients or the object itself). When the data is reordered in k-space, the signal decay makes a 2D function in k-space that is an effective filter, as shown *bottom left*. The Fourier transform of this filter determines the point spread function, which describes the blurring of the data from each voxel

pulse sequences that split the readout into shorter segments without requiring multishots (Bornert and Jensen 1994; Carmichael et al. 2005; Feinberg et al. 2002; Priest et al. 2004; Rzedzian 1987) and parallel imaging (PI) methods (Carlson and Minemura 1993; Griswold et al. 2002; Hutchinson and Raff 1988; Pruessmann et al. 1999; Sodickson and Manning 1997). Alternatively, improved shimming (Cusack et al. 2005; Gruetter 1993; Gruetter and Tkac 2000; Mackenzie et al. 1987; van Gelderen et al. 2007; Ward et al. 2002; Wilson et al. 2003; Wilson and Jezzard 2003) can also locally decrease blurring by increasing local field homogeneity. In most fMRI experiments, including EEG–fMRI, blurring is not a primary consideration for pulse sequence optimisation. This is due to the usual spatial extent of activation exceeding the voxel size and because the optimisation of SNR, temporal resolution and image dropout is usually more critical. However, it is important to remember that the resolution is degraded, especially in the phase-encoding direction in GE-EPI, and in some cases where small structures are interrogated—such as high-resolution mapping of cortical columns within visual areas—some minimisation of blurring may be beneficial.

2.2
Geometric Distortion

Due to the time difference between the acquisition of adjacent k-space data points in the phase-encoding direction (or correspondingly the low (PE) bandwidth, which is simply the reciprocal), local magnetic field perturbations from various sources (Jezzard and Clare 1999; Wielopolski et al. 1998) have the time to cause significant local phase accumulation relative to that produced by the phase-encoding gradients (i.e. the local magnetic field gradient area is large relative to the size of the phase-encoding blips). This causes an apparent shift in the data from the local position in the image, with the shift in position proportional to the size of the local difference in the local static magnetic field (B_0) (Jezzard and Balaban 1995). In addition to a simple shift of data from one position to another, data from one position may be stretched over a larger area or squashed into a smaller area. In Fig. 3, the process is described in terms of k-space coverage. At different positions within the brain, there is a local magnetic field gradient that has an additive effect, positive or negative, on the phase-encoding gradients. This can be conceptualised as causing a different k-space trajectory for magnetisation at a different spatial position. In one spatial position, the phase encoding (Ky) covers a greater effective k-space area and the lines are further apart. This corresponds to squeezing the data into a smaller area. Alternatively, the lines are forced closer together, with the effect of stretching the data in the image. Distortion will be increased where stronger local susceptibility-related magnetic fields are produced by EEG equipment.

The simplest method of reducing distortion is to shorten the time between the phase-encoding blips by switching the read gradients faster and with greater amplitude, thereby requiring an increased readout bandwidth (with a concomitant reduction in SNR). This corresponds to reducing the time taken to travel through the k-space trajectory in Fig. 1. Unfortunately, the rate and maximum amplitude of the read gradient switching is limited by physiological constraints; rapidly varying magnetic fields can induce currents in nerves large enough to cause stimulation (Cohen et al. 1990; Mansfield and Harvey 1993). In addition, the desired gradient waveform is only accurately produced when both its amplitude and switching rate lie within certain limits. Therefore, one option that is available is to reduce the number and increase the size of the phase-encoding steps in the acquisition window, necessitating the recovery of a full set of image information by some other means. There are a number of different techniques that are used to perform this function, and they can be classified into two approaches. First, there is interleaved segmented EPI (Butts et al. 1994; Hennel and Nedelec 1995) (for two segments, every other line of the standard k-space coverage is read out, and then the remaining lines are read out in a separate acquisition), although this entails a penalty in temporal resolution that would be unacceptable for many fMRI applications. Various strategies have been suggested to read out the segments consecutively. One of the simplest is to use a 45° RF pulse and acquisition followed directly by a 90° RF pulse and acquisition (Rzedzian 1987), or to take pairs of images with different spatial profiles imposed and then reconstruct the data (Carmichael et al. 2005; Feinberg et al. 2002; Priest et al. 2004). The second approach uses differing degrees of prior information to recreate full images from reduced data sets. Partial Fourier methods that exploit the conjugate symmetry of k-space have been used (Feinberg et al. 1986), but

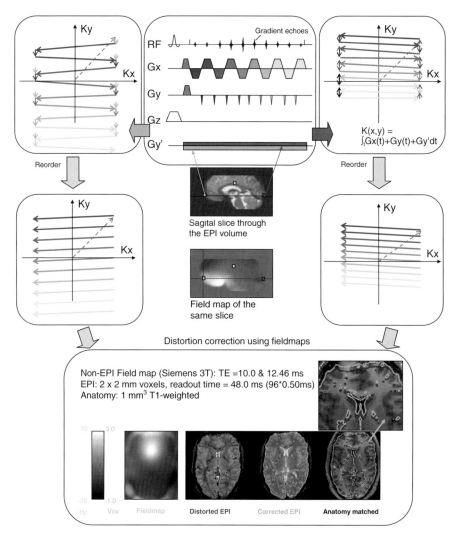

Fig. 3 Distortion in EPI images. When an extra local in-plane gradient is present in the phase-encoding direction due to susceptibility artefacts, the effective local k-space trajectory is altered. If the local gradient adds to the PE blips (as on the *left*), then the distance between the lines and k-space area covered is increased and this will cause the data to be spread over a larger area. This will make the local image data appear stretched. Alternatively, if local gradients have opposite polarity to the PE blips (as on the *right*), the k-space trajectory has less distance between the lines and covers a smaller area, and so the local image data will appear squashed. Fieldmap-based distortion correction is shown at the *bottom*. The fieldmap was obtained using a standard gradient echo sequence and two complex images at different echo times, which were masked, phase unwrapped and smoothed. This can be converted into units of displacement (here in voxels), and then the EPI image can be unwarped using the voxel displacement. This improves the match to the anatomical image that does not suffer from distortion

they do not always significantly reduce distortion and can introduce increased blurring. In recent years, a new group of methods, collectively known as parallel imaging (PI) have allowed a considerable increase in acquisition speed (Carlson and Minemura 1993; Hutchinson and Raff 1988; Pruessmann et al. 1999; Sodickson and Manning 1997). These all rely on the parallel use of receiver coils with different spatially varying sensitivities. Some calibration of the sensitivity functions of these coils gives information that is complementary to standard Fourier encoding. This allows a reduction in the density with which k-space must be sampled, reducing the distortion by the factor of speed-up (reduction in sampling density) employed in the PE direction. The penalty for all of these methods is a reduction in SNR and a potential increase in image reconstruction artefacts that can outweigh the benefits (Lutcke et al. 2006). Lastly, there are methods for correcting the distortion. These rely on mapping the underlying B_0 field, which means that the distortion can be spatially calibrated and corrected. Methods for B_0 mapping are numerous (e.g. Gruetter and Tkac 2000; Lamberton et al. 2007; Mansfield 1984; Poser et al. 2006; Priest et al. 2006), but most simply perform two scans at different TEs. The local phase difference between the images is proportional to the local magnetic field. The phase difference can then be translated into a pixel shift map to visualise and correct these distortions, as shown in Fig. 3 (Chen and Wyrwicz 1999; Hutton et al. 2002; Jezzard and Balaban 1995; Munger et al. 2000; Reber et al. 1998; Schmithorst et al. 2001; Zaitsev et al. 2004). The main limitation of this method is that information from regions where the data is squashed into a smaller area cannot be fully recovered. This can be overcome if images are obtained with alternate directions for k-space traversal (in the PE direction), effectively switching the areas that are squashed to being stretched and vice versa (Morgan et al. 2004; Weiskopf et al. 2005). However, differences between alternate volumes can be hard to eliminate, and an effective reduction in temporal resolution or volume coverage is likely. Distortions can still pose a problem for standard fMRI and EEG–fMRI studies, particularly when high structural fidelity is required, such as when fMRI is used to assist in presurgical mapping of eloquent cortex, or where presurgical EEG–fMRI results from epilepsy patients are evaluated against structural images obtained postresection.

2.3
Signal Dropout

Dropout, like distortion, is due to strong local magnetic field gradients interfering with the image acquisition process. There are two related but distinct mechanisms by which signal dropout can occur. The primary mechanism is due to local fields across the slice (through the imaging plane). The local magnetic fields cause magnetisation at different positions across the slice width to produce signals with corresponding frequencies. These signals from different positions will, with time, accumulate differing phases and so cancel; the net effect is more rapid signal decay (see Fig. 4). If the signal decays substantially before the centre of k-space has been traversed, where the main low-frequency components of the signal are encoded, the majority of the signal is not sampled and so the region will appear dark. The second mechanism is dropout due to in-plane gradients; if the in-plane gradients are strong enough, they will alter the k-space trajectory (i.e. an

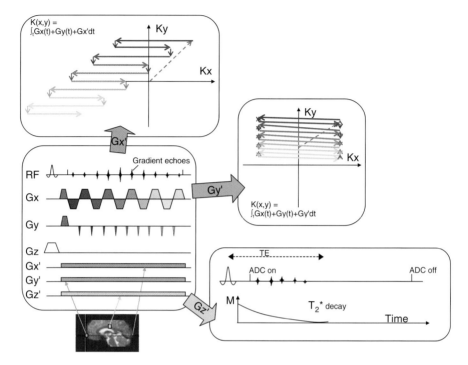

Fig. 4 Dropout in EPI images. Different mechanisms that cause signal dropout in EPI images are shown. An extra local gradient is present due to susceptibility artefacts (Gx', Gy' or Gz'). In the case of a local gradient Gz' from one particular position, this causes faster T_2^* decay via through-plane dephasing, such that the signal has decayed before the centre of k-space has been sampled. Dropout can also occur when the local in-plane gradients Gx' or Gy' cause an alteration in the k-space trajectory such that the centre of k-space is not sampled. Note that even if the k-space centre is sampled, this will occur either much earlier or later in the echo train, leading to a greatly reduced BOLD sensitivity

extreme example of what we saw previously for distortion). For dropout to occur, the trajectory must be altered radically such that the central region of k-space is not covered (see Fig. 4) (Deichmann et al. 2002, 2003; Weiskopf et al. 2006, 2007). It must also be remembered that in-plane gradients are still problematic even when dropout does not occur. This is because the effective TE (the point at which the centre of k-space is sampled) is shifted in time to earlier or later in the readout. An earlier TE will mean that there is strong signal but little BOLD contrast, whereas a later TE will have strong contrast but the signal will have decayed too much. Both in-plane and through-plane local susceptibility-related gradients can be increased where stronger magnetic fields are produced by EEG equipment.

There are a number of approaches that can be adopted to minimise dropout, primarily concerned with through-slice effects. The first consideration is the TE; reducing the TE means that the centre of k-space will be covered sooner, before the signal has largely decayed, and so reduces dropout. However, the BOLD sensitivity is reduced with TE.

The balance required is to minimise the TE without strongly reducing the BOLD sensitivity (Deichmann et al. 2002). At 1.5 T, this means that a TE of around 50 ms is typically used, shortening to around 30 ms at 3 T. Another initial very simple approach is to decrease the slice thickness, reducing the frequency range across the slice, and hence the degree of phase dispersion that will occur (Frahm et al. 1993; Merboldt et al. 2000). Some penalty is incurred in terms of signal for well-shimmed areas (i.e. areas with a uniform local magnetic field) due to decreased voxel volume, whereas poorly shimmed areas will benefit from a large increase in signal. There is also a penalty in terms of volume coverage, although gaps between slices can be increased. The balance between these different factors will depend on the particular experiment, regions of primary interest, the sequence and the scanner. In addition to making the slices thinner, the orientation of the slices can also be altered to minimise dropout (Cho et al. 1988; Deichmann et al. 2002; Weiskopf et al. 2006). Since the primary loss is due to gradients across the slice, by changing the slice tilt the size of the local gradients perpendicular to the slice plane can be reduced. However, slice tilting is often used to reduce the size of in-plane gradients that are causing dropout or reduced BOLD sensitivity. The increased through-plane gradients are then compensated with a z-shim (discussed below).

Despite optimising TE, slice thickness and slice tilt, significant dropout can still occur, particularly in orbitofrontal regions and the temporal poles (Deichmann et al. 2003). The local B_0 gradients produced by putting a subject into the magnet field can be compensated for by using a pulse sequence with an additional preparatory gradient of opposite polarity but similar area, which is generally referred to as a z-shim (Constable and Spencer 1999; Frahm et al. 1988; Ordidge et al. 1994a). There are two main effects from utilising a z-shim. Firstly, in areas of the brain that are not affected by strong local gradients, the $T_2{}^*$ is effectively increased and so this can reduce the BOLD sensitivity when using the same TE sequence. This suggests that only a moderate z-shim can be used without a significant penalty in sensitivity over much of the brain (Deichmann et al. 2002). Secondly, in areas where the z-shim compensates for local gradients, a large improvement in dropout is achieved with a correspondingly large improvement in sensitivity to BOLD signal changes. Unfortunately, it is normally difficult to achieve a z-shim improvement in one area without a decrease of performance in another, and so the optimal choice of z-shim (and slice tilt combination) will depend on the regions of most interest for a particular study (Deichmann et al. 2002; Weiskopf et al. 2006, 2007). One way to achieve a more optimal z-shim for a greater range of areas is to use a multiecho EPI readout (Poser et al. 2006). This means that images can be obtained at several different TEs and with different compensation gradient polarities or directions. The images can then be combined very simply (e.g. by addition), or by a weighting scheme devised from calibrating BOLD sensitivity to maximise the benefits (Constable and Spencer 1999; Poser et al. 2006). There can be some cost in terms of the time taken to obtain the data from each slice, which in turn may reduce volume coverage, making a simple reduction in slice width an attractive and simpler choice. However, multiecho EPI sequences have a very high ratio of data acquisition time over scan time and so can offer a very efficient alternative strategy. Dropout is often the greatest problem in both fMRI and EEG–fMRI studies. Dropouts can be made worse (or at least BOLD sensitivity may be reduced) where EEG equipment produces increased magnetic field inhomogeneity within the brain.

2.4
Image Ghosting

In EPI, ghosting is normally produced by a mismatch between echoes formed by read gradients of opposite polarity. In Fig. 1, the process of reordering k-space is demonstrated; alternate lines are reversed (flipped about the origin) in order to have traversed k-space in the same direction for each line. Any inconsistency between lines acquired under positive- or negative-polarity gradients will cause an error in the image reconstruction (i.e. a flipped positive gradient line should be the same as a negative line if the phase encoding is the same). As alternate lines are affected, a ghost (a partial repeat of the image) will appear displaced in the phase-encoding direction by half the field of view. While this is often referred to as the "Nyquist ghost", this is misleading as it is not a data undersampling error but a mismatch between alternate PE k-space lines, and thus the term N/2 ghost is more accurate. Gradient inconsistencies, eddy currents and susceptibility gradients can all contribute to this mismatch (Feinberg and Oshio 1994; Fischer and Ladebeck 1998; Reeder et al. 1997; Wan et al. 1997; Wielopolski et al. 1998). Ghosting can be affected by EEG equipment where susceptibility-related fields are responsible. Hardware improvements to increase gradient shape accuracy and reduce eddy currents, for example, or corrections to account for these inconsistencies can all reduce the artefact level (Fischer and Ladebeck 1998). One method frequently employed to correct these mismatches in alternate lines is to employ a reference scan (or navigator echo) (Hu and Le 1996; Ordidge et al. 1994b; Wan et al. 1997). The echo train used for the EPI acquisition is performed without PE gradients. A series of echoes is formed that can alternately be reversed in time. Any shift in the TE between them (in k-space) will produce a corresponding linear phase shift in image space. This allows the phase of the Fourier-transformed echoes to be compared and the difference between them used to correct all subsequent acquisitions. A further improvement can often be made to ghosting performance if the actual k-space trajectory is measured (Duyn et al. 1998; Josephs et al. 2000). One key consideration for fMRI is the stability of the ghost, because temporal changes due to drift or correction of imaging hardware can lead to false positive activation and a reduction in temporal SNR (TSNR) (see Sect. 4.1). Ghosting can still provide significant image artefacts, particularly at higher field strengths and where EEG equipment decreases magnetic field homogeneity.

2.5
RF Interference

MRI systems are specifically designed to be maximally sensitive to RF signals around a particular frequency called the Larmor frequency of the system. RF signals are highly prevalent, particularly in the typical environment of a scanner in a busy hospital or research laboratory surrounded by a wide range of electronic equipment. To record the relatively weak RF signals from the sample without any of these confounding signals from the local RF background, the magnet is placed within a Faraday cage. This is an enclosed conductive metal sheet or fine mesh that is connected to earth, and when external static or electromagnetic radiation is incident on the cage, electric currents are generated (and dissipated via the earth) which nullify the signal within the enclosed region. To make this approach effective, a good earth and complete enclosure of a room is required. This suggests an obvious weakness of MRI systems: access in and out of the room is essential, necessitating a door; gradient and RF systems require connection through the cage. The two weak points of the Faraday cage are thus the door and filter panel. Typically, attenuation of RF to 100 dB is specified, although in practice this can be difficult to achieve. Finally, equipment for stimulus presentation, physiological monitoring, or indeed EEG equipment within the scanner room requires extra consideration. Firstly, by introducing these extra active components within the cage, any RF or electrostatic discharges they may produce will cause interference and degrade image quality. Secondly, equipment with any kind of highly conductive wire or cable crossing from outside to inside the cage (i.e. via a waveguide) is a potential route for RF to be brought into the room. A more detailed description of methods for addressing these issues is given in the chapter "EEG Instrumentation and Safety". RF interference is generally visible in one of two forms in images: an increase in the overall background noise in an image more easily quantified as a corresponding decrease in SNR, attributable to incoherent broadband RF; and/or spatially localised bright spots in the image, attributable to coherent RF at distinct frequencies, as in Fig. 8C. In most structural imaging, the RF, due to its (slice-independent) constant frequency, will appear at the same position on each slice. For EPI, this is somewhat complicated by the fact that each readout direction is reversed, resulting in the N/2 ghost of the RF artefact due to local phase inconsistencies. A repeat of the artefact in the readout direction is often produced. fMRI is particularly sensitive to RF interference because it causes a local fluctuation in the signal intensity, which can dramatically increase the temporal variance and thus severely affect sensitivity to activation. This may result in false positive activation, particularly if any of the equipment is switched on during image acquisition. We address detection and monitoring of RF performance in more detail in Sect. 5.3.

3
Other Sources of Image Artefact in fMRI

3.1
Bulk Head Motion

The recorded EEG and fMRI time series are both highly sensitive to motion. The greatest effort should be put into minimising subject movement via better head restraint and increased comfort (Laufs et al. 2008). This is especially important for patient studies in general (Hamandi et al. 2004; Salek-Haddadi et al. 2003) and when recording the highly motion-sensitive EMG. The use of a vacuum head cushion (Benar et al. 2003) has been found to minimise both motion-induced artefacts on the images and motion-induced currents contaminating the electrophysiological signal. Additionally, bite bars, inflating cuffs and subject-specific moulded cushions are also used in some centres. The use of sedative agents to suppress motion needs careful consideration, as "neuroactive" substances can alter net synaptic activity in a region-specific manner and thus fMRI signal intensity

(Kleinschmidt et al. 1999). Under certain circumstances, sedation must be considered, such as when studying very young children with fMRI (Jacobs et al. 2007).

MRI motion correction via image realignment typically entails affine coregistration, and is normally effective at dealing with small differences in head position through a scan (Ashburner and Friston 2004). However, it should be remembered that the effects of motion can last longer than the period of movement itself; for example, the effective TR seen by tissue moved into a different slice will be different, leading to signal fluctuations lasting for several TR periods (Friston et al. 1996). By including the motion realignment parameters, and preferably an expansion to take into account these extra effects, motion-related variance can be effectively modelled within general linear model (GLM) analyses (Friston et al. 1996; Lund et al. 2005). If large motion events occur, it is worth considering nulling their effects. Again, the preferred method is to include extra regressors (one for each large motion event) into the GLM to account for this variance (Lemieux et al. 2007; Salek-Haddadi et al. 2006) (as opposed to removal of data from the time series). Valuable data sets can often be recovered if motion effects are modelled sufficiently at the analysis stage (Lemieux et al. 2007). Motion correction can also be performed using navigator echoes (Ordidge et al. 1994b), which relies on the Fourier shift theorem whereby a spatial shift of the image can be detected and corrected by measurement of the phase shift within MRI k-space data.

3.2
Physiological Noise

Some "noise" is physiological and related to global or local changes in brain state that happen spontaneously. These signals were previously considered as being purely noise in terms of cognitive, paradigm-driven experiments. However, increasingly, these spontaneous changes are being treated as signals of interest (Biswal et al. 1995; Fox and Raichle 2007; Laufs et al. 2003). EEG–fMRI allows some interpretation of these spatial patterns in terms of brain state (Laufs et al. 2008), and this will be addressed in more detail in subsequent chapters.

Cardiac and respiratory cycles also can cause confounding signal changes. These occur due to motion of the whole head and from changes in pressure within the skull resulting in pulsatile motion of the brain. Due to the temporal resolution of fMRI normally being below that of the cardiac signals, aliasing occurs and must be accounted for; otherwise these effects can look like low-frequency BOLD-related signal changes. Methods are available to derive regressors from EEG/EOG/ECG signals for subsequent entry into standard GLM analysis to remove any confounding signal variance from these sources (Glover et al. 2000; Liston et al. 2006).

4
The Impact of EEG Recording on MR Image Quality

In the chapters "EEG Quality: Origin and Reduction of the EEG Cardiac-Related Artefact" and "EEG Quality: The Image Acquisition Artefact", the effects of MRI on the EEG signal were discussed; here, we instead look at the potential influence of the EEG system on MRI image quality. As previously described, fMRI relies on good SNR, a high degree of temporal stability, and can be affected by artefacts due to the way that GE-EPI data is acquired. The presence of an EEG system can interact with both the static and rotating magnetic fields required for signal excitation and reception (Mullinger et al. 2007), which can have a subsequent impact on image quality (Krakow et al. 2000), as described below. Fortunately, these effects can be minimised by careful design of the EEG equipment.

4.1
Main Static Magnetic Field (B_0) Effects

MRI utilises a very strong, highly uniform main magnetic field, which is perturbed by the presence of any material with a magnetic susceptibility (χ). This degree of disturbance depends on the main field strength and the magnetic susceptibility ($\Delta B_0 = \chi B_0$). The high strength of the main field dictates that even weakly magnetic material such as water ($\chi = \sim 1 \times 10^{-7}$) can cause a local change in the magnetic field that can increase the distortion, dropout and ghosting described above. The main magnetic field can be readily measured from two gradient echo images with a different TE. The local difference between the phase of the images is due to the local magnetic fields, and so the offset of the field in Hz can be calculated (as for distortion correction). Even the weakly magnetic materials typically used in an MRI-compatible EEG cap have susceptibility values capable of introducing artefacts. The effect of two different commercially available MRI caps (both employing Ag/AgCl ring electrodes, 5 kΩ resistors, copper-braided wires and Abralyte 200 conductive gel) on the B_0 field in a uniform phantom taken from Mullinger et al. is shown in Fig. 5. There are clear localised regions of decreased homogeneity caused by the electrodes of the cap that are made worse with higher field strength. Taken over the volume, there is an increase in the number of pixels with a large field offset (Mullinger et al. 2007). However, in the same study, a similar measurement over the human brain at 3 T did not yield such a clear difference between cap on/cap off. A range of materials are available for the electrode heads, connecting wires, current-limiting resistors added for safety reasons (Lemieux et al. 1997), adhesives and gels, although a balance must be struck between EEG performance and the imaging requirements. Two factors determine the severity and impact of artefact caused by these components at a given field strength: its susceptibility and its position relative to both imaging and brain geometry. The relative geometry of the head and the electrodes is fixed by the experimental requirement of good EEG coverage (Debener et al. 2008). The available evidence suggests that plastic AgCl-coated electrodes can yield a small improvement in B_0 performance, although Ag/AgCl electrodes can also perform similarly in terms of image quality (Stevens et al. 2007) and may provide improved EEG quality. Both of these electrode types caused B_0 field perturbations over 10–15 mm at 4 T (Stevens et al. 2007) and so should not unduly affect signals from the brain when imaging the human head. Alternatives to the commonly used metallic EEG electrode materials (silver, silver chloride, gold) such as carbon may also yield low artefact levels (Krakow et al. 2000), while Sn or brass plated with Ni then Au can cause greater problems (Baumann and Noll 1999; Stevens et al. 2007). The susceptibility of most electrode gels is broadly similar to tissue (due to the conductivity required for EEG), giving limited scope for improvement in susceptibility-related artefacts caused by the gel/air interface. The choice of material for

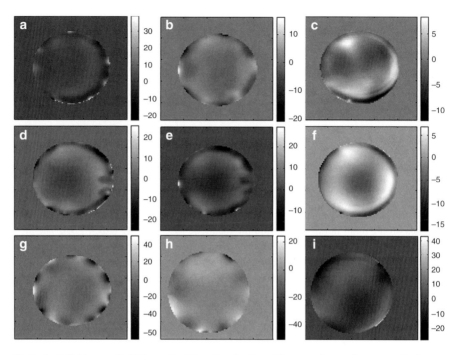

Fig. 5a–i B_0 field maps (in Hz) acquired from the phantom. Maps are shown after removal of large-scale field variations (due to the global shim) to view primarily the effect of the EEG cap at 1.5 T (**a–c**), 3 T (**d–f**) and 7 T (**g–i**) with the 64-electrode cap (*left*), 32-electrode cap (*centre*) and no cap (*right*) on. Reproduced with permission from Mullinger et al. (2007)

the safety resistors needs more careful selection, as many resistors use ferro- or diamagnetic materials, for example in the end caps connecting the terminating wires to the resistive material (Krakow et al. 2000). In the tests of Mullinger et al. (2007), the interface between the plastic surface of the phantom and the EEG electrodes and gel is likely to be the source of the greater variance in B_0. This interface is not present in the human head (see Fig. 6), where B_0 variation appears to be reduced compared to within the phantom. Increased inhomogeneity in B_0 will be seen as increased EPI image artefacts, with dropout, distortion and potentially ghosting produced. However, provided that the materials used for EEG electrodes and gel are carefully chosen and tested, there is only a small increase in B_0 inhomogeneity within the human brain, limiting the impact on image quality.

4.2
Transverse Rotational Magnetic Field (B_1) Effects

MRI signal excitation and reception uses a rotating RF field at the Larmor frequency, as described in Sect. 3.1.2. To excite the sample, an RF field is applied that causes the magnetisation to be rotated from the longitudinal axis into the transverse plane. This magnetisation then subsequently creates a rotating RF field that can then be detected by the RF coil. Any nonuniformity in the excitation profile makes it difficult to excite all of the magnetisa-

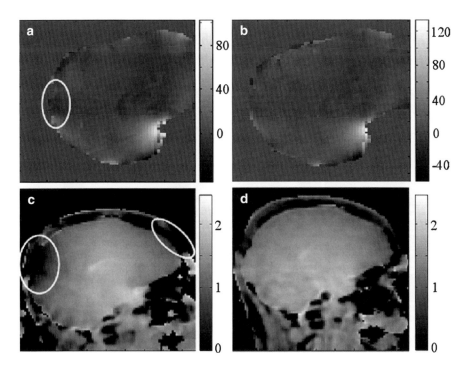

Fig. 6a–d B_0 and B_1 maps obtained in the human head. Effects of 32-electrode cap at 3 T on B_0 maps (in Hz) (**a**, **b**) and flip angle maps (normalised to average flip angle) (**c**, **d**). **a**, **c** Acquired with the cap on (regions affected are *highlighted*); **b**, **d** with no cap. Reproduced with permission from Mullinger et al (2007)

tion within the object (i.e. the flip angle will not be uniformly 90° across the object), and so some regions will suffer a corresponding signal reduction. Via the principle of reciprocity (Hoult and Lauterbur 1976), the B_1 field created by the coil for signal excitation is the same as the sensitivity of the coil (the MRI correlate of an EEG gain matrix) for signal detection. This means that the object will have a spatial variation in signal detection performance with the same pattern as for signal excitation.[2] Furthermore, the introduction of any conductive or dielectric material (i.e. the head or an EEG electrode) causes a change in the B_1 field (Sled and Pike 1998). This is because the field induces surface currents in the material that act to minimise the field produced within the object (i.e. they shield the object from the field). It is useful to consider the effects on two length scales: firstly, a global effect from the introduction of the EEG system that can generally be considered a loss of coil efficiency, and so SNR (see the section on the impact on SNR); secondly, local changes in the B_1 field are produced by local current flow which acts to reduce the B_1 field. This will produce areas with a reduced flip angle for signal excitation, and so a reduced signal and a corresponding drop in sensitivity for signal reception.

---

[2]This assumes that the same coil is used for both signal excitation and reception. It is increasingly common for different coils to be used for each purpose, with each imposing a different pattern.

The B_1 performance for the two EEG caps described in the previous section in a phantom can be seen in Fig. 7. The EEG cap has an effect on B_1 that appears to increase with field strength and is worse around the ECG wire. This is likely to be due to the increased

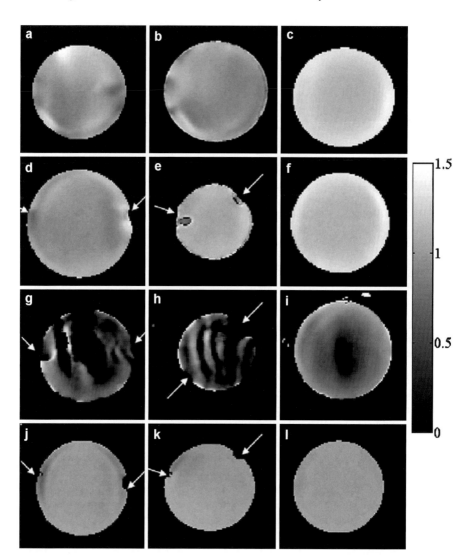

Fig. 7a–l Flip angle maps (B_1) acquired from a phantom. Flip angle maps of the phantom (normalised to average flip angle) with the 64-electrode cap (*left*), the 32-electrode cap (*centre*) and no cap (*right*). **a–c** show maps acquired at 3 T from similar slices to those shown in Fig. 1. The maps shown in the rest of the figure are taken from more inferior slices and show the effect of B_1 perturbations occurring in proximity to the ECG and EOG wires (*arrowed*) at 3 T (**d–f**), 7 T (**g–i**) and 1.5 T (**j–l**). A more inferior slice is shown for the 64-electrode cap compared with the 32-electrode cap, as the paths of the EOG and ECG wires were different on these caps. Thresholding in low-signal areas leads to the generation of significantly sized areas in the 7 T maps where the flip angle can not be characterised. Reproduced with permission from Mullinger et al (2007)

coupling of the longer length ECG wire to the RF field, with the induction of greater currents than for the shorter EEG wires. The B_1 perturbation produced by the electrodes themselves appears weak, at least at the lower field strengths. Increased electrode impedance decreases the perturbation in the B_1 field: Krakow et al. demonstrated that both plastic coated with AgCl and carbon electrodes, which offer greater impedance than metallic electrode materials, gave less artefact (Krakow et al. 2000). However, in a different comparison of electrodes at 4 T, where B_1 was independently assessed, similar shielding was produced by three different electrode types, with shielding reduced to 5% at 10–11 mm from the electrode (Stevens et al. 2007). In addition, secondary currents can flow in the safety resistors and cause artefacts, so these must be chosen carefully. Electrode wires can cause B_1 perturbations, even when safety resistors are present (Mullinger et al. 2007); higher-impedance alternatives such as carbon can reduce this artefact (Krakow et al. 2000).

RF pulses that aim to produce a uniform flip angle despite local variation in B_1 (frequently referred to as "adiabatic" pulses) do exist (Garwood et al. 1989; Garwood and Delabarre 2001), but are more commonly employed for global signal inversion or refocusing, and normally require greater RF power than standard excitation pulses (de Graaf et al. 1996). Certainly, investigation of EEG–fMRI performance with spatially selective 90° pulses that exhibit acceptable off-resonance behaviour such as derivatives of the BIR4 pulse (de Graaf et al. 1996; Shen and Rothman 1997) are merited, and may be essential to limit artefacts at higher field strengths. B_1 perturbations will produce regional intensity variation in EPI images without increased distortion. One simple method to determine whether B_1 or B_0 field effects are responsible for regionally reduced performance (where B_0 and B_1 mapping sequences are not available) is to compare spin echo 2DFT images with the EPI; where both exhibit changes in image intensity, the problem can be assigned to a local B_1 effect.

4.3
Impact on SNR

The overall effect of the introduction of the EEG system is a reduction in SNR. Locally this can be due to reduced signal related to decreased B_0 and B_1 homogeneity. Globally, there will be an average reduction in B_1 sensitivity due to the introduction of EEG equipment from shielding effects, and increased noise from increased RF coil impedance, with a concomitant global reduction in SNR. The shielding effect is a reduction in B_1 in the head from induced current flow in the EEG electrodes. To understand the increase in noise, the system can be considered as a whole with a highly resonant RF coil circuit having its impedance increased by the introduction of the head, and then further increased by the introduction of EEG components. While the increase in impedance (a reduction in the coil efficiency usually measured by the Q factor) is one effect, it is also possible that the whole system (coil with head and EEG system inside) suffers from a split or shifted resonant frequency. In this case, a quite dramatic reduction in coil performance can result. A reduction in SNR within the images will be seen, but, where the same coil is used for RF transmission, there will also be a large increase in the transmitted power required for a particular RF excitation, and increased local electric fields with the associated safety risks (Lemieux et al. 1997).

In the image quality study of Krakow et al. (2000), only the increase in electronic noise due to the introduction of the EEG amplifier was investigated, and no noise increase was detected when properly shielded. While this approach will detect any RF interference, it does not determine the amount of SNR loss due to a reduction in the RF coil performance via the mechanisms described above. One previous study observed a reduction in SNR that was proportional to the number of electrodes in the cap (Scarff et al. 2004), while an innovative ink cap that uses conductive ink rather than conventional wires had little apparent effect on the SNR (Vasios et al. 2006). More recently, tests of two commercially available caps at different field strengths on five subjects found a reduction of 4–28% in the TSNR. A smaller SNR reduction was found on the 3 T system, although this could be due to cap design and may not lead to a large difference in detected activation (Bonmassar et al. 2001). While some decrease in TSNR (see Sect. 5.1) could be caused by increased movement due to the greater discomfort of wearing an EEG cap, it is likely that this is also because of cap–coil interaction. It is worth noting that reducing the appearance of B_1-related artefacts is worthwhile even when they do not appear to greatly affect signal from the brain, because reducing this interaction will improve the overall SNR performance via reduced loading/detuning of the RF coil.

5
fMRI Quality Assurance (QA)

The large demands placed on MRI hardware by scanning at close to the maximum gradient switching rate and amplitude for extended periods, coupled with the sensitivity of fMRI to any temporal signal changes, means that careful, regular fMRI QA is important to ensure that scanner performance is maximised and any faults are quickly detected. In this section, some of the key QA measurements are described. In many respects, the principle is more important than any specific tests; the more that careful, regular, quantitative monitoring of the system is performed, the better. In particular, we focus on tests aimed more generally at fMRI QA, but which constitute a good basic set of tests of fMRI data quality that can be performed both with and without the EEG equipment. A summary of this can be found in Table 1.

5.1
Quantification of SNR and Temporal SNR

The receiver bandwidth determines the frequencies and levels of signal and noise obtained (given a certain object imaged at a specified resolution), since most of the signal is normally concentrated at low frequencies, whereas the noise is distributed across the frequency range. However, given that a certain bandwidth is used for a specific scan protocol, then the SNR describes the quality of the data and can be very sensitive, if nonspecific, to the performance of most components of the system. A phantom should be used that

Table 1 Examples of QA procedures

Scans	Suggested frequency	Example parameters	Example measurements	What to look out for	Possible cause
Spin echo 2DFT	Daily	192×128 matrix, TE = minimum, TR = 3 s, 5 central slices	SNR	Change or fluctuations in value	Nonspecific
EPI (as used for EEG–fMRI)	Weekly	TR = 2000 ms, TE = 30 ms, 200 volumes, 27 slices	Temporal mean	Strong repeats of the image (ghosts)	Gradient performance, timing and pre-emphasis, phase correction errors
			Temporal SD reformatted as coronal sections	Lines in the slice direction / strong images	RF interference / B0 and possible gradient drift
			Weisskoff plot	Change in plot	Nonspecific
			RDC	Change in value	Nonspecific
EPI (as used for EEG–fMRI) with and without EEG cap	Monthly	TR = 2000 ms, TE = 30 ms, 200 volumes, 27 slices		Compare with the measurements without EEG equipment	EEG system fault
Repeat run	Monthly	Place slices outside the phantom and set the transmit gain to zero. Run for >10 min, i.e. 400 volumes	Play the images back as a movie with a volume in each frame	Changes in background noise level, any structure in the noise	Coherent noise patterns within certain slices suggests spiking from the gradients or electrostatic discharges from another source. Higher signal in a consistent spatial position indicates RF interference

approximates the size and loading (RF interaction) of the human head. A phantom made of gel to eliminate flow effects is also desirable for testing fMRI temporal stability. Highly accurate and easily reproducible positioning of the phantom is important within both the RF coil and the main magnetic field isocentres (i.e. the SNR measured should not change when the test is performed by a different person!). Where different RF coils are routinely employed, each should be regularly tested. Different methods can be used to take a measurement of the signal and noise. However, most simple SNR tests (such as those described here) make the assumptions that the background noise follows a Raleigh distribution in the magnitude image and that the spatial distribution of noise is homogeneous. These criteria are not met in most images from array receiver coils, or where image filtering or corrections have been applied (Constantinides et al. 1997; Dietrich et al. 2007). To sample the signal, an image of the object must be obtained and the average signal within it calculated, typically by averaging the signal over a large (>75%) area. Noise can be measured in a similar manner by taking several background regions in the image and averaging them, although care must be taken to avoid regions exhibiting any artefact from the object, such as Gibbs ringing (Haacke et al. 1999), ghosting, or if any correction or filter is applied. An alternative approach to measure the noise is to obtain a further image using identical parameters, take the difference, and calculate the standard deviation within the same region of interest (ROI) (i.e. the area defined on the first image for the signal). This method can be affected by any temporal instability and, as such, is usefully viewed to detect any structure in the noise; if edges are visible, centre frequency or gradient drift may be indicated, or if a low SNR version of the object is apparent, RF/receiver instabilities can be responsible. Also, the value obtained from each SNR measurement method will be different by a constant factor due to the rectification of Gaussian noise when a background noise region is used. Different sequences may be employed for SNR calculation, but a fully relaxed 2DFT spin echo sequence is a highly reliable method, and is complimentary to an fMRI-specific EPI run. While standard SNR measurement is sensitive to many aspects of scanner performance, it does not generally test temporal fluctuations that can affect fMRI. In contrast to the static SNR, the TSNR includes contributions from fluctuations from scanner drift from the gradients as they heat, and from the main magnetic field, ghost fluctuations due to timing errors, etc. The TSNR is simply the mean signal in a voxel divided by its variance over time. This measure of SNR can be more reliable where PI reconstruction methods and/or image filters are applied (Dietrich et al. 2007). A number of values in addition to the TSNR can be calculated and monitored from an EPI time series obtained from a phantom. One such standardised set of measurements (used by the FBIRN consortium) that can be automated is freely available (http://www.nbirn.net) and well described (Friedman and Glover 2006). These standardised QA measurements are important for cross-centre comparison (Friedman et al. 2007).

5.2
The Weisskoff Test

The Weisskoff test is a simple method for assessing scanner stability (Weisskoff 1996) and is included within the FBIRN procedure (Friedman and Glover 2006). In its original formulation, two ROIs are obtained inside and outside the phantom for each point in time and compared as the region is linearly changed in size. Taking the average mean and standard deviation produced, the standard deviation should be reduced with the square root of number of voxels in the ROI if purely Johnson noise is present from the scanner hardware and sample. The calculation can then be repeated only where the relative fluctuation from time point to time point is calculated again as the regions are linearly changed in size. Any difference between the two curves generated is attributable to extra temporal fluctuations in the images from scanner instabilities. The performance of the scanner can thus be characterised for a particular phantom and scanning sequence and the performance assessed over time. A derivative single value measure can also be obtained from this test called the radius of decorrelation (RDC), which can be thought of as being the point at which statistical independence between voxels is lost; practically speaking, it is where the two curves described above begin to deviate (see Fig. 8).

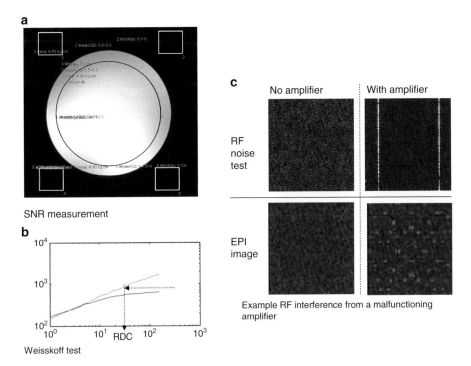

a

SNR measurement

b

Weisskoff test

c

	No amplifier	With amplifier
RF noise test		
EPI image		

Example RF interference from a malfunctioning amplifier

Fig. 8a–c Examples of QA measurements. An example SNR measurement is shown (**a**) with the mean and standard deviation in the regions of the signal and noise compared. An example Weisskoff plot is shown (**b**), including the radius of decorrelation. Finally, an example of the appearance of RF noise in images obtained with the RF transmitter effectively turned off is shown (**c**)

5.3
Coherent Noise Testing

While RF interference can affect other measurements such as SNR and the RDC, specific testing is useful because the introduction of EEG equipment into the scanner environment increases the potential for this problem to occur. As an additional test to those suggested above, viewing a 3D volume of the temporal variance (e.g. taking the magnitude image time series and calculating the temporal standard deviation for each voxel) is highly instructive. With the data displayed such that the slice direction is in the image plane (e.g. axial images reformatted as coronal sections), RF interference will be seen as stripes running along the slice direction because the source of the signal is the same frequency independent of the RF or imaging gradients and so it will appear in the same place. Very few other artefacts have a similar appearance (apart from possibly some flow effects). Another useful and simple test for detecting noise changes is to simply scan while not receiving signal from the object. This is normally achieved by setting the RF transmit gain to zero, and/or from imaging slices outside the object, and often requires any automated prescanning to be skipped or performed manually (because most clinical scanners will detect that no signal is present and the centre frequency setting, for example, will fail). By looking at a long time series of images containing pure noise, any transient increases or changes in time due to RF interference or electrostatic discharges (often called spike noise) can be relatively easily detected visually. Finally, the equipment should be tested in all possible states. For example, where different gain settings, sampling frequencies or numbers of channels may be used in an EEG amplifier, it is worthwhile checking each operational state because RF noise might be generated or its frequency shifted in one particular configuration. An example of RF noise from a malfunctioning EEG amplifier is shown in Fig. 8.

6
Summary and Conclusions

Image quality is at the core of any successful investigation of brain activity using fMRI. Therefore, it is crucial to understand the mechanisms of the image formation process and its possible pitfalls, particularly when special equipment is in the vicinity of the MRI instrument, such as that used for EEG recording. In general, properly designed and tested EEG equipment should not adversely degrade image quality. The optimisation of fMRI sequences and the application of rigorous QA protocols will ensure optimal image acquisition and minimise the risks of false-negative or false-positive findings.

Acknowledgements   I would like to thank the following contributors to this chapter: Ralf Deichmann (Brain Imaging Centre, Frankfurt) for his useful comments about EPI artefacts; Jack Wells (Department for Medical Physics, UCL, London), Philip Allen (Department of Clinical Neurophysiology, National Hospital for Neurology and Neurosurgery, London) and Nikolaus Weiskopf for careful reading of the manuscript; Chloe Hutton and Nikolaus Weiskopf (Wellcome Trust Centre for Neuroimaging, UCL, London) for providing the distortion correction part of Fig. 3 and the Weisskoff plot script for Fig. 8b; Alison Duncan (AMRIG, UCL, London) for providing Fig. a; Richard Bowtell (Sir Peter Mansfield Magnetic Resonance Centre, Nottingham, UK) and the International Journal of Psychophysiology (doi:10.1016/j.ijpsycho.2007.06.008) for allowing the reproduction of Figs. 5–7.

References

Ahn CB, Kim JH, Cho ZH (1986) High speed spiral scan echo planar imaging. IEEE Trans Med Imaging 5(1):2–5
Ashburner J, Friston K (2004) Rigid body registration. In: Frackowiak RSJ, Friston KJ, Frith CD, Dolan RJ, Price CJ, Zeki S, Ashburner J, Penny W (eds) Human brain function. Elsevier, Amsterdam, pp 635–653
Bandettini PA, Wong EC, Jesmanowicz A, Hinks RS, Hyde JS (1994) Spin-echo and gradient-echo EPI of human brain activation using BOLD contrast: a comparative study at 1.5 T. NMR Biomed 7:12–20
Baumann SB, Noll DC (1999) A modified electrode cap for EEG recordings in MRI scanners. Clin Neurophysiol 110:2189–2193

Benar C, Aghakhani Y, Wang Y, Izenberg A, Al Asmi A, Dubeau F, Gotman J (2003) Quality of EEG in simultaneous EEG–fMRI for epilepsy. Clin Neurophysiol 114:569–580

Biswal B, Yetkin FZ, Haughton VM, Hyde JS (1995) Functional connectivity in the motor cortex of resting human brain using echo-planar MRI. Magn Reson Med 34:537–541

Block KT, Frahm J (2005) Spiral imaging: a critical appraisal. J Magn Reson Imaging 21:657–668

Bonmassar G, Hadjikhani N, Ives JR, Hinton D, Belliveau JW (2001) Influence of EEG electrodes on the BOLD fMRI signal. Hum Brain Mapp 14:108–115

Bornert P, Jensen D (1994) Single-shot-double-echo EPI. Magn Reson Imaging 12:1033–1038

Butts K, Riederer SJ, Ehman RL, Thompson RM, Jack CR (1994) Interleaved echo planar imaging on a standard MRI system. Magn Reson Med 31:67–72

Carlson JW, Minemura T (1993) Imaging time reduction through multiple receiver coil data acquisition and image reconstruction. Magn Reson Med 29:681–687

Carmichael DW, Priest AN, De Vita E, Ordidge RJ (2005) Common SENSE (sensitivity encoding using hardware common to all MR scanners): a new method for single-shot segmented echo planar imaging. Magn Reson Med 54:402–410

Chen NK, Wyrwicz AM (1999) Correction for EPI distortions using multi-echo gradient-echo imaging. Magn Reson Med 41:1206–1213

Cho ZH, Kim DJ, Kim YK (1988) Total inhomogeneity correction including chemical shifts and susceptibility by view angle tilting. Med Phys 15:7–11

Cohen MS, Weisskoff RM, Rzedzian RR, Kantor HL (1990) Sensory stimulation by time-varying magnetic fields. Magn Reson Med 14:409–414

Constable RT, Spencer DD (1999) Composite image formation in z-shimmed functional MR imaging. Magn Reson Med 42:110–117

Constantinides CD, Atalar E, McVeigh ER (1997) Signal-to-noise measurements in magnitude images from NMR phased arrays. Magn Reson Med 38:852–857

Cusack R, Russell B, Cox SM, De Panfilis C, Schwarzbauer C, Ansorge R (2005) An evaluation of the use of passive shimming to improve frontal sensitivity in fMRI. Neuroimage 24:82–91

de Graaf RA, Nicolay K, Garwood M (1996) Single-shot, B1-insensitive slice selection with a gradient-modulated adiabatic pulse, BISS-8. Magn Reson Med 35:652–657

Debener S, Mullinger KJ, Niazy RK, Bowtell RW (2008) Properties of the ballistocardiogram artefact as revealed by EEG recordings at 1.5, 3 and 7 T static magnetic field strength. Int J Psychophysiol 67:189–199

Deichmann R, Gottfried JA, Hutton C, Turner R (2003) Optimized EPI for fMRI studies of the orbitofrontal cortex. Neuroimage 19:430–441

Deichmann R, Josephs O, Hutton C, Corfield DR, Turner R (2002) Compensation of susceptibility-induced BOLD sensitivity losses in echo-planar fMRI imaging. Neuroimage 15:120–135

Dietrich O, Raya JG, Reeder SB, Reiser MF, Schoenberg SO (2007) Measurement of signal-to-noise ratios in MR images: influence of multichannel coils, parallel imaging, and reconstruction filters. J Magn Reson Imaging 26:375–385

Duong TQ, Yacoub E, Adriany G, Hu X, Ugurbil K, Vaughan JT, Merkle H, Kim SG (2002) High-resolution, spin-echo BOLD, and CBF fMRI at 4 and 7 T. Magn Reson Med 48:589–593

Duyn JH, Yang Y, Frank JA, van der Veen JW (1998) Simple correction method for k-space trajectory deviations in MRI. J Magn Reson 132:150–153

Feinberg DA, Hale JD, Watts JC, Kaufman L, Mark A (1986) Halving MR imaging time by conjugation: demonstration at 3.5 kG. Radiology 161:527–531

Feinberg DA, Kiefer B, Johnson G (1995) GRASE improves spatial resolution in single shot imaging. Magn Reson Med 33:529–533

Feinberg DA, Oshio K (1994) Phase errors in multi-shot echo planar imaging. Magn Reson Med 32:535–539

Feinberg DA, Reese TG, Wedeen VJ (2002) Simultaneous echo refocusing in EPI. Magn Reson Med 48:1–5

Fernandez-Seara MA, Wang Z, Wang J, Rao HY, Guenther M, Feinberg DA, Detre JA (2005) Continuous arterial spin labeling perfusion measurements using single shot 3D GRASE at 3 T. Magn Reson Med 54:1241–1247

Fischer H, Ladebeck R (1998) Echo-planar imaging image artefacts. In: Schmitt F, Stehling MK, Turner R (eds) Echo-planar imaging. Springer, Berlin, pp 180–200

Fox MD, Raichle ME (2007) Spontaneous fluctuations in brain activity observed with functional magnetic resonance imaging. Nat Rev Neurosci 8:700–711

Frahm J, Merboldt KD, Hanicke W (1993) Functional MRI of human brain activation at high spatial resolution. Magn Reson Med 29:139–144

Frahm J, Merboldt KD, Hanicke W (1988) Direct FLASH MR imaging of magnetic field inhomogeneities by gradient compensation. Magn Reson Med 6:474–480

Friedman L, Glover GH (2006) Report on a multicenter fMRI quality assurance protocol. J Magn Reson Imaging 23:827–839

Friedman L, Stern H, Brown GG, Mathalon DH, Turner J, Glover GH, Gollub RL, Lauriello J, Lim KO, Cannon T, Greve DN, Bockholt HJ, Belger A, Mueller B, Doty MJ, He J, Wells W, Smyth P, Pieper S, Kim S, Kubicki M, Vangel M, Potkin SG (2007) Test-retest and between-site reliability in a multicenter fMRI study. Hum Brain Mapp 29:958–972

Friston KJ, Williams S, Howard R, Frackowiak RS, Turner R (1996) Movement-related effects in fMRI time-series. Magn Reson Med 35:346–355

Garwood M, Delabarre L (2001) The return of the frequency sweep: designing adiabatic pulses for contemporary NMR. J Magn Reson 153:155–177

Garwood M, Ugurbil K, Rath AR, Bendall MR, Ross BD, Mitchell SL, Merkle H (1989) Magnetic resonance imaging with adiabatic pulses using a single surface coil for RF transmission and signal detection. Magn Reson Med 9:25–34

Glover GH, Law CS (2001) Spiral-in/out BOLD fMRI for increased SNR and reduced susceptibility artifacts. Magn Reson Med 46:515–522

Glover GH, Li TQ, Ress D (2000) Image-based method for retrospective correction of physiological motion effects in fMRI: RETROICOR. Magn Reson Med 44:162–167

Griswold MA, Jakob PM, Heidemann RM, Nittka M, Jellus V, Wang J, Kiefer B, Haase A (2002) Generalized autocalibrating partially parallel acquisitions (GRAPPA) 121. Magn Reson Med 47:1202–1210

Gruetter R (1993) Automatic, localized in vivo adjustment of all first- and second-order shim coils. Magn Reson Med 29:804–811

Gruetter R, Tkac I (2000) Field mapping without reference scan using asymmetric echo-planar techniques. Magn Reson Med 43:319–323

Haacke EM, Brown RW, Thompson MR, Venkatesan R (1999) The continuous and discrete Fourier transforms. In: Magnetic resonance imaging: physical principles and sequence design. Wiley, New York, pp 207–230

Hamandi K, Salek-Haddadi A, Fish DR, Lemieux L (2004) EEG/functional MRI in epilepsy: the Queen Square Experience. J Clin Neurophysiol 21:241–248

Hennel F, Nedelec JF (1995) Interleaved asymmetric echo-planar imaging. Magn Reson Med 34:520–524

Hoult DI, Lauterbur PC (1976) The signal to noise ratio of the nuclear magnetic resonance experiment. J Magn Reson 34:425–433

Hu X, Le TH (1996) Artifact reduction in EPI with phase-encoded reference scan. Magn Reson Med 36:166–171

Hutchinson M, Raff U (1988) Fast MRI data acquisition using multiple detectors. Magn Reson Med 6:87–91

Hutton C, Bork A, Josephs O, Deichmann R, Ashburner J, Turner R (2002) Image distortion correction in fMRI: a quantitative evaluation. Neuroimage 16:217–240

Jacobs J, Kobayashi E, Boor R, Muhle H, Stephan W, Hawco C, Dubeau F, Jansen O, Stephani U, Gotman J, Siniatchkin M (2007) Hemodynamic responses to interictal epileptiform discharges in children with symptomatic epilepsy. Epilepsia 48:2068–2078

Jezzard P, Balaban RS (1995) Correction for geometric distortion in echo planar images from B0 field variations 50. Magn Reson Med 34:65–73

Jezzard P, Clare S (1999) Sources of distortion in functional MRI data. Hum Brain Mapp 8:80–85

Josephs O, Weiskopf N, Deichmann R, Turner R (2000) Trajectory measurement and generalised reconstruction in rectilinear EPI. In: Proc 8th Int Meet ISMRM, Denver, CO, USA, 1–7 April 2000

Kleinschmidt A, Bruhn H, Kruger G, Merboldt KD, Stoppe G, Frahm J (1999) Effects of sedation, stimulation, and placebo on cerebral blood oxygenation: a magnetic resonance neuroimaging study of psychotropic drug action. NMR Biomed 12:286–292

Krakow K, Allen PJ, Symms MR, Lemieux L, Josephs O, Fish DR (2000) EEG recording during fMRI experiments: image quality. Hum Brain Mapp 10:10–15

Lamberton F, Delcroix N, Grenier D, Mazoyer B, Joliot M (2007) A new EPI-based dynamic field mapping method: application to retrospective geometrical distortion corrections. J Magn Reson Imaging 26:747–755

Laufs H, Daunizeau J, Carmichael DW, Kleinschmidt A (2008) Recent advances in recording electrophysiological data simultaneously with magnetic resonance imaging. Neuroimage 40:515–528

Laufs H, Krakow K, Sterzer P, Eger E, Beyerle A, Salek-Haddadi A, Kleinschmidt A (2003) Electroencephalographic signatures of attentional and cognitive default modes in spontaneous brain activity fluctuations at rest. Proc Natl Acad Sci USA 100:11053–11058

Lemieux L, Allen PJ, Franconi F, Symms MR, Fish DR (1997) Recording of EEG during fMRI experiments: patient safety. Magn Reson Med 38:943–952

Lemieux L, Salek-Haddadi A, Lund TE, Laufs H, Carmichael D (2007) Modelling large motion events in fMRI studies of patients with epilepsy. Magn Reson Imaging 25:894–901

Liston AD, Lund TE, Salek-Haddadi A, Hamandi K, Friston KJ, Lemieux L (2006) Modelling cardiac signal as a confound in EEG–fMRI and its application in focal epilepsy studies. Neuroimage 30:827–834

Lund TE, Norgaard MD, Rostrup E, Rowe JB, Paulson OB (2005) Motion or activity: their role in intra- and inter-subject variation in fMRI. Neuroimage 26:960–964

Lutcke H, Merboldt KD, Frahm J (2006) The cost of parallel imaging in functional MRI of the human brain. Magn Reson Imaging 24:1–5

Mackenzie IS, Robinson EM, Wells AN, Wood B (1987) A simple field map for shimming. Magn Reson Med 5:262–268

Mansfield P (1977) Multi-planar image formation using NMR spin echoes. J Phys C 10:L55–L58

Mansfield P (1984) Spatial mapping of the chemical shift in NMR. Magn Reson Med 1:370–386

Mansfield P, Harvey PR (1993) Limits to neural stimulation in echo-planar imaging. Magn Reson Med 29:746–758

Menon RS, Thomas CG, Gati JS (1997) Investigation of BOLD contrast in fMRI using multi-shot EPI. NMR Biomed 10:179–182

Merboldt KD, Finsterbusch J, Frahm J (2000) Reducing inhomogeneity artifacts in functional MRI of human brain activation-thin sections vs gradient compensation. J Magn Reson 145: 184–191

Miller KL, Hargreaves BA, Lee J, Ress D, deCharms RC, Pauly JM (2003) Functional brain imaging using a blood oxygenation sensitive steady state. Magn Reson Med 50:675–683

Miller KL, Hargreaves BA, Lee J, Ress D, deCharms RC, Pauly JM (2004) Functional brain imaging with BOSS FMRI. Conf Proc IEEE Eng Med Biol Soc 7:5234–5237

Miller KL, Smith SM, Jezzard P, Pauly JM (2006) High-resolution FMRI at 1.5T using balanced SSFP. Magn Reson Med 55:161–170

Morgan PS, Bowtell RW, McIntyre DJ, Worthington BS (2004) Correction of spatial distortion in EPI due to inhomogeneous static magnetic fields using the reversed gradient method. J Magn Reson Imaging 19:499–507

Mullinger K, Debener S, Coxon R, Bowtell R (2007) Effects of simultaneous EEG recording on MRI data quality at 1.5, 3 and 7 tesla. Int J Psychophysiol 67:178–188

Munger P, Crelier GR, Peters TM, Pike GB (2000) An inverse problem approach to the correction of distortion in EPI images. IEEE Trans Med Imaging 19:681–689

Nair G, Duong TQ (2004) Echo-planar BOLD fMRI of mice on a narrow-bore 9.4 T magnet. Magn Reson Med 52:430–434

Norris DG, Zysset S, Mildner T, Wiggins CJ (2002) An investigation of the value of spin-echo-based fMRI using a Stroop color-word matching task and EPI at 3 T. Neuroimage 15:719–726

Ordidge R (1999) The development of echo-planar imaging (EPI): 1977–1982. MAGMA 9;117–121

Ordidge RJ, Gorell JM, Deniau JC, Knight RA, Helpern JA (1994a) Assessment of relative brain iron concentrations using T2-weighted and T2*-weighted MRI at 3 Tesla. Magn Reson Med 32:335–341

Ordidge RJ, Helpern JA, Qing ZX, Knight RA, Nagesh V (1994b) Correction of motional artifacts in diffusion-weighted MR images using navigator echoes. Magn Reson Imaging 12:455–460

Parkes LM, Schwarzbach JV, Bouts AA, Deckers RH, Pullens P, Kerskens CM, Norris DG (2005) Quantifying the spatial resolution of the gradient echo and spin echo BOLD response at 3 Tesla. Magn Reson Med 54:1465–1472

Poser BA, Versluis MJ, Hoogduin JM, Norris DG (2006) BOLD contrast sensitivity enhancement and artifact reduction with multiecho EPI: parallel-acquired inhomogeneity-desensitized fMRI. Magn Reson Med 55:1227–1235

Preston AR, Thomason ME, Ochsner KN, Cooper JC, Glover GH (2004) Comparison of spiral-in/out and spiral-out BOLD fMRI at 1.5 and 3 T. Neuroimage 21:291–301

Priest AN, Carmichael DW, De Vita E, Ordidge RJ (2004) Method for spatially interleaving two images to halve EPI readout times: two reduced acquisitions interleaved (TRAIL) Magn Reson Med 51:1212–1222

Priest AN, De Vita E, Thomas DL, Ordidge RJ (2006) EPI distortion correction from a simultaneously acquired distortion map using TRAIL. J Magn Reson Imaging 23:597–603

Pruessmann KP, Weiger M, Scheidegger MB, Boesiger P (1999) SENSE: sensitivity encoding for fast MRI 18. Magn Reson Med 42;952–962

Reber PJ, Wong EC, Buxton RB, Frank LR (1998) Correction of off resonance-related distortion in echo-planar imaging using EPI-based field maps. Magn Reson Med 39:328–330

Reeder SB, Atalar E, Bolster BD Jr, McVeigh ER (1997) Quantification and reduction of ghosting artifacts in interleaved echo-planar imaging. Magn Reson Med 38:429–439

Rzedzian R (1987) High speed, high resolution, spin echo imaging by mosaic scan and MESH. In: Proc 6th Annu Meet SMRM, New York, 17–21 Aug 1987

Salek-Haddadi A, Diehl B, Hamandi K, Merschhemke M, Liston A, Friston K, Duncan JS, Fish DR, Lemieux L (2006) Hemodynamic correlates of epileptiform discharges: an EEG–fMRI study of 63 patients with focal epilepsy. Brain Res 1088:148–166

Salek-Haddadi A, Lemieux L, Merschhemke M, Diehl B, Allen PJ, Fish DR (2003) EEG quality during simultaneous functional MRI of interictal epileptiform discharges. Magn Reson Imaging 21:1159–1166

Sangill R, Wallentin M, Ostergaard L, Vestergaard-Poulsen P (2006) The impact of susceptibility gradients on cartesian and spiral EPI for BOLD fMRI. MAGMA 19:105–114

Scarff CJ, Reynolds A, Goodyear BG, Ponton CW, Dort JC, Eggermont JJ (2004) Simultaneous 3-T fMRI and high-density recording of human auditory evoked potentials. Neuroimage 23:1129–1142

Schmidt CF, Boesiger P, Ishai A (2005) Comparison of fMRI activation as measured with gradient- and spin-echo EPI during visual perception. Neuroimage 26:852–859

Schmithorst VJ, Dardzinski BJ, Holland SK (2001) Simultaneous correction of ghost and geometric distortion artifacts in EPI using a multiecho reference scan. IEEE Trans Med Imaging 20:535–539

Schmitt F, Stehling MK, Turner R (eds) (1998) Echo-planar imaging. Springer, Berlin

Shen J, Rothman DL (1997) Adiabatic slice-selective excitation for surface coils. J Magn Reson 124:72–79

Sled JG, Pike GB (1998) Standing-wave and RF penetration artifacts caused by elliptic geometry: an electrodynamic analysis of MRI. IEEE Trans Med Imaging 17:653–662

Sodickson DK, Manning WJ (1997) Simultaneous acquisition of spatial harmonics (SMASH): fast imaging with radiofrequency coil arrays. Magn Reson Med 38:591–603

Stevens TK, Ives JR, Klassen LM, Bartha R (2007) MR compatibility of EEG scalp electrodes at 4 Tesla. J Magn Reson Imaging 25:872–877

Turner R, Ordidge RJ (2000) Technical challenges of functional magnetic resonance imaging. IEEE Eng Med Biol Mag 19:42–54

van Gelderen P, de Zwart JA, Starewicz P, Hinks RS, Duyn JH (2007) Real-time shimming to compensate for respiration-induced B0 fluctuations. Magn Reson Med 57:362–368

Vasios CE, Angelone LM, Purdon PL, Ahveninen J, Belliveau JW, Bonmassar G (2006) EEG/(f) MRI measurements at 7 Tesla using a new EEG cap ("InkCap"). Neuroimage 33:1082–1092

Wan X, Gullberg GT, Parker DL, Zeng GL (1997) Reduction of geometric and intensity distortions in echo-planar imaging using a multireference scan. Magn Reson Med 37:932–942

Ward HA, Riederer SJ, Jack CR Jr. (2002) Real-time autoshimming for echo planar timecourse imaging. Magn Reson Med 48:771–780

Weiskopf N, Hutton C, Josephs O, Deichmann R (2006) Optimal EPI parameters for reduction of susceptibility-induced BOLD sensitivity losses: a whole-brain analysis at 3 T and 1.5 T. Neuroimage 33:493–504

Weiskopf N, Hutton C, Josephs O, Turner R, Deichmann R (2007) Optimized EPI for fMRI studies of the orbitofrontal cortex: compensation of susceptibility-induced gradients in the readout direction. MAGMA 20:39–49

Weiskopf N, Klose U, Birbaumer N, Mathiak K (2005) Single-shot compensation of image distortions and BOLD contrast optimization using multi-echo EPI for real-time fMRI. Neuroimage 24:1068–1079

Weisskoff RM (1996) Simple measurement of scanner stability for functional NMR imaging of activation in the brain. Magn Reson Med 36:643–645

Wielopolski PA, Schmitt F, Stehling MK (1998) Echo-planar pulse sequences. In: Schmitt F, Stehling MK, Turner R (eds) Echo-planar imaging. Springer, Berlin, pp 65–134

Wilson JL, Jenkinson M, Jezzard P (2003) Protocol to determine the optimal intraoral passive shim for minimisation of susceptibility artifact in human inferior frontal cortex 3. Neuroimage 19:1802–1811

Wilson JL, Jezzard P (2003) Utilization of an intra-oral diamagnetic passive shim in functional MRI of the inferior frontal cortex. Magn Reson Med 50:1089–1094

Zaitsev M, Hennig J, Speck O (2004) Point spread function mapping with parallel imaging techniques and high acceleration factors: fast, robust, and flexible method for echo-planar imaging distortion correction. Magn Reson Med 52:1156–1166

Zhong K, Leupold J, Hennig J, Speck O (2007) Systematic investigation of balanced steady-state free precession for functional MRI in the human visual cortex at 3 Tesla. Magn Reson Med 57:67–73

Specific Issues Related to EEG–fMRI at $B_0 > 3\,T$

11

Giorgio Bonmassar and Karen J. Mullinger

1
Introduction

Functional MRI (fMRI) can be used to map regional changes in cerebral blood flow and the level of haemoglobin oxygenation (BOLD) associated with neuronal activity (Belliveau et al. 1991; Kwong et al. 1992; Ogawa et al. 1992). In 2003 the US Food and Drug Administration raised the value of the static field of "no significant risk" for MRI to 8 Tesla (T), potentially opening up this technology to large numbers of laboratories in the USA. Regulatory agencies in Europe and Asia reached similar conclusions, and as a result the number of high-field systems worldwide is growing rapidly. The increased static field B_0 allows the potential for improved signal-to-noise ratio (SNR), offering the possibility of increasing spatial resolution and reducing scan times (Wiesinger et al. 2006; Harel et al. 2006). In this chapter, we outline the safety issues raised and the challenges involved in performing EEG at high-field MRI or at static magnetic fields greater than 3 T.

2
Safety Considerations

2.1
Physical Principles and Relevant Safety Guidelines

The physical principles and mechanisms that arise from the interaction of EEG and MRI data acquisition systems are described in the chapter "EEG Instrumentation and Safety", where the reader will also find the safety guidelines that should be taken in consideration

G. Bonmassar
AbiLab, Athinoula A. Martinos Center for Biomedical Imaging, Massachusetts General Hospital, Charlestown, MA, USA
e-mail: giorgio@nmr.mgh.harvard.edu

C. Mulert and L. Lemieux (eds.), *EEG– fMRI*
DOI: 10.1007/978-3-540-87919-0_11, © Springer Verlag Berlin Heidelberg 2010

for the simultaneous recording of EEG and fMRI data. In summary, those guidelines concern: heat deposition inside the body (FDA 2003; IEC 2002); heating of objects, such as EEG electrodes, placed in contact with the body; and tissue contact currents, such as those induced in conducting objects placed in contact with or close proximity to the body. This chapter focuses on safety considerations at high field; while the mechanisms that may result in health hazards are the same as for more standard field strengths, some of the effects are amplified by the stronger field. While the allowed SAR is constant across field strengths, the SAR of sequences employed in high-field MRI scanning is generally higher than that at lower field strengths. Moreover, although the safety record to date at standard field strengths has been good, with no reported incidents to our knowledge, the experience at high field is much more limited.

At high static magnetic fields (B_0 > 3 T), MRI employs a correspondingly higher RF frequency for signal excitation and reception because of the linear relation between Larmor frequency and B_0 field strength. Since SAR increases as the square of the Larmor frequency, problems associated with exposure to RF may worsen (Hoult et al. 2008). In addition, at B_0 = 7 T the Larmor frequency for water protons is 300 MHz (i.e. approximately corresponding to a 1-m wavelength in empty space). Hence, at higher frequencies or in different media, the size of the biological object can be comparable to or larger than the effective wavelength; this may cause problems because dielectric resonant effects cause an inhomogeneous excitation field B_1^+ (i.e. the circularly polarized component of the transverse magnetic field) (Sled and Pike 1998). As is the case at lower field strengths, localized peaks in SAR caused by interactions between the RF coil and tissue/sample properties may be a safety issue when using sequences close to volume-average SAR limits and depending on how the scanner-reported SAR is estimated. Analytical studies using homogeneous spheres to simulate the human head (Bottomley and Andrew 1978; Bottomley et al. 1985; Mansfield and Morris 1982; Glover et al. 1985; Keltner et al. 1991) have shown that as the frequency of the B_1^+ field increases homogeneity tends to decrease, and correspondingly the peak (local) SAR may be increased.

2.2
Safety Studies at High Fields

MRI-compatible temperature probes have been used for in vitro measurements (Sharan et al. 2003; Kangarlu et al. 2003), sometimes in the presence of metallic implants (Chou et al. 1997; Carmichael et al. 2008). Temperature measurements have also been carried out to specifically test the safety of EEG caps at high field. These tests have included investigating the effect of different wire lengths on RF heating (Stevens 2007a). This study showed that the extent of heating at the tip of a wire was dependent on the ratio of the wire length to the RF wavelength and that care must be taken not to set up a resonance effect in the wires of the EEG system. A commercially available 32-channel EEG cap has also been tested for heating effects at 7 T by Mullinger (2008). The results of this study showed that for the particular setup used in this case it was safe to record EEG at 7 T, although the authors highlighted the need to test new combinations of equipment, as heating effects may vary depending on the experimental setup. Vasios et al. (2006) also investigated the heating effects of a custom-made EEG cap, the "InkCap", which was designed to reduce potential RF heating effects by using distributed impedance in the conductive structures of the cap, thus reducing RF interactions. They compared the heating effects observed with this cap to those produced by commercially available EEG caps at 7 T. This study demonstrated that, at all of the locations considered, the InkCap exhibited lower or equal heating effects to those recorded from the commercially available caps.

While measurements are useful and necessary for a direct evaluation of RF heating, they do have limitations. For example, in vitro models are not always anatomically accurate (e.g. they may be based on spherical phantoms); also, temperature probes such as the fluoroscopic optical fibers are only able to provide measurements at a small number of locations (determined by the number of channels on the instrument) and only over a limited part of the test object or body (on the order of 1 mm^3) (Nitz et al. 2005). This limitation can be partly addressed using simulations that can provide estimates of the electromagnetic fields and SAR.

SAR simulation studies on anatomically accurate head models have been performed using the finite difference time domain (FDTD) method (Jin 1999), and several numerical head models have been presented in the literature (Kainz et al. 2005; Gandhi and Chen 1999). While $2 \times 2 \times 2.5$ mm^3 volume elements provide sufficient accuracy when evaluating whole-head SAR in MRI (Collins and Smith 2003), this approximation is no longer valid when peak 10 g averaged SAR is considered the main dosimetric parameter. Moreover, the spatial resolution limits proper modeling of the anatomical structures of the human head (Angelone et al. 2006), which can result in a lack of or limitations in the accuracy of EM estimation at radiofrequency in those anatomical structures. A model of human head tissue with isotropic 1 mm^3 voxels (Fig. 1), representing 21 brain and 28 non-brain anatomically accurate tissue types (Filipek et al. 1994) each associated with its electrical properties defined for that frequency according to the literature, was used to simulate the EM fields from a birdcage RF coil (Jin 1999) (Fig. 2). Simulations were carried out for a frequency of 300 MHz with perfectly matched layer boundary conditions (Berenger 1994) using the FDTD technique (Gabriel et al. 1996a, b; Dimbylow and Gandhi 1991; Cangellaris and Wright 1991). The resulting B_1-field maps reproduced the typical central brightening observed at 7 T (Fig. 2). The amount of exposure to electromagnetic fields is determined using computational models of dosimetry tested with direct measurements. Numerical simulations and measurements have also been performed using medical implants (Gangarosa et al. 1987; Chou and Guy 1979) and EEG electrodes during MRI (Carmichael et al. 2007, 2008; Angelone et al. 2004; Mirsattari et al. 2004; Ho 2001; Rezai et al. 2002). These studies show the presence of local heating, usually concentrated near the implant/electrode, and a dependence on the dimensions, orientation, shape, and location of the implant/electrode. Safety studies (Mirsattari et al. 2004; Armenean et al. 2004; Lazeyras et al. 2001; Lemieux et al. 1997) specifically designed to address the safety of EEG–fMRI have been performed at 1.5 T on human subjects, and these demonstrate that any temperature increase and induced currents can be limited to the allowed limit if adequate measures are taken and protocols followed (e.g. limiting scanning to low-SAR sequences such as gradient echo EPI, using only head RF coils, fMRI acquisition, and preselect MR instrumentation). Some studies have addressed these issues at higher field strength, with Angelone et al. (2006, 2004) investigating these effects through simulations (as detailed below), and Mullinger (2008) and Vasios et al. (2006) investigating these effects through direct temperature measurements at 7 T; both studies used a head transmit coil.

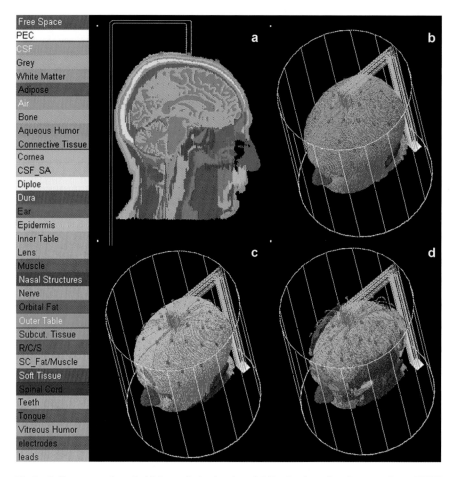

Fig. 1a–d Representation of a high-resolution head model (1 × 1 × 1 mm³) and a co-registered EEG electrode set. (**a**) The sagittal view shows the 29 tissues manually segmented. The corresponding color code for each tissue is to the left of the image. (**b**) 3D view of the head model and the EEG electrodes/leads. View of the internal tissues, where the epidermis (**c**) and the epidermis and subcutaneous fat (**d**) have been removed for illustrative purposes (*bottom*). (Reprinted from Angelone et al. 2006)

As a result of the same mechanism that leads to inhomogeneous RF excitation, enhanced local E fields are a common feature at high fields (Bottomley and Andrew 1978; Mansfield and Morris 1982; Glover et al. 1985), and so there is potentially a greater risk of extreme peaks in SAR near the electrodes/leads (Angelone 2004). In simulations at 7 T it was noticed that local SAR depends on the number of electrodes, the lead layout (e.g. different ways for the EEG wires to escape the coil), pulse sequences, the RF transmit coil type, and the head morphology.

A study using an eight-tissue model showed that whole-head SAR can increase by a factor of up to four when EEG is recorded using copper leads and 128 EEG electrodes compared to without EEG (see also the chapter "EEG Instrumentation and Safety") (Angelone

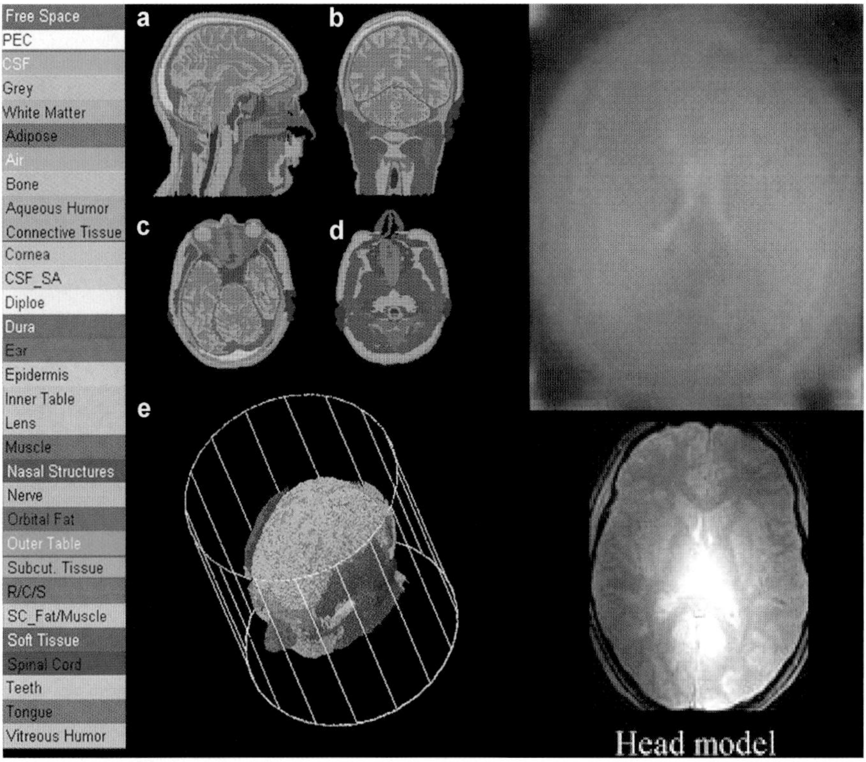

Fig. 2a–e Central brightening effect (CBE) and human head model at 7 T. *Left*: 29-structure head model with birdcage coil used for simulation at 7 T (*center*) MRI image taken on human subject at 7 T. *Right*: B_1^+ field distribution calculated using the head model. The model properly estimates the CBE distribution in the MRI images. The (**a**) sagittal, (**b**) coronal, and (**c, d**) axial views of the 29 structures segmented without and (**e**) with the birdcage head model. (Reprinted from Angelone et al. 2005)

et al. 2004) due to a large increase in the resistive load experienced by the RF coil. However, this study also showed (Fig. 3) the absence of a local hot spot irrespective of RF coil type or number of EEG electrodes used. Furthermore, it is well known (Wiggins et al. 2005) that leads or cables with lengths of the same order as the RF wavelength may result in excessive heating associated with resonance effects and coil detuning (Konings et al. 2000). This was demonstrated by Stevens (2007a), who showed that if the wire length was equal to a quarter of the RF wavelength then a resonant effect could be set up and image artifacts created. The use of RF chokes on longer wires may be an effective way to overcome this problem (Stevens 2007b). When the number of EEG leads is very high, the dense array of wires may even reduce the local SAR (Angelone et al. 2004), typically in the occipital lobe.

The effect of electrode and of lead resistivity on tissue EM fields has also been investigated, demonstrating that the material of the EEG electrodes alone has a small influence compared to the overall EEG electrode/lead configuration (Fig. 4) and that the use of current-limiting resistors between EEG electrodes and leads, which are designed to reduce the risk of RF burns due to contact currents at the skin/electrode interface (Lemieux

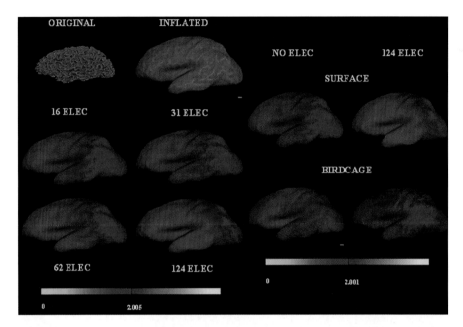

Fig. 3 *Top left*: The original pial and inflated surface of a human brain automatically segmented from MRI images. *Bottom left*: SAR distribution in the inflated cortical surface with a different number of electrodes using a surface coil. *Right*: SAR distribution for a surface (*top*) and for a birdcage coil (*bottom*) using 124 electrodes compared with a no-electrodes configuration. (Reprinted from Angelone et al. 2004)

et al. 1997), does not have a significant impact on the electric field inside the body (Angelone et al. 2006). However, it may be that at higher fields with decreasing resonant lengths the use of distributed impedance becomes more important.

While it has been shown that scanner-supplied SAR estimates are not a reliable indicator of localized heating due to conductive objects such as implants across scanners, temperature change has been shown to be proportionally related to SAR for a fixed scanning configuration (Baker et al. 2004). Furthermore, SAR is currently the only available relevant index for practical use (Shellock 2007). A possible solution is to use large safety margins in combination with carefully defined experimental protocols, for example by using MR sequences with the SAR well below power levels that cause heating close to safety guideline limits (Lemieux et al. 1997; Vasios 2006; Carmichael et al. 2007, 2008).

3
EEG Recording and Quality

While the methods described in the chapter "EEG Quality: Origin and Reduction of the EEG Cardiac-Related Artifact" that are used to minimize pulse or motion-related artifacts on EEG at the source should be employed, the laws of physics tell us that the residual artifact will be amplified in high-field conditions.

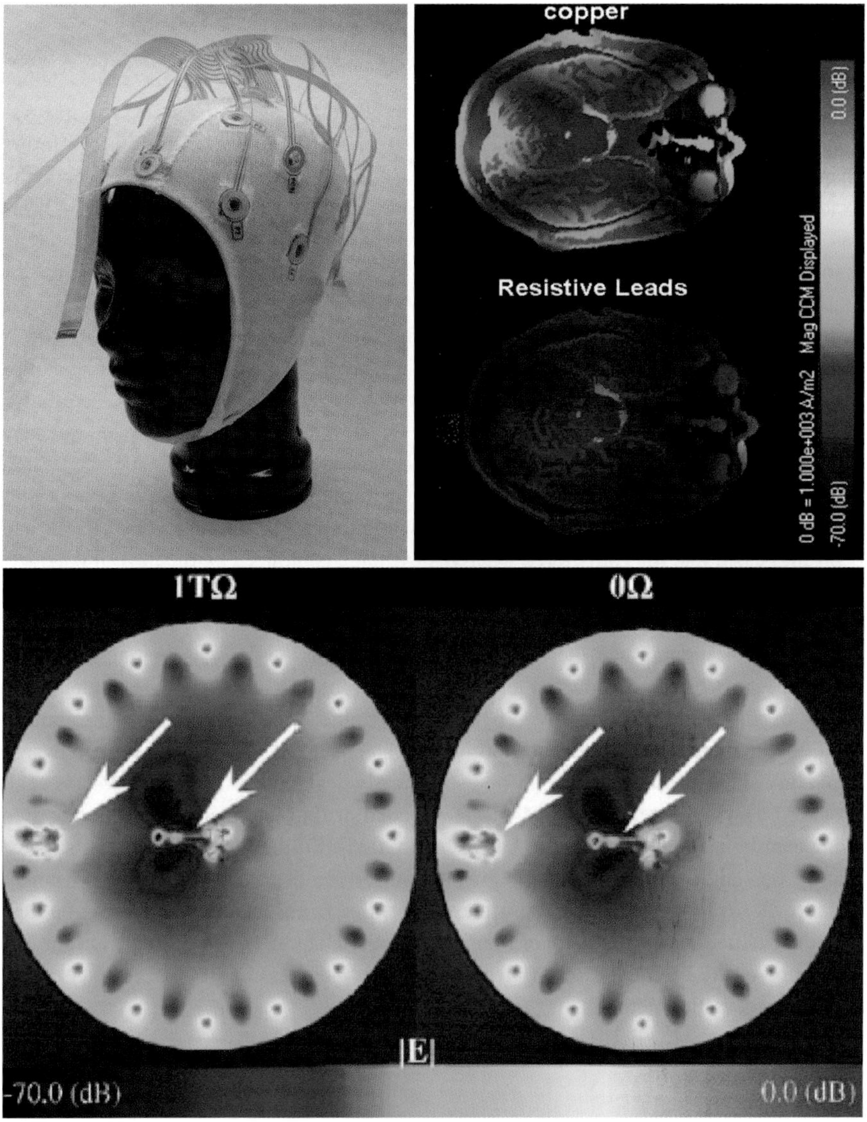

Fig. 4 *Top*: The InkCap (*left*), a high-resistive 32-electrode EEG cap based on conductive ink technology and tested for safety with magnetic fields up to 7 T. (*Right*) Induced currents simulated for standard copper (*top right*) and resistive (*bottom right*) leads using an FDTD algorithm with the 29-tissue high-resolution head model and a standard birdcage coil. The color bar codes red to 0 dB = 1,000 A/m². (Reprinted from Vasios. et al. 2006.) *Bottom*: Magnitude of the electric field distribution for two models with 1 TΩ (*left*) and 0 V resistors (*right*). Axial slice corresponding to the plane on top of the head model. The electric field distribution is clearly modified along the copper leads (*arrows*), but is not affected by the presence of the resistors and is the same even in these two extreme cases (scale: 0–70 dB with 0 dB = 10^4 V/m). (Reprinted from Angelone et al. 2006)

3.1
Pulse-Related Artifact

Pulse artifact noise removal is one of the most important steps for the successful integration of simultaneously recorded EEG and fMRI data at high field. As discussed in the chapter "EEG Quality: Origin and Reduction of the EEG Cardiac-Related Artifact", the exact origin of the pulse artifact is still poorly understood. The ballistocardiogram (BCG) has been recognized for over 50 years: it is produced when blood from the heart is pumped upwards along the ascending aorta. When the heart pumps blood, the major motion is along the axis parallel to the spine as a rocking movement of the patient's body at each heart beat (Reilly 1992). This type of noise is of small amplitude, is not present in every subject, and is easy to eliminate outside of the MRI environment by using damping foam or by placing the subject in a position other than supine during EEG recordings. The first EEG recordings obtained inside MRI scanners were also characterized by pulse related noise (Huang-Hellinger et al. 1995); this was interpreted as being due to pulsatile whole-body, head or scalp motion, time locked to the cardiac cycle (Ives et al. 1993; Nakamura et al. 2006; Schomer et al. 2000). In addition to the ballistic effect, it has also been suggested that the Hall effect, whereby a voltage is induced by the flow of conducting blood in the proximity of electrodes, may contribute to the artifact (Wendt et al. 1998; Debener et al. 2008). The variation of the BCG artifact at 1.5, 3 and 7 T showed that the artifact magnitude increases with field strength, as does its spatial variability (Debener et al. 2008). Although a tentative suggestion for a more accurate model of the causes of the pulse artifact is given by the authors, more research is required to understand the interaction of all the contributing mechanisms fully. Using a novel cap design based on conductive ink technology and specifically designed for use at 7 T, Vasios et al. observed a 3.5-fold reduction of the pulse-related artifact compared to EEG recorded using a carbon fiber electrode set (Vasios et al. 2005). Furthermore, the authors suggest that the design of the new cap offers greater comfort, tends to reduce subject movement and allows for longer measurement times. Appendix 1 presents the principles of a new filtering method based on Kalman filtering. See the chapter "EEG Quality: Origin and Reduction of the EEG Cardiac-Related Artifact" for a discussion of pulse artifact reduction postprocessing methods.

3.2
Other Noise Sources at High Field

Electromotive forces induced in loops formed by the EEG recording system and subject by body movement are proportional to field strength, so it is particularly important to keep subjects as still as possible during combined EEG–fMRI experiments carried out at high field. This increase also underlies an issue discussed by Mullinger (2008): that the amplifiers and cables within the magnetic field must be isolated from any vibration. In addition, switching off cryogenic cooling compression pumps during EEG recording may reduce vibrations and resulting induced noise.

4
Image Quality

As described in the chapter "EEG Quality: The Image Acquisition Artifact", EEG equipment placed inside or close to the field of view may degrade image quality through two mechanisms: perturbation of the fields used for image generation (RF, gradient and static), causing image distortion or signal loss, and the introduction of RF interference by the EEG amplification and digitization electronics, resulting in noise in the images. The former may be more problematic in high-field scanners, particularly the effects resulting from interactions with the static field. In addition, RF shielding can occur due to the interaction of the electromagnetic field from the wires and EEG electrodes, and may depend on the wires' radii and orientations, the surrounding tissue conductivity, and the total number of wire leads (Row 1955; Young and Wait 1989). Shielding and B_1 nonuniformity may get worse if the leads or electrode electrical lengths approach resonance, which may be more likely as the field strength increases. These effects may reduce the electric field in one location while increasing it in others, with possible image quality and safety implications (Angelone et al. 2004).

The interaction of copper EEG leads with the B_1^+ field has been investigated at 1.5, 3 and 7 T using 32- and 64-channel EEG systems with braided copper wire leads (Mullinger 2008). Significant artifact were only observed close to the wires leading to the ECG and EOG electrodes, which are longer than the EEG leads. Even with signal loss problems that arise from the presence of the longer copper leads, the same group has demonstrated that it is possible to record BOLD signals from areas affected (Mullinger 2008). However, most of the B_0 distortions observed were limited to the outer 1 cm of the phantom and human head, and were thus outside the brain, and these artifact were mainly caused by the EEG electrodes. Although the field perturbations increased with field strength, due to their localized nature it was concluded that fMRI data would not be significantly degraded, even at high field, as the skull and scalp are ~1 cm thick on average (Lu et al. 2005). The B_1^+ distortions due to the longer leads on the cap posed a more significant problem since they were observed at all field strengths, though they were significantly worse at higher field strengths. The precise cause of this artifact remains to be investigated, although the longer lead lengths are believed to be a contributing factor and RF chokes such as those described by Stevens (2007b) may alleviate this problem. Importantly, the temporal SNR in the presence of the 64-channel cap at 7 T was shown to be greater than that of images collected with no cap present at 3 T.

A detailed study of the effect of electrode composition on B_0 and B_1 artifact at 4 T has been carried out by Stevens et al. (2007), and it showed that electrodes containing any ferromagnetic material unsurprisingly produce large magnetic susceptibility artifact. However, the spatial extent of the artifact produced when diamagnetic materials are used is generally small, with Ag/AgCl producing the smallest artifact, in line with the findings of Mullinger and colleagues suggesting adequate EPI image quality even at 7 T (Mullinger et al. 2008). A special EEG cap has been developed specifically for application at high field (Angelone et al. 2006). The cap is based on conductive ink microstrips which have a resistance per unit length of 2 kΩ/m, with electrodes made of Ag/AgCl-printed rings and two motion sensors placed on the temporal regions of the cap. Performance was assessed by FDTD simulations, temperature measurements and EEG recordings during structural and functional MRI recordings at 7 T using 12 healthy human volunteers. EM field and SAR estimates were obtained by simulation for different values of the microstrip resistivity (Fig. 4) with a circularly polarized 16-rod birdcage coil (Angelone et al. 2004). Measurements on a phantom and human subjects (Angelone et al. 2006) demonstrated superior EEG and image quality compared to a cap based on carbon fiber at 7 T (Angelone et al. 2004).

5
Example of an Application of EEG–fMRI at 7 T: Auditory Steady State Response (ASSR)

In the field of audiology, electrophysiological measurements play an important role when tests designed to obtain behavioral measurements are performed on individuals who are unable to respond to audible stimuli. In particular, newborns, very young children, elderly people or incapacitated patients benefit from the use of such measurements. Although auditory brainstem responses (ABR) are considered the gold standard in diagnostic testing, a recent review presented a collection of studies linking the ASSR threshold in infants and children to the pure-tone hearing threshold (Cone-Wesson et al. 2002). The ASSR stimulation frequency may reflect the activity of underlying generators (Stach 2002): low frequency (0–20 Hz) with late-latency responses, middle frequency (20–60 Hz) stimuli are associated with middle-latency responses, and high frequency (>60 Hz) stimuli with brainstem responses. The ASSR is an evoked response modulated by pure tones in amplitude (AM) or frequency (FM). Commonly, the tones are switched ON and OFF repeatedly during the course of the session in order to determine an average reading. In adults, the strongest responses occur at a rate of approximately 40/s (Galambos et al. 1981). The ASSR amplitude at 40 Hz is usually much larger than any component of the ABR, and is therefore easier to record, especially in noisy environments such as MRI. For example, a 40-Hz modulation frequency sets off an increase of EEG activity in the delta (up to 3 Hz) and theta (4–7 Hz) bands during periods of sleep, and correlates significantly with decreased amplitude. In this section we present high-field ERP-fMRI physiological recordings from eight healthy volunteers performed by Purdon et al. (Fig. 5).

In this study, stimuli consisted of 1-ms clicks or noise bursts at 40 Hz in a 30-s ON/OFF pattern for a total of 15 min per run. A laptop computer running Presentation 0.76 (Neurobehavioral Systems, Albany, CA, USA) delivered all the auditory stimuli and by a custom-built, electrically shielded electrostatic headphone system with a frequency response to 20 kHz and an acoustic noise attenuation of >30 dB above 800 Hz. Functional MRI acquisitions were arranged according to a "long-TR" auditory fMRI design, with TR = 1 s (fifteen 4 mm slices, 1 mm skip, coronal orientation) and a 9-s gap between volumes, allowing Hemodynamic responses elicited by acoustic scanner noise to subside before the next volume acquisition. EEG acquisitions were interleaved with image acquisitions using the High-Field One EEG recording system (see Appendix 2 in this chapter) with a high dynamic range to prevent saturation during imaging (1-kHz sampling rate; DC to 500 Hz bandwidth). EEG electrodes were placed in adjacent bipolar pairs along a coronal

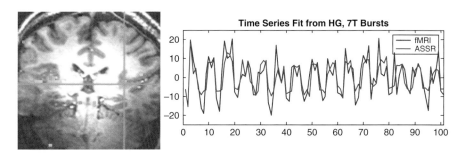

Fig. 5   EEG–fMRI study of auditory steady-state responses (*ASSR*) at 7 T. *Left*: Activation map. *Right*: Time series fit from Heschl's gyrus (*HG*). Spontaneous fluctuations in ASSR match spontaneous fluctuations in the BOLD signal. (Reprinted from Purdon et al. 2005)

plane (M2 ≥ T8, T8 ≥ C6, C6 ≥ C4, C4 ≥ Cz, Cz ≥ C3, C3 ≥ C5, C5 ≥ T7, T7 ≥ M1) using resistive carbon fiber leads (Angelone et al. 2004). Motion sensors were placed above preauricular points for motion artifact rejection. ASSRs were computed from M2 ≥ Cz in the frequency domain using multitaper spectral analysis (Percival and Walden 1993) (bandwidth = 0.4 Hz) from 4 s windows centered 4 s prior to each volume acquisition (Black et al. 1999). For each EEG recording window, the amplitude (square root of the power) at 40 Hz was computed to produce a 40 Hz amplitude time-series. The fMRI time series were then analyzed using a linear model consisting of the 40 Hz amplitude time series plus a sixth order polynomial (nuisance effect), fitted using the *3d Deconvolve* method in AFNI (Boundy et al. 1996). The fluctuations in 40 Hz amplitude were found to be correlated with (4 s delayed) BOLD changes throughout the auditory system, including the cochlear nucleus, the inferior colliculus (IC), the medial geniculate nucleus, and Heschl's gyrus (HG), suggesting that brainstem structures play an important role in generating or modulating the 40 Hz ASSR. Figure 5 shows the BOLD fMRI activity at 7 T in HG and IC, along with the time series fit between fMRI (blue) and ASSR amplitude (red) for the indicated voxel. These studies demonstrate that time-varying ERP measurements can be made concurrently with fMRI, and that these time-varying measurements can be correlated with the BOLD signal at 7 T.

6
Conclusions

In this chapter we have presented the issues and challenges brought about by using EEG/MRI at high fields, including safety, noise reduction, and hardware considerations.

In relation to safety, we have seen that investigators have mostly focused on RF-induced heating, reflecting the MR regulatory guidelines on maximum SAR exposure. While the results of investigations on the safety of recording EEG while scanning at high field suggests that it can be done safely, it is important to limit those conclusions to the specific experimental conditions described in those studies, and site-specific assessments are always advised prior to application, whether using commercially marketed or "homemade" equipment. We can therefore expect the body of evidence on the safety and data quality aspects to increase with growing interest in combining the two modalities at high field to ensure that its promise of greater signal is fully exploited. These remarks equally apply to the issues of EEG and MRI data quality, which—although promising results have already been obtained—remain a technical challenge.

Acknowledgements Thanks to Prof Richard Bowtell, of the Sir Peter Mansfield Magnetic Resonance Centre, University of Nottingham, and Dr David Carmichael of the UCL Institute of Neurology, for their input.

Appendix 1:
The Multidimensional Kalman Adaptive Filtering Method

We provide an outline of a 3D extension of the Kalman filter for pulse-related noise cancellation in multiple channels simultaneously based on the adaptive Kalman filter algorithm (Haykin 1996). The adaptive algorithm makes use of any correlation between each of the motion sensor signals $m_i(t)$ and the observed signal $y(t, c)$ to estimate the finite impulse response (FIR) kernel $w_i^t(k,c)$ and to remove the noise signals $n_i(t, c)$. Since the true underlying (neuronal) EEG signal $s(t,c)$ is uncorrelated with the motion signals $m_i(t)$, it is unaffected by the adaptive algorithm and, on average, the result of the noise cancellation process $\hat{s}(t, c)$ will be the true underlying EEG.

Each channel "c" of the EEG signal $y(t, c)$ is modeled as the sum of a "true" underlying EEG signal $s(t, c)$ and a sum of 3D signals $n_x(t, c)$, $n_y(t, c)$ and $n_z(t, c)$ containing motion and ballistocardiogram components along the three cardinal directions:

$$y(t,c) = s(t,c) + n_x(t,c) + n_y(t,c) + n_z(t,c) \quad c = 1,...,32 \tag{1}$$

Next, we enumerate the spatial components of both the noise $n_i(t,c)$, $i = 1, 2, 3$ (i.e. $n_x(t,c)$, $n_y(t,c)$ and $n_z(t,c)$) and the motion sensor signals $m_i(t)$. The relationship between the noise signals $n_i(t,c)$ and the motion sensor signals $m_i(t)$ is modeled linearly using a time-varying, FIR kernel $w_i^t(k)$ with the equation:

$$n_i(t,c) = \sum_{k=0}^{N_i-1} w_i^t(k,c)m_i(t-k) \quad i = 1, 2, 3, \tag{2}$$

where N_i is the order of the FIR kernel $w_i^t(k, c)$, chosen to be the same for all channels. An adaptive filtering algorithm is used to produce an estimate of the FIR kernel $w_i^t(k, c)$, which in turn is used to estimate the noise signal $n_i(t, c)$. The sum of estimated noise components signals is then subtracted from the recorded signal $y(t, c)$ to reveal the underlying EEG signal $s(t, c)$,

$$\hat{n}_i(t,c) = \sum_{k=0}^{N-1} \hat{w}_i^t(k)m_i(t-k),$$
$$\hat{s}(t,c) = y(t,c) - \sum_{i=1}^{3} \hat{n}_i(t,c). \tag{3}$$

In previous studies (Schomer et al. 2000), we showed that the ballistocardiogram is spatially smooth and that the first eigenvalue of the principal component analysis (PCA) alone accounts for over 90% of the variance. Building on those results, we consider adaptive filtering on the first Q components of the PCA of $y(t,c)$ (i.e. $\hat{y}_q(t)$: $q = 1,\ldots,Q$), and select Q according to the desired resulting minimum fractional variance. Figure 6 shows the filtering scheme, which includes: (a) the dimensionality reduction for the 32-channel

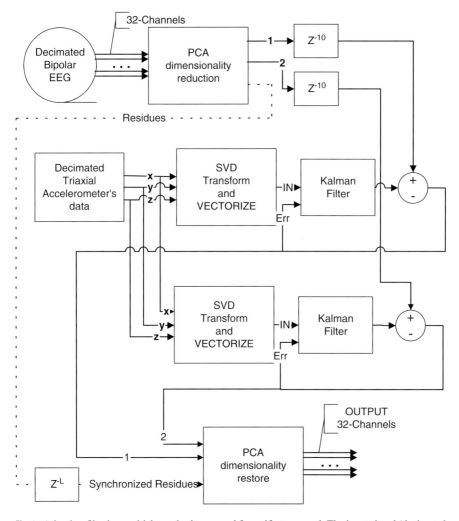

Fig. 6 Adaptive-filtering multichannel scheme used for artifact removal. The input signal (decimated bipolar EEG), after band pass and decimation, is a signal of 32 channels that is first transformed into two principal component analysis (PCA) components. Each component is then separately filtered using the proposed Kalman filter. According to this filtering scheme, three motion sensor signals are first singular value decomposition (SVD) transformed and vectorized before Kalman filtering. After filtering, each "clean" PCA component is used to reconstruct the 32-channel EEG signal. There is a module of Z-10 for causality, given that the motion sensors have an intrinsic delay due to mechanical inertia. Z-L is used to compensate for the Z-10 and the delay in the FIR filter

EEG signals by means of PCA, and (b) singular value decomposition (SVD) transformation along the principal direction of the 3D motion. Figure 6 also illustrates the algorithm with the simplified value of $Q = 2$, which is a remarkable reduction in computation time: 16 times faster than when $Q = 2$.

The synchronization in Fig. 6 occurs because every channel contains a certain mixture of the two filtered PCA components. $m_1(t)$ is the vector composed of the N samples from the first motion sensor prior to and equal to "t", $m_2(t)$ are the data from the second motion sensor, and $m_3(t)$ are data from the third motion sensor. The matrix $m(t) = [m_1(t)\ m_2(t)\ m_3(t)]$ is then separated into three components which are approximately mutually orthogonal, and the final result is obtained by diagonalizing the new motion-sensor covariance matrix $\overline{m}(t)$:

$$w(t + 1, q) = aw(t,q) + v_3(t)$$

$$y_q(t) = \tilde{m}^T(t) \cdot w(t,q) + s_q(t)$$

$$w(t,q) = [w_1^t(0,q)w_2^t(0,q)\ w_3^t(0,q)\ w_1^t(1,q)\ w_2^t(1,q)\ w_3^t(1,q)\ ...\ w_1^t(N,q)\ w_2^t(N,q)\ w_3^t(N,q)]$$

$$\tilde{m}(t) = [\tilde{m}_1(t)\ \tilde{m}_2(t)\ \tilde{m}_3(t)\ \tilde{m}_1(t-1)\ \tilde{m}_2(t-1)\ \tilde{m}_3(t-1)\ ...\ \tilde{m}_3(t-N+1)]^T. \tag{4}$$

The proposed transformation (i.e. rotation) is found by taking the SVD of the original motion-sensor matrix, $m(t) = U \cdot S \cdot VT$, and transforming $m(t)$ into a new matrix: $\tilde{m}(t) = m(t) \cdot V^T$. $\tilde{m}(t)$ is created by concatenating every row of $\overline{m}(t)$ in a vector of $3N$ elements. Furthermore, we have expressed the filter tap weights $w_i^t(k,q)$ and the three components of the motion sensor $m_i(t)$ in vector form, with T denoting matrix transposition, and where $v_3(t)$ can be a singular white noise matrix with the covariance matrix $\Lambda i,j = qi \oplus 3\delta i \oplus 3,j \oplus 3I$, where $\oplus 3$ denotes addition modulus 3, $\delta_{i,j}$ is the Kronecker delta, a is a scalar state-transition parameter, and $s(t)$ is the underlying "true" EEG signal, modeled as a white noise with variance λ. We can then recursively estimate the filter taps using the Kalman filter with updated equations (Haykin 2002).

Appendix 2:
The Open Hardware and Software Project. The High-Field One System for Real-Time EEG–fMRI

While many commercial and academic systems have been developed to perform EEG recordings during fMRI, rapidly evolving technical, clinical, and scientific requirements have created an opportunity for hardware and software systems that can be customized for specific electrophysiology-fMRI applications. Hardware platforms may require customization to enable a variety of recording types (e.g. electroencephalogram, local field potentials, or multiunit activity) while meeting the stringent and costly requirements of MRI safety and compatibility. *Real-time* signal processing tools are an enabling technology for electrophysiology-fMRI studies, particularly for application areas such as sleep, epilepsy, neurofeedback, and drug studies, yet real-time signal processing tools are difficult to develop. See the chapter "EEG Quality: The Image Acquisition Artifact" for a discussion of existing hardware solutions. In this section we outline this system, which we call

High-Field One [i.e. HF-1 (Purdon et al.2008)]. Since high-field MRI is a very challenging environment, it imposes the following requirements: (a) a high dynamic range to avoid saturation during scanning, (b) low RF emissions, and (c) low eddy currents.

RF noise immunity was obtained in HF-1 despite the EEG-MRI requirements of: (1) an absence of ferromagnetic components, (2) resolution of input signals down to 100 nV (exceeding the requirements described in the chapter "The Added Value of EEG–fMRI in Imaging Neuroscience"), and (3) RF noise immunity in the link with the computer system outside the MRI. HF-1 has a bandwidth from DC to 4 kHz (no high-pass filter is needed thanks to the large dynamic range), and a 24-bit sampling rate of 20,833 S/s. It also has a complete set of digital circuits for analogue-to-digital conversion, storage, and USB connection with an external PC. HF-1 is connected to a laptop via a USB optical interface. Furthermore, an optical digital line is used to synchronize EEG acquisition with the PCMCIA digital acquisition card (National Instruments, Austin, TX, USA), enabling us to record the trigger signals from a parallel port of a stimulus PC in order to do real-time averaging of epochs.

Although the system (Fig. 7) has been successfully used at 1.5 and 3 T fields, it was specifically designed for very high fields and was therefore tested on humans and animals at 7 T with the following specifications for the gradient coils: maximum gradient strength 40 mT/m (whole-body) and 60 mT/m (head); slew rate of 200 T/m/s (whole body) and 333 T/m/s (head).

Main Design Features

The first stage of the system increases the EEG SNR by amplifying the signals before relaying them to the rest of the system. The purpose of this first stage is twofold: (1) to further attenuate (Aw) the fraction of the RF pulse picked up by the Ink Cap, and (2) to amplify the EEG signal in order to improve its SNR, which is given by:

$$\text{SNR} = \frac{P^s}{P^n + \lambda\rho_1}. \tag{5}$$

where P^s is the power of the observed signal (i.e. EEG), $\lambda = (Ri + R)/Ri$, Ri is the input resistance of the second-stage amplifier, $P^n = |V_{rms}^n|2/(4RB)$, and $\rho 1$ is the intrinsic noise power of the first stage amplifier in the band of interest, B. Hence, the SNR is linearly dependent on the first-stage gain.

The third and last stage (Fig. 7) consists of a microcontroller unit (MCU) that is used to supervise all of the functions of the instruments and the clock management circuit, which generates three clocks: (a) an MCU clock (i.e. 48 MHz), (b) an analogue-to-digital conversion (ADC) clock (i.e. 8 MHz), and (c) a USB clock (i.e. 6 MHz). The MCU synchronises, communicates through a handshake protocol, and controls the input of each ADC. The MCU also controls the internal USB section. The data from the ADC is streamed in a FIFO controller using an internal bus controlled by a line driver. The USB serial port section consists of a USB controller connected to the internal data bus. The USB section is

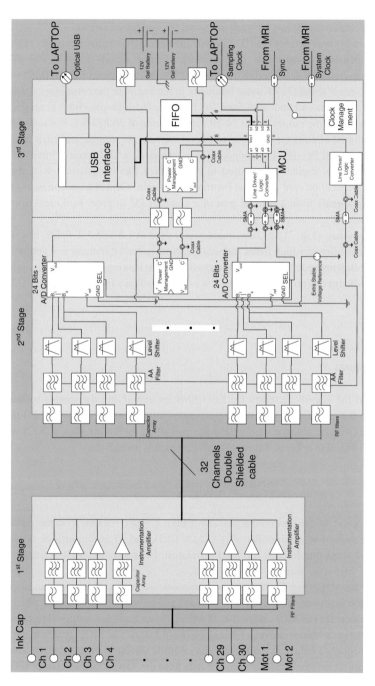

Fig. 7 High-Field One (HF-1) hardware overview. The hardware is organized into three main stages: (1) an amplification system, (2) an analogue-to-digital converter (ADC), and (3) a programmable microcontroller unit (MCU) for controlling ADC functions. The EEG data are relayed outside the MRI via a USB-based optical link. A laptop system is used for data display, recording, integration with external signals such as event triggers and physiological monitoring, and real-time signal processing. The HF-1 hardware is compatible with MRI systems, has been tested at field strengths of up to 7 T, and can be used for both EEG and more general electrophysiological recordings such as local field potential or multiunit activity

connected to an external custom-shielded USB optical extension. The optical sampling clock section informs the acquisition computer of the sampling frequency and is connected to the MCU; it can be located up to 120 m away and is connected to a DAQ card in the acquisition computer for acquisition of the ERP trigger. A PC runs the Labview code and allows monitoring of the electrophysiological traces in real time. It also performs band-pass filtering, saves this large set of data in real time (Rector and George 2001), and computes steady-state responses and spectrograms, also in real time. Complete synchronisation of the MRI and EEG systems was achieved by generating a 48 MHz clock from the 10 MHz master clock of the Siemens Trio (Siemens AG, Erlangen, Germany) scanner using a direct digital synthesizer.

The HF-1 software and hardware designs are freely available at http://nmr.mgh.harvard.edu/abilab/, subject to a free licensing agreement. The HF-1 hardware system can be constructed based on the complete specifications provided. These specifications include circuit diagrams in Orcad (Cadence, San Jose, CA, USA) format, print circuit board layouts in both Orcad and Gerber (Gerber Systems Corporation) formats, and bills for materials specifying all required components and part numbers. Print circuit board layouts were designed to permit both automated pick-and-place assembly and soldering, as well as hand assembly and soldering. With these specifications, it is possible to achieve turnkey production of the complete hardware system, or components of it, as desired by the end-user.

References

Angelone LM, and G. Bonmassar. Use of resistances and resistive leads: implications on computed electric field and SAR values. in ISMRM Twelfth Scientific Meeting. 2004

Angelone LM, et al. (2004) Metallic electrodes and leads in simultaneous EEG-MRI: specific absorption rate (SAR) simulation studies. Bioelectromagnetics 25(4):285–295

Angelone LM, et al, (2005) New high resolution head model for accurate electromagnetic field computation. Proc 13th ISMRM Sci Meet, Miami, FL, USA, 7–13 May 2005, p 881

Angelone LM, et al. (2006) On the effect of resistive EEG electrodes and leads during 7 Tesla MRI: simulation and temperature measurement studies. Magn Reson Imaging 24(6):801–812

Armenean C, et al. (2004) RF-induced temperature elevation along metallic wires in clinical magnetic resonance imaging: influence of diameter and length. Magn Reson Med 52(5):1200–1206

Baker KB, et al. (2004) Evaluation of specific absorption rate as a dosimeter of MRI-related implant heating. J Magn Reson Imaging 20(2):315–320

Belliveau JW, et al. (1991) Functional mapping of the human visual cortex by magnetic resonance imaging. Science 254:716–719

Berenger JP (1994) A perfectly matched layer for the absorption of electromagnetic waves. Comput Phys 114:185–200

Black PM, et al. (1999) Craniotomy for tumor treatment in an intraoperative magnetic resonance imaging unit. Neurosurgery 45(3):423–431; discussion 431–433

Bottomley PA, Andrew ER (1978) RF magnetic field penetration, phase shift and power dissipation in biological tissue: Implications for NMR imaging. Phys Med Biol 23:630–643

Bottomley P, Redington R, Edelstein W (1985) Estimating radiofrequency power deposition in body NMR imaging. Magn Reson Med 2:336–349

Boundy KL, et al. (1996) Localization of temporal lobe epileptic foci with iodine-123 iododexetimide cholinergic neuroreceptor single-photon emission computed tomography. Neurology 47(4):1015–1020

Carmichael DW, et al. Functional MRI with active, fully implanted, deep brain stimulation systems: safety and experimental confounds. Neuroimage, 2007. 37(2): p. 508–517

Carmichael DW, et al. Safety of localizing epilepsy monitoring intracranial electroencephalograph electrodes using MRI: radiofrequency-induced heating. J Magn Reson Imaging, 2008. 28(5): p. 1233–1244

Cangellaris AC, Wright SM (1991) Analysis of the numerical error caused by the stair-stepped approximation of a conducting boundary in FDTD simulations of electromagnetic phenomena. IEEE Trans Antennas Propagat 39:1518–1525

Chou CK, Guy AW (1979) Carbon-loaded teflon electrodes for chronic EEG recordings in microwave research. J Microw Power 14(4):399–404

Chou CK, McDougall JA, Chan KW (1997) RF heating of implanted spinal fusion stimulator during magnetic resonance imaging. IEEE Trans Biomed Eng 44(5):367–373

Collins CM, Smith MB (2003) Spatial resolution of numerical models of man and calculated specific absorption rate using the FDTD method: a study at 64 MHz in a magnetic resonance imaging coil. J Magn Reson Imaging 18(3):383–388

Cone-Wesson B, et al. (2002) The auditory steady-state response: comparisons with the auditory brainstem response. J Am Acad Audiol 13(4):173–187; quiz 225–226

Debener S, et al. (2008) Properties of the ballistocardiogram artifact as revealed by EEG recordings at 1.5, 3 and 7 Tesla. Int J Psychophysiol 67:189–199

Dimbylow PJ, Gandhi OP (1991) Finite-difference time-domain calculations of SAR in a realistic heterogeneous model of the head for plane-wave exposure from 600 MHz to 3 GHz. Phys Med Biol 36(8):1075–1089

FDA (2003) Criteria for significant risk investigations of magnetic resonance diagnostic devices. Center for Devices and Radiological Health, US FDA, Silver Spring

Filipek PA, et al. (1994) The young adult human brain: an MRI-based morphometric analysis. Cereb Cortex 4(4): 344–360

Gabriel C, Gabriel S, Corthout E (1996a) The dielectric properties of biological tissues: I. Literature survey. Phys Med Biol 41:2231–2249

Gabriel C, Gabriel S, Corthout E (1996b) The dielectric properties of biological tissues: II. Measurements in the frequency range 10 Hz to 20 GHz. Phys Med Biol 41:2251–2269

Galambos R, Makeig S, Talmachoff P (1981) A 40-Hz auditory potential recorded from the human scalp. Proc Natl Acad Sci USA 78:2643–2647

Gandhi OP, Chen XB (1999) Specific absorption rates and induced current densities for an anatomy-based model of the human for exposure to time-varying magnetic fields of MRI. Magn Reson Med 41(4):816–823

Gangarosa RE, et al. (1987) Operational safety issues in MRI. Magn Reson Imaging 5(4):287–292

Glover GH, et al. (1985) Comparison of linear and circular polarization for magnetic resonance imaging. J Magn Reson 64:255–270

Harel N, et al. (2006) Frontiers of brain mapping using MRI. J Magn Reson Imaging 23(6):945–957

Haykin S (1996) Adaptive filter theory, 3rd edn. Prentice Hall, Upper Saddle River

Haykin S (2002) Adaptive filter theory, 4th edn. Prentice Hall, Upper Saddle River

Ho HS (2001) Safety of metallic implants in magnetic resonance imaging. J Magn Reson Imaging 14(4):472–477

Hoult DI, Foreman D, Kolansky G, Kripiakevich D (2008) Overcoming high-field RF problems with non-magnetic cartesian feedback transceivers. MAGMA 21(1–2):15–29

Huang-Hellinger FR, et al. (1995) Simultaneous functional magnetic resonance imaging and electrophysiological recording. Hum Brain Mapp 3:13–23

IEC (2002) International standard, medical equipment, part 2-33: particular requirements for the safety of the magnetic resonance equipment for medical diagnosis, 2nd revision. International Electrotechnical Commission 601-2-33: Geneva, pp 29–31

Ives JR, et al. (1993) Monitoring the patient's EEG during echo-planar MRI. Electroenceph Clin Neurophysiol 87:417–420

Jin J-M (1999) Electromagnetic analysis and design in magnetic resonance imaging (Biomedical Engineering Series). CRC Press, Boca Raton

Kainz W, et al. (2005) Dosimetric comparison of the specific anthropomorphic mannequin (SAM) to 14 anatomical head models using a novel definition for the mobile phone positioning. Phys Med Biol 50(14):3423–3445

Kangarlu A, Shellock FG, Chakeres DW (2003) 8.0-Tesla human MR system: temperature changes associated with radiofrequency-induced heating of a head phantom. J Magn Reson Imaging 17(2):220–226

Keltner JR, et al. (1991) Electromagnetic fields of surface coil in vivo NMR at high frequencies. Magn Reson Med 22:467–480

Konings MK, Bartels LW, Smits HFM, Bakker CJG (2000) Heating around intravascular guidewires by resonating RF waves. JMRI 12:79–85

Kwong KK, et al. (1992) Functional MR imaging of primary visual and motor cortex. In: 10th Annu Meet Soc Magnetic Resonance Imaging, New York, 25–29 April 1992

Lazeyras F, et al. (2001) Functional MRI with simultaneous EEG recording: Feasibility and application to motor and visual activation. J Magn Reson Imaging 13(6):943–948

Lemieux L, et al. (1997) Recording of EEG during fMRI experiments: patient safety. Magn Reson Med 38(6):943–952

Lu, H, et al. Routine clinical brain MRI sequences for use at 3.0 Tesla. J Magn Reson Imaging, 2005. 22(1): p. 13–22

Lu HZ, et al. (2005) Routine clinical brain MRI sequences for use at 3.0 Tesla. J Magn Reson Imaging 22:13–22

Mansfield P, Morris PG (1982) NMR imaging in biomedicine (Advances in Magnetic Resonance, Suppl 2). Academic, New York

Mirsattari SM, et al. (2004) MRI compatible EEG electrode system for routine use in the epilepsy monitoring unit and intensive care unit. Clin Neurophysiol 115(9):2175–2180

Mullinger K (2008) Exploring the feasibility of simultaneous EEG/fMRI at 7T. Magn Reson Imaging 26(7):607–616

Mullinger KJ, et al. (2008) Effects of simultaneous EEG recording on MRI data quality at 1.5, 3 and 7 Tesla. Int J Psychophysiol 67:178–188

Nakamura W, et al. (2006) Removal of ballistocardiogram artifacts from simultaneously recorded EEG and fMRI data using independent component analysis. IEEE Trans Biomed Eng 53(7):1294–1308

Nitz WR, et al. (2005) Specific absorption rate as a poor indicator of magnetic resonance-related implant heating. Invest Radiol 40(12):773–776

Ogawa, S., et al. (1992) Intrinsic signal changes accompanying sensory stimulation: Functional brain mapping with magnetic resonance imaging. Proc Natl Acad Sci USA 89:5951–5955

Percival DB, Walden AT (1993) Spectral analysis for physical applications: multitaper and conventional univariate techniques. Cambridge University Press, Cambridge

Purdon PL, et al. (2005) Concurrent EEG/fMRI of temporal fluctuations in the 40-Hz auditory steady state response. Proc Intl Soc Magn Reson Med 13:1421

Purdon PL, et al. (2008) High-Field One: an open-source hardware and software platform for acquisition and real-time processing of electrophysiology during MRI. J Neurosci Methods 175(2):165–186

Purdon PL, et al. Concurrent Recording of 40-Hz Auditory Steady State Response and Functional MR. in 10th Annual Meeting of the Organization for Human Brain Mapping. 2004. Budapest, Hungary: Neuroimage

Rector DM, George JS (2001) Continuous image and electrophysiological recording with real-time processing and control. Methods 25(2):151–163

Reilly JP (1992) Electrical stimulation and electropathology. Cambridge University Press, New York

Rezai AR, Finelli D, Nyenhuis JA, Hrdlicka G, Tkach J, Sharan A, Rugieri P, Stypulkowski PH, Shellock FG (2002) Neurostimulation systems for deep brain stimulation: in vitro evaluation of magnetic resonance imaging-related heating at 1.5 Tesla. J Magn Reson Imaging 15(3):241–250

Row R (1955) Theoretical and experimental study of electromagnetic scattering by two identical conducting cylinders. J Appl Phys 26(6):666–675

Schomer LD, et al. (2000) EEG linked functional magnetic resonance imaging in epilepsy and cognitive neurophysiology. J Clin Neurophysiol 17(1):43–58

Sharan A, et al. (2003) MR safety in patients with implanted deep brain stimulation systems (DBS). Acta Neurochir Suppl 87:141–145

Shellock FG (2007) Comments on MR heating tests of critical implants. J Magn Reson Imaging 26(5):1182–1185

Sled JG, Pike GB (1998) Standing-wave and RF penetration artifacts caused by elliptic geometry: an electrodynamic analysis of MRI. IEEE Trans Med Imaging 17(4):653–662

Stach BA (2002) The auditory steady-state response: a primer. Hearing J 55(9):10–14

Stevens, T., J. Ives, and R. Bartha. Energy Coupling between RF Electric Fields and Conductive Wires: Image Artifacts and Heating. in International Society for Magnetic Resonance in Medicine. 2007. Berlin, Germany

Stevens, T., J. Ives, and R. Bartha. Avoiding Resonant Lengths of Wire with RF Chokes at 4 Tesla. in International Society for Magnetic Resonance in Medicine. 2007. Berlin, Germany

Stevens TK, et al. (2007) MR compatibility of EEG scalp electrodes at 4 Tesla. J Magn Reson Imaging 25:872–877

Vasios CE, et al. (2005) An ink cap for recording EEG during 7 Tesla MRI. In: 35th Annu Meet Soc Neuroscience, Washington, DC, USA, 12–16 Nov 2005

Vasios CE, et al. (2006) EEG/(f)MRI measurements at 7 Tesla using a new EEG cap ("InkCap"). Neuroimage 33(4):1082–1092

Wendt M, et al. Dynamic tracking in interventional MRI using wavelet-encoded gradient-echo sequences. IEEE Trans Med Imaging, 1998. 17(5): p. 803–809

Wiesinger F, et al. (2006) Potential and feasibility of parallel MRI at high field. NMR Biomed 19(3):368–378

Wiggins GC, et al. (2005) Eight-channel phased array coil and detunable TEM volume coil for 7 T brain imaging. Magn Reson Med 54(1):235–240

Young J, Wait J (1989) Shielding properties of an ensemble of thin, infinitely long, parallel wires over a lossy half space. IEEE Trans Electromagn Compat 31(3):238–244

Experimental Design and Data Analysis Strategies

12

Christian-G. Bénar, Andrew P. Bagshaw, and Louis Lemieux

1
Introduction

As described in earlier chapters, EEG and fMRI are two powerful, noninvasive tools for studying human brain activity. Since they have complementary spatiotemporal properties, with EEG providing millisecond temporal resolution and fMRI millimetre spatial resolution, there has been a drive over the last decade to record them simultaneously, a technique referred to as simultaneous EEG–fMRI or simply EEG–fMRI. The combined data promise to provide a more complete view of brain activity and hopefully improve understanding of the spatiotemporal dynamics of brain processes.

The earliest attempts to combine EEG and fMRI avoided the technical issues of recording EEG in the MRI scanner by acquiring the two data sets separately and combining the results, with fMRI providing relatively good spatial information, and EEG a finer level of temporal resolution. As discussed in the chapter "Principles of Multimodal Functional Imaging and Data Integration", this approach is particularly suitable when the brain phenomenon or effects of interest are predictable in time (e.g. externally triggered) and reproducible across sessions (i.e. the expected signal changes are unaffected by the experimental conditions). Furthermore, serially acquired multi-modal data are best suited for analyses of effects averaged across sessions. Conversely, the data obtained from simultaneous acquisitions is devoid of any such constraints and can be used to study individual events, on the condition that data quality is not compromised by possible interactions between the EEG and MR systems. Simultaneous recordings generally add an extra layer of complexity to the experimental setup (see the chapters "EEG Quality: Origin and Reduction of the EEG Cardiac-Related Artefact", "EEG Quality: The Image Acquisition Artefact", and "Image Quality Issues") but there is a potential time saving compared to serial acquisitions.

The applications of simultaneous EEG–fMRI can be grouped into two categories, according to the nature of brain activity under study: first, the technique has been used to study

C.-G. Bénar (✉)
INSERM U751, Université de la Méditerranée, Marseille, France
e-mail: Christianbenar@univmed.fr

C. Mulert and L. Lemieux (eds.), *EEG–fMRI*
DOI: 10.1007/978-3-540-87919-0_12, © Springer Verlag Berlin Heidelberg 2010

spontaneous transient events or fluctuations in EEG power, for example interictal epileptic discharges, sleep spindles or the alpha rhythm. In this case, simultaneous recordings are necessary, since the activity of interest varies unpredictably (lack of experimental control) and without external manifestation other than in the EEG or fMRI, and therefore comparable datasets could not be obtained with certainty across separate unimodal sessions.

Second, EEG–fMRI has been used in cognitive and sensory neuroscience applications where the activity of interest is induced by an experimental stimulus. In this situation, EEG–fMRI is necessary if one is interested in the part of the signal that varies unpredictably, i.e. interevent variation, or to eliminate potential intersession confounds such as habituation, learning, attention, fatigue, etc.

This chapter's starting assumption is the availability, in the mind of the potential user of EEG–fMRI, of a hypothesis or question regarding the link between a particular feature or set of features of the EEG signal and haemodynamic changes. This chapter's main purpose is therefore to give the reader an overview of the different ways in which EEG–fMRI data can be acquired and analysed to address this type of question. While there is now a consensus on the most efficient way in which EEG–fMRI can be acquired, i.e. via continuous recording in contrast to interleaved acquisitions, the most effective way in which to integrate the data remains an active area of research.

2
Data Acquisition and Experimental Design

Ignoring any technical consideration, all multimodal data acquisitions should be performed simultaneously. However, data quality is a crucial issue in determining degree of multimodal acquisition synchrony. The MR scanner is a very challenging environment for EEG recordings, and both data acquisition processes can severely affect the other's performance through electromagnetic interactions (see the chapters "EEG Instrumentation and Safety", "EEG Quality: Origin and Reduction of the EEG Cardiac-Related Artefact", "EEG Quality: The Image Acquisition Artefact", and "Image Quality Issues"). Recording good-quality EEG inside the scanner and during scanning requires special measures to be taken to minimise any effect on MR image quality (Krakow et al. 2000; see the chapter "Image Quality Issues") and patient safety (Lemieux et al. 1997; see the chapter "EEG Instrumentation and Safety").

As highlighted in the chapter "EEG Instrumentation and Safety", and as identified in the initial work of Ives and colleagues (Ives et al. 1993), EEG data recorded during fMRI scanning suffers from two major artefacts. The MR image acquisition artefact obscures the physiological EEG whenever scanning occurs, and the pulse-related artefact (often called ballistocardiogram or BCG, although the mechanism is not known precisely) is continuously present in most subjects placed within the scanner's static magnetic field (Allen et al. 1998; see the chapter "EEG Quality: Origin and Reduction of the EEG Cardiac-Related Artefact"). These two artefacts constitute important practical barriers to recording continuous EEG data during fMRI.

The first recordings used triggered or sparse recordings, and relied only on periods during which the EEG was uncontaminated by the artefact resulting from gradient switching.

We will discuss this strategy in greater detail in Sect. 2.1 (see also the chapter "EEG–fMRI in Adults with Focal Epilepsy"). When it was shown that this artefact (even though it is impressively large) could be reduced significantly using signal processing methods, this launched the current interest in continuous recordings and increased the possibilities offered by simultaneous EEG–fMRI. This is discussed in Sect. 2.2. Both acquisition modes permit the investigation of two main types of activity, spontaneous and stimulus-related, although there can be constraints imposed by the data acquisition strategy on the experimental design. This issue is discussed in Sect. 2.3, "Experimental Protocol".

2.1
Interleaved EEG and fMRI Acquisitions: Triggered and Sparse Scanning

In the first report of EEG recorded in the MRI scanner, Ives and colleagues identified some of the major technical issues associated with the technique, namely the presence of artefacts on EEG associated with the heartbeat and scanning (Ives et al. 1993) (see the chapters "EEG Quality: Origin and Reduction of the EEG Cardiac-Related Artefact" and "EEG Quality: The Image Acquisition Artefact"). The first application of EEG–fMRI in two patients with epilepsy used an interleaved data acquisition scheme to minimise the impact of the scanning artefact on EEG, by triggering an echo planar image (EPI) acquisition a few seconds after the observation of a paroxysmal discharge on the EEG (Warach et al. 1996). The trigger delay was chosen to capture images at the presumed peak time of the spike-related haemodynamic response (see Fig. 1). This resulted in a set of post-spike images (epileptic activity image set). Following the general approach of contrasting brain states in fMRI, images are also acquired following periods devoid of epileptiform

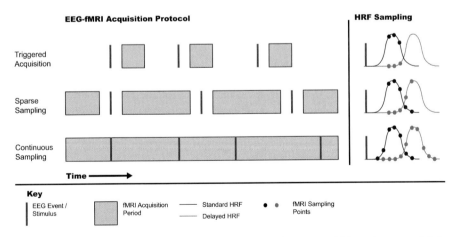

Fig. 1 Illustration of triggered, sparse (interleaved) and continuous acquisition schemes, and their effect on the sampling of the event-related BOLD change. *Left*: relationship between the fMRI acquisition strategy and the EEG events of interest. *Right*: BOLD change sampling for each of the acquisition techniques, for standard and delayed HRF

discharges (normal background or control image set), and activation maps obtained by comparing the mean control image to the mean epileptic activity image (voxel-wise t tests; see Sect. 2.1) or cross-correlation analysis (Bandettini et al. 1993). The sequence of acquisition of the post-spike and control images can be random, according to the spontaneous EEG (Symms et al. 1999), or sequential blocks of post-spike and control images, with the administration of spike-suppressing drug in-between (Seeck et al. 1998). This acquisition technique, called spike-triggered fMRI, is a form of *interleaved multimodal imaging*.

The application of on-line pulse artefact reduction can lead to an increase in spike detection reliability (Allen et al. 1998; Salek-Haddadi et al. 2003b). Spike-triggered fMRI went on to be used by a number of groups who were interested in revealing the haemodynamic correlates of epileptic activity (Seeck et al. 1998; Krakow et al. 1999; Patel et al. 1999; Symms et al. 1999; Al-Asmi et al. 2003). However, although spike-triggered fMRI represented a technical breakthrough, it has a number of drawbacks. Firstly, it is only applicable to the study of large, clear EEG events that can easily be detected visually in the EEG, allowing scan acquisition to be initiated reliably. Secondly, it required a highly trained observer to monitor the EEG for the duration of the scanning session to identify events of interest. Thirdly, degradation of the EEG quality during scanning and the resulting lack of information on the subject's state means that only a short train of images (slices or volumes) could be acquired per event, limiting the total amount of data that can be acquired (per unit time), with a resulting impact on the statistical power (Krakow et al. 2001). Moreover, detection power relies entirely on the assumption that the post-discharge scans sample the peak of the spike-related BOLD change. Finally, this acquisition mode does not provide continuous sampling of the MR signal, making impossible to model slow drifts in the fMRI signal, which can lead to reduced detection power.

An alternative interleaved acquisition mode that we will refer to as *interleaved periodic EEG–fMRI* was subsequently implemented to study other EEG phenomena, for example evoked potentials and spontaneous activity such as the alpha rhythm. By having a relatively long scan repetition time (TR) but acquiring a few slices spaced evenly within each TR (e.g. six slices with a TR of 4 s), the majority of each scan period is free from gradient switching, resulting in periods of clean EEG (Goldman et al. 2000). A similar strategy is to acquire all slices at the beginning of each TR, leaving a silent period with artefact-free EEG (Bonmassar et al. 1999; Kruggel et al. 2000; Feige et al. 2005). A final variant is to acquire a prolonged period of fMRI, for example 30 s, followed by an equivalent period without fMRI during which EEG is acquired and is particularly suited for slowly varying phenomena, such as sleep patterns (Portas et al. 2000; Bonmassar et al. 2001). Periodic interleaved schemes are not suitable for the study of spontaneous brief discharges, which can occur undetected during periods of scanning.

While sparse sampling techniques opened up the use of EEG–fMRI to the study of a wider range of EEG phenomena, they still had a number of disadvantages. Although statistical power was increased relative to spike triggering, sampling of the haemodynamic time course is limited (see Fig. 1). For example, if the stimulation is time-locked to the fMRI, the same points on the HR would be sampled at each TR, leading to suboptimal characterisation of the time course. Similarly, if the time course of the BOLD changes differs markedly from the presumed (e.g. canonical) response, detection power would be considerably reduced, a problem that also affects the spike-triggered approach (Fig. 1).

Perhaps the greatest disadvantage of sparse sampling protocols is the constraint on the experimental method in terms of timing of the stimuli and fMRI acquisition. Typically, considerably fewer slices are acquired compared to a conventional fMRI acquisition, effectively reducing the efficiency of the experimental design.

Given these disadvantages, sparse sampling and spike-triggered protocols have now been superseded with the advent of continuous EEG–fMRI, although they are still sometimes employed (e.g. Christmann et al. 2007), particularly in the investigation of auditory stimuli when a silent period is beneficial (Belin et al. 1999; Scarff et al. 2004).

2.2
Simultaneous EEG and fMRI Acquisitions: Continuous Scanning

Continuous scanning—i.e. uninterrupted acquisition of fMRI volumes, as is the case in conventional fMRI experiments—is the preferred option in terms of fMRI data acquisition strategy in the majority of experimental situations. By acquiring the maximum amount of data per unit time, statistical (detection) power and characterisation of the HRF are optimised (see Fig. 1). A number of hardware and software technical developments allow adequate EEG quality recording during MR scanning for most applications. The most widely used techniques for the removal of artefacts on the EEG are based on modifications of the template subtraction method developed by Allen and colleagues for pulse and scanning artefact reduction (Allen et al. 1998, 2000; see the chapters "EEG Quality: Origin and Reduction of the EEG Cardiac-Related Artefact" and "EEG Quality: The Image Acquisition Artefact"). A number of commercially available EEG recording and artefact correction systems allow continuous scanning. Studies have demonstrated that EEG data quality from continuous recording can be as good as that from sparse sampling paradigms, at least at low frequencies (<20 Hz), thereby allowing analysis of a wide range of EEG phenomena (Salek-Haddadi et al. 2003b; Becker et al. 2005; Comi et al. 2005; Sammer et al. 2005; Im et al. 2006; Bénar et al. 2007b; Debener et al. 2007; Warbrick and Bagshaw 2008).

2.3
Experimental Protocol

EEG–fMRI experimental protocols reflect the two main types of EEG phenomena, namely spontaneous brain activity in the resting state (i.e. in the absence of any experimental manipulation or stimulation) and stimulus-driven paradigms, where the interest is focussed on the brain response to particular stimuli.

2.3.1
Resting State EEG–fMRI: Spontaneous Brain Activity

The first simultaneous EEG–fMRI studies concentrated on two types of spontaneous activity, interictal epileptic spikes (Ives et al. 1993; Warach et al. 1996; Seeck et al. 1998;

Krakow et al. 1999; Al-Asmi et al. 2003) and alpha waves (Goldman et al. 2002; Laufs et al. 2003a; Moosmann et al. 2003). EEG–fMRI has also found application in the study of a number of other types of spontaneous activity: generalised spike-and-wave discharges (Archer et al. 2003; Aghakhani et al. 2004; Gotman et al. 2005; Laufs et al. 2006b; Hamandi et al. 2008), ictal epileptic discharges (Jackson and Opdam 2000; Salek-Haddadi et al. 2002; Federico et al. 2005; Kobayashi et al. 2006) and sleep spindles (Laufs et al. 2006c; Schabus et al. 2007). For reviews, see Salek-Haddadi et al. (2003a); Gotman et al. (2006); Stern (2006); Laufs and Duncan (2007). EEG–fMRI has also been used to study the neural correlates of sleep (Lovblad et al. 1999; Portas et al. 2000; Czisch et al. 2002; Tanaka et al. 2003; Czisch et al. 2004; Fukunaga et al. 2006; Horovitz et al. 2007) or arousal level (Matsuda et al. 2002; Foucher et al. 2004), and has been applied to the investigation of "resting state" networks (Laufs et al. 2003b; Mantini et al. 2007b; Scheeringa et al. 2008).

In such studies subjects are usually asked to keep their eyes closed and to stay still. Keeping the eyes closed is clearly relevant for alpha-wave studies, and also permits eye blink artefacts on the EEG to be avoided. The advantage of keeping the eyes closed is not so straightforward for the study of other brain rhythms. This is a parameter of the protocol that needs consideration, as there could be interactions between having eyes open/closed, arousal level and the activity of interest. For example, for epileptic spikes, there can be a higher spike yield in low arousal or sleep states (Malow et al. 1997), which can be a confounding effect as the response could originate from regions involved in the fluctuation of the arousal level, in the generation of alpha waves or in visual areas.

2.3.2
Stimulus-Driven Paradigms

While the advantages of simultaneous EEG–fMRI are obvious for the study of spontaneous activity, this is not so for paradigms involving experimental manipulation of the subject's brain state (Josephs et al. 1997), for example in evoked response studies involving repetitions of the same set of stimuli. As noted in the chapter "Principles of Multimodal Functional Imaging and Data Integration", one must consider the possibility of separate EEG and fMRI recording sessions before embarking on simultaneous acquisitions in such situations. In particular, one must consider whether the EEG recording could take place in a separate session by replicating the experimental protocol performed in the scanner. Moreover, simultaneous recordings have major drawbacks relative to separate EEG and fMRI sessions. For example, simultaneous recording significantly lengthens the fMRI session because of the time needed to apply the EEG cap or electrodes and to set up the EEG system in the fMRI environment (even though simultaneous recording shortens the total acquisition time for a given subject). In addition, simultaneous recording results in a less comfortable setup for the subject, which may limit the total scanning time and in extreme cases can result in premature termination of the session.

However, as noted in the chapter "Principles of Multimodal Functional Imaging and Data Integration", there are situations where simultaneous recordings are necessary. Firstly, to ensure that signals correspond to the same conditions and brain states, for example in terms of lighting, ambient noise, confinement, arousal, emotional state, strategy, etc.

This can be of particular interest for memory and learning protocols, as well as for auditory paradigms (Mulert et al. 2004). Secondly, for the study of individual events (Fell 2007), which are the only "true" events (in contrast to averages), allowing a deeper study of the relationship between fMRI and EEG (Debener et al. 2005; Eichele et al. 2005; Bénar et al. 2007b). Thirdly, monitoring of EEG markers of general brain state (e.g. arousal) may inform the analysis of responses to stimuli (Matsuda et al. 2002). Finally, the EEG can serve as a "control" modality when one needs to compare the fMRI recordings with other modalities that can also be recorded simultaneously with EEG, such as MEG, intracranial EEG, near-infrared spectroscopy, etc. The simultaneously acquired EEG signals can then serve to assess the extent to which the activity of interest (e.g. evoked potentials or background activity) is reproducible across sessions.

3
Analysis of Simultaneously Acquired EEG–fMRI Data

Since it is a relatively new instrument, EEG–fMRI studies have often had an exploratory flavour, although they are hypothesis-driven at the level of each dataset. This is particularly the case in the study of spontaneous brain activity (epileptic discharges, rhythms, etc.) aimed at identifying the spatiotemporal patterns of haemodynamic change related to the EEG phenomena of interest, with the primary question generally being "do any parts of the brain activate/deactivate in relation to a specific EEG phenomenon?" This has mainly been done through analyses of the correlation of the BOLD time series with a postulated EEG-derived model of haemodynamic changes, implemented in the form of general linear models (GLM). In the language of the chapter "Principles of Multimodal Functional Imaging and Data Integration", this analytical approach can be characterised as being asymmetric and hypothesis-driven (EEG-derived GLM). The above question can be rephrased to be more specific as: "assuming a fixed and well-characterised response to a brief neuronal (EEG) event, what are the brain regions, if any, which activate/deactivate in relation to the observed EEG events?" and can be answered using the spike-triggered acquisition mode discussed previously and in analyses of EEG–fMRI data that assume a fixed HRF (see below).

Another question that has often been explored is "what is the 'optimal' EEG-derived model of haemodynamic changes?" Interest in this question has been motivated by the suspicion that the relationship between neuronal activity and haemodynamic changes for spontaneous brain activity reflected on the EEG may deviate from the norm (represented by the "canonical" HRF), particularly in pathological systems. Unfortunately, no ground truth against which models can be formally evaluated is generally available in human studies, and in practice this question has been explored by using relatively flexible HRF basis sets or families of GLMs to map out the spatiotemporal variability of the EEG-related BOLD changes, including the shape of the HRF. For stimulus-based studies, the analysis of EEG–fMRI has focused on exploring the relationship between specific details of the EEG responses and the time-locked BOLD signal. These can be addressed within the GLM framework using parametric designs. Even more exploratory approaches have also been proposed that rely on the identification of patterns in the multivariate data based on general assumptions relating to the statistical properties of the signals, such as principal component analysis (PCA) and independent component analysis (ICA). The above relates to the analysis of individual datasets and will be discussed in more detail in the remainder of this section.

Note that the methods available for group studies where anatomically consistent effects can be hypothesized across subjects, such as evoked responses and EEG rhythms, will not be reviewed here since the details are not specific to EEG–fMRI, and we refer the reader to the chapter "Brain Rhythms" for further reading. However, there is one aspect of the analysis of group EEG–fMRI data that demands particular attention, namely the potential for exceedingly unbalanced designs from widely varying experimental efficiencies of recordings of spontaneous brain activity. A discussion of this point can be found in Friston et al. (2005), and an example application in generalised epilepsy in Hamandi et al. (2008).

3.1
Model-Based Analysis of fMRI Time-Series Data

The basic strategy for the analysis of fMRI data aims at identifying the voxels at which the BOLD signal is significantly correlated with a postulated time course, and therefore can be reframed as the problem of identifying the sources of signal variance.

3.1.1
Preprocessing

It has been shown that a large proportion of the variance in fMRI time series can be attributed to head motion (Friston et al. 1996). Therefore, the first step of the fMRI processing pipeline usually consists of the spatial realignment of the serially acquired scans (Friston et al. 1995). This step is commonly followed by spatial smoothing to boost the signal of interest according to the matched filter theorem and to make the data conform better to the assumptions of Gaussian random field (GRF) theory, which is used to make inferences in the classical statistical framework (see below). The amount of smoothing must be chosen by considering the expected spatial scale of the expected haemodynamic changes and the need for the degree of data smoothness to be substantially greater than the voxel size (see Penny and Friston, Classical and Bayesian Inference in fMRI, in: Human Brain Function; see Josephs and Henson 1999 for a detailed discussion of event-related fMRI data analysis).

The rest of the analysis pipeline focuses on the derivation of maps consisting of voxels for which changes in the BOLD signal can be related to the aspect of brain activity, which is of interest to the investigator.

3.1.2
The General Linear Model (GLM) and Statistical Inference

The most commonly used fMRI data analysis strategy relies on fitting a general linear model (GLM) to the data (Friston et al. 1994). A GLM consists of a set of equations expressing the predicted fMRI signal time course as a weighted sum of linear terms representing the effects of interest and confounds. The GLM is therefore an expression of the assumption that fMRI changes can be linearly related to the experimental effects at every voxel. In the absence of prior localisation-related hypotheses about this relationship, as is commonly the case in most fMRI studies, the same GLM (set of linear equations) is estimated (i.e. fitted to the data) at every brain voxel, resulting in estimated weights. The localising information provided by fMRI derives from the variability of resulting weights across voxels.

This section provides a brief introduction to the GLM, focusing on model specification and statistical inference; explanations of model estimation and statistical models can be found in Worsley et al. (2002) or in the Statistical Parametric Mapping (SPM) software manual (available at http://www.fil.ion.ucl.ac.uk/spm/doc/manual.pdf). Note that the GLM approach is closely related to the often-used correlation analysis and represents a generalisation of the latter that is capable of handling multiple linear regressions corresponding to multiple effects of interest.

In the following we will focus exclusively on classical estimation and inference; the reader is invited to consult Penny and Friston (2003) for a comparative discussion of the classical and Bayesian approaches to fMRI data analysis.

Building a GLM

The fMRI signal at any given voxel is represented as a vector of serial observations, y_i, $i = 1...N$, where N is the total number of observations (scans). Each observation y_i is modelled as a weighted sum of x_k ($k = 1...K$) "regressors", where K is the number of effects represented in the model, and the residual (zero mean) error,

$$e: y_i = \beta_1 x_{i1} + \beta_2 x_{i2} + ... + \beta_K x_{iK} + e_i, \tag{1}$$

where β_j are the unknown weights for each of the K effects; the β's are usually referred to as the model parameters. Expressed in vector and matrix form, we have:

$$Y = X\beta + e. \tag{2}$$

The matrix **X** represents the modelled effects and is known as the design matrix. The aim of the GLM estimation procedure is to estimate the model parameters, i.e. vector β, at every voxel.

Regressors are usually categorised as effects of interest or effects of no interest (i.e. confounds). The dichotomy relates to the desire to separate signal from noise in all its forms, such as associated with instrumental, physiological or other effects (body motion) not related to the effects of interest.

Regressors of interest therefore model the part of the fMRI signal that relates to the experimental events or conditions (stimuli, responses, epileptic spikes, EEG alpha power, etc). Regressors representing the effects of interest are typically obtained by convolving impulses or boxcar functions, which are mathematical representations of the events or conditions of interest, with a model of the even-related fMRI response such as the canonical haemodynamic response function (HRF) or other basis set (e.g. inclusion of additional time and dispersion derivatives; Fourier expansion; finite impulse response). The choice of a specific mathematical representation for the events of interest is dictated by the nature of the events. In the case of a very brief external stimuli or spontaneous epileptic spikes,[1] the events are typically represented by a stick (delta) function. In contrast, runs (or bursts) of epileptic spikes may be represented as series of individual stick functions, each presenting a spike, or as variable-duration blocks. For continually varying brain activity, such as brain rhythms, the EEG signal power may be used as a mathematical representation of the neuronal activity. The choice of haemodynamic basis set reflects a number of considerations: for example, one may wish to estimate the shape of the event-related BOLD change rather than assume any particular shape, in which case a flexible model is required using a basis set consisting of multiple functions over a shorter or longer time window than the canonical HRF; alternatively, by restricting the basis set to a single function, effects that match this function can be detected with maximum sensitivity; see Josephs and Henson 1999. Each of these choices corresponds to a model to be tested, expressing a specific set of assumptions about the relationship between stimulus (when present), neuronal response and haemodynamic signal. This will be the subject of further discussion in forthcoming sections on specific EEG-derived modelling strategies.

Regressors of no interest are introduced to attempt to model the remainder of the fMRI signal. Important examples are: structured noise, which may include movement-related signal changes, and can be modelled using the realignment parameters of the fMRI time series; and slow fluctuations due to drift in scanner sensitivity, which can be modelled as a sum of low-frequency sine and cosine waves. When modelled accurately, the inclusion of such effects can be important, as it permits a more reliable estimation of the coefficients of the GLM corresponding to the effects of interest, and increases the level of confidence in the findings (Lund et al. 2005). For example, if the regressor of interest varies slowly and is not orthogonal to the slow drifts, part of the energy of the slow drift could be wrongly attributed to the regressor of interest (i.e. the corresponding coefficient would be overestimated).

Within the classical framework, parameter estimation proceeds using *ordinary least squares*, a standard methodology which aims to minimise the residual sum of squares, i.e. the sum of the squared difference between the predicted signal change and the observations (sum of *e* terms in Eq. 1). For the GLM, this procedure guarantees maximum likelihood estimates, which is an important, often-cited statistical concept. It means that the estimated parameter values are the most probable given the data.

An important issue when building a GLM is that of correlation (i.e. nonorthogonality) between regressors, which can result in loss of sensitivity. This may be particularly problematic in models that contain several event-related parametric factors, and require an orthogonalisation procedure (Eichele et al. 2005). Another issue concerns the linearity between EEG and fMRI that is implied in the construction of a parametric regressor. Such linearity may not be guaranteed (Vazquez and Noll 1998; Wager et al. 2005; Wan et al. 2006), but the large literature using the linear model suggests that it is a reasonable assumption. Moreover, linear analysis may still capture some nonlinear effects (Deneux and

---

[1]Epileptic spikes span approximately 100 ms, which is very short in terms of fMRI; although this duration can vary in a subject, the effect of spike length has not yet been explored and spikes are typically represented as "'zero-duration'" events.

Faugeras 2006). Additional regressors can also be added to a GLM (with the parameters elevated to the power of 2, 3, etc.) in order to model nonlinear effects (Friston et al. 1998).

Statistics

The goal of statistical inference in fMRI within the GLM framework is to test whether the amplitude of β (or a combination of coefficients) is significantly different from zero. A linear combination of coefficients is called a contrast. For example, in a task involving an active condition (corresponding to β_1) and a reference condition (corresponding to β_2), the contrast would be $(\beta_1 - \beta_2)$.[2] The statistical significance of such a contrast can be tested with a t statistic:

$$T = (\beta_1 - \beta_2)/\mathrm{std}\,(\beta_1 - \beta_2) \sim (\beta_1 - \beta_2)/S(\beta_1 - \beta_2) \tag{3}$$

where $\mathrm{std}(\beta)$ is the estimated standard deviation of β, which is proportional to the sum of the squares of the residuals, $S(\beta)$. Taking the simple case of a GLM with a single regressor of interest and its corresponding parameter, β, we can use such a t statistic

$$T = \beta/\mathrm{std}\,(\beta) \tag{4}$$

to test the hypothesis, $\beta > 0$. This is the simplest contrast and is commonly used to test whether a predicted experimental effect (e.g. associated with a simple ON-OFF stimulus) is likely to be present in the data.

Another option is to test whether at least one coefficient within a set is different from zero. This can be necessary when the activity of interest is modelled by several regressors, such as in models using a basis set consisting of more than one function. For example, in order to test for departures of the haemodynamic response from the canonical HRF, it can be useful to include the derivative of the HRF into the model in addition to the canonical HRF to map brain regions for which the BOLD signal can be represented by any linear combination of the canonical HRF and its temporal derivative. This can be accomplished using an F test, which is essentially a generalisation of the t test that allows us to test a hypothesis on a subset, β_1, of the parameters β; for example, that $\beta_1 = 0$. An F statistic can be devised by considering the full model and the reduced version of the model that is obtained if the hypothesis is true ($\beta_1 = 0$). Representing the reduced model by the subset of parameters, β_2, the appropriate F statistic is:

$$F = \frac{\dfrac{[S(\beta_2) - S(\beta)]}{p - p_2}}{\dfrac{S(\beta)}{N - p}}, \tag{5}$$

where $S(\beta)$ is the squares of the residuals for the full model (and $S(\beta_2)$ for the reduced model), p is the rank of the design matrix for the full model (and p_2 for the reduced model),

---

[2] Corresponding to contrast vector [1, -1] in the language of the SPM software.

and N is the number of scans. An explanation of the implementation of Eq. 5 in the SPM software using contrast matrices can be found in (see Penny and Friston, 2003). An example of its application using a Fourier basis set can be found in the chapter "EEG–fMRI in Adults with Focal Epilepsy" (Fig. 1).

Significance of BOLD Changes

The above process results in 3D maps representing the t or F statistic of the effect of interest at every voxel: the so-called "statistical parametric maps" or SPMs. The statistics are derived independently for each voxel, which can easily number in the tens of thousands in the brain—hence the "massively univariate analysis" terminology often used in the context of fMRI. However, the significance of the deviations from the null hypothesis (i.e. the conversion of t statistics to Z scores) must be assessed in relation to the maximum score or the size of an activated region. Crucially, only the false-positive rate (type I errors) can be controlled. Type II error control is generally neglected since it is difficult to specify a quantitative alternative hypothesis in fMRI as is required for a power calculation. To put it simply, the lack of activation does not prove that there is no underlying brain activity.

Numerous means of calculating significance thresholds for functional MR images have been developed, the most important of which is based on the theory of random Gaussian fields (Worsley et al. 1992). This is a parametric framework that controls for the fact that, in the null hypothesis of no significant effect, the maximum value of the map can be above the threshold with a p value of α (typically, $\alpha = 0.05$). Such a threshold is corrected for the large multiple comparison problem that arises when simultaneously testing a large number of voxels, and corresponds to the family-wise error rate (FWE). Another option, within the same framework, is to use a threshold based on the extent of a given cluster of activated voxels above an uncorrected threshold with a low p value (typically, $\alpha = 0.001$) (Poline et al. 1997; Cao 1999). The thresholds obtained with random field theory are typically high and require a large level of image smoothing (typically with a filter FWHM of 10–15 mm). A second alternative is to use the threshold that allows a given portion of activated voxels to be false detections. This is the "false detection rate" (FDR), which is a less conservative than the family-wise statistic on the maximum (Genovese et al. 2002). We note that the classical interpretation of FDR has recently been challenged (Chumbley and Friston 2009). A third alternative is to derive the distribution of the statistic in the null hypothesis directly from the data, for example by shuffling the labels of active and control conditions (Bullmore et al. 2001). This is the nonparametric framework, which allows the structure of the data (spatiotemporal correlations) to be taken into account explicitly, and which handles the multiple comparison issue in a straightforward manner (Nichols and Holmes 2002; Meriaux et al. 2006).

3.2
EEG-Derived GLM: Use of Event Onsets and Illustration in Epilepsy

The study of the haemodynamic correlates of spontaneous brain activity using EEG–fMRI is particularly interesting, as it raises a number of important issues related to GLM building,

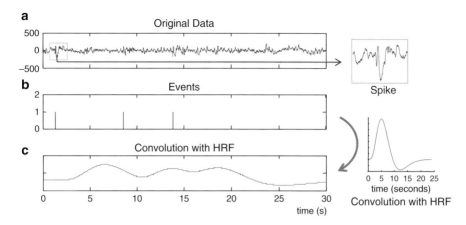

Fig. 2a–c Modelling of fMRI signal time course using event timing alone and basis set consisting of a single function. **a** Each event (here, interictal epileptic spikes) is marked by visual inspection of the EEG data recorded in the scanner. **b** Onset vector: series of identical impulse ("delta") functions. **c** Corresponding regressor for a general linear model (GLM) obtained by convolving the events with a canonical HRF

namely the identification and categorisation of events of interest, the mathematical representation of those events and the choice of a basis set for the HRF, and model comparison. Due to fluctuations in the background EEG, defining the baseline (control state) is also a challenge.

Since the first applications of EEG–fMRI were in patients with epilepsy, the first attempts at data integration were geared towards the study of subclinical (without behavioural manifestations), randomly occurring, epileptic discharges (for reviews, see Salek-Haddadi et al. 2003a; Gotman et al. 2004, 2006; Lemieux 2004). The aim of this strategy is to find regions of BOLD change linked to the discharges. The timing of interictal epileptiform discharges (IED) is used in an event-related fMRI analysis to create regressors representing the effects of interest, by convolving the event onsets represented as delta functions[3] with a model of the event-related haemodynamic change in the form of a haemodynamic basis set (Fig. 2).

Readers less familiar with EEG in epilepsy should be made aware that the spatiotemporal aspects of IED vary greatly between patients and can also vary in time for any given patient. Therefore, although conceptually simple, this approach relies on the detection of those events—a subjective process—and their categorisation. The latter point is important because each regressor corresponds to a hypothesis that can be phrased as follows: there are brain regions in which the BOLD signal change *averaged across the events* is nonzero. This implies that the events grouped into each regressor are haemodynamically consistent. More sophisticated approaches can take into account various morphological aspects of the IED, such as duration and amplitude.

The haemodynamic basis set can consist of a single function such as the canonical or standard HRF, or a multiplicity of functions such as sets of time-shifted standard HRF, the finite impulse response (FIR) and Fourier basis sets (Bagshaw et al. 2004; Josephs et al. 1997;

---

[3]Usually implemented as a stick function of unitary amplitude.

Josephs and Henson 1999). As alluded to in the previous section, models based on a single function are optimal for the detection of BOLD changes that match that function, whereas models based on basis sets with multiple functions can be used to assess the shape of the event-related BOLD changes and to map inter-regional variations in the time course of the changes.

The degree of variability in the time course of the IED-related BOLD changes and the potential effect on detection efficiency remains the subject of investigation (Kang et al. 2003; Bagshaw et al. 2004; Lu et al. 2006; Salek-Haddadi et al. 2006; Lemieux et al. 2008). It has been shown that BOLD changes time-locked with EEG events may appear earlier or later than predicted by the standard model, in epilepsy and normal brain rhythms (Feige et al. 2005; de Munck et al. 2007; Lemieux et al. 2008), sometimes even prior to scalp EEG changes (Hawco et al. 2007). Such observations may be seen as highlighting a limitation of the scalp EEG as a basis for modelling whole-brain brain activity, but also as an example of the added value of the combined method. However, the lack of a proper assessment of response variability using the specific modelling approaches used in the above studies in relation to event-related BOLD effects in healthy brains limits our ability to interpret the observed deviations as being specifically related to epilepsy. In particular, the often-cited study by Aguirre on the variability of the response to a reaction-time motor task is based on a Fourier basis set consisting of only three sines and three cosines, which is less flexible than most models used in the above epilepsy studies (Aguirre et al. 1998).

The above issues are ultimately related to model selection, which is a fundamental problem of science and is particularly troublesome in the classical statistical framework, which usually favours complex models over simple models since the former tend to explain a greater proportion of the variance.[4] Nonetheless, it is relatively common practice to compare models in EEG–fMRI, particularly when exploring the relationship between EEG and fMRI. This is often done by selecting the way in which regressors expressing different model variants are incorporated into GLMs. By incorporating all effects of interest within a single, embedded model, one can test for the significance of the variance explained by specific factors through appropriate F contrasts (see Salek-Haddadi et al. 2006 and Liston et al. 2006 for illustrations). An alternative is to build a set of alternative GLMs. In this approach, statistical correction factors must be applied to account for multiple models, and selection of the result ("best" model and associated map) requires the application of an additional criterion, such as the extent of activation or t score (Bagshaw et al. 2005).

Evidently, the data acquisition and analysis strategies described above are fundamentally different from conventional "activation" fMRI experiments in that there is no explicit reference or control state. In the resting state, fluctuations in brain rhythms are accompanied by typical BOLD patterns (Goldman et al. 2002; Laufs et al. 2003a, 2003b; Mantini et al. 2007b). Therefore, it is conceivable that background EEG may be used to improve models of the baseline fMRI signal fluctuations in addition to the usual confounding effects of respiration, the cardiac cycle, motion and instrument-related effects (e.g. low-frequency drifts).

The exquisite temporal resolution of EEG recorded simultaneously with fMRI offers the possibility of modelling MR signal changes in the latter at a much faster timescale than the BOLD effect, namely the neuroelectric MR effect (sometimes referred to as neuronal

---

[4]The Bayesian approach is probably preferable as it allows inclusion of an "Occam factor" in the comparison.

current MR imaging) (Bodurka and Bandettini 2002; Hagberg et al. 2006). By precisely identifying the onset of generalised spike-wave discharges in relation to the acquisition of individual MR slices, Liston et al. employed a basis set consisting of a series of FIRs to study MR signal changes at a 30-ms timescale (Liston et al. 2004).

3.3
EEG-Derived GLM: Parametric Design and Single Trial

The use of single-trial and spectral information, which are widely applied in sensory and cognitive neuroscience applications, leads to event-related designs similar to those described above in epilepsy, differing mainly in the nature of the EEG information that is included in the GLM analysis.

A strategy employed to investigate the coupling between the EEG and fMRI signals is the manipulation of one or several parameters within the protocol and the comparison of the corresponding fluctuations in the EEG and fMRI signals. As described in the chapter "Principles of Multimodal Functional Imaging and Data Integration", this type of study may be done in separate or simultaneous data acquisition sessions depending on the experimental conditions and the type of inference that one wishes to make. For example, by varying the intertrial interval or stimulation intensity, one is able to divide the trials into groups, resulting in one EEG and one fMRI analysis per group. One can then test whether the two signals fluctuate similarly across groups (Horovitz 2004). This approach has been applied for evoked potentials (Liebenthal et al. 2003), high frequency (gamma activity) (Foucher et al. 2003), and even recently to ultrahigh (600 Hz) responses (Ritter et al. 2008).

The inclusion of parameters derived from a single-trial analysis of the EEG data, i.e. from the individual EEG responses to the stimuli, offers the possibility of exploring the relationship between EEG and haemodynamic signals much more deeply; for example, the BOLD correlates of the ERP amplitude (Debener et al. 2005; Eichele et al. 2005), latency (Bénar et al. 2007b), or the amplitude of high-frequency oscillations (Mulert et al. 2007). See Fig. 3 for a description of parametric analysis and Fig. 4 for an application.

The analysis of single-trial data is hampered by a low signal-to-noise ratio, reflecting a lack of neuronal specificity (the signal is a mixture of different processes because of volume-conduction effects) compared to averaged responses. Single-trial analysis techniques designed to improve signal-to-noise ratio based on feature extraction are receiving increasing attention in combined EEG–fMRI analysis (Mayhew et al. 2006; Philiastides and Sajda 2006), as well as in all fields of EEG processing, for example brain–computer interfaces (Cincotti et al. 2003). Several aspects of the activity can help to characterise intertrial fluctuations: temporal structure, its time–frequency structure (Quian Quiroga and Garcia 2003; Bénar et al. 2007a; Wang et al. 2007), its spatial configuration across sensors, or a combination of these (Ranta-aho et al. 2003; Li et al. 2007).

Spatial processing techniques can also be used to help separate the activity from different sources, and also provide a form of denoising by gathering the information arising from different sensors. The main method of spatial unmixing that has been applied so far in EEG–fMRI is ICA (see the section on multivariate analysis). Source localisation or spatial filtering can also serve this purpose, with the additional potential advantage, given

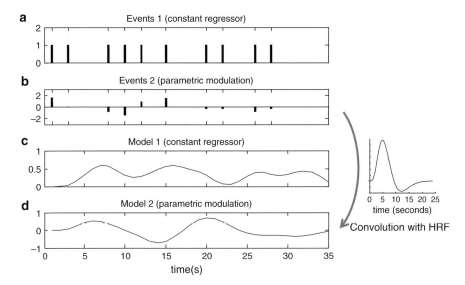

Fig. 3a–d Modelling of fMRI data using parametric modulation. **a** Vector of event onsets as in Fig. 2; **b** EEG event feature vector (e.g. amplitude, duration). **c, d** Corresponding regressor obtained by convolution of (**a**) and (**b**) respectively with the canonical HRF. When combined in a single GLM, statistical maps can be obtained showing voxels for which each effect explains a significant amount of additional variance by defining appropriate contrasts (Salek-Haddadi et al. 2006)

an appropriate model, of providing spatial information on the processes of interest (Brookes et al. 2008). This is a very promising approach, as it would permit the fMRI signal to be correlated with the source of EEG data originating from the same region.

3.4
EEG-Derived GLM: EEG Spectrum

One of the most important uses of EEG–fMRI to date has been in identifying the brain regions that co-vary with changes in brain rhythms and more generally EEG spectral power. Although oscillatory activity has been studied since the earliest days of EEG (Berger 1929), locating the cortical generators of this activity using EEG alone is difficult because of the ill-posed nature of the inverse problem (Hadamard 1902; Geselowitz 1967; Helmholtz 1853). fMRI provides an alternative method that has the potential advantage over EEG source localisation of being capable of detecting activity in subcortical structures.

Studies of spectral power can be split into two basic categories: those which examine spontaneous fluctuations and those which use an experimental manipulation to modify spectral power in a specific frequency range. The analytical approach is essentially the same for both types of data, and is conceptually similar to what was discussed previously. Typically, EEG data are filtered in short epochs of the order of a second, and power in one or more frequency bands is quantified for each epoch. In most applications, the power time

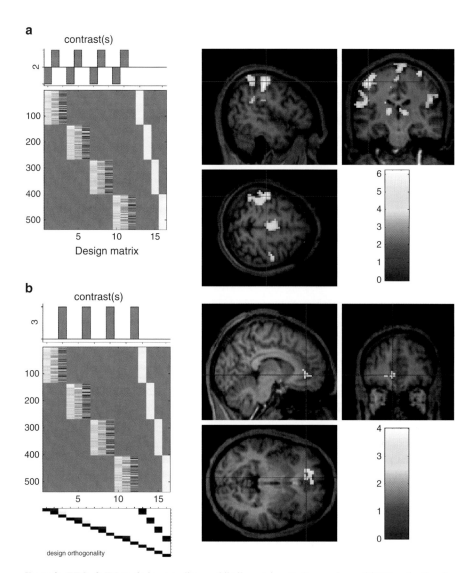

Fig. 4a–b EEG–fMRI study in an auditory oddball experiment. Comparison of fMRI activation for (**a**) rare events and (**b**) parametric modulation based on P300 amplitude at Cz (subject 1 of Bénar et al. 2007b). The detailed design matrix is presented on the left column. There are four runs and three regressors per run: frequent events, rare events and parametric modulation (see Fig. 3). In (**a**) the contrast is "rare–frequent". In (**b**) the contrast only includes the parametric regressor

series is convolved with a postulated kernel function representing the BOLD change per impulse input (usually the standard haemodynamic response function) and entered as a regressor in a GLM analysis (Fig. 5). The choice of EEG channel or group of channels for the power calculation requires careful consideration (e.g. see Laufs et al. 2003a). This kind

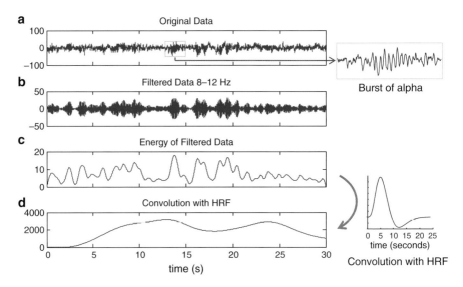

Fig. 5a–d Modelling of fMRI time series using the energy within a frequency band. **a** Original EEG data, where several alpha wave bursts can be seen. **b, c** Energy in the 8–12 Hz band, using a sliding-window Fourier transform (Goldman et al. 2002). **d** Regressor obtained by convolving energy with canonical HRF

of study is particularly demanding on EEG quality (see the chapters "EEG Quality: Origin and Reduction of the EEG Cardiac-Related Artefact" and "EEG Quality: The Image Acquisition Artefact").

Early examples of this type of study were based on interleaved acquisitions, with posterior alpha power extracted from simultaneously acquired EEG–fMRI data (Goldman et al. 2002; Laufs et al. 2003a). Although to date this technique has mostly been applied to the study of the alpha rhythm (Moosmann et al. 2003; Feige et al. 2005; Goncalves et al. 2006; Laufs et al. 2006a; de Munck et al. 2007), it can also be used to examine oscillations at higher or lower frequency. For example, Laufs and colleagues (Laufs et al. 2003b) also quantified beta power and included that as a regressor in the fMRI analysis, and noted the similarity between the regions identified and those associated with the default mode network (DMN) (Raichle and Snyder 2007). Recent work on event-related synchronisation and desynchronisation (ERD/ERS, Pfurtscheller and Lopes da Silva 1999) using EEG–fMRI has focussed on the BOLD correlates of low-frequency oscillations in the theta and delta range (<7 Hz) during hyperventilation (Makiranta et al. 2004) and mental arithmetic (Mizuhara et al. 2004; Sammer et al. 2007). Some work has also been done at even lower frequencies of the order of 1 Hz or less (see Khader et al. 2008 for a review). Parkes and colleagues attempted to use the same methodology to examine the BOLD correlates of the post-movement beta rebound (Parkes et al. 2006). See the chapter "Brain Rhythms" for a review of the findings.

Using an approach similar to Liston et al. (2006), Mandelkow et al. attempted to detect fast (neuronal current-related) signal changes linked to alpha power, but were hampered by the pulse artefact (Mandelkow et al. 2007). More generally, difficulties that can arise from narrow band filtering are presented in 5.3.2.

3.5
Multivariate Analysis

The analysis technique outlined above is based on the interrogation of the fMRI signal through the same EEG-derived model at each and every voxel, and is therefore often referred to as a *massively univariate* approach. An alternative approach is the identification of meaningful patterns (e.g. across multiple voxels or EEG channels) based on more generic assumptions for the properties of signals and their generators (Martinez-Montes et al. 2004).

Several multivariate techniques have been proposed for the analysis of biophysical signals: PCA (Rosler and Manzey 1981; Lai and Fang 1999; Dien et al. 2007), singular value decomposition (SVD), nonlinear PCA (Friston et al. 1999; Thirion and Faugeras 2003), canonical component analysis (Vitrai et al. 1984; De Clercq et al. 2006), partial least squares (PLS) analysis (McIntosh and Lobaugh 2004), ICA (Makeig et al. 1997; Kobayashi et al. 1999; Vigario et al. 2000; Jung et al. 2001; James and Gibson 2003; Tang et al. 2005), and parallel factor analysis (Miwakeichi et al. 2004).

ICA can be used to decompose EEG signals (N channels $\times$ P time points) into a set of fixed topographies (across the N channels) and a corresponding time course, with the constraint that the time courses are maximally independent (temporal ICA). Spatial ICA, whereby a constraint of maximally independent spatial patterns is employed, has been used successfully to identify "sources" in fMRI. Several algorithms have been proposed for computing such decompositions (Bell and Sejnowski 1995; Cardoso 1999; Hyvarinen and Oja 2000).

ICA can be used to remove the artefact on the EEG traces (Bénar et al. 2003; Srivastava et al. 2005; Briselli et al. 2006; Nakamura et al. 2006; Bagshaw and Warbrick 2007; Debener et al. 2007; Mantini et al. 2007a), or on the fMRI signal (McKeown et al. 2005; Bagshaw and Warbrick 2007). The artefacts thus identified can be subsequently removed from the data for further analysis. This approach is potentially very useful, but one of the major difficulties is the identification of the components of interest (LeVan et al. 2006; Ting et al. 2006; Perlbarg et al. 2007; Tohka et al. 2008). Moreover, the activity of interest (e.g. the pulse-related artefact) may not have a stable spatiotemporal pattern, which violates one of the basic assumptions of ICA, rendering the process suboptimal (Wallstrom et al. 2004; Debener et al. 2008). Conversely, ICA has also been used to identify signals representing activity of interest (McKeown et al. 1998; Jung et al. 2001; Duann et al. 2002; Rodionov et al. 2007). This has two attractions: signal denoising, which is very useful for single-trial analysis (Bagshaw and Warbrick 2007), and it separates the activity from different sources. Such an approach has been used for single-trial EEG–fMRI studies (Debener et al. 2005). Recently, a joint ICA approach was proposed with both EEG and fMRI signals considered together (Kraut et al. 2003; Stevens et al. 2005; Calhoun et al. 2006; Eichele et al. 2008; Moosmann et al. 2008; Pearlson and Calhoun 2007).

4
EEG and fMRI Localisation: Modes of Integration

We have already seen how EEG and fMRI can be correlated using EEG-derived GLMs and how multivariate methods are beginning to be used to extract further spatial and temporal information from the signals. In this approach, the EEG is used purely as a time marker of brain state, in the same way as external stimuli or responses in conventional cognitive fMRI studies. We now step back from simultaneous acquisitions to explore further how the two modalities can be integrated with the specific aim of localising the generators of the underlying brain activity. For example, how can EEG source imaging be combined with fMRI to enhance localisation?

As discussed in the chapter "Principles of Multimodal Functional Imaging and Data Integration", methods for the fusion of localisation information obtained from EEG and fMRI analysis can be categorised according to the degree to which the relationship between the two signals forms part of a model and the role that each modality plays in the model. Coregistration of independently derived EEG and fMRI localisation probably represents the least model-dependent mode of data fusion. In the preceding sections we have already described the mechanics of a more "intimate" though asymmetric form of integration, namely the prediction of fMRI signal changes based on EEG. Finally, we find "symmetric" source reconstruction algorithms.

4.1
Comparison of Independently Derived Results

One of the most common strategies for multimodal integration has been to treat the EEG and fMRI data sets separately and compare the results in space (fusion a posteriori; Kruggel et al. 2000, 2001; Liebenthal et al. 2003; Foucher et al. 2004; Makiranta et al. 2004; Becker et al. 2005; Henning et al. 2005; Otzenberger et al. 2005; Sammer et al. 2005). The simplest way to combine EEG source reconstruction and fMRI data is to compare the localisation results obtained separately (e.g. from the analysis of averaged events) by coregistration and projection onto a common anatomical space (Opitz et al. 1999).

Prior to any attempt at further integration it is probably wise to use this approach as a first step. Spatial concordance cannot be expected in many circumstances due to the fundamentally different natures of the two signals (Nunez and Silberstein 2000; Disbrow et al. 2000; Ritter and Villringer 2006). Nonetheless, a good degree of spatial concordance can provide cross-validation (Lemieux 2001a; Bénar et al. 2006).

In situations with few well-separated activated regions, good spatial concordance (see Fig. 6) allows one to consider the use of the time course of the EEG sources to estimate the chronometry of activation (Rossell et al. 2003; O'Hare et al. 2008). However, the EEG inverse problem can become ambiguous for a small number of electrodes, a large number of activated regions, for spatially extended sources, for regions close to one another, or those with highly correlated time courses (Supek and Aine 1993; Huang et al. 1998; Sekihara et al. 2002). As a consequence, it seems intuitively obvious that guiding the EEG inverse problem with information coming from fMRI, as presented in the next sections, will be helpful.

4.2
fMRI as a Spatial Constraint for EEG Source Reconstruction

The good spatial coverage and localising capability of fMRI on the one hand and the ambiguity of the EEG inverse problem on the other have inspired some investigators to develop

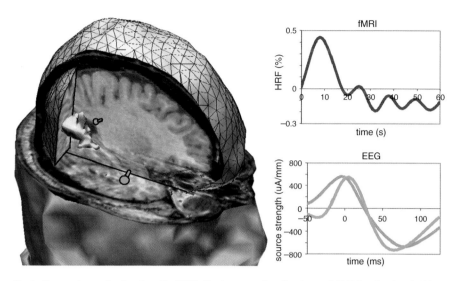

Fig. 6 Comparison of epileptic spike EEG dipole source localisation and fMRI activation (subject 1 of Bénar et al. 2002). Here, only one of the two dipoles (*blue*) matches the fMRI cluster. The evolution of the dipole strength at the concordant dipole location may provide additional time resolution

methods based on the use of fMRI information as a prior constraint that informs EEG source localisation.

In a dipolar framework, this can be done by applying constraints based on the fMRI activation clusters, in the form of either solution space masks or initialisation of the estimates (Menon et al. 1997; Ahlfors et al. 1999; Toma et al. 2002; Bledowski et al. 2004). In a distributed sources framework, it is possible to give more weight to regions with fMRI activation (Liu et al. 1998; Babiloni et al. 2000), although tuning of the weighting parameter is not straightforward. The strength of the fMRI-derived constraints on source modelling is an important consideration: a hard constraint whereby solution dipoles are limited to the region of activation is probably inappropriate in most situations due to the potential discrepancy between EEG generator and BOLD localisation—for example, in cases with regions that respond selectively to one or other of the modalities, perhaps because the task induces a change in neuronal synchrony that does not result in altered metabolic demand.

Careful consideration of the effect of constraints on the solution requires validation when possible. This is a potentially difficult problem, as the number of sources is a very sensitive parameter in EEG dipolar source localisation: for example, placing a model dipole in a region that is silent on fMRI could capture part of the signal from other sources. Conversely, not placing a dipole in an actual EEG source that is not seen by fMRI could result in a "spilling" of its activity to the other dipoles. Similarly, in a distributed sources framework, an fMRI source in an EEG silent area could capture some of the EEG activity. It is therefore necessary to carefully quantify the effects of mismatches over EEG–fMRI integration techniques (Liu et al. 2006).

By enabling the fMRI constraint to be incorporated probabilistically, Bayesian modelling (Baillet and Garnero 1997; Schmidt et al. 1999; Trujillo-Barreto et al. 2001; Phillips et al. 2005) integrates fMRI-activated regions in the form of statistical *priors*, which also forms a natural framework for the evaluation of distributed sources. Moreover, the Bayesian formalism provides a mechanism for model comparison (Trujillo-Barreto et al. 2004), and to assess whether a given fMRI constraint is compatible with the EEG data, for example (Daunizeau et al. 2005; Grova et al. 2008).

4.3
Towards Symmetrical Models of EEG and fMRI Fusion

There have been a few examples of alternatives to the "classical" model of EEG-derived fMRI modelling employed in the vast majority of studies of spontaneous brain activity (see the chapters "Brain Rhythms", "Sleep", "EEG–fMRI in Adults with Focal Epilepsy", "EEG–fMRI in Idiopathic Generalised Epilepsy (Adults)", and "EEG–fMRI in Children with Epilepsy") and evoked responses. For example, fMRI has been used to inform the interpretation of spontaneously occurring events or patterns in simultaneously recorded EEG. Liston et al. (2006b) used a spike clustering method and projection of the entire EEG record onto a set of equivalent sources. They were able to provide additional evidence that spike-like events, not previously identified by expert observers, were probably low-amplitude spikes, since their BOLD signature matched that of the visually identified spikes. Outside the field of epilepsy, Mantini et al. were able to demonstrate the electrophysiological signatures of six spatially characterised resting-state networks (identified using data-driven fMRI analysis) by studying the correlation between the BOLD signal in those networks and the simultaneously recorded EEG across frequency bands (Mantini et al. 2007).

The asymmetry in the role of each modality may reflect a historical bias towards better characterisation of scalp EEG. The ultimate aim of neuroimaging is a model of all neuro-signals and their relationship to neuronal activity, upon which an assessment of the true value of any given modality (in relation to specific brain activity) could be based. A path to such a model has been proposed that removes this asymmetry in biophysical models of neurosignals, with neural activity as input. A symmetrical Bayesian source estimation framework has been introduced that integrates fMRI and EEG data (Trujillo-Barreto et al. 2001). The theoretical promise is that such models would take full advantage of the available information, with resulting improved sensitivity. For example, a weak prediction from each modality may reach significance in the joint analysis.

Such models rely on accurate coupling models, which remain the subject of investigation. In its current implementation, heuristic forms of the coupling function have been used and the Bayesian approach can be used to account for discordant EEG and fMRI-activated regions (Daunizeau et al. 2007) (see the chapter "EEG–fMRI in Animal Models" for further discussion of this approach).

5
Unresolved Problems and Caveats

Ultimately, the entire EEG–fMRI enterprise aims to improve our ability to characterise neuronal activity and in the process improve our understanding of the relationship between the two types of signals. We have explored a range of data acquisition and analysis strategies that allow the investigator to investigate the BOLD correlates of certain aspects of the EEG and more generally the sources of the EEG and fMRI signals. Despite some success at revealing novel information, there are unresolved issues, both conceptual and practical, which need addressing.

5.1
Relationship Between Neuronal Activity, EEG and fMRI Signals

As discussed in the chapter "EEG: Origin and Measurement", scalp EEG is primarily a measure of the synchronous postsynaptic activity of cortical pyramidal neurones (Lopes da Silva and Van Rotterdam 2005; Nunez and Srinivasan 2005), and is largely insensitive to deep structures such as the hippocampus (Merlet and Gotman 2001; Gavaret et al. 2004). Changes in synchrony can have a large effect on the scalp EEG signal even if the overall neuronal firing rate is not altered. Moreover, the closed morphology of certain deep structures such as amygdala or thalamus greatly reduces the measurable external field. However, several studies report findings from deep structures, and the final word may not have been said about the ability of EEG to record from deep structures (Schnitzler et al. 2006). Therefore, scalp EEG is a biased measure of brain activity, dependent not only on the location of the generating region but also the exact temporal relationship between cell populations. As discussed in the chapter "The Basics of Functional Magnetic Resonance Imaging", fMRI reflects changes in blood flow, oxygenation and volume. Indirectly, BOLD fMRI is a measure of energy consumption or metabolic demand (Arthurs and Boniface 2002; Logothetis and Wandell 2004). Combined intracerebral microelectrode and fMRI measurements have shown that the BOLD signal is correlated with variations in neuronal firing rate, and to a greater extent with variations in local field potentials. In particular, strong correlations have been reported between gamma band electrical activity (>35 Hz) and BOLD signals (Logothetis et al. 2001; Niessing et al. 2005; Lachaux et al. 2007; see the chapter "Locally Measured Neuronal Correlates of Functional MRI Signals"). Based on such observations and heuristic arguments, Kilner et al. postulated a linear relationship between the ratio of high- to low-frequency EEG signal power and BOLD (Kilner et al. 2005). However, the observation of haemodynamic signals locked to stimulus timing but without sensory input or expression in the form of the local measures of neuronal activity potentially raises questions about the causal assumptions implied in the GLM and the relationship between neural activity and BOLD (Sirotin and Das 2009).

The linear nature of most fMRI modelling strategies requires the identification of aspects of the EEG signal that are predicted to vary linearly in relation to the BOLD signal to be most efficient, an assumption that has not been investigated to any great extent. Evidently, this is a simple starting assumption in most cases, and has been the subject of much work in relation to evoked or event-related responses. Nonlinear effects have been observed in response to sensory stimuli (Birn and Bandettini 2005; Wan et al. 2006), and epilepsy using the Volterra series in the GLM framework (Salek-Haddadi et al. 2006), and there is certainly considerable scope for more investigation of this issue, particularly in relation to the relative nonlinearities of EEG and fMRI (Arthurs et al. 2007).

5.2
Specific Issues Related to Spontaneous Brain Activity

5.2.1
HRF

In conventional event-related cognitive fMRI experiments in healthy subjects, models based on the standard or canonical HRF (possibly with the addition of extra terms to allow for some variability) have proven successful. Nonetheless, as noted earlier, significant variability has been observed in responses to normal stimuli in healthy brains.

Spontaneous brain activity may be associated with neurophysiological processes that have no correlates on scalp EEG (in deep structures, or too weak to be detected on the scalp, or lacking sufficient synchrony). For example, imagine that a certain brain state involves two processes, both associated with haemodynamic change: one reflected on scalp EEG, and the other not reflected on EEG. A fixed temporal relationship between the two processes would lead to an apparent time shift in the HRF. The relationship between the synchronous activity of cortical pyramidal cells in pathological areas and blood flow deviates from the norm (see Salek-Haddadi et al. 2006 for a detailed discussion of this issue).

A number of studies have investigated the haemodynamic changes related to interictal epileptiform activity, and revealed considerable variability in this response across subjects (Lemieux et al. 2001b; Bénar et al. 2002; Gotman et al. 2004), with some evidence of delayed responses (Bagshaw et al. 2004; Grouiller et al. 2007; Lu et al. 2006, 2007) and superlinearity at short event durations (Bagshaw et al. 2005). For the alpha rhythm, the presence of a travelling wave was suggested by flexible HRF modelling (de Munck et al. 2007). One interesting observation has been BOLD changes consistent with occurring prior to the observation of the discharge on scalp EEG (Hawco et al. 2007; Lemieux et al. 2008) something that has also been seen in relation to the alpha rhythm (Feige et al.) and epileptic seizures in humans and animal models (Makiranta et al. 2004; Federico et al. 2005).

Nonetheless, these observations highlight the potential limitations of using EEG as a basis to model BOLD fMRI and the issue of the choice of optimal basis set. Multivariate techniques such as ICA have the advantage that there is no need to define a model of the BOLD response, and are therefore useful tools for exploratory data analysis, and they allow the assumptions of the HRF model to be directly tested.

5.2.2
Experimental Efficiency of Paradigmless fMRI

In conventional, paradigm-driven fMRI studies, such as cognitive studies, one has the opportunity to optimise the experimental design (Dale 1999; Friston et al. 1999). Moreover, the classical procedure is to rely on a contrast between an active and a baseline condition. For spontaneous activity, the time course of the activity of interest is essentially random, with important consequences for experimental efficiency and consequently the technique's yield and clinical potential. For example, in focal epilepsy, localising information is obtained in roughly 60% of cases in whom interictal spikes are observed over EEG–fMRI sessions lasting between 20 and 60 min (see the chapters "EEG–fMRI in Adults with Focal Epilepsy", "EEG–fMRI in Idiopathic Generalised Epilepsy (Adults)", and "EEG–fMRI in Children with Epilepsy"), even though these are cases selected for their relatively high levels of EEG activity.

The lack of experimental control has also highlighted the question of fMRI baseline by blurring the boundary between "activated" and control state. Despite the fundamental difficulties associated with a lack of experimental control, we anticipate that the study of the brain's resting state using functional imaging will continue to constitute an active area of investigation.

5.3
The Impact of Data Acquisition and Processing Artefacts on fMRI Data Analysis

5.3.1
Artefacts in the Signals

A prudent approach to fMRI analysis is to devise models that incorporate as much knowledge of the factors that may influence the signal as possible. In this regard, the EEG and ECG can provide information not normally available in conventional fMRI experiments. Although movements pose a considerable problem in simultaneous EEG–fMRI, by giving rise to artefacts in both the EEG and the fMRI time series, the combination of EEG and fMRI makes it possible to assess the occurrence of motion events in a way that is not normally possible in fMRI without EEG, through the inspection of the EEG traces in relation to the fMRI scan realignment parameters. This can be useful in cases where motion is expected to be correlated with events of interest, such as seizures, and can be an important form of bias assessment (Salek-Haddadi et al. 2003c).

Other important potential sources of fMRI signal variance are respiration and heartbeat-related artefacts. Recent work has been done to remove these, which are generally aliased in the fMRI signal but can be captured to a large extent in the ECG and incorporated into models of the fMRI signal (Gary et al. 2000; Liston et al. 2006; Perlbarg et al. 2007).

A very important pitfall is that some of these artefacts can be correlated (e.g. heartbeat and respiration artefacts) (Mandelkow et al. 2007), or, even worse, correlated with the protocol itself. For example, the subject can move the head when responding, or close the eyes after the response. This can lead to signal changes in both EEG and fMRI that will be correlated with the protocol and may be mistaken for a brain activation in response to the protocol. The net result of stimulus (or effect of interest)-related confounds is a reduction of sensitivity when properly incorporated into the fMRI model or possible false activation otherwise (Lund et al. 2005). Again, the availability of simultaneous physiological recordings can help to devise models that account for effects related to such confounds.

5.3.2
Artefacts Introduced by EEG Preprocessing

The results of any signal processing method must always be considered very carefully, as every method can produce spurious results if its assumptions are not fulfilled. As a consequence, such confounds must be tracked down at every step. A generally misleading effect is the fact that each EEG channel is recorded with respect to a reference electrode (Lehmann and Skrandies 1984). This means that any measure of relation between channels (coherence, phase locking, etc.) can be confounded by this common signal.

Another major source of confounding is the fact that transient activity filtered in a limited bandwidth can be mistaken for actual oscillatory data (see Fig. 7). This means that if one wants to perform a frequency-band-related analysis in EEG–fMRI, the data has to be checked carefully for artefacts. This can be quite easy for bands corresponding to low frequencies, but can prove more difficult for small artefacts (i.e. small spikes) that can be hidden in the data but produce a disastrous effect on high-frequency activity estimation.

Similarly, as mentioned in the section on multivariate analysis, there can be cross-talk issues in ICA decomposition. Indeed, if part of the signal of interest is not captured by its own component but rather spills onto artefact-related components, it will be removed in the ICA procedure (Wallstrom et al. 2004). This can in theory also happen for

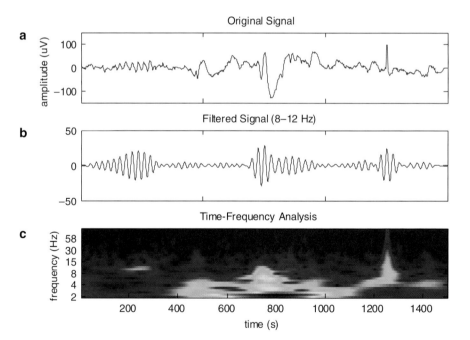

Fig. 7a-c Pitfall of narrow-band filtering. **a** Original composite signal, with an alpha oscillation (around 200 ms), an epileptic spike (around 800 ms) and a synthetic spiky artefact (around 1,300 ms). **b** All signals seem oscillatory when filtered in a narrow band. **c** Time-frequency analysis allows the different signals to be differentiated

high-frequency activity, which corresponds to a weak signal in EEG, or for protocol-related activity that is only present in a small time window in each trial.

6
Summary and Outlook

The possibility of recording EEG inside the MRI scanner allows one to introduce fine temporal information from the EEG into the analysis of the fMRI signal at the single-trial level and allows the investigation of the haemodynamic correlates of spontaneous phenomena best observed on EEG, such as epileptic discharges or fluctuations in brain rhythms. The technique's limitations reflect those of EEG and fMRI taken individually. While the most widely used analysis method to date has been the general linear model, data-driven techniques such as ICA provide a framework for further exploratory studies. Given the uncertainties related to the choice of model, the Bayesian framework offers a promising way forward. Finally, we anticipate that increasing efforts will be directed into solving the "inverse problem" of EEG–fMRI.

Acknowledgements The authors wish to thank Jean Gotman and Christophe Grova for their comments and corrections to the manuscript.

References

Aguirre GK, Zarahn E, D'Esposito M (1998) The variability of human, BOLD hemodynamic responses. Neuroimage 8:360–369

Aghakhani Y, Bagshaw AP, Bénar CG, Hawco C, Andermann F, Dubeau F, Gotman J (2004) fMRI activation during spike and wave discharges in idiopathic generalized epilepsy. Brain 127:1127–1144

Ahlfors SP, Simpson GV, Dale AM, Belliveau JW, Liu AK, Korvenoja A, Virtanen J, Huotilainen M, Tootell RB, Aronen HJ, Ilmoniemi RJ (1999) Spatiotemporal activity of a cortical network for processing visual motion revealed by MEG and fMRI. J Neurophysiol 82:2545–2555

Al-Asmi A, Bénar CG, Gross DW, Khani YA, Andermann F, Pike B, Dubeau F, Gotman J (2003) fMRI activation in continuous and spike-triggered EEG-fMRI studies of epileptic spikes. Epilepsia 44:1328–1339

Allen PJ, Josephs O, Turner R (2000) A method for removing imaging artifact from continuous EEG recorded during functional MRI. Neuroimage 12:230–239

Allen PJ, Polizzi G, Krakow K, Fish DR, Lemieux L (1998) Identification of EEG events in the MR scanner: the problem of pulse artifact and a method for its subtraction. Neuroimage 8:229–239

Archer JS, Abbott DF, Waites AB, Jackson GD (2003) fMRI "deactivation" of the posterior cingulate during generalized spike and wave. Neuroimage 20:1915–1922

Arthurs OJ, Boniface S (2002) How well do we understand the neural origins of the fMRI BOLD signal? Trends Neurosci 25:27–31

Arthurs OJ, Donovan T, Spiegelhalter DJ, Pickard JD, Boniface SJ (2007) Intracortically distributed neurovascular coupling relationships within and between human somatosensory cortices. Cereb Cortex 17:661–668

Babiloni F, Carducci F, Cincotti F, Del Gratta C, Roberti GM, Romani GL, Rossini PM, Babiloni C (2000) Integration of high resolution EEG and functional magnetic resonance in the study of human movement-related potentials. Methods Inf Med 39:179–182

Bodurka J, Bandettini PA (2002) Toward direct mapping of neuronal activity: MRI detection of ultraweak, transient magnetic field changes. Magn Reson Med 47:1052–1058

Bagshaw AP, Aghakhani Y, Benar CG, Kobayashi E, Hawco C, Dubeau F, Pike GB, Gotman J (2004) EEG-fMRI of focal epileptic spikes: analysis with multiple haemodynamic functions and comparison with gadolinium-enhanced MR angiograms. Hum Brain Mapp 22:179–192

Bagshaw AP, Hawco C, Benar CG, Kobayashi E, Aghakhani Y, Dubeau F, Pike GB, Gotman J (2005) Analysis of the EEG-fMRI response to prolonged bursts of interictal epileptiform activity. Neuroimage 24:1099–1112

Bagshaw AP, Warbrick T (2007) Single trial variability of EEG and fMRI responses to visual stimuli. Neuroimage 38:280–292

Baillet S, Garnero L (1997) A bayesian approach to introducing anatomo-functional priors in the EEG/MEG inverse problem. IEEE Trans Biomed Eng 44:374–385

Bandettini PA, Jesmanowicz A, Wong EC, Hyde JS (1993) Processing strategies for time-course data sets in functional MRI of the human brain. Magn Reson Med 30:161–173

Becker R, Ritter P, Moosmann M, Villringer A (2005) Visual evoked potentials recovered from fMRI scan periods. Hum Brain Mapp 26:221–230

Belin P, Zatorre RJ, Hoge R, Evans AC, Pike B (1999) Event-related fMRI of the auditory cortex. Neuroimage 10:417–429

Bell AJ, Sejnowski TJ (1995) An information-maximization approach to blind separation and blind deconvolution. Neural Comput 7:1129–1159

Bénar C, Aghakhani Y, Wang Y, Izenberg A, Al-Asmi A, Dubeau F, Gotman J (2003) Quality of EEG in simultaneous EEG-fMRI for epilepsy. Clin Neurophysiol 114:569–580

Bénar C, Clerc M, Papadopoulo T (2007a) Adaptive time-frequency models for single-trial M/EEG analysis. Inf Process Med Imaging 20:458–469

Bénar CG, Gross DW, Wang Y, Petre V, Pike B, Dubeau F, Gotman J (2002) The BOLD response to interictal epileptiform discharges. Neuroimage 17:1182–1192

Bénar CG, Grova C, Kobayashi E, Bagshaw AP, Aghakhani Y, Dubeau F, Gotman J (2006) EEG-fMRI of epileptic spikes: concordance with EEG source localization and intracranial EEG. Neuroimage 30:1161–1170

Bénar CG, Schon D, Grimault S, Nazarian B, Burle B, Roth M, Badier JM, Marquis P, Liegeois-Chauvel C, Anton JL (2007b) Single-trial analysis of oddball event-related potentials in simultaneous EEG-fMRI. Hum Brain Mapp 28:602–613

Berger H (1929) Über das Elektroenkephalogramm des Menschen. Archiv für Psychiatrie und Nervenkrankheiten 87:527–570

Birn RM, Bandettini PA (2005) The effect of stimulus duty cycle and "off" duration on BOLD response linearity. Neuroimage 27:70–82

Bledowski C, Prvulovic D, Hoechstetter K, Scherg M, Wibral M, Goebel R, Linden DE (2004) Localizing P300 generators in visual target and distractor processing: a combined event-related potential and functional magnetic resonance imaging study. J Neurosci 24: 9353–9360

Bonmassar G, Anami K, Ives J, Belliveau JW (1999) Visual evoked potential (VEP) measured by simultaneous 64-channel EEG and 3T fMRI. Neuroreport 10:1893–1897

Bonmassar G, Schwartz DP, Liu AK, Kwong KK, Dale AM, Belliveau JW (2001) Spatiotemporal brain imaging of visual-evoked activity using interleaved EEG and fMRI recordings. Neuroimage 13:1035–1043

Briselli E, Garreffa G, Bianchi L, Bianciardi M, Macaluso E, Abbafati M, Grazia Marciani M, Maraviglia B (2006) An independent component analysis-based approach on ballistocardiogram artifact removing. Magn Reson Imaging 24:393–400

Brookes MJ, Mullinger KJ, Stevenson CM, Morris PG, Bowtell R (2008) Simultaneous EEG source localisation and artifact rejection during concurrent fMRI by means of spatial filtering. Neuroimage 40:1090–1104

Bullmore E, Long C, Suckling J, Fadili J, Calvert G, Zelaya F, Carpenter TA, Brammer M (2001) Colored noise and computational inference in neurophysiological (fMRI) time series analysis: resampling methods in time and wavelet domains. Hum Brain Mapp 12(2):61–78

Calhoun VD, Adali T, Pearlson GD, Kiehl KA (2006) Neuronal chronometry of target detection: fusion of hemodynamic and event-related potential data. Neuroimage 30:544–553

Cao J (1999) The size of the connected components of excursion sets of chi2, t and F fields. Adv Appl Probab 31:577–593

Cardoso JF (1999) High-order contrasts for independent component analysis. Neural Comput 11:157–192

Christmann C, Koeppe C, Braus DF, Ruf M, Flor H (2007) A simultaneous EEG-fMRI study of painful electric stimulation. Neuroimage 34:1428–1437

Chumbley JR, Friston KJ (2009) False discovery rate revisited: FDR and topological inference using Gaussian random fields. Neuroimag 44:62–70

Cincotti F, Mattia D, Babiloni C, Carducci F, Salinari S, Bianchi L, Marciani MG, Babiloni F (2003) The use of EEG modifications due to motor imagery for brain-computer interfaces. IEEE Trans Neural Syst Rehabil Eng 11:131–133

Comi E, Annovazzi P, Silva AM, Cursi M, Blasi V, Cadioli M, Inuggi A, Falini A, Comi G, Leocani L (2005) Visual evoked potentials may be recorded simultaneously with fMRI scanning: a validation study. Hum Brain Mapp 24:291–298

Czisch M, Wehrle R, Kaufmann C, Wetter TC, Holsboer F, Pollmacher T, Auer DP (2004) Functional MRI during sleep: BOLD signal decreases and their electrophysiological correlates. Eur J Neurosci 20:566–574

Czisch M, Wetter TC, Kaufmann C, Pollmacher T, Holsboer F, Auer DP (2002) Altered processing of acoustic stimuli during sleep: reduced auditory activation and visual deactivation detected by a combined fMRI/EEG study. Neuroimage 16:251–258

Dale AM (1999) Optimal experimental design for event-related fMRI. Hum Brain Mapp 8: 109–114

Daunizeau J, Grova C, Marrelec G, Mattout J, Jbabdi S, Pelegrini-Issac M, Lina JM, Benali H (2007) Symmetrical event-related EEG/fMRI information fusion in a variational bayesian framework. Neuroimage 36:69–87

Daunizeau J, Grova C, Mattout J, Marrelec G, Clonda D, Goulard B, Pelegrini-Issac M, Lina JM, Benali H (2005) Assessing the relevance of fMRI-based prior in the EEG inverse problem: a Bayesian model comparison approach. IEEE Tran Signal Process 53:3461–3472

Debener S, Mullinger KJ, Niazy RK, Bowtell RW (2008) Properties of the ballistocardiogram artefact as revealed by EEG recordings at 1.5, 3 and 7 T static magnetic field strength. Int J Psychophysiol 67(3):189–199

Debener S, Strobel A, Sorger B, Peters J, Kranczioch C, Engel AK, Goebel R (2007) Improved quality of auditory event-related potentials recorded simultaneously with 3-T fMRI: removal of the ballistocardiogram artefact. Neuroimage 34:587–597

Debener S, Ullsperger M, Siegel M, Fiehler K, von Cramon DY, Engel AK (2005) Trial-by-trial coupling of concurrent electroencephalogram and functional magnetic resonance imaging identifies the dynamics of performance monitoring. J Neurosci 25:11730–11737

De Clercq W, Vergult A, Vanrumste B, Van Paesschen W, Van Huffel S (2006) Canonical correlation analysis applied to remove muscle artifacts from the electroencephalogram. IEEE Trans Biomed Eng 53:2583–2587

de Munck JC, Goncalves SI, Huijboom L, Kuijer JP, Pouwels PJ, Heethaar RM, Lopes da Silva FH (2007) The hemodynamic response of the alpha rhythm: an EEG/fMRI study. Neuroimage 35:1142–1151

Deneux T, Faugeras O (2006) Using nonlinear models in fMRI data analysis: model selection and activation detection. Neuroimage 32:1669–1689

Dien J, Khoe W, Mangun GR (2007) Evaluation of PCA and ICA of simulated ERPs: promax vs. infomax rotations. Hum Brain Mapp 28:742–763

Disbrow EA, Slutsky DA, Roberts TP, Krubitzer LA (2000) Functional MRI at 1.5 tesla: a comparison of the blood oxygenation level-dependent signal and electrophysiology. Proc Natl Acad Sci USA 97:9718–9723

Duann JR, Jung TP, Kuo WJ, Yeh TC, Makeig S, Hsieh JC, Sejnowski TJ (2002) Single-trial variability in event-related BOLD signals. Neuroimage 15:823–835

Eichele T, Calhoun VD, Moosmann M, Specht K, Jongsma ML, Quiroga RQ, Nordby H, Hugdahl K (2008) Unmixing concurrent EEG-fMRI with parallel independent component analysis. Int J Psychophysiol 67(3):222–234

Eichele T, Specht K, Moosmann M, Jongsma ML, Quiroga RQ, Nordby H, Hugdahl K (2005) Assessing the spatiotemporal evolution of neuronal activation with single-trial event-related potentials and functional MRI. Proc Natl Acad Sci USA 102:17798–17803

Federico P, Abbott DF, Briellmann RS, Harvey AS, Jackson GD (2005) Functional MRI of the pre-ictal state. Brain 128:1811–1817

Feige B, Scheffler K, Esposito F, Di Salle F, Hennig J, Seifritz E (2005) Cortical and subcortical correlates of electroencephalographic alpha rhythm modulation. J Neurophysiol 93:2864–2872

Fell J (2007) Cognitive neurophysiology: beyond averaging. Neuroimage 37:1069–1072

Foucher JR, Otzenberger H, Gounot D (2003) The BOLD response and the gamma oscillations respond differently than evoked potentials: an interleaved EEG-fMRI study. BMC Neurosci 4:22

Foucher JR, Otzenberger H, Gounot D (2004) Where arousal meets attention: a simultaneous fMRI and EEG recording study. Neuroimage 22:688–697

Friston KJ, Holmes AP, Worsley KJ, Poline JP, Firth CD, Frackowiak RSJ (1994) Statistical parametric maps in functional imaging: a general linear approach. Human Brain Mapping, 2(4): 189–210

Friston K, Phillips J, Chawla D, Buchel C (1999) Revealing interactions among brain systems with nonlinear PCA. Hum Brain Mapp 8:92–97

Friston KJ, Ashburner J, Poline JB, Frith CD, Heather JD, Frackowiak RS (1995) Spatial registration and normalization of images. Hum Brain Mapp 2:165–189

Friston KJ, Josephs O, Rees G, Turner R (1998) Nonlinear event-related responses in fMRI. Magn Reson Med 39:41–52

Friston KJ, Stephan KE, Lund TE, Morcom A, Kiebel S (2005) Mixed-effects and fMRI studies. Neuroimage 24:244–252

Friston KJ, Williams S, Howard R, Frackowiak RS, Turner R (1996) Movement-related effects in fMRI time-series. Magn Reson Med 35:346–355

Fukunaga M, Horovitz SG, van Gelderen P, de Zwart JA, Jansma JM, Ikonomidou VN, Chu R, Deckers RH, Leopold DA, Duyn JH (2006) Large-amplitude, spatially correlated fluctuations in BOLD fMRI signals during extended rest and early sleep stages. Magn Reson Imaging 24: 979–992

Gavaret M, Badier JM, Marquis P, Bartolomei F, Chauvel P (2004) Electric source imaging in temporal lobe epilepsy. J Clin Neurophysiol 21:267–282

Genovese CR, Lazar NA, Nichols T (2002) Thresholding of statistical maps in functional neuroimaging using the false discovery rate. Neuroimage 15:870–878

Geselowitz DB (1967) On bioelectric potentials in an inhomogeneous volume conductor. Biophys J 1967, vol 7, pp. 1–11

Glover GH, Li TQ, Ress D (2000) Image-based method for retrospective correction of physiological motion effects in fMRI: RETROICOR. Magnet Reson Med 44(1):162–167

Goldman RI, Stern JM, Engel J Jr., Cohen MS (2000) Acquiring simultaneous EEG and functional MRI. Clin Neurophysiol 111:1974–1980

Goldman RI, Stern JM, Engel J Jr., Cohen MS (2002) Simultaneous EEG and fMRI of the alpha rhythm. Neuroreport 13:2487–2492

Goncalves SI, de Munck JC, Pouwels PJ, Schoonhoven R, Kuijer JP, Maurits NM, Hoogduin JM, Van Someren EJ, Heethaar RM, Lopes da Silva FH (2006) Correlating the alpha rhythm to BOLD using simultaneous EEG/fMRI: inter-subject variability. Neuroimage 30:203–213

Gotman J, Bénar CG, Dubeau F (2004) Combining EEG and FMRI in epilepsy: methodological challenges and clinical results. J Clin Neurophysiol 21:229–240

Gotman J, Grova C, Bagshaw A, Kobayashi E, Aghakhani Y, Dubeau F (2005) Generalized epileptic discharges show thalamocortical activation and suspension of the default state of the brain. Proc Natl Acad Sci USA 102:15236–15240

Gotman J, Kobayashi E, Bagshaw AP, Benar CG, Dubeau F (2006) Combining EEG and fMRI: a multimodal tool for epilepsy research. J Magn Reson Imaging 23:906–920

Grouiller F, Vercueil L, Krainik A, Segebarth C, Kahane P, David O (2007) Evaluation of the hemodynamic response function for interictal epileptiform discharges. In: Proceedings of 13th Annual Meeting of the Organization for Human Brain Mapping, Chicago, IL, USA, 10–14 June 2007

Grova C, Daunizeau J, Kobayashi E, Bagshaw AP, Lina JM, Dubeau F, Gotman J (2008) Concordance between distributed EEG source localization and simultaneous EEG-fMRI studies of epileptic spikes. Neuroimage 39:755–774

Hadamard J (1902) Sur les problèmes aux dérivées partielles et leur signification physique. Princeton Uni Bull 13:49–52

Hagberg GE, Bianciardi M, Maraviglia B (2006) Challenges for detection of neuronal currents by MRI. Magn Reson Imaging 24:483–493

Hamandi K, Laufs H, Noth U, Carmichael DW, Duncan JS, Lemieux L (2008) BOLD and perfusion changes during epileptic generalised spike wave activity. Neuroimage 39:608–618

Hawco CS, Bagshaw AP, Lu Y, Dubeau F, Gotman J (2007) BOLD changes occur prior to epileptic spikes seen on scalp EEG. Neuroimage 35:1450–1458

von Helmholtz H (1853) Uber einige gesetzeder verbeitung elektrischer strome in koperlichen leitern mit anwendung auf die theorischelektrischen versuche, Ann.Physik.u Chem. 89, pp. 211–233

Henning S, Merboldt KD, Frahm J (2005) Simultaneous recordings of visual evoked potentials and BOLD MRI activations in response to visual motion processing. NMR Biomed 18:543–552

Horovitz SG, Rossion B, Skudlarski P, Gore JC (2004) Parametric design and correlational analyses help integrating fMRI and electrophysiological data during face processing. Neuroimage 22:1587–1595

Horovitz SG, Fukunaga M, de Zwart JA, van Gelderen P, Fulton SC, Balkin TJ, Duyn JH (2008) Low frequency BOLD fluctuations during resting wakefulness and light sleep: a simultaneous EEG-fMRI study. Hum Brain Mapp 29(6):671–682

Huang M, Aine CJ, Supek S, Best E, Ranken D, Flynn ER (1998) Multi-start downhill simplex method for spatio-temporal source localization in magnetoencephalography. Electroencephalogr Clin Neurophysiol 108:32–44

Hyvarinen A, Oja E (2000) Independent component analysis: algorithms and applications. Neural Netw 13:411–430

Im CH, Liu Z, Zhang N, Chen W, He B (2006) Functional cortical source imaging from simultaneously recorded ERP and fMRI. J Neurosci Methods 157:118–123

Ives JR, Warach S, Schmitt F, Edelman RR, Schomer DL (1993) Monitoring the patient's EEG during echo planar MRI. Electroencephalogr Clin Neurophysiol 87:417–420

Jackson GD, Opdam HI (2000) Ictal fMRI: methods and models. Adv Neurol 83:203–211

James CJ, Gibson OJ (2003) Temporally constrained ICA: an application to artifact rejection in electromagnetic brain signal analysis. IEEE Trans Biomed Eng 50:1108–1116

Josephs O, Turner R, Friston K (1997) Event-related fMRI. Hum Brain Mapp 5:243–248

Josephs O, Henson RN (1999) Event-related functional magnetic resonance imaging: modelling, inference and optimization. Philos Trans R Soc Lond B Biol Sci 354:1215–1228

Jung TP, Makeig S, Westerfield M, Townsend J, Courchesne E, Sejnowski TJ (2001) Analysis and visualization of single-trial event-related potentials. Hum Brain Mapp 14:166–185

Kang JK, Benar C, Al-Asmi A, Khani YA, Pike GB, Dubeau F, Gotman J (2003) Using patient-specific hemodynamic response functions in combined EEG-fMRI studies in epilepsy. Neuroimage 20:1162–1170

Khader P, Schicke T, Roder B, Rosler F (2008) On the relationship between slow cortical potentials and BOLD signal changes in humans. Int J Psychophysiol 67(3):252–261

Kilner JM, Mattout J, Henson R, Friston KJ (2005) Hemodynamic correlates of EEG: a heuristic. Neuroimage 28:280–286

Kobayashi E, Hawco CS, Grova C, Dubeau F, Gotman J (2006) Widespread and intense BOLD changes during brief focal electrographic seizures. Neurology 66:1049–1055

Kobayashi K, James CJ, Nakahori T, Akiyama T, Gotman J (1999) Isolation of epileptiform discharges from unaveraged EEG by independent component analysis. Clin Neurophysiol 110:1755–1763

Krakow K, Allen PJ, Symms MR, Lemieux L, Josephs O, Fish DR (2000) EEG recording during fMRI experiments: image quality. Hum Brain Mapp 10:10–15

Krakow K, Lemieux L, Messina D, Scott CA, Symms MR, Duncan JS, Fish DR (2001) Spatio-temporal imaging of focal interictal epileptiform activity using EEG-triggered functional MRI. Epileptic Disord 3(2):67–73

Krakow K, Woermann FG, Symms MR, Allen PJ, Lemieux L, Barker GJ, Duncan JS, Fish DR (1999) EEG-triggered functional MRI of interictal epileptiform activity in patients with partial seizures. Brain 122 (Pt 9):1679–1688

Kraut MA, Calhoun V, Pitcock JA, Cusick C, Hart J Jr. (2003) Neural hybrid model of semantic object memory: implications from event-related timing using fMRI. J Int Neuropsychol Soc 9:1031–1040

Kruggel F, Herrmann CS, Wiggins CJ, von Cramon DY (2001) Hemodynamic and electroencephalographic responses to illusory figures: recording of the evoked potentials during functional MRI. Neuroimage 14:1327–1336

Kruggel F, Wiggins CJ, Herrmann CS, von Cramon DY (2000) Recording of the event-related potentials during functional MRI at 3.0 Tesla field strength. Magn Reson Med 44:277–282

Lachaux JP, Fonlupt P, Kahane P, Minotti L, Hoffmann D, Bertrand O, Baciu M (2007) Relationship between task-related gamma oscillations and BOLD signal: new insights from combined fMRI and intracranial EEG. Hum Brain Mapp 28:1368–1375

Lai SH, Fang M (1999) A novel local PCA-based method for detecting activation signals in fMRI. Magn Reson Imaging 17:827–836

Laufs H, Duncan JS (2007) Electroencephalography/functional MRI in human epilepsy: what it currently can and cannot do. Curr Opin Neurol 20:417–423

Laufs H, Holt JL, Elfont R, Krams M, Paul JS, Krakow K, Kleinschmidt A (2006a) Where the BOLD signal goes when alpha EEG leaves. Neuroimage 31:1408–1418

Laufs H, Kleinschmidt A, Beyerle A, Eger E, Salek-Haddadi A, Preibisch C, Krakow K (2003a) EEG-correlated fMRI of human alpha activity. Neuroimage 19:1463–1476

Laufs H, Krakow K, Sterzer P, Eger E, Beyerle A, Salek-Haddadi A, Kleinschmidt A (2003b) Electroencephalographic signatures of attentional and cognitive default modes in spontaneous brain activity fluctuations at rest. Proc Natl Acad Sci USA 100:11053–11058

Laufs H, Lengler U, Hamandi K, Kleinschmidt A, Krakow K (2006b) Linking generalized spike-and-wave discharges and resting state brain activity by using EEG/fMRI in a patient with absence seizures. Epilepsia 47:444–448

Laufs H, Walker MC, Lund TE (2006c) EEG-fMRI of sleep spindles and K-complexes at 3T. Clin Neurophysiol 117:148–149

Lehmann D, Skrandies W (1984) Spatial analysis of evoked potentials in man: a review. Prog Neurobiol 23:227–250

Lemieux L, Allen PJ, Franconi F, Symms MR, Fish DR (1997) Recording of EEG during fMRI experiments: patient safety. Magn Reson Med 38:943–952

Lemieux L (2004) Electroencephalography-correlated functional MR imaging studies of epileptic activity. Neuroimaging Clin N Am 14:487–506

Lemieux L, Krakow K, Fish DR (2001a) Comparison of spike-triggered functional MRI BOLD activation and EEG dipole model localization. Neuroimage 14:1097–1104

Lemieux L, Laufs H, Carmichael D, Paul JS, Walker MC, Duncan JS (2008) Noncanonical spike-related BOLD responses in focal epilepsy. Hum Brain Mapp 29:329–345

Lemieux L, Salek-Haddadi A, Josephs O, Allen P, Toms N, Scott C, Krakow K, Turner R, Fish DR (2001b) Event-related fMRI with simultaneous and continuous EEG: description of the method and initial case report. Neuroimage 14:780–787

LeVan P, Urrestarazu E, Gotman J (2006) A system for automatic artifact removal in ictal scalp EEG based on independent component analysis and Bayesian classification. Clin Neurophysiol 117:912–927

Li R, Principe JC, Bradley M, Ferrari V (2007) Robust single-trial ERP estimation based on spatiotemporal filtering. Conf Proc IEEE Eng Med Biol Soc 1:5206–5209

Liebenthal E, Ellingson ML, Spanaki MV, Prieto TE, Ropella KM, Binder JR (2003) Simultaneous ERP and fMRI of the auditory cortex in a passive oddball paradigm. Neuroimage 19:1395–1404

Liston AD, Lund TE, Salek-Haddadi A, Hamandi K, Friston KJ, Lemieux L (2006) Modelling cardiac signal as a confound in EEG-fMRI and its application in focal epilepsy studies. Neuroimage 30(3):827–834

Liston AD, Salek-Haddadi A, Kiebel SJ, Hamandi K, Turner R, Lemieux L (2004) The MR detection of neuronal depolarization during 3-Hz spike-and-wave complexes in generalized epilepsy. Magn Reson Imaging 22:1441–1444

Liu AK, Belliveau JW, Dale AM (1998) Spatiotemporal imaging of human brain activity using functional MRI constrained magnetoencephalography data: Monte Carlo simulations. Proc Natl Acad Sci U S A 95:8945–8950

Liu Z, Kecman F, He B (2006) Effects of fMRI-EEG mismatches in cortical current density estimation integrating fMRI and EEG: a simulation study. Clin Neurophysiol 117:1610–1622

Logothetis NK, Pauls J, Augath M, Trinath T, Oeltermann A (2001) Neurophysiological investigation of the basis of the fMRI signal. Nature 412:150–157

Logothetis NK, Wandell BA (2004) Interpreting the BOLD signal. Annu Rev Physiol 66:735–769

Lopes da Silva FH, Van Rotterdam A (2005) Biophysical spects of EEG and magnetoencephalogram generation. In: Niedermeyer E, Lopes da Silva FH (eds) Electroencephalography: basic principles, clinical applications, and related fields. Lippincott Williams & Wilkins, Baltimore

Lovblad KO, Thomas R, Jakob PM, Scammell T, Bassetti C, Griswold M, Ives J, Matheson J, Edelman RR, Warach S (1999) Silent functional magnetic resonance imaging demonstrates focal activation in rapid eye movement sleep. Neurology 53:2193–2195

Lu Y, Bagshaw AP, Grova C, Kobayashi E, Dubeau F, Gotman J (2006) Using voxel-specific hemodynamic response function in EEG-fMRI data analysis. Neuroimage 32:238–247

Lu Y, Grova C, Kobayashi E, Dubeau F, Gotman J (2007) Using voxel-specific hemodynamic response function in EEG-fMRI data analysis: an estimation and detection model. Neuroimage 34:195–203

Lund TE, Norgaard MD, Rostrup E, Rowe JB, Paulson OB (2005) Motion or activity: their role in intra- and inter-subject variation in fMRI. Neuroimage 26:960–964

Makeig S, Jung TP, Bell AJ, Ghahremani D, Sejnowski TJ (1997) Blind separation of auditory event-related brain responses into independent components. Proc Natl Acad Sci USA 94:10979–10984

Makiranta MJ, Ruohonen J, Suominen K, Sonkajarvi E, Salomaki T, Kiviniemi V, Seppanen T, Alahuhta S, Jantti V, Tervonen O (2004) BOLD-contrast functional MRI signal changes related to intermittent rhythmic delta activity in EEG during voluntary hyperventilation-simultaneous EEG and fMRI study. Neuroimage 22:222–231

Malow BA, Kushwaha R, Lin X, Morton KJ, Aldrich MS (1997) Relationship of interictal epileptiform discharges to sleep depth in partial epilepsy. Electroencephalogr Clin Neurophysiol 102:20–26

Mandelkow H, Halder P, Brandeis D, Soellinger M, de Zanche N, Luechinger R, Boesiger P (2007) Heart beats brain: the problem of detecting alpha waves by neuronal current imaging in joint EEG-MRI experiments. Neuroimage 37:149–163

Mantini D, Perrucci MG, Cugini S, Ferretti A, Romani GL, Del Gratta C (2007a) Complete artifact removal for EEG recorded during continuous fMRI using independent component analysis. Neuroimage 34:598–607

Mantini D, Perrucci MG, Del Gratta C, Romani GL, Corbetta M (2007b) Electrophysiological signatures of resting state networks in the human brain. Proc Natl Acad Sci USA 104:13170–13175

Martinez-Montes E, Valdes-Sosa PA, Miwakeichi F, Goldman RI, Cohen MS (2004) Concurrent EEG/fMRI analysis by multiway partial least squares. Neuroimage 22:1023–1034

Matsuda T, Matsuura M, Ohkubo T, Ohkubo H, Atsumi Y, Tamaki M, Takahashi K, Matsushima E, Kojima T (2002) Influence of arousal level for functional magnetic resonance imaging (fMRI) study: simultaneous recording of fMRI and electroencephalogram. Psychiatry Clin Neurosci 56:289–290

Mayhew SD, Iannetti GD, Woolrich MW, Wise RG (2006) Automated single-trial measurement of amplitude and latency of laser-evoked potentials (LEPs) using multiple linear regression. Clin Neurophysiol 117:1331–1344

McIntosh AR, Lobaugh NJ (2004) Partial least squares analysis of neuroimaging data: applications and advances. Neuroimage 23(Suppl 1):S250–S263

McKeown M, Hu YJ, Jane Wang Z (2005) ICA denoising for event-related fMRI studies. Conf Proc IEEE Eng Med Biol Soc 1:157–161

McKeown MJ, Makeig S, Brown GG, Jung TP, Kindermann SS, Bell AJ, Sejnowski TJ (1998) Analysis of fMRI data by blind separation into independent spatial components. Hum Brain Mapp 6:160–188

Menon V, Ford JM, Lim KO, Glover GH, Pfefferbaum A (1997) Combined event-related fMRI and EEG evidence for temporal-parietal cortex activation during target detection. Neuroreport 8:3029–3037

Meriaux S, Roche A, Dehaene-Lambertz G, Thirion B, Poline JB (2006) Combined permutation test and mixed-effect model for group average analysis in fMRI. Hum Brain Mapp 27:402–410

Merlet I, Gotman J (2001) Dipole modeling of scalp electroencephalogram epileptic discharges: correlation with intracerebral fields. Clin Neurophysiol 112:414–430

Miwakeichi F, Martinez-Montes E, Valdes-Sosa PA, Nishiyama N, Mizuhara H, Yamaguchi Y (2004) Decomposing EEG data into space-time-frequency components using parallel factor analysis. Neuroimage 22:1035–1045

Mizuhara H, Wang LQ, Kobayashi K, Yamaguchi Y (2004) A long-range cortical network emerging with theta oscillation in a mental task. Neuroreport 15:1233–1238

Moosmann M, Eichele T, Nordby H, Hugdahl K, Calhoun VD (2008) Joint independent component analysis for simultaneous EEG-fMRI: principle and simulation. Int J Psychophysiol 68(1):81

Moosmann M, Ritter P, Krastel I, Brink A, Thees S, Blankenburg F, Taskin B, Obrig H, Villringer A (2003) Correlates of alpha rhythm in functional magnetic resonance imaging and near infrared spectroscopy. Neuroimage 20:145–158

Mulert C, Hepp P, Leicht G, Karch S, Lutz J, Moosmann M, Reiser M, Hegerl U, Pogarell O, Möller H-J, Jäger L (2007) High frequency oscillations in the gamma-band and the corresponding BOLD signal: trial-by-trial coupling of EEG and fMRI reveals the involvement of the thalamic reticular nucleus (TRN). In: 13th Annu Meet Organization for Human Brain Mapping, Chicago, IL, USA, 10–14 June 2007

Mulert C, Jager L, Schmitt R, Bussfeld P, Pogarell O, Moller HJ, Juckel G, Hegerl U (2004) Integration of fMRI and simultaneous EEG: towards a comprehensive understanding of localization and time-course of brain activity in target detection. Neuroimage 22:83–94

Nakamura W, Anami K, Mori T, Saitoh O, Cichocki A, Amari S (2006) Removal of ballistocardiogram artifacts from simultaneously recorded EEG and fMRI data using independent component analysis. IEEE Trans Biomed Eng 53:1294–1308

Nichols TE, Holmes AP (2002) Nonparametric permutation tests for functional neuroimaging: a primer with examples. Hum Brain Mapp 15:1–25

Niessing J, Ebisch B, Schmidt KE, Niessing M, Singer W, Galuske RA (2005) Hemodynamic signals correlate tightly with synchronized gamma oscillations. Science 309:948–951

Nunez P, Srinivasan R (2005) Electric fields of the brain. Oxford University Press, New York

Nunez PL, Silberstein RB (2000) On the relationship of synaptic activity to macroscopic measurements: does co-registration of EEG with fMRI make sense? Brain Topogr 13:79–96

O'Hare AJ, Dien J, Waterson LD, Savage CR (2008) Activation of the posterior cingulate by semantic priming: a co-registered ERP/fMRI study. Brain Res 1189:97–114

Opitz B, Mecklinger A, Friederici AD, von Cramon DY (1999) The functional neuroanatomy of novelty processing: integrating ERP and fMRI results. Cereb Cortex 9:379–391

Otzenberger H, Gounot D, Foucher JR (2005) P300 recordings during event-related fMRI: a feasibility study. Brain Res Cogn Brain Res 23:306–315

Parkes LM, Bastiaansen MC, Norris DG (2006) Combining EEG and fMRI to investigate the post-movement beta rebound. Neuroimage 29:685–696

Patel MR, Blum A, Pearlman JD, Yousuf N, Ives JR, Saeteng S, Schomer DL, Edelman RR (1999) Echo-planar functional MR imaging of epilepsy with concurrent EEG monitoring. AJNR Am J Neuroradiol 20:1916–1919

Pearlson GD, Calhoun V (2007) Structural and functional magnetic resonance imaging in psychiatric disorders. Can J Psychiatry 52:158–166

Perlbarg V, Bellec P, Anton JL, Pelegrini-Issac M, Doyon J, Benali H (2007) CORSICA: correction of structured noise in fMRI by automatic identification of ICA components. Magn Reson Imaging 25:35–46

Pfurtscheller G, Lopes da Silva FH (1999) Event-related EEG/MEG synchronization and desynchronization: basic principles. Clin Neurophysiol 110:1842–1857

Philiastides MG, Sajda P (2006) Temporal characterization of the neural correlates of perceptual decision making in the human brain. Cereb Cortex 16:509–518

Phillips C, Mattout J, Rugg MD, Maquet P, Friston KJ (2005) An empirical bayesian solution to the source reconstruction problem in EEG. Neuroimage 24:997–1011

Poline JB, Worsley KJ, Evans AC, Friston KJ (1997) Combining spatial extent and peak intensity to test for activations in functional imaging. Neuroimage 5:83–96

Portas CM, Krakow K, Allen P, Josephs O, Armony JL, Frith CD (2000) Auditory processing across the sleep-wake cycle: simultaneous EEG and fMRI monitoring in humans. Neuron 28:991–999

Quian Quiroga R, Garcia H (2003) Single-trial event-related potentials with wavelet denoising. Clin Neurophysiol 114:376–390

Raichle ME, Snyder AZ (2007) A default mode of brain function: a brief history of an evolving idea. Neuroimage 37:1083–1090; discussion 1097–1089

Ranta-aho PO, Koistinen AS, Ollikainen JO, Kaipio JP, Partanen J, Karjalainen PA (2003) Single-trial estimation of multichannel evoked-potential measurements. IEEE Trans Biomed Eng 50:189–196

Ritter P, Freyer F, Curio G, Villringer A (2008) High-frequency (600 Hz) population spikes in human EEG delineate thalamic and cortical fMRI activation sites. Neuroimage 42:483–490

Ritter P, Villringer A (2006) Simultaneous EEG-fMRI. Neurosci Biobehav Rev 30:823–838

Rodionov R, De Martino F, Laufs H, Carmichael DW, Formisano E, Walker M, Duncan JS, Lemieux L (2007) Independent component analysis of interictal fMRI in focal epilepsy: comparison with general linear model-based EEG-correlated fMRI. Neuroimage 38:488–500

Rosler F, Manzey D (1981) Principal components and varimax-rotated components in event-related potential research: some remarks on their interpretation. Biol Psychol 13:3–26

Rossell SL, Price CJ, Nobre AC (2003) The anatomy and time course of semantic priming investigated by fMRI and ERPs. Neuropsychologia 41:550–564

Salek-Haddadi A, Diehl B, Hamandi K, Merschhemke M, Liston A, Friston K, Duncan JS, Fish DR, Lemieux L (2006) Hemodynamic correlates of epileptiform discharges: an EEG-fMRI study of 63 patients with focal epilepsy. Brain Res 1088:148–166

Salek-Haddadi A, Friston KJ, Lemieux L, Fish DR (2003a) Studying spontaneous EEG activity with fMRI. Brain Res Brain Res Rev 43:110–133

Salek-Haddadi A, Lemieux L, Fish DR (2002) Role of functional magnetic resonance imaging in the evaluation of patients with malformations caused by cortical development. Neurosurg Clin N Am 13:63–69, viii

Salek-Haddadi A, Lemieux L, Merschhemke M, Diehl B, Allen PJ, Fish DR (2003b) EEG quality during simultaneous functional MRI of interictal epileptiform discharges. Magn Reson Imaging 21:1159–1166

Salek-Haddadi A, Lemieux L, Merschhemke M, Friston KJ, Duncan JS, Fish DR (2003c) Functional magnetic resonance imaging of human absence seizures. Ann Neurol 53:663–667

Sammer G, Blecker C, Gebhardt H, Bischoff M, Stark R, Morgen K, Vaitl D (2007) Relationship between regional hemodynamic activity and simultaneously recorded EEG-theta associated with mental arithmetic-induced workload. Hum Brain Mapp 28:793–803

Sammer G, Blecker C, Gebhardt H, Kirsch P, Stark R, Vaitl D (2005) Acquisition of typical EEG waveforms during fMRI: SSVEP, LRP, and frontal theta. Neuroimage 24:1012–1024

Scarff CJ, Reynolds A, Goodyear BG, Ponton CW, Dort JC, Eggermont JJ (2004) Simultaneous 3-T fMRI and high-density recording of human auditory evoked potentials. Neuroimage 23:1129–1142

Schabus M, Dang-Vu TT, Albouy G, Balteau E, Boly M, Carrier J, Darsaud A, Degueldre C, Desseilles M, Gais S, Phillips C, Rauchs G, Schnakers C, Sterpenich V, Vandewalle G, Luxen A, Maquet P (2007) Hemodynamic cerebral correlates of sleep spindles during human non-rapid eye movement sleep. Proc Natl Acad Sci USA 104:13164–13169

Scheeringa R, Bastiaansen MC, Petersson KM, Oostenveld R, Norris DG, Hagoort P (2008) Frontal theta EEG activity correlates negatively with the default mode network in resting state. Int J Psychophysiol 67(3):242–251

Schmidt DM, George JS, Wood CC (1999) Bayesian inference applied to the electromagnetic inverse problem. Hum Brain Mapp 7:195–212

Schnitzler A, Timmermann L, Gross J (2006) Physiological and pathological oscillatory networks in the human motor system. J Physiol Paris 99:3–7

Seeck M, Lazeyras F, Michel CM, Blanke O, Gericke CA, Ives J, Delavelle J, Golay X, Haenggeli CA, de Tribolet N, Landis T (1998) Non-invasive epileptic focus localization using EEG-triggered functional MRI and electromagnetic tomography. Electroencephalogr Clin Neurophysiol 106:508–512

Sekihara K, Nagarajan SS, Poeppel D, Marantz A (2002) Performance of an MEG adaptive-beamformer technique in the presence of correlated neural activities: effects on signal intensity and time-course estimates. IEEE Trans Biomed Eng 49:1534–1546

Srivastava G, Crottaz-Herbette S, Lau KM, Glover GH, Menon V (2005) ICA-based procedures for removing ballistocardiogram artifacts from EEG data acquired in the MRI scanner. Neuroimage 24:50–60

Stern JM (2006) Simultaneous electroencephalography and functional magnetic resonance imaging applied to epilepsy. Epilepsy Behav 8:683–692

Stevens MC, Calhoun VD, Kiehl KA (2005) fMRI in an oddball task: effects of target-to-target interval. Psychophysiology 42:636–642

Supek S, Aine CJ (1993) Simulation studies of multiple dipole neuromagnetic source localization: model order and limits of source resolution. IEEE Trans Biomed Eng 40:529–540

Symms MR, Allen PJ, Woermann FG, Polizzi G, Krakow K, Barker GJ, Fish DR, Duncan JS (1999) Reproducible localization of interictal epileptiform discharges using EEG-triggered fMRI. Phys Med Biol 44:N161–168

Tanaka H, Fujita N, Takanashi M, Hirabuki N, Yoshimura H, Abe K, Nakamura H (2003) Effect of stage 1 sleep on auditory cortex during pure tone stimulation: evaluation by functional magnetic resonance imaging with simultaneous EEG monitoring. AJNR Am J Neuroradiol 24:1982–1988

Tang AC, Sutherland MT, McKinney CJ (2005) Validation of SOBI components from high-density EEG. Neuroimage 25:539–553

Thirion B, Faugeras O (2003) Dynamical components analysis of fMRI data through kernel PCA. Neuroimage 20:34–49

Ting KH, Fung PC, Chang CQ, Chan FH (2006) Automatic correction of artifact from single-trial event-related potentials by blind source separation using second order statistics only. Med Eng Phys 28:780–794

Tohka J, Foerde K, Aron AR, Tom SM, Toga AW, Poldrack RA (2008) Automatic independent component labeling for artifact removal in fMRI. Neuroimage 39:1227–1245

Toma K, Matsuoka T, Immisch I, Mima T, Waldvogel D, Koshy B, Hanakawa T, Shill H, Hallett M (2002) Generators of movement-related cortical potentials: fMRI-constrained EEG dipole source analysis. Neuroimage 17:161–173

Trujillo-Barreto NJ, Aubert-Vazquez E, Valdes-Sosa PA (2004) Bayesian model averaging in EEG/MEG imaging. Neuroimage 21:1300–1319

Trujillo-Barreto NJ, Martínez-Montes E, Melie-García L, Valdés-Sosa PA (2001) A symmetrical bayesian model for fMRI and EEG/MEG neuroimage fusion. Int J Bioelectromag 3:1

Vazquez AL, Noll DC (1998) Nonlinear aspects of the BOLD response in functional MRI. Neuroimage 7:108–118

Vigario R, Sarela J, Jousmaki V, Hamalainen M, Oja E (2000) Independent component approach to the analysis of EEG and MEG recordings. IEEE Trans Biomed Eng 47:589–593

Vitrai J, Czobor P, Simon G, Varga L, Marosfi S (1984) Beyond principal component analysis: canonical component analysis for data reduction in classification of EPs. Int J Biomed Comput 15:93–111

Wager TD, Vazquez A, Hernandez L, Noll DC (2005) Accounting for nonlinear BOLD effects in fMRI: parameter estimates and a model for prediction in rapid event-related studies. Neuroimage 25:206–218

Wallstrom GL, Kass RE, Miller A, Cohn JF, Fox NA (2004) Automatic correction of ocular artifacts in the EEG: a comparison of regression-based and component-based methods. Int J Psychophysiol 53:105–119

Wang Z, Maier A, Leopold DA, Logothetis NK, Liang H (2007) Single-trial evoked potential estimation using wavelets. Comput Biol Med 37:463–473

Wan X, Riera J, Iwata K, Takahashi M, Wakabayashi T, Kawashima R (2006) The neural basis of the hemodynamic response nonlinearity in human primary visual cortex: implications for neurovascular coupling mechanism. Neuroimage 32:616–625

Warach S, Ives JR, Schlaug G, Patel MR, Darby DG, Thangaraj V, Edelman RR, Schomer DL (1996) EEG-triggered echo-planar functional MRI in epilepsy. Neurology 47:89–93

Warbrick T, Bagshaw AP (2008) Scanning strategies for simultaneous EEG-fMRI evoked potential studies at 3 T. Int J Psychophysiol 67(3):169–177

Worsley KJ, Evans AC, Marrett S, Neelin P (1992) A three-dimensional statistical analysis for CBF activation studies in human brain. J Cereb Blood Flow Metab 12:900–918

Worsley KJ, Liao CH, Aston J, Petre V, Duncan GH, Morales F, Evans AC (2002) A general statistical analysis for fMRI data. Neuroimage 15:1–15

Part III

Applications of EEG–fMRI

Resting State

Brain Rhythms

13

Helmut Laufs

1
Considerations for the Study of Rest

Accurately determining the temperature of whiskey in a shot glass is not a trivial task. Lowering the tip of the thermometer into the fluid will introduce both thermal and kinetic energy, thus biasing the measurement. Additionally, the alcohol is volatile and hence the volume not constant. Similarly, experimentally assessing spontaneous resting brain activity is a virtually impossible task. The general scientific approach of externally manipulating (independent variable) the system under observation in order to obtain informative measurements (dependent variable) about the object of interest may suspend the resting state; in other words, it may cause the object of interest to change and evade. In any case, the alive brain obviously never truly remains at rest, as this would prohibit (re)active functioning. In this chapter, the term "resting state" will refer to a state of "endogenous brain activity" that is spontaneously ongoing, not intentionally induced externally nor voluntarily generated by the subject.

1.1
Why Study the Resting State?

The study of resting state brain activity becomes especially interesting if one perceives neural processes as being mainly intrinsic—weighting, gating and subsequently integrating new and external information into the brain—as opposed to a rather absolute resting state that contrasts with momentary activity driven by external demands (Raichle and Snyder 2007). Unless one is creating a contextual setting with respect to which "rest" is defined (Fair et al. 2007; Raichle et al. 2001; Raichle and Snyder 2007), then paradigmatic, repetitive stimulation

H. Laufs (✉)
Department of Neurology and Brain Imaging Center, Johann Wolfgang Goethe-Universität, Theodor-Stern-Kai 7, 60590 Frankfurt am Main, Germany
e-mail: helmut@laufs.com

C. Mulert and L. Lemieux (eds.), *EEG–fMRI*
DOI: 10.1007/978-3-540-87919-0_13, © Springer Verlag Berlin Heidelberg 2010

by definition precludes rest. This suggests that the method of choice is the analysis of ongoing spontaneous brain activity rather than averaged or induced brain activity. The most prominent property of this activity are neuronal ensemble oscillations, or "rhythms".

These resting state oscillations can be perturbed by spontaneous, brief pathological or physiological interruptions, the study of which further nourishes interest in the resting state and spontaneous variations of it. Conversely, knowledge of resting state brain activity can improve our understanding of task-induced brain activity. This may need to be seen in the context of the underlying spontaneous brain activity: perceiving rest as a momentary state (i.e. a brief epoch of ongoing endogenous activity), it has been proposed that intrinsic fluctuations within cortical systems can account for (intertrial) variability in human behaviour through its addition to the purely task-induced activity (Fox et al. 2007).

Also, there is evidence that sets of brain regions, "networks", which typically exhibit coherent activity in a task context, facilitating binding (Mesulam 1990, 1998; Munk and Neuenschwander 2000), are also intermittently active during rest (see the first paragraph of this section). Their degree of prominence or even absence during rest is related to the (patho) physiological brain state on both short ("microstate") and long (psychiatric condition) timescales (Lehmann et al. 2005). In Alzheimer's disease, for example, both electrophysiological and imaging experiments of spontaneous brain activity have pointed to disease-associated variability of resting-state networks (Sorg et al. 2007; Stam et al. 2005).

2
A Multimodal Approach to the Resting State

Endogenous changes in resting state activity can be observed across vigilance and sleep stages, but also as pathologic activity in the form of epileptic activity. Both types of activity (changes) can be detected and characterised using electroencephalography (EEG), the gold standard method for determining sleep stages (Rechtschaffen and Kales 1968) and epileptiform activity noninvasively (Gibbs et al. 1935). While the EEG indicates the occurrence of a state, it does not reveal much about its nature.

Concurrent measurements of EEG and blood oxygenation level dependent (BOLD) functional magnetic resonance imaging (fMRI) allow us to simultaneously assess brain activity from two angles (see the chapter "Experimental Design and Data Analysis Strategies"). One modality can be used to inform the other. In this manner, spontaneous neural oscillations can be studied without external manipulation. For example, the EEG data can describe endogenous modulations of vigilance or can serve to identify spontaneous events such as sleep spindles and epileptic discharges (see the chapters "Sleep", "EEG–fMRI in Adults with Focal Epilepsy", "EEG–fMRI in Idiopathic Generalised Epilepsy (Adults)" and "EEG–fMRI in Children with Epilepsy"). The EEG can be treated as the independent variable, forming a regressor that can be used to interrogate the fMRI data, the dependent variable. The reverse is also possible, and attempts at data fusion are also being made where all of the data are used equally as dependent and independent variables simultaneously (see the chapter "EEG–fMRI Information Fusion: Biophysics and Data Analysis").

In the following, examples of simultaneous EEG–fMRI studies performed in humans will be discussed. Among a variety of proposed resting-state networks, this chapter will focus mainly on two for which functional interpretations already exist: the default mode network (DMN) and the dorsal attentional network. It will be shown that one EEG feature can correlate with different fMRI activation maps, and that a single resting-state network can be associated with a variety of EEG patterns. An explanation will be proposed as an aid to interpreting results in the context of the nontrivial EEG–fMRI relationship.

2.1
From Unimodal to Multimodal Studies of Rest

2.1.1
Electrophysiological Studies of "Brain Oscillations"

"Brain oscillations" relate to the rhythmicity of neuronal firing, indicating organised activity. However, this organisation does not guarantee normality, and less obvious oscillations do not imply pathology. Studying the origin of neuronal oscillations thus allows insight into healthy and pathological brain function. Many EEG studies (too numerous to mention) have been performed for over a century; these have mainly been resting-state examinations in a clinical context and in sleep research. A methodological milestone was achieved in the form of invasive, single-cell and multiunit recordings (Steriade 1995). In crude summary, human EEG activity within a certain frequency band cannot be directly linked to specific (mal)function without taking into account its amplitude, spatial distribution, reactivity, intra- and interindividual variability, and generally speaking the context in which it is observed (Laufs et al. 2006c; Nunez et al. 2001; Urrestarazu et al. 2007). Accordingly, a variety of EEG oscillations, from ultraslow (direct current/below 0.1 Hz) to ultrafast (around 1,000 Hz), have been observed and mostly assigned Greek letters ranging from alpha to omega (Curio 2000). Invasive EEG experiments (Steriade 2005) and noninvasive source localisation methods (Lopes da Silva 2004; Michel et al. 2004) have shed light on specific brain regions involved in the generation and maintenance of various brain oscillations.

2.1.2
Functional Imaging Studies of "Brain Oscillations"

Unimodal fMRI studies of rest are primarily based on data-driven analysis approaches (functional connectivity; principal or independent component analysis, PCA/ICA). Over a dozen consistent resting-state networks have been identified (Fox and Raichle 2007). The interpretation of signal changes in these resting-state networks remains difficult when assessed unimodally and (necessarily) in the absence of a task and distinct context. Objectively assessing a subject's state during data acquisition (e.g. via external observation or a post hoc interview) remains a difficult and inaccurate task, especially when subjects drift between wakefulness and drowsiness. An additional perspective on brain activity at rest can be obtained via a second measure, that of EEG. This can give information on the subject's "state of mind", especially the level of vigilance. If functionally well-established EEG features can be correlated with fMRI, then the associated fMRI maps can be better interpreted. The meaning of the fMRI maps will most likely parallel the meaning of the associated EEG (Laufs et al. 2006c). On the other hand, EEG–fMRI can help to elucidate the brain processes that underlie specific, less-understood EEG phenomena if the related fMRI signal changes have been observed and interpreted previously, for example in the context of a task (Laufs et al. 2007; Schabus et al. 2007). Finally, hypotheses that were initially developed exclusively in the EEG domain can be confirmed by associated congruent fMRI patterns (Giraud et al. 2007).

2.2
Endogenous Brain Oscillations in Healthy Subjects

Neuronal oscillations in different EEG frequency bands and associated topographies have been identified in the context of different types of active mental activity. Spontaneous brain activity during relaxed wakefulness ("awake rest") has inherently been less well characterised, despite the fact that it is recorded in day-to-day clinical practice and was the first condition to have been assessed with EEG (Berger 1929). The most prominent EEG rhythm during the awake resting state was described by Hans Berger: he termed the posterior 8–12 Hz oscillations the "alpha rhythm" and noticed its desynchronisation with ceasing vigilance on the one hand and with engagement in an attention-demanding task on the other (Berger 1929).

Unsurprisingly, the first EEG–fMRI investigations studying healthy volunteers at rest were concerned with the BOLD correlates of this very prominent EEG alpha rhythm. In line with neurophysiological animal studies, Goldman et al., Moosmann et al. and (similarly) later Mantini et al. noted that thalamic BOLD activity was positively correlated with posterior alpha oscillations on scalp EEG. They identified an inverse correlation of the alpha EEG with the occipital-parietal areas, reflecting the alpha oscillations' scalp topography (Goldman et al. 2002; Mantini et al. 2007; Moosmann et al. 2003). Laufs et al., and again similarly Mantini et al., also found that a frontal-parietal network was associated with alpha desynchronisation (Laufs et al. 2003a; Mantini et al. 2007). In line with Berger's observations, they claimed to have visualised endogenously waxing and waning attention with fluctuating alpha desynchronisation indexed by activity changes in a frontal-parietal network, which had previously and independently been established as being an attentional system (Laufs et al. 2003a, 2006c). An almost identical network had been found to be engaged during a variety of attention-demanding tasks, especially mental arithmetic (Gruber et al. 2001): a form of brain activity that is also classically known to suppress the alpha rhythm (Berger 1929); see Fig. 1.

In a strict sense, apart from any (thalamic) activation associated with alpha power increases (Feige et al. 2005; Goldman et al. 2002; Mantini et al. 2007; Moosmann et al. 2003), none of the studies mentioned above revealed notable coherent (cortical) correlates of scalp EEG alpha oscillations; instead, by identifying inverse relationships, brain regions that increase their activity in the *absence* of marked alpha activity were identified (Laufs et al. 2006c). Once again, in congruence with Hans Berger's observations, when they reanalysed their data, Laufs et al. found indications that the occipitally pronounced, inversely alpha-associated pattern occurred in association with a decline in vigilance. This finding was supported by a corresponding enhanced spectral density in the theta (4–7 Hz) band, as typically observed during drowsiness. Furthermore, positron emission

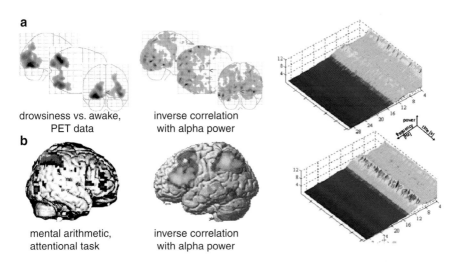

Fig. 1a–b Functionally characterised imaging patterns (*left*), inversely alpha-correlated fMRI maps (*middle*) and associated averaged EEG spectra (*right*). A single EEG feature can be associated with a variety of fMRI maps. **a** Using PET, Kjaer et al. found higher signals in bilateral occipital brain regions during drowsiness compared to at rest (Kjaer et al. 2002). Similar occipital and additional parietal fMRI signal changes were inversely associated with alpha power in a group of resting subjects showing EEG features of drowsiness (Laufs et al. 2006c). **b** A bilateral frontal-parietal network is known to support attention-demanding tasks, especially mental arithmetic (Gruber et al. 2001). In awake, resting subjects, the fMRI signals in a set of brain regions very similar to that involved during mental arithmetic increase with desynchronised alpha oscillations (Laufs et al. 2003a; Mantini et al. 2007)

tomography (PET) data had shown activation in occipital brain regions during light sleep when contrasted against wakefulness (Kjaer et al. 2002). The absence of a single average cortical BOLD signal pattern correlated positively with alpha power across studies may be explained by (spatially) nonuniform brain activity at the population level during periods of prominent alpha oscillations, which fMRI group analysis must fail to detect (Friston et al. 1999; Laufs et al. 2006c).

2.3
Similar Electrical Oscillations, Different fMRI Networks

The example discussed in the previous section showed that endogenous electrical oscillations, namely posterior alpha power during relaxed wakefulness, can be associated with different fMRI maps (haemodynamic networks). Slight methodological or analytic differences between the cited studies can only partially explain this effect. It is more likely that different (dynamic) brain states were studied and reflected in several EEG features, among which only one, the suppression of occipital alpha oscillations, was included in the above-mentioned analyses. This feature must be common to the different identified brain states and represents only an indirect measure. This suggests that, for a more detailed assessment of neural oscillations, broader EEG spectral properties and more comprehensive EEG spatial information must be incorporated into such analyses. Statistical considerations also require the parallel evaluation of, for example, multiple EEG frequency bands, especially if the bands are correlated with one another (Laufs et al. 2006c; Mantini et al. 2007): if only one of several correlated EEG features is used as a regressor in a general linear model (GLM), the attribution of the associated fMRI variance to a frequency band will be unspecific. For instance, if alpha and theta power are highly correlated, then the utilisation of either the theta or the alpha regressor in an fMRI analysis may yield very similar fMRI maps.

In an attempt to analyse a broader EEG frequency content (although not across space), Laufs et al. simultaneously correlated occipital theta, alpha and different beta frequency bands with fMRI data in a GLM (Laufs et al. 2003b). They found that activity in the beta2 (17–23 Hz) frequency band correlates with the DMN (Raichle et al. 2001). No significant theta band correlations were found in the fMRI data in that study (Laufs et al. 2003b). PET meta-analyses had originally identified the DMN (see Fig. 2) (Mazoyer et al. 2001). This describes a set of brain regions that show greater activity at rest than during states of reduced

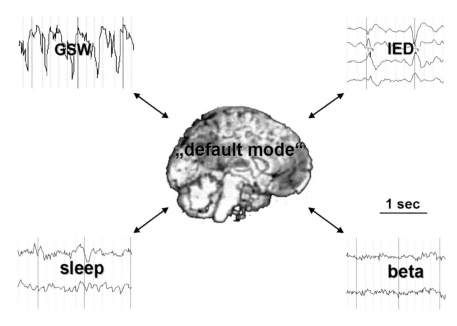

Fig. 2 A single fMRI map can be associated with a variety of EEG features at rest. Generalised *spike* and *wave* (*GSW*) discharges on EEG, typical rhythmic EEG oscillations during absence seizures with loss of consciousness, are associated with decreased fMRI signal in the precuneus, dorsal prefrontal cortices and the temporoparietal junction, regions of the "default mode network" (Archer et al. 2003; De Tiege et al. 2007; Gotman et al. 2005; Hamandi et al. 2006; Laufs et al. 2006a; Salek-Haddadi et al. 2003). Interictal epileptic discharges (*IEDs*) occurring frequently on EEG in temporal lobe epilepsy, characterised by complex partial seizures during which consciousness is impaired, are associated with fMRI signal decreases in "default mode" brain regions (Kobayashi et al. 2006b; Laufs et al. 2006a). During *sleep*, especially sleep stage II, central alpha power was found to be inversely associated with fMRI signal changes in regions constituting the DMN (Laufs et al. 2007). *Beta*-band EEG oscillations are associated with fMRI signal fluctuations in "default mode" brain regions (Laufs et al. 2003b; Mantini et al. 2007)

consciousness and states of extroverted perception and action. Thus, their activities are highest during an idling or intermediate-activity state following which the brain can then either engage in more activity (e.g. a task) or less activity (e.g. sleep)—hence its name (Raichle et al. 2001). While most resting state networks were later identified by data-driven fMRI experiments, the DMN was described in PET and fMRI meta analyses as a group of areas that consistently exhibited decreases from relative baselines of a wide variety of goal-directed behavioural tasks (Raichle et al. 2001). This allowed a meaning to be assigned to this network.

The identification of the "default mode" regions via a regressor derived from spontaneous EEG (beta-2 power) oscillations during wakefulness suggested that this network is dynamically active even when "at rest". Band specificity was demonstrated by making EEG the dependent variable: an fMRI signal time course taken from a representative region within the DMN (left temporoparietal junction) was correlated with specific EEG sub-bands and best fitted to the beta-2 oscillations (Laufs et al. 2003b).

Mantini et al. further extended this EEG–fMRI integration to an awake and at rest condition. They incorporated EEG bands between 1 and 50 Hz, averaged across the entire scalp, into their analysis. They correlated the fMRI time courses of resting state networks (identified by means of ICA) with these bands (Mantini et al. 2007). There was again an almost exclusively inverse correlation between the fMRI signals and the EEG frequency band (delta, theta, alpha, beta, gamma) power for four out of six identified resting-state networks. This may indicate that at the group level, a commonality of brain states could only be detected in the form of desynchronisation of brain oscillations at different frequencies. The most specific and positive EEG–fMRI correlation was revealed for the 30–50 Hz gamma band. This will require validation given that the BOLD signal changes occurred in the frontal lobe near areas typically bound to EPI signal dropout, and that 30–50 Hz EEG may contain increased noise. Once confirmed, this finding will support previous studies on the relationship between neural oscillations reflected in intracranial electrophysiological measurements and the BOLD signal (Lachaux et al. 2007; Logothetis et al. 2001; Niessing et al. 2005). However, fast intracranial oscillations do not necessarily translate one-to-one to scalp EEG.

As discussed above, occipital beta-2 power was found to correlate positively with the DMN (Laufs et al. 2003b). Mantini et al. additionally found that spatially averaged alpha power co-varied with BOLD activity in the resting state network (Mantini et al. 2007). Finally, Scheeringa et al. identified a very similar network during eyes-open rest that was inversely correlated with frontal theta power, the latter derived by applying ICA on the EEG data (Scheeringa et al. 2007). This latter example demonstrates once again how the state of the subject (eyes open, resting in the context of a cognitive task) as well as the analytical strategy pursued (frontal EEG power, single frequency band) can affect EEG–fMRI correspondence. If an inherent and possibly conscious processing-independent physiological principle is studied, this danger will be limited (Giraud et al. 2007).

2.4
Similar fMRI Networks, Different Electrical Oscillations

As argued in the section above, similar electrical oscillations can correlate with different fMRI oscillations. On the other hand, the "default mode" fMRI resting-state oscillations have been found to correlate with power in different EEG frequency bands, including (during eyes-closed rest) with spatially averaged alpha and beta (Mantini et al. 2007), posterior beta-2 (Laufs et al. 2003b), and (during eyes open rest) inversely with frontal theta oscillations (Scheeringa et al. 2007); see Fig. 2.

Based on fMRI functional connectivity analysis, Horovitz et al. suggested that the dynamic resting state activity persists in this network during reduced vigilance (Horovitz et al. 2007). A single-case EEG–fMRI study related activity in the DMN during sleep stage II (Rechtschaffen and Kales 1968) primarily to decreased central alpha power (Laufs et al. 2007). While PET data (Maquet 2000) congruent with the "default mode" concept (Raichle et al. 2001) identified a relative decrease in activity in that network during sleep compared to wakefulness, it is now clear that this network sustains its activity despite decreasing vigilance, and possibly functions at a lower energy level. The association of decreased activity in the DMN with other EEG features (focal and generalised epileptic activity) will be discussed below.

2.5
Brain Oscillations and Networks During Sleep

EEG is the central tool in sleep research, and oscillations serve to define sleep stages (Rechtschaffen and Kales 1968). EEG–fMRI is therefore an ideal tool to extend investigations of awake, resting brain oscillations to states of reduced vigilance. This will only be briefly touched on here because a separate chapter of this book is dedicated to EEG–fMRI and sleep (see the chapter "Sleep"). Due to their limited temporal resolution, EEG–PET studies have to assess sleep stage-related mean brain activity over many minutes (Maquet 2000), but cannot identify within-state activity or metabolic correlates of brief sleep-specific oscillations and events such as sleep spindles, vertex sharp waves or K-complexes. While the first EEG–fMRI study of spontaneous sleep without visual or acoustic stimulation was still performed in the spirit of these PET studies (Kaufmann et al. 2006), since then, sleep stage-specific EEG frequency patterns have been studied in a single case alongside an event-related analysis of sleep spindles and K-complexes (Laufs et al. 2007). A larger study confirmed and extended the findings of sleep spindle-associated bilateral thalamic, superior temporal and sensorimotor cortical activations (Schabus et al. 2007). Both studies discussed temporal lobe activation as a possible indication of memory processing during sleep, but due to the nature of resting-state investigations there was no probing task, and so this interpretation presently remains speculative. This is an example of a shortcoming of resting-state studies, even when concurrent EEG information is available.

Delta oscillations are a prominent and characteristic feature of deeper non rapid eye movement sleep stages (Rechtschaffen and Kales 1968), but correlating these EEGs with fMRI oscillations during sleep stages III and IV in the single-case study did not reveal significant fMRI networks. Possible explanations for this include ignoring the phase of the oscillations and inappropriately limited exploitation of their spatial distribution, and it indicates that more sophisticated analysis strategies should be used in future studies (Laufs et al. 2007).

2.6
Endogenous Brain Oscillations in Patients with Epilepsy

Epilepsy is a special case of EEG–fMRI resting-state studies, and three chapters of this book are dedicated to it ("EEG–fMRI in Adults with Focal Epilepsy", "EEG–fMRI in Idiopathic Generalised Epilepsy (Adults)" and "EEG–fMRI in Children with Epilepsy"). This is why this chapter restricts itself to pathology-specific brain rhythms as well as further examples of EEG patterns associated with the brain networks discussed above.

Historically, the development of EEG recording during fMRI was driven by the motivation to localise the source of epileptic activity via haemodynamic correlates of the spontaneously occurring, unpredictable EEG events. Patients at rest were examined in order to create an event-related model for interrogating the fMRI data, and additional paradigms appeared dispensable at the time (Gotman et al. 2006; Laufs and Duncan 2007). The objective of the studies was not the resting state but to contrast epileptic activity against an implicit baseline. As it turned out, however, generalised epileptic activity in the form of 3/s spike and wave complexes affects activity in the DMN (Archer et al. 2003; De Tiege et al. 2007; Gotman et al. 2005; Hamandi et al. 2006; Laufs et al. 2006a; Salek-Haddadi et al. 2003). The behavioural correlate of the prototype for such generalised discharges are absence seizures, which are characterised by impaired consciousness. Other conditions of impaired consciousness have already been associated with a decrease in activity in default mode brain regions (Laureys et al. 2004), and the fMRI maps associated with absence seizures can be interpreted in an analogous way (Gotman et al. 2005; Laufs et al. 2006d). Surprisingly, even frequent focal interictal epileptic discharges in patients with temporal lobe epilepsy were associated with a relative signal decrease in the DMN, although behavioural changes are not obvious during focal interictal epileptic activity (Kobayashi et al. 2006a; Laufs et al. 2006a). Assuming that decreased activity in the DMN during focal epileptic activity represents another instance of impaired consciousness, this may explain cognitive deficits observed in epilepsy patients with frequent interictal discharges and complex partial seizures characterised by a loss of consciousness (Laufs et al. 2006a). Thus, resting-state EEG–fMRI can identify impaired brain function. Altered brain rhythms—changes in ongoing EEG activity such as focal theta or delta slowing—may indicate pathology and can be used to localise the epileptogenic area in EEG–fMRI analyses (Laufs et al. 2006b; Siniatchkin et al. 2007). Studies relating ongoing brain activity itself to epileptic pathology are underway.

3
Linking Neuronal Oscillations to Haemodynamic Changes

At present, noninvasive scalp EEG–fMRI experiments still provide the best opportunity to study the relationship between neural and haemodynamic oscillations in humans because simultaneous, invasive intracranial EEG–fMRI measurements are still on the horizon (Carmichael et al. 2007; Laufs et al. 2008).

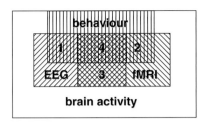

Fig.3 Analytical perspective on the interpretation of simultaneous EEG–fMRI studies. A subset of the entire brain activity manifests itself in observable behaviour (*vertical bars*), parts of which can be measured by either EEG (*1*), fMRI (*2*), or both (*4*). Some neuronal changes not reflected in overt behaviour may also be detected by either EEG (*forward slash*), fMRI (*backward slash*), or both (*3*). In cases *3* and *4*, the correlation between EEG and fMRI is direct in that there is a common substrate of neural activity. Excitingly, if behaviour is related to neural processes that also manifest themselves in EEG (*1*) and fMRI (*2*) independently, but which are not the same processes that are the source of the EEG and fMRI effects, this situation can still result in meaningful, indirect correlation between fMRI and EEG. Simultaneous multimodal experiments benefit from situations where common neural processes result in EEG and fMRI signals, but the most benefit is derived when these neural processes cannot be monitored in the form of behaviour (*3*). The difficulty involved in interpreting the results of EEG–fMRI studies is the uncertainty over whether a modality is recording data from situations *3* or *4* or data from a joint situation of *1* and *2*. In the latter case, prediction and constraint are not justified because the neural processes recorded in the two modalities are not identical

Given the examples above, when drawing conclusions from scalp EEG–fMRI experiments regarding the neurophysiology of the BOLD signal, it should be carefully assessed as to whether the EEG–BOLD correlation can be considered "direct" (see Fig. 3); in other words, whether the sources of the scalp electrical oscillations overlap significantly with those of the fMRI signal. More studies are needed to identify the factors that influence the quality of the relationship between neural oscillations measured with scalp EEG and the brain networks identified via BOLD–fMRI. For example, the experimental design and analysis strategy pursued in an experiment and the state of vigilance of the subject studied are relevant factors. An appropriate and flexible forward model combining EEG and fMRI should be chosen in order to accommodate interregional or otherwise induced variability in the EEG–fMRI correspondence in both healthy volunteers (de Munck et al. 2007; Laufs et al. 2006c, 2007, 2008) and patients (Aghakhani et al. 2006; Jacobs et al. 2007; Lemieux et al. 2007).

4
Conclusion

Neural and haemodynamic oscillations are the measurable correlate of "brain rhythms". They can be recorded via (surface) EEG and BOLD–fMRI, which are often only indirectly linked: very similar electrical oscillations in the brain can be associated with different fMRI-derived spatial maps, while haemodynamic oscillations of a distinct single network may correspond to diverse EEG patterns. BOLD and surface EEG signals are generated differently and exhibit different temporospatial properties, which is the fundamental reason for this observation. Also, in a fixed experimental setup, the EEG–fMRI overlap is still influenced by the brain state, or context, in which the multimodal data are acquired. This has implications for the interpretation of any EEG–fMRI-based finding, and highlights caveats concerning the integration of the two signal types, especially in the form of data fusion models assuming multimodal symmetry (Laufs et al. 2008); see also the chapter "EEG–fMRI Information Fusion: Biophysics and Data Analysis".

Terms like "rest" and "state" semantically imply inertness, while dynamic endogenous neural oscillations can in fact be visualised within so-called different resting states. The terminology is nonetheless acceptable, as it appears that distinct neural network configurations with certain properties exist "at rest", and these modes can be characterised using EEG–fMRI. The identification of such configurations and the transitions between them in healthy and pathologic conditions promises to advance our understanding of basic neurophysiology and disease.

The studies reviewed in this chapter can be seen as an overture to EEG–fMRI research into resting-state brain activity. Even during the production phase of this book, the number of publications and research groups that are focussing on this topic has risen exponentially. Because of this and increasing methodological finesse, both the depth and differentiation of the EEG–fMRI studies attempting to dissect resting-state brain activity are increasing: Olbrich et al. (2009) have analysed the fMRI correlates of brain states from wakefulness to sleep onset that are subdivided into five different states based on electrophysiological measures. Jann et al. (2009) extended the analysis of alpha-correlated fMRI resting-state network analysis by taking into account high-density EEG, allowing to the phase locking of alpha oscillations across the scalp to be assessed. Horovitz et al. explored new ground in lower vigilance states, focussing on both the distribution and the amplitude of spontaneous BOLD signal fluctuations. With decreasing vigilance, they found that some resting-state patterns persist and that the amplitude of BOLD signal variations increase in certain brain areas. Last but not least, the "alpha rhythm" itself was functionally examined more closely by Ben-Simon et al. (2008), who proposed different fMRI correlates for an induced type of alpha rhythm vs. a spontaneous type. Tyvaert et al. (2008) have tried to increase the sensitivity of EEG–fMRI epilepsy studies by taking into account the correlation of EEG oscillations with BOLD signal changes across the brain. These studies are again only a subsection of studies preluding the next generation of research into the organisation of the human brain at "rest".

References

Aghakhani Y, Kobayashi E, Bagshaw AP, Hawco C, Benar CG, Dubeau F, Gotman J (2006) Cortical and thalamic fMRI responses in partial epilepsy with focal and bilateral synchronous spikes. Clin Neurophysiol 117(1):177–91
Archer JS, Abbott DF, Waites AB, Jackson GD (2003) fMRI "deactivation" of the posterior cingulate during generalized spike and wave. Neuroimage 20(4):1915–22

Ben-Simon E, Podlipsky I, Arieli A, Zhdanov A, Hendler T (2008) Never resting brain: simultaneous representation of two alpha related processes in humans. PLoS One. 3(12):e3984. Epub 2008 Dec 19. PubMed PMID: 19096714; PubMed Central PMCID: PMC2602982.

Berger H (1929) Über das elektrenkephalogramm des menschen. Archiv für Psychiatrie und Nervenkrankheiten 87:527–70

Carmichael DW, Pinto S, Limousin-Dowsey P, Thobois S, Allen PJ, Lemieux L, Yousry T, Thornton JS (2007) Functional MRI with active, fully implanted, deep brain stimulation systems: safety and experimental confounds. Neuroimage 37(2):508–17

Curio G (2000) Ain't no rhythm fast enough: EEG bands beyond beta. J Clin Neurophysiol 17(4):339–40

de Munck JC, Goncalves SI, Huijboom L, Kuijer JP, Pouwels PJ, Heethaar RM, Lopes da Silva FH (2007) The hemodynamic response of the alpha rhythm: an EEG/fMRI study. Neuroimage 35(3):1142–51

De Tiege X, Harrison S, Laufs H, Boyd SG, Clark CA, Gadian DG, Neville BG, Vargha-Khadem F, Cross HJ (2007) Impact of interictal secondary-generalized activity on brain function in epileptic encephalopathy: an EEG–fMRI study. Epilepsy Behav 11(3):460–5

Fair DA, Schlaggar BL, Cohen AL, Miezin FM, Dosenbach NU, Wenger KK, Fox MD, Snyder AZ, Raichle ME, Petersen SE (2007) A method for using blocked and event-related fMRI data to study "resting state" functional connectivity. Neuroimage 35(1):396–405

Feige B, Scheffler K, Esposito F, Di Salle F, Hennig J, Seifritz E (2005) Cortical and subcortical correlates of electroencephalographic alpha rhythm modulation. J Neurophysiol 93(5):2864–72

Fox MD, Raichle ME (2007) Spontaneous fluctuations in brain activity observed with functional magnetic resonance imaging. Nat Rev Neurosci 8(9):700–11

Fox MD, Snyder AZ, Vincent JL, Raichle ME (2007) Intrinsic fluctuations within cortical systems account for intertrial variability in human behavior. Neuron 56(1):171–84

Friston KJ, Holmes AP, Price CJ, Buchel C, Worsley KJ (1999) Multisubject fMRI studies and conjunction analyses. Neuroimage 10(4):385–96

Gibbs FA, Davis H, Lennox WG (1935) The electro-encephalogram in epilepsy and in conditions of impaired consciousness. Arch Neurol Psychiatry 34:1133

Giraud AL, Kleinschmidt A, Poeppel D, Lund TE, Frackowiak RS, Laufs H (2007) Endogenous cortical rhythms determine cerebral specialization for speech perception and production. Neuron 56(6):1127–34

Goldman RI, Stern JM, Engel J Jr., Cohen MS (2002) Simultaneous EEG and fMRI of the alpha rhythm. Neuroreport 13(18):2487–92

Gotman J, Grova C, Bagshaw A, Kobayashi E, Aghakhani Y, Dubeau F (2005) Generalized epileptic discharges show thalamocortical activation and suspension of the default state of the brain. Proc Natl Acad Sci USA 102(42):15236–40

Gotman J, Kobayashi E, Bagshaw AP, Benar CG, Dubeau F (2006) Combining EEG and fMRI: A multimodal tool for epilepsy research. J Magn Reson Imaging 23(6):906–20

Gruber O, Indefrey P, Steinmetz H, Kleinschmidt A (2001) Dissociating neural correlates of cognitive components in mental calculation. Cereb Cortex 11(4):350–9

Hamandi K, Salek-Haddadi A, Laufs H, Liston A, Friston K, Fish DR, Duncan JS, Lemieux L (2006) EEG–fMRI of idiopathic and secondarily generalized epilepsies. Neuroimage 31(4): 1700–10

Horovitz SG, Fukunaga M, de Zwart JA, van Gelderen P, Fulton SC, Balkin TJ, Duyn JH (2008 Jun) Low frequency BOLD fluctuations during resting wakefulness and light sleep: a simultaneous EEG-fMRI study. Hum Brain Mapp. 29(6):671–82. PubMed PMID: 17598166.

Jacobs J, Kobayashi E, Boor R, Muhle H, Stephan W, Hawco C, Dubeau F, Jansen O, Stephani U, Gotman J, et al. (2007) Hemodynamic responses to interictal epileptiform discharges in children with symptomatic epilepsy. Epilepsia 48(11):2068–78

Jann K, Dierks T, Boesch C, Kottlow M, Strik W, Koenig T (2009 Apr 15) BOLD correlates of EEG alpha phase-locking and the fMRI default mode network. Neuroimage. 45(3):903–16. PubMed PMID: 19280706.

Kaufmann C, Wehrle R, Wetter TC, Holsboer F, Auer DP, Pollmacher T, Czisch M (2006) Brain activation and hypothalamic functional connectivity during human non-rapid eye movement sleep: an EEG/fMRI study. Brain 129(Pt 3):655–67

Kjaer TW, Law I, Wiltschiotz G, Paulson OB, Madsen PL (2002) Regional cerebral blood flow during light sleep: a H(2)(15)O-PET study. J Sleep Res 11(3):201–7

Kobayashi E, Bagshaw AP, Benar CG, Aghakhani Y, Andermann F, Dubeau F, Gotman J (2006a) Temporal and extratemporal BOLD responses to temporal lobe interictal spikes. Epilepsia 47(2):343–54

Kobayashi E, Bagshaw AP, Grova C, Dubeau F, Gotman J (2006b) Negative BOLD responses to epileptic spikes. Hum Brain Mapp 27(6):488–97

Lachaux JP, Fonlupt P, Kahane P, Minotti L, Hoffmann D, Bertrand O, Baciu M (2007) Relationship between task-related gamma oscillations and BOLD signal: new insights from combined fMRI and intracranial EEG. Hum Brain Mapp 28(12):1368–75

Laufs H, Daunizeau J, Carmichael DW, Kleinschmidt A (2008 Apr 1) Recent advances in recording electrophysiological data simultaneously with magnetic resonance imaging. Neuroimage. 40(2):515–28. Epub 2007 Dec 7. Review. PubMed PMID: 18201910.

Laufs H, Duncan JS (2007) Electroencephalography/functional MRI in human epilepsy: what it currently can and cannot do. Curr Opin Neurol 20(4):417–23

Laufs H, Hamandi K, Salek-Haddadi A, Kleinschmidt AK, Duncan JS, Lemieux L (2006a) Temporal lobe interictal epileptic discharges affect cerebral activity in "default mode" brain regions. Hum Brain Mapp 28(10):1923–32

Laufs H, Hamandi K, Walker MC, Scott C, Smith S, Duncan JS, Lemieux L (2006b) EEG–fMRI mapping of asymmetrical delta activity in a patient with refractory epilepsy is concordant with the epileptogenic region determined by intracranial EEG. Magn Reson Imaging 24(4):367–71

Laufs H, Holt JL, Elfont R, Krams M, Paul JS, Krakow K, Kleinschmidt A (2006c) Where the BOLD signal goes when alpha EEG leaves. Neuroimage 31(4):1408–18

Laufs H, Kleinschmidt A, Beyerle A, Eger E, Salek-Haddadi A, Preibisch C, Krakow K (2003a) EEG-correlated fMRI of human alpha activity. Neuroimage 19(4):1463–76

Laufs H, Krakow K, Sterzer P, Eger E, Beyerle A, Salek-Haddadi A, Kleinschmidt A (2003b) Electroencephalographic signatures of attentional and cognitive default modes in spontaneous brain activity fluctuations at rest. Proc Natl Acad Sci USA 100(19):11053–8

Laufs H, Lengler U, Hamandi K, Kleinschmidt A, Krakow K (2006d) Linking generalized spike-and-wave discharges and resting state brain activity by using EEG/fMRI in a patient with absence seizures. Epilepsia 47(2):444–8

Laufs H, Walker MC, Lund TE (2007) "Brain activation and hypothalamic functional connectivity during human non-rapid eye movement sleep: an EEG/fMRI study"—its limitations and an alternative approach. Brain 130(Pt 7):e75

Laureys S, Owen AM, Schiff ND (2004) Brain function in coma, vegetative state, and related disorders. Lancet Neurol 3(9):537–46

Lehmann D, Faber PL, Galderisi S, Herrmann WM, Kinoshita T, Koukkou M, Mucci A, Pascual-Marqui RD, Saito N, Wackermann J et al. (2005) EEG microstate duration and syntax in acute, medication-naive, first-episode schizophrenia: a multi-center study. Psychiatry Res 138(2):141–56

Lemieux L, Laufs H, Carmichael D, Paul JS, Walker MC, Duncan JS (2008 Mar) Noncanonical spike-related BOLD responses in focal epilepsy. Hum Brain Mapp. 29(3):329–45. PubMed PMID: 17510926.

Logothetis NK, Pauls J, Augath M, Trinath T, Oeltermann A (2001) Neurophysiological investigation of the basis of the fMRI signal. Nature 412(6843):150–7

Lopes da Silva F (2004) Functional localization of brain sources using EEG and/or MEG data: volume conductor and source models. Magn Reson Imaging 22(10):1533–8

Mantini D, Perrucci MG, Del Gratta C, Romani GL, Corbetta M (2007) Electrophysiological signatures of resting state networks in the human brain. Proc Natl Acad Sci USA 104(32):13170–5

Maquet P (2000) Functional neuroimaging of normal human sleep by positron emission tomography. J Sleep Res 9(3):207–31

Mazoyer B, Zago L, Mellet E, Bricogne S, Etard O, Houde O, Crivello F, Joliot M, Petit L, Tzourio-Mazoyer N (2001) Cortical networks for working memory and executive functions sustain the conscious resting state in man. Brain Res Bull 54(3):287–98

Mesulam MM (1990) Large-scale neurocognitive networks and distributed processing for attention, language, and memory. Ann Neurol 28(5):597–613

Mesulam MM (1998) From sensation to cognition. Brain 121(Pt 6):1013–52

Michel CM, Murray MM, Lantz G, Gonzalez S, Spinelli L, Grave de Peralta R (2004) EEG source imaging. Clin Neurophysiol 115(10):2195–222

Moosmann M, Ritter P, Krastel I, Brink A, Thees S, Blankenburg F, Taskin B, Obrig H, Villringer A (2003) Correlates of alpha rhythm in functional magnetic resonance imaging and near infrared spectroscopy. Neuroimage 20(1):145–58

Munk MH, Neuenschwander S (2000) High-frequency oscillations (20 to 120 Hz) and their role in visual processing. J Clin Neurophysiol 17(4):341–60

Niessing J, Ebisch B, Schmidt KE, Niessing M, Singer W, Galuske RA (2005) Hemodynamic signals correlate tightly with synchronized gamma oscillations. Science 309(5736):948–51

Nunez PL, Wingeier BM, Silberstein RB (2001) Spatial-temporal structures of human alpha rhythms: theory, microcurrent sources, multiscale measurements, and global binding of local networks. Hum Brain Mapp 13(3):125–64

Olbrich S, Mulert C, Karch S, Trenner M, Leicht G, Pogarell O, Hegerl U (2009 Apr 1) EEG-vigilance and BOLD effect during simultaneous EEG/fMRI measurement. Neuroimage. 45(2):319–32. Epub 2008 Nov 28. PubMed PMID: 19110062.

Raichle ME, MacLeod AM, Snyder AZ, Powers WJ, Gusnard DA, Shulman GL (2001) A default mode of brain function. Proc Natl Acad Sci USA 98(2):676–82

Raichle ME, Snyder AZ (2007) A default mode of brain function: a brief history of an evolving idea. Neuroimage 37(4):1083–90; discussion 1097–9

Rechtschaffen A, Kales AA (1968) A manual of standardized terminology, techniques and scoring system for sleep stages of human subjects. US Government Printing Office, US Public Health Service, Washington, DC, pp 1463–76

Salek-Haddadi A, Lemieux L, Merschhemke M, Friston KJ, Duncan JS, Fish DR (2003) Functional magnetic resonance imaging of human absence seizures. Ann Neurol 53(5):663–7

Schabus M, Dang-Vu TT, Albouy G, Balteau E, Boly M, Carrier J, Darsaud A, Degueldre C, Desseilles M, Gais S, et al. (2007) Hemodynamic cerebral correlates of sleep spindles during human non-rapid eye movement sleep. Proc Natl Acad Sci USA 104(32):13164–9

Scheeringa R, Bastiaansen MC, Petersson KM, Oostenveld R, Norris DG, Hagoort P (2008 Mar) Frontal theta EEG activity correlates negatively with the default mode network in resting state. Int J Psychophysiol. 67(3):242–51. Epub 2007 Jul 12. PubMed PMID: 17707538.

Siniatchkin M, van Baalen A, Jacobs J, Moeller F, Moehring J, Boor R, Wolff S, Jansen O, Stephani U (2007) Different neuronal networks are associated with spikes and slow activity in hypsarrhythmia. Epilepsia 48(12):2312–21. doi:10.1111/j.1528-1167.2007.01195.x

Sorg C, Riedl V, Muhlau M, Calhoun VD, Eichele T, Laer L, Drzezga A, Forstl H, Kurz A, Zimmer C et al. (2007) Selective changes of resting-state networks in individuals at risk for Alzheimer's disease. Proc Natl Acad Sci USA 104(47):18760–5

Stam CJ, Montez T, Jones BF, Rombouts SA, van der Made Y, Pijnenburg YA, Scheltens P (2005) Disturbed fluctuations of resting state EEG synchronization in Alzheimers disease. Clin Neurophysiol 116(3):708–15

Steriade M (1995) Brain activation, then (1949) and now: coherent fast rhythms in corticothalamic networks. Arch Ital Biol 134(1):5–20

Steriade M (2005) Sleep, epilepsy and thalamic reticular inhibitory neurons. Trends Neurosci 28(6):317–24

Tyvaert L, Levan P, Grova C, Dubeau F, Gotman J (2008 Dec) Effects of fluctuating physiological rhythms during prolonged EEG-fMRI studies. Clin Neurophysiol. 119(12):2762–74. Epub 2008 Nov 1. PubMed PMID: 18977169.

Urrestarazu E, Chander R, Dubeau F, Gotman J (2007) Interictal high-frequency oscillations (100–500 Hz) in the intracerebral EEG of epileptic patients. Brain 130(Pt 9):2354–66

Sleep

14

Michael Czisch and Renate Wehrle

Abbreviations

ACC   Anterior cingulate cortex
BOLD   Blood oxygenation level dependent
(r)CBF   (Regional) cerebral blood flow
EMG   Electromyography
EOG   Electrooculography
EPI   Echo planar imaging
KC   K-complex
MEG   Magnetoencephalography
NBR   Negative BOLD response
PET   Positron emission tomography
PCC   Posterior cingulate cortex
PFC   Prefrontal cortex
PGO   Ponto-geniculo-occipital (waves)
PSG   Polysomnography
SPECT   Single photon emission computed tomography
SWS   Slow-wave sleep

1
FMRI in Sleep Research

1.1
Sleep

The time spent asleep consumes about one third of our lifetimes. In contrast to anaesthesia or a comatose state, the perceptual disengagement from the environment and alteration ("loss") of consciousness can be reversed during sleep upon intense stimulation. A large

M. Czisch (✉)
Max Planck Institute of Psychiatry, Kraepelinstr. 2-10, 80804, Munich, Germany
e-mail: czisch@mpipsykl.mpg.de

C. Mulert and L. Lemieux (eds.), *EEG– fMRI*   279
DOI: 10.1007/978-3-540-87919-0_14, © Springer Verlag Berlin Heidelberg 2010

body of knowledge on sleep-related processes has accumulated in the last few decades, but the precise functions of sleep are yet to be disclosed.

Most of our current understanding of cortical activity across the different stages of vigilance is derived from EEG recordings. Concomitant to falling asleep, the changes in brain activity on a cellular level—namely switching from tonic to burst mode firing with increased periods of hyperpolarisation—induce typical changes in EEG (Steriade 2003; Carskadon and Dement 2005). Altered surface EEG during sleep in humans was first documented as far back as 1929 by Hans Berger (Berger 1929). This was later followed by Loomis' description of specific characteristics in sleep recordings, like K-complexes (KCs) and sleep spindles (Loomis et al. 1938). The misconception of sleep as a cessation of brain activity as compared to the reticular activation during wakefulness was finally overthrown in 1953, when Eugene Aserinsky and Nathaniel Kleitman first described an active brain state accompanied by rapid eye movements (REM) that recurs at regular intervals during sleep (Aserinsky and Kleitman 1953). Awakenings from this state of high cortical activity correspond with higher incidences of vivid dream reports, which putatively accompany the activated cortical states. REM sleep shares many features with wakefulness, and is therefore also referred to as "paradoxical sleep". A further characteristic of REM sleep is the loss of voluntary muscle control. Based on these distinct features, international standards for scoring sleep stages have been established that rely not only on EEG, but also include electrooculogram (EOG) and electromyogram (EMG) criteria (Rechtschaffen and Kales 1968). For clinical purposes, this electrophysiological triad is usually extended by acquiring data on cardiovascular activity (electrocardiogram, pulsoximetry), breathing parameters (thoracic and abdominal movements, effective breathing), snoring, and EMG recordings of particular muscle groups (e.g. anterior tibialis muscle). This multimodal recording approach (polysomnography, PSG) represents the standard way of registering sleep in humans.

The depth of sleep is conventionally subdivided into stages characterised by specific EEG criteria, switching from the predominance of high-frequency rhythms (gamma, beta, and alpha) during active wakefulness to the slowing of the frequency towards theta, delta and slow oscillations, including distinct graphoelements like KCs and sleep spindles (Fig. 1).

The four stages of NREM sleep are paralleled by increasing arousal thresholds. NREM sleep makes up about 80% of the total sleep time, and about 50% of the night is spent in light NREM sleep stage 2.

The timing and amount of sleep is regulated by a homeostatic process (increased sleep pressure after prolonged wakefulness) and by a circadian process (tendency to fall asleep according to constantly fluctuating physiological rhythms). Based on these rhythms, paced by the suprachiasmatic nucleus, sleep is organised into progressive alternations of the sleep stages (NREM sleep stages 1–4 and REM sleep) in cycles lasting about 90 min on average. Sleep stages 3 and 4, which are termed slow-wave sleep (SWS) because of the prevailing delta EEG activity, predominate in the first sleep cycles, whereas REM sleep episodes prevail in the second half of the night (Pace-Schott and Hobson 2002; Carskadon and Dement 2005).

The spectral EEG composition during sleep shows characteristic topographic (Finelli et al. 2001b; De Gennaro et al. 2005) and coherence patterns (Achermann and Borbely 1998; Cantero et al. 2004). A prominent example of typical regional-specific patterns is

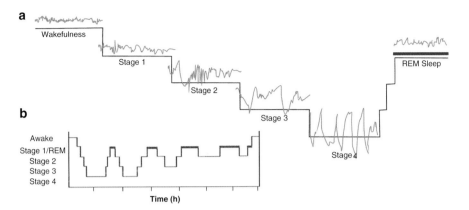

Fig. 1a–b Sleep EEG and sleep cycles in human sleep. **a** Typical EEG activity during the different vigilance stages: wakefulness is characterised by high-frequency (gamma, beta) activity that is shifting towards slower theta rhythms in sleep stage one. Theta is also the background activity during sleep stage two, which in addition is interspersed with sleep spindles (12–15 Hz) and K-complexes (KCs). Sleep stages three and four, also termed slow-wave sleep (SWS), are dominated by increasing amounts of delta activity. During REM sleep, cortical activation with high-frequency activity similar to wakefulness prevails. **b** The continuous alternation of sleep cycles during the course of the night, with typical decreases in SWS and increases in REM sleep

given by the hyperfrontality of slow oscillations. Additionally, homeostatic sleep pressure and individual genetic factors (Finelli et al. 2001a; Retey et al. 2005; Tucker et al. 2007) influence the spectral power distribution.

While sleep changes the rhythmic neuronal activity, the processing of information and consciousness states are dramatically altered during sleep too: the reduced responsiveness to environmental stimuli that is observed in parallel with the first sleep oscillations is partially mediated by attenuated transmission via the thalamus, which serves as central input gate for sensory stimuli. Inhibition of sensory information has been further linked to NREM sleep spindles, which can reduce postsynaptic potentials of thalamic neurons. External stimulation may elicit KCs as a typical sleep-related expression of stimulus–response. The functional significance of KCs as arousal or antiarousal reactions is still debated (Colrain 2005; Halasz 2005). As NREM sleep deepens and cortical cells "join in" with the rhythms, widespread synchronous, slow oscillations dominate and thus alter neuronal functionality (Steriade 2003) (Fig. 2).

Event-related potentials (ERP) represent a method of studying information processing by stimulus-related neuronal responses. Applied during human sleep (for reviews, see Bastuji and Garcia-Larrea 1999; Colrain and Campbell 2007), ERP studies report enormous changes, especially for late cortical potentials. Components typical of more complex information processing during wakefulness are mostly absent during NREM sleep (e.g. the P300 component), and are replaced by waveforms with similar behaviour and longer latencies (e.g. a P450 component). Some large-amplitude ERP components specifically appear in NREM sleep and possibly reflect inhibitory processes. Still, strongly deviant or highly relevant stimuli may lead to awakenings. In contrast to NREM sleep, most late cortical

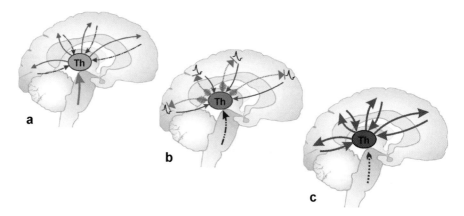

Fig. 2a–c Information processing during wakefulness, NREM sleep and REM sleep. Schematic sketches of thalamocortical information flow: during wakefulness, the thalamus (*Th*) plays a central role in conveying incoming afferent signals to the cortex, and cortical cells reciprocally communicate with the thalamus (**a**). During NREM sleep, thalamic and cortical cells change their neuronal firing patterns, inducing strongly altered modes of information processing. Here, prominent elements are the thalamically generated sleep spindles and cortically generated slow oscillations (**b**). During REM sleep, the activities of thalamic and cortical cells resemble wakefulness but are putatively dominated by intrinsic thalamocortical loops, without appropriate integration of external stimulation (**c**)

potentials and the ability to discriminate complex stimuli are partially restored during REM sleep. The apparent lack of integration of external information in REM sleep is not mediated by thalamocortical inhibition, but is assumed to occur due to altered prefrontal activity and generally altered connectivity patterns, possibly dominated by intrinsic loops (Llinas and Paré 1991).

1.2
Imaging Sleep

Neuroimaging during sleep is a relatively new research area. Various methods are utilised to address sleep-specific questions, and each method has its own advantages and drawbacks. Several excellent reviews condense recent findings and illustrate their impact on sleep research and the characterisation of sleep disorders (Maquet 2000; Drummond et al. 2004; Nofzinger 2004; Dang-Vu et al. 2007a). In brief, the first studies (performed about 20 years ago) applied positron emission tomography using radioactively labelled fluordeoxyglucose (FDG-PET), averaging neuronal glucose uptake over about half an hour. The long decay times allow for the application of the tracer in the general setting of a common sleep laboratory, with a delayed read-out in the PET scanner during which the subject could even be awake. The temporal resolution of the neuroimaging procedure was later enhanced by the application of $H_2{}^{15}O$-PET. This tracer also opened the possibility of repeatedly scanning an individual, but introduced the drawback that participants need to sleep inside the PET scanner. A related method, single photon emission computed tomography (SPECT), provides similar information to PET and can, for example, document dissociated states of motor arousal and persistent cortical sleep during sleepwalking (Bassetti et al. 2000).

A further method, high-density EEG, can reveal important spatial information on, for example, the site of origin and the travel of slow oscillations, or on experience-dependent local alterations in slow-wave activity (Massimini et al. 2003; Huber et al. 2006). Closely related to EEG, magnetoencephalography (MEG) measures the magnetic fields induced by the electrical neuronal currents that form the EEG response. The temporal resolution of MEG is in the millisecond range, but signals from deep brain structures cannot be recorded straightforwardly. MEG was applied in sleep research to investigate, for example, REM sleep saccades (Ioannides et al. 2004) and brain rhythms such as sleep spindles (Manshanden et al. 2002).

Taken together, PET, SPECT, MEG and high-density EEG studies have consistently confirmed hypotheses from animal studies that sleep is not a single invariable brain state: compared to wakefulness, NREM sleep is characterised by a global decrease in cerebral metabolism and blood flow, and furthermore by regional CBF decreases in the pons, the mesencephalon, thalamus, basal ganglia and basal forebrain, hypothalamus, and various other cortical regions, including the prefrontal cortex (PFC) and anterior cingulate cortex (ACC). For REM sleep, on the other hand, high neuronal activity has consistently been reported. Activity is increased in, for example, the pontine tegmentum, thalamus, amygdala, hippocampus and ACC as compared to both wakefulness and NREM sleep, but less activity compared to wakefulness has been reported for the dorsolateral PFC, posterior cingulate cortex (PCC), precuneus and inferior parietal cortex.

1.3
EEG and fMRI in Sleep Research

In previous fMRI experiments performed during sleep without unequivocal concomitant EEG recordings, an absence of behavioural reactions was used to determine that the participant had fallen asleep. Only the recent introduction of nonmagnetic EEG recording systems that can operate in strong magnetic fields and improvements in EEG postprocessing techniques (Benar et al. 2003) have made it possible to obtain fMRI data during verified, unambiguous sleep (Table 1).

1.3.1
The Need for and Advantages of a Combined Approach

New and impressive ways of targeting sleep-related phenomena that have previously only been investigated via invasive measurements in animal models are now possible due to the high spatial and temporal resolution offered by simultaneous fMRI and EEG measurements:

- Classic sleep scoring

Sleep is defined by EEG criteria. The acquisition of simultaneous EEG recordings during fMRI is therefore mandatory to differentiate the characteristics of altered brain activity during sleep. Additional EOG and EMG recordings are needed to allow for classical scoring of all sleep stages according to international guidelines (Rechtschaffen and Kales 1968).

Table 1 Main characteristics of simultaneous EEG–fMRI studies during sleep

Author	Year	No. of subjects	fMRI Method	Duration (hrs)	EEG	Sleep stages	Stimu-lation	Analysis of BOLD response
Løvblad	1999	2 (5)	silent BURST	5–7	Y	REM, NREM	–	REM vs. NREM, cross-correlations
Portas	2000	7 (12)	interleaved	2	N	NREM	ac	17s blocks (tones, names) fixed GLM with factors state × event + interactions
Czisch	2002	9 (14)	silent GEFI	n.g. (>1)	Y	NREM st 1–4	ac	30 s blocks (text) cross-correlations within stages; ROI (aud + vis cortex)
Born	2002	5 (10)	dummy, inter-leaved	n.g. (>1)	N	NREM	vis	15 s blocks (flashlight) fixed GLM within stages; additional $H_2^{15}O$ PET
Tanaka	2003	6 (6)	GEFI	<1	N	NREM st 1	ac	36 s blocks (tone) fixed GLM with state × habituation; ROI (aud ctx)
Czisch	2004	8 (13)	replay	1–3	Y	NREM st 2–4	ac	30 s blocks (tones, text, music) fixed GLM within stages, relation to EEG delta activity
Wehrle	2005	7 (11)	replay	3	Y	REM	ac	Eye movements as reference function, fixed GLM
Khub-chandani	2005	5 (8)	continuous	4–5	Y	NREM	–	NREM vs. wakefulness, Subtraction method
Kaufmann	2006	9 (14)	replay	1–3	Y	NREM st 1–4, W	–	Sleep stages as reference function, rfx GLM, correlates to hypothalamus
Wehrle	2007	3 (11)	replay	3	Y	REM tonic, phasic	ac	30 s blocks (tones, text, music) fixed + rfx GLM within stages, correlates to thalamus
Rasch	2007	12 (14)	continuous	~1.5	Y	NREM SWS	od	30 s blocks (replay of odor cues) during SWS, GLM, ROI (hippocampus)
Schabus	2007	14 (25)	continuous	<3	Y	NREM spindles	–	Event-related design to onset of slow and fast spindles, rfx GLM; several ROIs
Horovitz	2008	11 (14)	interleaved	1	Y	NREM st 1-2	–	Percent signal change related to sleep stages and EEG index of wakefulness; several ROIs

No. of subjects: number of subjects with successful trials given (number of subjects participating); fMRI Method: MRI acquisition applied for feasibility of multimodal sleep studies, GEFI – gradient echo fast imaging; Duration (hrs): estimated duration of overall fMRI session, n.g – not given; EEG: information on EEG simultaneous to fMRI available; Sleep stages: stages according to Rechtschaffen & Kales (1968) covered in analysis; Stimulation: kind of sensory stimulation applied in study protocol, ac – acoustic, vis – visual, od – odor; Analysis of BOLD response: main statistical approach used in study, rfx – random effects analysis, GLM – general linear model, ROI – region of interest, aud – auditory, ctx – cortex.

- Special features within sleep/characteristics of sleep

Sleep electrophysiology contains a variety of valuable information: characteristic EEG graphoelements like KCs and sleep spindles; arousals and fluctuating microstates; changing spectral compositions; evoked potentials; REM; and much more. Studying the associated brain networks with fMRI is only feasible with the aid of simultaneous electrophysiological recordings of a sufficiently high quality.

1.3.2
Advantages of Separate Measurements

Nevertheless, as the simultaneous fMRI and EEG approach is still somewhat technically demanding, it cannot yet be considered a full substitute for classical recording methods. Some research questions may profit from utilising each method separately:

- Focussing on EEG and PSG

Given the remaining technical constraints, the actual target aimed at—the state of sleep itself—is hampered in the fMRI environment. Studies focussing only on electrophysiological measures might be preferable when looking at:

- Alterations within the progression of sleep stages
- Continuous all-night recordings
- Participants who are not good sleepers
- Effects of interventions on sleep, especially on sleep structure
- Sleep disorders, especially when they involve increased motor activity
- Focussing on fMRI

The interplay of brain areas that disclose aspects of the functional significance of sleep can also be usefully studied via fMRI without simultaneous EEG acquisition. Utilising fMRI alone appears more feasible and advantageous when targeting:

- Specific cerebral functions that are possibly influenced by sleep, e.g. memory consolidation (Walker et al. 2005; Gais et al. 2007)
- The influence of sleep restriction or sleep deprivation (Drummond and Brown 2001)
- Dysfunctional states related to sleep disorders (Bucher et al. 1997; Schwartz et al. 2008).

2
fMRI During Sleep: Technical Challenges

Many aspects of polysomnographic sleep fMRI experiments share common problems with simultaneous EEG–fMRI recordings in general, and are described extensively elsewhere in this book (see the chapters "Principles of Multimodal Functional Imaging and

Data Integration", "Origin and Reduction of the EEG Cardiac-Related Artefact", "EEG Instrumentation and Safety", "EEG Quality: The Image Acquisition Artefact", and "Experimental Design and Data Analysis Strategies"). Nevertheless, specific difficulties emerge when investigating sleep. Depending on the hardware and software facilities and the specific research questions involved, the topics discussed in the following sections may arise.

2.1
General Issues with Sleep fMRI

- Multimodality of sleep recording

As outlined in the introduction to this chapter, the proper definition of sleep in humans is based not only on EEG but on EOG and EMG criteria too. This places additional requirements on the hardware facilities, like availability of additional electrodes and channels, or special wiring for longer cables. A potential benefit can be gained from bipolar recordings of, say, EMG. Furthermore, postprocessing techniques must offer solutions that allow high-quality electrophysiological data to be recorded; otherwise, events of interest cannot be unambiguously distinguished. Effective solutions for eliminating ECG distortions are of major importance, or special requirements for high-frequency signals like EMG may be needed (Wehrle et al. 2005; van Duinen et al. 2005) (Fig. 3).

- Reference system

Classical sleep recording or ERP studies tend to use mastoid electrodes as a reference site. However, it may be difficult to get sufficiently high-quality recordings at this electrode

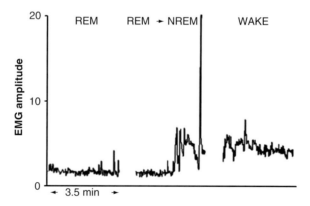

Fig. 3 EMG recordings during REM sleep. The amplitude of chin EMG recordings during fMRI scanning is shown for three consecutive scans of the same participant. In contrast to the elevated EMG levels during NREM sleep (*middle*, after arousal) and wakefulness (*right*), unambiguous REM sleep displays muscle atonia (*left*), with only short muscle twitches

position because of a high susceptibility to cardioballistic artefacts. In addition, headphones needed for proper sound protection often cover these sites, and may cause subjective discomfort or pain. It is therefore advisable to use a different site as the primary reference during data acquisition. EOG recordings may additionally benefit from the use of different reference schemes instead of the mastoid reference as recommended by Rechtschaffen and Kales (1968).

- Participant not falling or staying asleep

fMRI procedures per se induce highly adverse effects on sleep. The inevitable strong head fixation that also forces the participant to stay in a supine position limits the chances of falling asleep, as does the noisy environment in the narrow tunnel. Noisy environments inherently deteriorate sleep architecture, resulting in increases in sleep latency, sleep fragmentation and sleep stage changes, and a reduction in the total amount of sleep (Muzet 2007). Waxing and waning of drowsiness can easily be obtained during extended recording sessions, but consolidated sleep is more difficult to record.

- Extended recording time: subjective discomfort

It is difficult to not only fall asleep but also to stay asleep in the scanner. Even if participants manage to achieve stable sleep, fMRI sessions cannot be extended endlessly to obtain whole-night recordings. The participant's comfort should be a particular consideration when the subject is placed in the scanner, as aching electrodes or strong head fixation will make it more difficult to fall or stay asleep. One should also be prepared for the participant to be disoriented or feel uneasy after awakening in the magnet. In such situations, the complex experimental setup hampers the rapid removal of the participant from the scanner.

- Extended recording time: electrophysiological recordings

For most electrophysiological recording devices, signal quality usually deteriorates over time. Increased sweating may negatively impact on electrode contact. Some electrode sites strongly deteriorate during extended sessions but cannot be reattached or replaced in sleeping subjects without awakening.

- Extended recording time: fMRI recordings

MR image quality is also affected when the scanner is operated for an extended period of time. In general, the field homogeneity is adjusted using shimming procedures once, at the very beginning of the session, but it may degrade over time due to participants' movements or hardware instabilities. The coils continuously deliver magnetic field gradients with extremely short rise times and large amplitudes for several hours. This leads to temperature instabilities in the coils. Furthermore, the stability of the main magnetic field cannot be guaranteed over an extended period of time, leading to intensity drifts in the images. This is especially true if the cryogenic helium compressor of the magnet is transiently switched off during the experiment to minimise artefacts on EEG. Depending on the imaging parameters, physiological artefacts with BOLD activity correlated to cardiac or respiratory noise may be increased and should be accounted for (Lund et al. 2006; Wehrle et al. 2007; Laufs et al. 2007; Kaufmann et al. 2007).

• Movement

Participants' movements tend to increase during sleep. Body movements, including myocloni, are a common phenomenon during the process of falling asleep, as well as around REM sleep. During these periods, a compelling urge to move may lead to the arousal and awakening of the subject or disrupt fMRI recordings.

• Drop-out rate

The issues listed above indicate that the overall drop-out rate in sleep studies is higher than for classical fMRI studies performed during daytime or without EEG. It is worth pointing out that expectations regarding the time needed to acquire reasonable data sets ought to be adjusted to these limiting factors.

2.2
More Specific Issues with Sleep fMRI

• Specific suppression of sleep stages

Drop-out rates also depend on the sleep stage under investigation, because while acoustic noise reduces the overall amount of sleep, it predominantly affects specific sleep stages, namely REM sleep (Fig. 4).

To test the detrimental influence of the scanning procedures on sleep architecture, the fMRI environment was mimicked in a sleep lab situation (Wehrle et al., unpublished). The participant's head was fixated inside a sham MR coil, restricting the body posture to the supine position, while repetitive scanner noise with comparable loudness level was replayed. Such procedures were shown to have severe effects on general sleep structure. Specifically, these conditions fragmented and reduced REM sleep. REM sleep with concomitant muscle atonia represents a vulnerable sleep stage, one that is highly sensitive to uncomfortable and apparently dangerous environments, and is thus difficult to achieve in the MR scanner (see also Khubchandani et al. 2005). Furthermore, body movements that occur before and during REM sleep are not possible in the scanner.

• Selection bias

So far, subjects who are not able to sleep on their back or who are sensitive to environmental disturbances have not been studied at all. The selection of individuals who are eventually able to sleep inside the scanner may introduce a bias due to the sole recruitment of subjects who may display specifically enhanced sleep patterns or sleep-protective mechanisms.

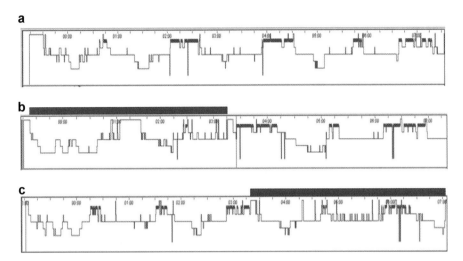

Fig. 4a–b Suppression of (REM) sleep during fMRI. Effect of fMRI procedures on sleep architecture. Head restraint and scanner noise were applied, without interference from magnetic fields, in the sleep lab during one half of the night. The distribution of sleep stages across a whole night for a single subject are shown: baseline night without any interference (**a**), MR simulation during the first half (**b**) and second half (**c**) of the night, indicated by the *red bar*. Adverse effects, especially for REM sleep, include prolonged onset of and strong fragmentation of REM sleep periods, thus decreasing the overall amount of REM sleep to less than 50% of the baseline condition

- No control over sleep state

There is no guarantee or control regarding whether participants do or do not fall asleep during scanning, and whether the sleep stage aimed at is reached for a sufficient long time. fMRI studies during sleep thus face a methodological drawback regarding possible within-subject effects based on repeated measurements, or intervention studies.

- No whole-night recordings

Information on sleep and sleep quality during a whole night of sleep such as that usually obtained in sleep laboratory recordings is rarely feasible in fMRI studies. If participants fall asleep, one or two sleep cycles can usually be recorded. Information on the entire sleep progression throughout the night, such as sleep stage latencies or stage distributions across a complete sleep period, is not reliably available.

- Fluctuation of microstates

Furthermore, fluctuating microstates within sleep cannot be voluntarily influenced. Baseline activity is presumably not even stable during wakefulness (Goncalves et al. 2006). All studies performed so far point to very prominent BOLD signal changes related to even short-lived EEG elements during sleep, and so continuous changes in baseline states must be expected to increase during sleep. Depending on the timescale of the fMRI recording during sleep, this methodological issue should be taken into account during analysis.

2.3
Possible Solutions

- Habituation

Habituation to noisy or uncomfortable sleeping environments is a common physiological adaptation process and can certainly be extended to the extreme situation of sleeping in an fMRI scanner. Subjects should be accustomed to the experimental setup in order to increase the probability of sleep.

- Sleep deprivation

One method of counteracting the arousing effects of fMRI procedures is to apply sleep deprivation previous to the fMRI experiment. The elevated sleep pressure will shorten sleep latency and increase sleep continuity. Total sleep deprivation also induces changes in the composition of EEG spectral power during recovery sleep; however, the spatial distributions that are typical of individual participants are basically preserved (Finelli et al. 2001a). Sleep deprivation also affects mood, possibly making subjects more sensitive to any experimental discomfort.

- MR recording techniques

Some of the first fMRI studies minimised gradient noise by applying pulse sequences and avoiding fast gradient switching. The BURST method (Hennig and Hodapp 1993) was successfully applied during REM sleep (Løvblad et al. 1999), and a "silent" gradient fast echo experiment was performed in NREM sleep (Czisch et al. 2002). Unfortunately, a drawback of these MR techniques lies in their lower signal-to-noise ratios as compared to echo planar imaging (EPI), and in the restriction to one or few slices due to sequence timing, which hampers group comparisons. However, reducing the slope of the gradient flanks reduced MR-induced artefacts in the EEG recordings. This made these methods especially interesting, as it allowed the correction of gradient artefacts through the elimination of discrete distorted EEG frequency bins (Hoffmann et al. 2000). New postprocessing correction algorithms relying on high sampling rates of synchronised EEG recordings (Mandelkow et al. 2006) and the subsequent subtraction of gradient artefacts are now commercially available.

Interleaved recordings, where EPI acquisitions are separated by periods of undisturbed EEG recordings during which the sleep stages can be assessed, represent another way to overcome the problems of gradient-induced artefacts. During the interleaved gradient-free periods, the EPI sound can be replayed in order to guarantee a constant acoustic background noise, which ensures that the subject is not repetitively aroused (Portas et al. 2000).

For some MR systems, limited data storage capacities may still make it necessary to run extended periods of continuously replayed scanner noise during sleep consolidation, or to run the scanner in a dummy mode with realistic gradient noise but without actual data sampling. Replayed sounds will not disturb the online EEG recordings but will never perfectly match the frequency characteristics of true gradient noise, thus including a risk of arousing the subject upon switching to data acquisition. Running the scanner in a dummy mode with actual gradient switching has the advantage that acoustic frequencies are matched and the scanner vibrations are also delivered to the sleeper. However, this procedure requires online EEG artefact correction to identify the beginning of the sleep stage of interest.

3
FMRI in Sleep: Results

The following section will focus on functional MRI studies performed during unambiguous sleep, based on the mandatory simultaneous use of polysomnographic recordings. With the exception of a few recent conference presentations, the experiments described here are limited to peer-reviewed articles published before January 2008. Related research lines like morphological MRI studies in sleep disorders (sleep apnea, narcolepsy, hypersomnia, etc.) and studies utilising fMRI to investigate cognitive functions related to sleep or sleep deprivation performed without parallel EEG measurements will not be discussed here. Reports on fMRI during sleep without polysomnographic verification, where the participants did not respond upon stimulation, did not show obvious movements during a paediatric scan, or were reported subjectively to have slept during the experiment, are only marginally addressed.

3.1
Spontaneous Sleep

fMRI was successfully applied in order to study the neurophysiology of unperturbed sleep, without additional external stimulation. These studies were an important milestone, as demonstrated the general applicability of fMRI measurements during sleep by replicating findings that were obtained previously using radioactive tracer-dependent neuroimaging. The fMRI approach allowed these findings to be broadened and extended due to improved resolution and better classification of sleep substates and associated neuronal activities. This is especially important when single EEG graphoelements like spindles or delta oscillations are investigated.

3.1.1
NREM Sleep

As the staging of sleep according to the Rechtschaffen and Kales scoring guidelines (1968) represents the gold standard in sleep research, Kaufmann et al. (2006) described specific activation changes in the process of falling asleep by setting the BOLD response in relation to the respective sleep stages. Technical limitations restricted the MR repetition time to a rather long duration of 10 s, but thus minimised cardiac artefacts in the fMRI analysis as compared to faster repetition rates (Kaufmann et al. 2006, 2007; Laufs et al. 2007).

Consistent with the majority of previously published findings, the cerebral activity as reflected in the BOLD signal decreased throughout NREM sleep as compared to wakefulness. The signal changes comprised cortical regions, the limbic lobe, the thalamus, the caudate nucleus and midbrain structures such as the hypothalamus. In an extension of previous reports, the fMRI approach allowed for a more detailed analysis of sleep-stage-specific patterns that are involved in the successive discontinuation of wakefulness, suggesting that a synchronised sleeping state can only be established if these regions interact in a well-balanced manner. Structures that showed reduced activation as compared to wakefulness even during sleep stage 1 were the anterior thalamic nuclei, the PCC and the cuneus. In addition, during sleep stage 2, which is usually associated with a loss of self-conscious awareness, signal reductions were obtained in frontal and more ACC areas, along with the inferior parietal and superior temporal gyri, the insula and the dorsal thalamic nuclei (Fig. 5).

Consolidated SWS showed a further reduction of activity in the frontal and inferior parietal gyri, the insula, the caudate nucleus and the ACC. This cascade of successive downregulation may be a prerequisite for establishing deep NREM sleep.

A promising approach that is yet to be further exploited in sleep research involves relating fMRI data to ongoing phenomena like spectral EEG power. Well in line with neuroimaging correlates of alpha activity found during wakefulness (Goldman et al. 2002; Moosmann et al. 2003; Feige et al. 2005), we obtained thalamic contributions associated with alpha activity during NREM sleep (Kaufmann et al. 2004). Equivalent signal decreases in occipital regions could not be obtained when evaluating alpha correlates against the EEG background of sleep.

One major advantage of fMRI as compared to PET imaging is its potential for analysing temporally coordinated network activity. As the hypothalamus is known to be of particular

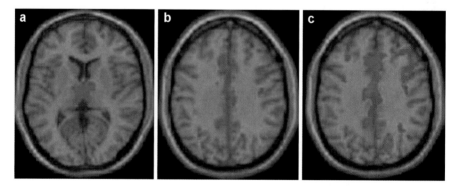

Fig. 5a–c Negative BOLD response in NREM sleep. Effect of sleep stages according to Rechtschaffen and Kales (1968) on relative BOLD signal changes when falling asleep. The transition from wakefulness to sleep stage 1 is accompanied by signal decreases in the thalamus (**a**). Further deepening of sleep towards sleep stage 2 is accompanied by prominent decreases in the anterior cingulate (**b**), which increases and includes other cortical areas when proceeding to SWS (**c**) (Kaufmann et al. 2006; reprinted with kind permission from Oxford University Press)

importance in the regulation of the sleep–wake cycle, cerebral network activity related to this seed area was investigated (Kaufmann et al. 2006). During NREM sleep, specific temporally correlated network activity of the hypothalamus and the cortex included limbic regions, parietal and frontal cortex, basal forebrain, as well as the brainstem. The network resembles the pathway of the ascending reticular activating system, projecting from the brainstem and posterior hypothalamus throughout the forebrain, thereby modulating the organism's arousal state. As this network analysis was based on the principle of temporal correlation of BOLD activity, it may be presumed that a higher degree of synchronisation of this network during NREM sleep as compared to wakefulness supposedly summarises both wake- and sleep-promoting alterations in this neuroanatomical functional unit. Both the medial PFC, involved in higher cognitive processes, and the PCC showed increased synchronicity with the hypothalamus. The PCC is known to be tonically active during wakefulness as part of the default mode brain network that is presumably responsible for collecting information about the external environment (Raichle et al. 2001). Therefore, sleep-related alterations may represent up- and downregulation of vigilance control regions with concurrent fading of integrative abilities when falling asleep.

Apart from relating BOLD signals to sleep stages, fMRI allows the study of BOLD correlates of characteristic graphoelements within sleep in event-related statistical designs. Although cerebral activity is generally decreased during NREM sleep as compared to wakefulness, distinct regional and temporal loci of increased activation with respect to the sleep-stage-specific baseline can be observed. A recent publication by Schabus and colleagues investigated the cerebral correlates of sleep spindles, transient oscillations in the beta frequency range defining NREM sleep stage 2 (Schabus et al. 2007). Two distinct types of spindles with presumably functional differences were described earlier, namely slow (<13 Hz) and fast (>13 Hz) spindles, with a predominance over frontal and centroparietal areas, respectively (Fig. 6).

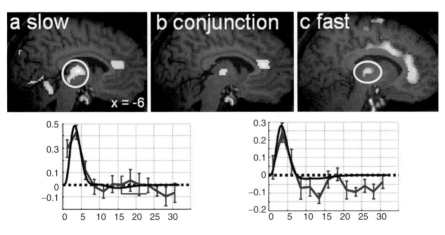

Fig. 6a–c NREM spindle correlates. BOLD correlates of the onset of slow (**a**) and fast (**c**) sleep spindles, and a conjunction of both spindle types (**b**). Note that thalamic activation characterises both types of spindles, whereas the fast spindle type is associated with an activation of the cingulate and somatosensory cortical areas (Schabus et al. 2007; reprinted with the kind permission of the National Academy of Sciences of the USA)

The authors first identified an activation pattern that was common for both spindle types, comprising the thalamus, ACC, left insula, and the bilateral superior temporal gyrus. When separating the spindle types, activity related to slow spindles largely corresponded to the common pattern, including activation of the superior frontal gyrus. In contrast, fast spindles showed additional recruitment in the supplementary motor area, sensorimotor and midcingulate cortex. Differential comparison to slow spindles revealed increased responses for fast spindles in the left hippocampus, frontal/PFC regions, sensorimotor cortex and anterior insula. Peak activation for slow spindles was located in the mediodorsal nucleus of the thalamus, and for fast spindles in the ventral posterior and pulvinar thalamic nuclei, which anatomically project to sensorimotor and posterior parietal cortices. Thalamic activation in both spindle types is well in line with neurophysiological evidence that spindles are generated in the thalamus and arise through the inhibition of thalamocortical neurons and postinhibitory rebound spiking in thalamocortical cells in large cortical regions.

Horovitz and colleagues recently presented fMRI data describing that, in the absence of external stimuli, distinct synchronous fluctuations of the BOLD signal can be observed when falling asleep (Horovitz et al. 2008). The authors investigated the spontaneous BOLD signal fluctuations using the EEG to classify drowsiness up to light NREM sleep. During this transition, significant increases in the fluctuation level of the BOLD signal were observed in several cortical areas, especially in the visual cortex. Further direct correlations to EEG characteristics were not reported. The authors report ongoing fluctuations in areas described as the default-mode network (Raichle et al. 2001) and primary sensory cortex that persist during light sleep, and are not restricted to the conscious waking state.

Animal cellular data show that NREM sleep is organised by slow oscillations (SO), derived from periods with intense neuronal firing alternating with hyperpolarisation phases (Steriade 2006). SOs were also demonstrated in humans (Achermann and Borbely 1997; Massimini et al. 2003). In a recent study, Dang-Vu et al. investigated fMRI during deep NREM sleep to assess the BOLD response associated with SO (Dang-Vu et al. 2007b). Negative BOLD responses were not observed. Positive brain responses associated with SO could be verified in subcortical structures, including brainstem, hypothalamus and thalamus. Significant activations were also located in primary and associative neocortical areas, and in limbic regions, including the hippocampus. These findings again highlight core structures underlying the organisation of NREM sleep phenomena.

3.1.2
REM Sleep

Circadian timing in the early morning hours, and REM-suppressing effects of the fMRI environment (as outlined in the introduction to this chapter), are among the main reasons why fMRI studies of REM sleep are performed less often.

Nevertheless, the first study to use truly combined EEG and fMRI methods in sleep research, published in 1999 by Løvblad and colleagues, reported REM sleep data (Løvblad et al. 1999). The authors investigated BOLD signal changes during REM sleep as compared to the NREM background preceding the REM sleep episode. They applied a silent BURST sequence to minimise acoustic noise and gradient-induced EEG artefacts, which

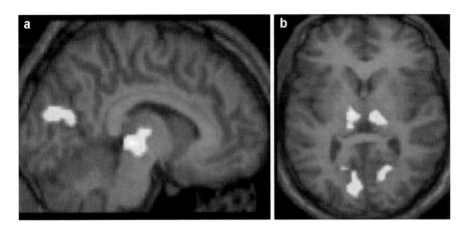

Fig.7a–b   Rapid eye movement correlates in REM sleep. BOLD activity correlated to rapid eye movements during REM sleep. Within REM sleep, the number of rapid eye movements per fMRI volume was calculated. BOLD signal intensity corresponding to eye movements in REM sleep shows activation in bilateral posterior thalamus and in occipital areas. (**a**) sagittal, (**b**) axial slice (Wehrle 2005; reprinted with kind permission of Lippincott, Williams & Wilkins)

permitted the continuous sampling of data over several hours. Muscle atonia could not be reliably detected and sleep-stage classification was modified focussing on presence of REMs, an absence of KCs to distinguish REM sleep from sleep stage 2, and a lack of response to calling the subject's name via the intercom system. In their study, Løvblad et al. successfully examined two (out of a total of five) participants during REM sleep. Increased activation of the occipital cortex and reduced activity in the frontal lobes during REM sleep as compared to BOLD amplitudes during NREM sleep was reported. These findings are in agreement with previous PET studies highlighting a deactivation in the frontal cortex and an increased activation in secondary, but not in primary, visual cortex during REM sleep (Maquet et al. 1996; Braun et al. 1997; Nofzinger et al. 1997; Braun et al. 1998).

Later, REM sleep data were also acquired using a regular EPI protocol, offering improved signal-to-noise ratios and spatial coverage (Wehrle et al. 2005, 2007). Technical amendments to the EEG recording hardware made it possible to define unambiguous REM sleep based on muscle atonia and the presence of REMs. By directly correlating the appearance of eye movements and BOLD signal fluctuations, it was possible to determine whether ponto-geniculate-occipital (PGO) waves can be directly visualised in human sleep (Wehrle et al. 2005) (Fig. 7).

PGO waves have long been described in animal models using invasive techniques, and have been proposed to precede eye movements and to be the generators of REM sleep in mammals. BOLD activation in a direct temporal relationship with REM during REM sleep revealed bilateral activation in the thalamus and the secondary visual cortex, a pattern remarkably consistent with PGO activity in animal models.

Taken together, these findings underscore that spontaneous sleep is not a state of brain quiescence, but is organised into exact progressions of highly specific brain network activities.

3.2
Sensory Processing During Sleep

During sleep we can be aroused by external stimuli, and so the brain's capacity to selectively process and evaluate stimuli according to their relevance must be preserved to a certain degree. Thalamocortical transmission is altered during sleep, and combined EEG–fMRI opens up the possibility of studying the underlying neuronal mechanisms of such changes in sensory processing in humans.

3.2.1
NREM Sleep

Several fMRI studies have investigated the reactivity of the human brain during sleep. In most cases acoustic stimuli were applied, as they appear best suited to exploring cerebral activation upon stimulation during sleep.

- Acoustic stimulation

Portas and colleagues used two types of acoustic stimuli, a neutral beep tone and the subject's own name, which carries high personal affective significance (Portas et al. 2000). Sleep was classified according to the criteria of Rechtschaffen and Kales, exploiting the undisturbed EEG traces before and after the fMRI blocks. As expected, the individual's own name provoked significantly more awakenings than neutral tones or baseline conditions, confirming the arousing capacity of this stimulus type. The fMRI analysis revealed a remarkable similar activation pattern when contrasting stimuli against resting baseline for both wakefulness and sleep, showing bilateral activation of the auditory cortex, thalamus and caudate nucleus. When comparing sleep to wakefulness, reduced activation was reported in several cortical, cingulate, thalamic and peri-amygdalic areas. Finally, an interaction analysis of stimulus type and sleep state revealed increased activation of the left amygdala and left PFC for name vs. tone stimuli, specifically during the trials where participants had been sleeping.

Text stimuli without arousing or affective components were applied in a block design using a silent sequence for data acquisition (Czisch et al. 2002). The single-slice gradient echo sequence produced relatively small EEG artefacts due to slow rising gradient flanks, allowing continuous and unambiguous sleep-stage classification throughout the complete data acquisition. fMRI was recorded during wakefulness and during all NREM sleep stages up to SWS. The BOLD response in the auditory cortex was significantly influenced by the sleep-wake cycle, with an almost abolished positive BOLD response during NREM sleep. Surprisingly, we additionally observed a negative BOLD response (NBR) upon acoustic stimulation during sleep, with a maximum amplitude and extent during sleep stage 2. Sleep stage 1 was characterised by a transition phase showing intermediate responses with positive BOLD signals in the auditory cortex, and emerging transmodal NBR in the occipital cortex. Analysis of the EEG revealed an increase in slow-wave activity (KCs and EEG delta waves) during stimulus presentation as compared to the resting baseline during light NREM sleep. This finding corroborates a presumed decreased neuronal activity, because increased sleep depth is characterised by growing EEG slow-wave activity that presumably reflects prolonged periods of neuronal hyperpolarisation. Similar findings were obtained during generalised epileptic seizures with slow EEG activity.

In order to investigate this phenomenon in more detail, we used a standard EPI sequence allowing for a better spatial coverage in a subsequent study (Czisch et al. 2004). Again, a block design with acoustic nonarousing stimuli was applied, and scanner sounds were replayed via headphones in-between the experimental runs (Fig. 8).

We were able to reproduce the NBR upon acoustic stimulation, especially during light NREM sleep stage 2. The amplitude of the NBR was best correlated to the relative increase in the KC density upon stimulation, whereas relative increases in total delta power showed closer association with the spatial extent of the NBR. Investigation of the regional BOLD time series revealed a stable NBR immediately following the stimulus onset in the auditory cortex. In contrast, the thalamic time curves indicated an initial positive BOLD response that (despite ongoing acoustic stimulation) returned to baseline levels after a few seconds. This effect was also most pronounced in the very first stimulation epoch, suggesting an initial thalamic reaction to sensory stimuli involving an assessment of the potential meaning of the stimuli, followed by reduced activity of the thalamus, probably due to habituation processes.

A further study investigated the effect of sleep stage 1 on auditory cortex reactivity upon presentation of pure tones (Tanaka et al. 2003). Here, subjects were measured during the process of falling asleep using an interleaved EPI sequence for unperturbed EEG recording between fMRI acquisitions. During sleep stage 1, the authors observed a significant decrease in the BOLD signal amplitudes as compared to wakefulness in the temporal

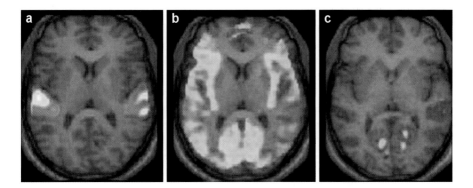

Fig. 8a–c Information processing during NREM sleep. Effects of acoustic stimulation on brain reactivity during sleep. Acoustic stimulation in a block design during wakefulness induces activation of the bilateral auditory cortex (**a**), which decreases during sleep stage 1 (data not shown). During light NREM sleep stage 2, acoustic stimulation elicits a relative decrease in BOLD signals in widespread cortical areas (**b**), which is accompanied by transient increases in slow EEG activity (including KCs). During SWS with ongoing slow EEG activity, no further changes are elicited upon acoustic stimulation (**c**) (partly reprinted from Czisch et al. 2004 with the kind permission of Blackwell Publishing)

gyrus. Their findings confirm a reduction of auditory activation upon external stimulation during drowsiness and falling asleep.

In this context, publications investigating sensory processing in sleeping infants and young children, which were performed without concomitant PSG, should be mentioned. Recently, Redcay and colleagues studied children during natural sleep while presenting vocal and nonvocal sounds as well as tones (Redcay et al. 2007). The authors report a positive BOLD response to different auditory stimuli in several areas including the bilateral superior temporal gyrus during sleep, with greater activation for nonvocal than for vocal sounds. Functional connectivity of superior temporal regions showed associated activity in further higher-order regions during sleep. Wilke et al. applied a passive listening task with vocal vs. nonvocal stimuli, and described preserved language processing in a six-year-old boy during sleep (Wilke et al. 2003). Here, stronger activation in receptive language areas was observed during sleep for vocal sounds.

- Visual stimulation

fMRI in children frequently requires sedation to minimise movement artefacts. To investigate the ability of infants to regulate their CBF responses, Born and colleagues used visual stimulation with a flashing stroboscopic light in sedated children (Born et al. 1998, 2002b). Upon stimulation, a consistent NBR in the occipital cortex was reported. NBR upon sensory stimulation has also been reported in other studies with sedated children (Martin et al. 1999; Altman and Bernal 2001). The findings of Born and colleagues were also supported by recently published data (Redcay et al. 2007) with significant NBR in occipital regions in sleeping children. Redcay et al. also analysed the functional connectivity of the sensory areas, and reported preserved networks during sleep. In 2002, Born and colleagues reported similar cortical stimulation-induced decreases while investigating healthy adult volunteers with simultaneous EEG recordings during natural SWS (Born et al. 2002a). Just like during sedation, a NBR was observed in the occipital cortex, which was located more rostrodorsally as compared to the BOLD increase regularly observed during wakefulness. In an independent sample, Born and colleagues successfully studied further subjects by applying $H_2^{15}O$-PET imaging under continuous stimulation (Born et al. 2002a). They were able to reproduce the fMRI results, detecting a reduced relative rCBF upon stimulation in the occipital cortex. These findings are discussed in the context of neuronal inhibition of the visual cortex upon stimulation. As our findings using acoustic stimuli during NREM sleep describe a similar reduced BOLD response in visual areas, this reduction may be regarded as a general or cross-modal sleep protective response independent of the modality of the stimuli.

- Olfactory stimulation

Another interesting aspect of sleep that may be investigated with fMRI is its putative role in consolidation of newly acquired memories. Olfactory stimuli that were associated with a learning session during daytime were applied by Rasch and colleagues during subsequent SWS in order to reactivate specific memories during sleep (Rasch et al. 2007). Olfactory afferents can project directly to higher-order regions including the hippocampus, and may thus putatively modulate hippocampus-dependent declarative memories. The re-application of olfactory stimuli during sleep was actually shown to enhance the recall of the hippocampus-dependent declarative memory, but not hippocampus-independent tasks like finger-tapping (Rasch et al. 2007). To test whether olfactory-induced reactivations are indeed related to increased activity in the hippocampal system, the authors re-exposed subjects to the same odour cues in fMRI sessions during SWS following the learning sessions. During sleep, renewed application of the olfactory stimulus induced a bilateral increase in the hippocampal region of interest, which exceeded the relative changes found during wakefulness, supporting data from animal studies that patterns of hippocampal neuronal activity associated with learning are reactivated in SWS.

3.2.2
REM Sleep

Most of the studies performed so far have investigated the processing of external stimuli during stages of NREM sleep. To study the altered processing of external stimulation during REM sleep with fMRI, acoustic stimulation using nonarousing stimuli was applied in healthy subjects (Wehrle et al. 2007). Neuroimaging as well as EEG recordings indicate high thalamocortical activity in both wakefulness and REM sleep; nevertheless, sensory integration of external stimuli does not occur during REM sleep (Maquet 2000; Hobson and Pace-Schott 2002). Upon contrasting acoustic stimulation with the resting baseline in unambiguous REM sleep, we observed two distinct patterns of activity when separating the fMRI sessions depending on the number of concomitant REMs. During the tonic REM sleep background with the classical high-frequency EEG and low muscle tone, but with only a limited number of phasic rapid eye movement bursts, the cortical activation obtained upon acoustic stimulation resembled the regular positive BOLD response as observed during wakefulness. The amplitudes of the respective increase in auditory cortex activation were however strongly reduced compared to the ones obtained during wakefulness. In contrast to these findings, acoustic stimulation during phasic REM sleep epochs with a high number of REMs showed a diffusive NBR including the thalamus. No activation of the auditory cortex was observed. This is in line with evoked potential studies during human REM sleep, where evoked responses are strongly suppressed and may differ depending on the actual presence or absence of REMs (Sallinen et al. 1996; Takahara et al. 2002). In addition, a parallel reduction in the number of REMs and in thalamocortical signal intensity upon external stimulation was observed. An investigation of temporal correlations of BOLD activity to time curves derived from thalamic regions of interest suggested highly synchronised activity of thalamocortical areas specific to periods with REMs (Fig. 9).

These findings support increased thalamocortical intrinsic activation associated with phasic REM sleep bursts. The high activity of the brain, especially during phasic REM sleep, may be regarded as a functionally isolated "closed loop", as proposed by Llinas and Paré (1991), reflecting an intrinsically highly active brain state. These phasic periods are embedded in a tonic REM sleep background which has an increased capacity to process external stimulation.

Fig. 9 Phasic REM sleep. Cortical activation correlated to—supposedly intrinsic—thalamic activity associated with phasic REM periods. During periods with a high number of REMs, the brain's reactivity to external stimulation is strongly suppressed (reprinted from Wehrle et al. 2007 with the kind permission of Blackwell Publishing)

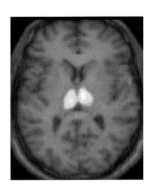

3.3
Animal Data

Our knowledge of the neurophysiology of sleep is for the most part based on experiments in animal models, where invasive protocols can be applied in order to derive detailed knowledge of the cellular mechanisms underlying sleep.

However, applying fMRI during natural sleep in animals is an extremely demanding task. Usually, animal welfare considerations allow the application of MRI only in anaesthetised animals. Sedation is also needed to minimise movements in addition to stereotactic fixation of the animal's head. Of course, anaesthesia prevents fMRI from being applied to complex behavioural tasks that can only be measured in conscious and cooperating animals. To study unsedated animals, lengthy training periods are necessary to habituate the animal to the experimental fMRI environment. This is even more true for natural sleep, since the animal needs to relax and fall asleep in the restricted and extremely loud experimental setup. These considerations make the application of fMRI in animal models less attractive, especially in rodents, where invasive recordings and histological analysis are easy to realise.

Nevertheless, Khubchandani and colleagues managed to conduct the only fMRI study on natural sleep in animals performed so far (Khubchandani et al. 2005). The authors used nonmagnetic silver wire electrodes implanted on the skulls of rats using polycarbonate screws for EEG measurements, sewn to the muscle of the external canthus of the eye for EOG, or implanted in the neck muscle for EMG. Sleep-wakefulness scoring was performed by taking low-frequency EEG with decreased EOG and EMG amplitudes to be the criteria for sleep, whereas high-frequency EEG with concomitant increased EOG and EMG classified wakefulness. To immobilise the animal during the MR procedure, a mould of dental cement was attached to the skull and fixed in the animal holder during measurements. Training consisted of habituation to the scanner noise as well as to the body restraint for up to several hours. Surprisingly, no gradient-induced artefacts or influences of the static magnetic field on the electrophysiological recordings were reported at 4.7 T (Khubchandani et al. 2003). Prior to the final sleep recording, the rats were sleep deprived for 24 h. The authors applied a gradient echo fast imaging method that was restricted to three planes passing through the preoptic area. Based on image subtraction, the authors describe increased signal intensities in the medial preoptic area during NREM sleep, interpreted as sleep-inducing action of this area. Consistent with imaging data from humans, concomitant signal decreases in the frontoparietal network as compared to images obtained during wakefulness were reported.

4
Summary and Outlook

The first pioneering works that applied simultaneous electrophysiological readings to characterise sleep in the MR environment were published as far back as 1999 (Løvblad et al. 1999; Portas et al. 2000; Born et al. 2002a). These studies proved the feasibility of this multimodal approach and its benefits for sleep research. Later studies made use of interleaved measurements with gradient-free periods between fMRI volumes (Tanaka et al. 2003), or of newly developed artefact correction algorithms, allowing for unambiguous sleep-stage scoring according to standard criteria during continuous fMRI acquisition (Czisch et al. 2002, 2004; Khubchandani et al. 2005; Kaufmann et al. 2006; Wehrle et al. 2007; Rasch et al. 2007). Recently, the focus has shifted towards specific graphoelements within sleep stages, like sleep spindles or REM, further exploiting the high temporospatial precision of this multimodal approach (Wehrle et al. 2005; Schabus et al. 2007). This progress was made possible by constant improvements in EEG hardware components, allowing for multimodal recordings, by the increased capacities of modern MR systems for continuous data collection, and by advanced online and postprocessing algorithms that simplify the identification of sleep.

fMRI, with its intrinsic methodological advantages, will continue to make essential contributions to sleep research. It can be expected that the classical sleep-stage scoring proposed by Rechtschaffen and Kales 40 years ago will be refined by a detailed analysis of functional substates, including the spectral composition and transient elements of drowsiness and sleep. fMRI associated with evoked neuronal activity will provide information on subtle changes in brain reactivity during sleep. Additional lines of research, e.g. focussing on the modulation of sleep-related functions throughout lifetime, on sleep deprivation and on pharmacological modulation, may also be addressed by these neuroimaging methods in the future. The proposed role of sleep in daytime functioning, such as memory consolidation and neuronal plasticity, may be further disclosed, probably differentiating processes based on NREM and REM sleep specific networks.

Access to information on sleep and sleepiness during fMRI will also help to disentangle signal fluctuations based on vigilance alterations from direct effects of interventional influences. The direct assessment of cerebral correlates linked to sleep-related disorders in the uncomfortable experimental environment may particularly benefit from improved noise cancellation methods and fewer restrictions on body posture. In the future, hardware and software developments will enable research groups to apply more demanding experimental designs, and will bring us new insights into spontaneous brain activity and successful or dysfunctional cerebral compensation processes associated with sleep-related disturbances.

Acknowledgements We gratefully thank all enduring participants. Part of the authors' work performed at the Max Planck Institute in Munich was supported by a grant from the Deutsche

Forschungsgemeinschaft (DFG WE 2250/6-I,II). We want to thank Florian Holsboer, Thomas Pollmächer, Dorothee P. Auer and Thomas Wetter for support. We owe special debts to C. Kaufmann for all his endless and engaged contributions, P. Sämann for fruitful discussions, and A. Mann and R. Schirmer for excellent technical support.

References

Achermann P, Borbely AA (1997) Low-frequency (< 1 Hz) oscillations in the human sleep electroencephalogram. Neuroscience 81:213–222

Achermann P, Borbely AA (1998) Temporal evolution of coherence and power in the human sleep electroencephalogram. J Sleep Res 7(Suppl 1):36–41

Altman NR, Bernal B (2001) Brain activation in sedated children: auditory and visual functional MR imaging. Radiology 221:56–63

Aserinsky E, Kleitman N (1953) Regularly occurring periods of eye motility, and concomitant phenomena, during sleep. Science 118:273–274

Bassetti C, Vella S, Donati F, et al. (2000) SPECT during sleepwalking. Lancet 356:484–485

Bastuji H, Garcia-Larrea L (1999) Evoked potentials as a tool for the investigation of human sleep. Sleep Med Rev 3:23–45

Benar C, Aghakhani Y, Wang Y, et al. (2003) Quality of EEG in simultaneous EEG–fMRI for epilepsy. Clin Neurophysiol 114:569–580

Berger H (1929) Über das Elektrenkephalogramm des Menschen. Arch Psychiatr Nervenkr 87:527–570

Born AP, Law I, Lund TE, et al. (2002a) Cortical deactivation induced by visual stimulation in human slow-wave sleep. Neuroimage 17:1325–1335

Born AP, Rostrup E, Miranda MJ, et al. (2002b) Visual cortex reactivity in sedated children examined with perfusion MRI (FAIR). Magn Reson Imaging 20:199–205

Born P, Leth H, Miranda MJ, et al. (1998) Visual activation in infants and young children studied by functional magnetic resonance imaging. Pediatr Res 44:578–583

Braun AR, Balkin TJ, Wesensten NJ, et al. (1997) Regional cerebral blood flow throughout the sleep-wake cycle. An H2(15)O PET study. Brain 120:1173–1197

Braun AR, Balkin TJ, Wesensten NJ, et al. (1998) Dissociated pattern of activity in visual cortices and their projections during human rapid eye movement sleep. Science 279:91–95

Bucher SF, Seelos KC, Oertel WH, et al. (1997) Cerebral generators involved in the pathogenesis of the restless legs syndrome. Ann Neurol 41:639–645

Cantero JL, Atienza M, Madsen JR, et al. (2004) Gamma EEG dynamics in neocortex and hippocampus during human wakefulness and sleep. Neuroimage 22:1271–1280

Carskadon MA, Dement WC (2005) Normal human sleep: an overview. In: Kryger MH, Roth T, Dement WC (eds) Principles and practice of sleep medicine. Elsevier, Philadelphia, pp 13–23

Colrain IM (2005) The K-complex: a 7-decade history. Sleep 28:255–273

Colrain IM, Campbell KB (2007) The use of evoked potentials in sleep research. Sleep Med Rev 11:277–293

Czisch M, Wehrle R, Kaufmann C, et al. (2004) Functional MRI during sleep: BOLD signal decreases and their electrophysiological correlates. Eur J Neurosci 20:566–574

Czisch M, Wetter TC, Kaufmann C, et al. (2002) Altered processing of acoustic stimuli during sleep: reduced auditory activation and visual deactivation detected by a combined fMRI/EEG study. Neuroimage 16:251–258

Dang-Vu TT, Desseilles M, Petit D, et al. (2007a) Neuroimaging in sleep medicine. Sleep Med 8:349–372

Dang-Vu TT, Schabus M, Desseilles M, et al. (2007b) Human brain is active during deep non-REM sleep. Sleep Biol Rhythms 5:A51

De Gennaro L, Ferrara M, Vecchio F, et al. (2005) An electroencephalographic fingerprint of human sleep. Neuroimage 26:114–122

Drummond SP, Brown GG (2001) The effects of total sleep deprivation on cerebral responses to cognitive performance. Neuropsychopharmacology 25:S68–S73

Drummond SP, Smith MT, Orff HJ, et al. (2004) Functional imaging of the sleeping brain: review of findings and implications for the study of insomnia. Sleep Med Rev 8:227–242

Feige B, Scheffler K, Esposito F, et al. (2005) Cortical and subcortical correlates of electroencephalographic alpha rhythm modulation. J Neurophysiol 93:2864–2872

Finelli LA, Achermann P, Borbely AA (2001a) Individual fingerprints in human sleep EEG topography. Neuropsychopharmacology 25:S57–S62

Finelli LA, Borbely AA, Achermann P (2001b) Functional topography of the human nonREM sleep electroencephalogram. Eur J Neurosci 13:2282–2290

Gais S, Albouy G, Boly M, et al. (2007) Sleep transforms the cerebral trace of declarative memories. Proc Natl Acad Sci USA 104:18778–18783

Goldman RI, Stern JM, Engel J Jr., et al. (2002) Simultaneous EEG and fMRI of the alpha rhythm. Neuroreport 13:2487–2492

Goncalves SI, de Munck JC, Pouwels PJ, et al. (2006) Correlating the alpha rhythm to BOLD using simultaneous EEG/fMRI: inter-subject variability. Neuroimage 30:203–213

Halasz P (2005) K-complex, a reactive EEG graphoelement of NREM sleep: an old chap in a new garment. Sleep Med Rev 9:391–412

Hennig J, Hodapp M (1993) Burst imaging. MAGMA 1:39–48

Hobson JA, Pace-Schott EF (2002) The cognitive neuroscience of sleep: neuronal systems, consciousness and learning. Nat Rev Neurosci 3:679–693

Hoffmann A, Jager L, Werhahn KJ, et al. (2000) Electroencephalography during functional echo-planar imaging: detection of epileptic spikes using post-processing methods. Magn Reson Med 44:791–798

Horovitz SG, Fukunaga M, de Zwart JA, et al. (2008) Low frequency BOLD fluctuations during resting wakefulness and light sleep: a simultaneous EEG–fMRI study. Hum Brain Mapp 29(6):671–682

Huber R, Ghilardi MF, Massimini M, et al. (2006) Arm immobilization causes cortical plastic changes and locally decreases sleep slow wave activity. Nat Neurosci 9:1169–1176

Ioannides AA, Corsi-Cabrera M, Fenwick PB, et al. (2004) MEG tomography of human cortex and brainstem activity in waking and REM sleep saccades. Cereb Cortex 14:56–72

Kaufmann C, Wehrle R, Wetter TC, et al. (2004) BOLD correlations with human sleep EEG spectra across sleep stages awake to S4. Neuroimage 22 (Suppl. 1), e1987

Kaufmann C, Wehrle R, Wetter TC, et al. (2007) Beyond noise: reply to Laufs et al. Brain 130:e76

Kaufmann C, Wehrle R, Wetter TC, et al. (2006) Brain activation and hypothalamic functional connectivity during human non-rapid eye movement sleep: an EEG/fMRI study. Brain 129: 655–667

Khubchandani M, Jagannathan NR, Mallick HN, et al. (2005) Functional MRI shows activation of the medial preoptic area during sleep. Neuroimage 26:29–35

Khubchandani M, Mallick HN, Jagannathan NR, et al. (2003) Stereotaxic assembly and procedures for simultaneous electrophysiological and MRI study of conscious rat. Magn Reson Med 49:962–967

Laufs H, Walker MC, Lund TE (2007) Brain activation and hypothalamic functional connectivity during human non-rapid eye movement sleep: an EEG/fMRI study—its limitations and an alternative approach. Brain 130:e75

Llinas RR, Paré D (1991) Of dreaming and wakefulness. Neuroscience 44:521–535

Loomis AL, Harvey N, Hobart GA (1938) Distribution of disturbance patterns in the human electroencephalogram, with special reference to sleep. J Neurophysiol 1:413–430

Løvblad KO, Thomas R, Jakob PM, et al. (1999) Silent functional magnetic resonance imaging demonstrates focal activation in rapid eye movement sleep. Neurology 53:2193–2195

Lund TE, Madsen KH, Sidaros K, et al. (2006) Non-white noise in fMRI: does modelling have an impact? Neuroimage 29:54–66

Mandelkow H, Halder P, Boesiger P, et al. (2006) Synchronization facilitates removal of MRI artefacts from concurrent EEG recordings and increases usable bandwidth. Neuroimage 32:1120–1126

Manshanden I, de Munck JC, Simon NR, et al. (2002) Source localization of MEG sleep spindles and the relation to sources of alpha band rhythms. Clin Neurophysiol 113:1937–1947

Maquet P (2000) Functional neuroimaging of normal human sleep by positron emission tomography. J Sleep Res 9:207–231

Maquet P, Peters J, Aerts J, et al. (1996) Functional neuroanatomy of human rapid-eye-movement sleep and dreaming. Nature 383:163–166

Martin E, Joeri P, Loenneker T, et al. (1999) Visual processing in infants and children studied using functional MRI. Pediatr Res 46:135–140

Massimini M, Rosanova M, Mariotti M (2003) EEG slow (approximately 1 Hz) waves are associated with nonstationarity of thalamo-cortical sensory processing in the sleeping human. J Neurophysiol 89:1205–1213

Moosmann M, Ritter P, Krastel I, et al. (2003) Correlates of alpha rhythm in functional magnetic resonance imaging and near infrared spectroscopy. Neuroimage 20:145–158

Muzet A (2007) Environmental noise, sleep and health. Sleep Med Rev 11:135–142

Nofzinger EA (2004) What can neuroimaging findings tell us about sleep disorders? Sleep Med 5(Suppl 1):S16–S22

Nofzinger EA, Mintun MA, Wiseman M, et al. (1997) Forebrain activation in REM sleep: an FDG PET study. Brain Res 770:192–201

Pace-Schott EF, Hobson JA (2002) The neurobiology of sleep: genetics, cellular physiology and subcortical networks. Nat Rev Neurosci 3:591–605

Portas CM, Krakow K, Allen P, et al. (2000) Auditory processing across the sleep-wake cycle: simultaneous EEG and fMRI monitoring in humans. Neuron 28:991–999

Raichle ME, MacLeod AM, Snyder AZ, et al. (2001) A default mode of brain function. Proc Natl Acad Sci USA 98:676–682

Rasch B, Buchel C, Gais S, et al. (2007) Odor cues during slow-wave sleep prompt declarative memory consolidation. Science 315:1426–1429

Rechtschaffen A, Kales A (1968) A manual of standardized terminology, techniques and scoring system for sleep stages of human subjects (Publ No 204). NIH, Washington, DC

Redcay E, Kennedy DP, Courchesne E (2007) fMRI during natural sleep as a method to study brain function during early childhood. Neuroimage 38:696–707

Retey JV, Adam M, Honegger E, et al. (2005) A functional genetic variation of adenosine deaminase affects the duration and intensity of deep sleep in humans. Proc Natl Acad Sci USA 102:15676–15681

Sallinen M, Kaartinen J, Lyytinen H (1996) Processing of auditory stimuli during tonic and phasic periods of REM sleep as revealed by event-related brain potentials. J Sleep Res 5:220–228

Schabus M, Dang-Vu TT, Albouy G, et al. (2007) Hemodynamic cerebral correlates of sleep spindles during human non-rapid eye movement sleep. Proc Natl Acad Sci USA 104:13164–13169

Schwartz S, Ponz A, Poryazova R, et al. (2008) Abnormal activity in hypothalamus and amygdala during humour processing in human narcolepsy with cataplexy. Brain 131(2):514–522

Steriade M (2003) The corticothalamic system in sleep. Front Biosci 8:d878–d899

Steriade M (2006) Grouping of brain rhythms in corticothalamic systems. Neuroscience 137:1087–1106

Takahara M, Nittono H, Hori T (2002) Comparison of the event-related potentials between tonic and phasic periods of rapid eye movement sleep. Psychiatry Clin Neurosci 56:257–258

Tanaka H, Fujita N, Takanashi M, et al. (2003) Effect of stage 1 sleep on auditory cortex during pure tone stimulation: evaluation by functional magnetic resonance imaging with simultaneous EEG monitoring. AJNR Am J Neuroradiol 24:1982–1988

Tucker AM, Dinges DF, Van Dongen HP (2007) Trait interindividual differences in the sleep physiology of healthy young adults. J Sleep Res 16:170–180

van Duinen H, Zijdewind I, Hoogduin H, et al. (2005) Surface EMG measurements during fMRI at 3T: accurate EMG recordings after artifact correction. Neuroimage 27:240–246

Walker MP, Stickgold R, Jolesz FA, et al. (2005) The functional anatomy of sleep-dependent visual skill learning. Cereb Cortex 15:1666–1675

Wehrle R, Czisch M, Kaufmann C, et al. (2005) Rapid eye movement-related brain activation in human sleep: a functional magnetic resonance imaging study. Neuroreport 16:853–857

Wehrle R, Kaufmann C, Wetter TC, et al. (2007) Functional microstates within human REM sleep: first evidence from fMRI of a thalamocortical network specific for phasic REM periods. Eur J Neurosci 25:863–871

Wilke M, Holland SK, Ball WS Jr. (2003) Language processing during natural sleep in a 6-year-old boy, as assessed with functional MR imaging. AJNR Am J Neuroradiol 24:42–44

Epilepsy

EEG–fMRI in Adults with Focal Epilepsy

15

Matthew C. Walker, Umair J. Chaudhary, and Louis Lemieux

1
Introduction

The application of EEG-correlated fMRI (EEG–fMRI) in adults with focal epilepsy has two principal aims: to improve our understanding of the generators of epileptiform activity and to improve the surgical treatment of epilepsy. EEG–fMRI, except in unusual circumstances (Salek-Haddadi et al. 2003; Kobayashi et al. 2006d), has been used to study scalp *interictal* epileptiform discharges (IEDs). The relative abundance of IEDs (and the lack of associated clinical manifestations) drove the initial development of EEG–fMRI with a view to studying the fMRI signal changes associated with epileptic activity (Ives et al. 1993; Hill et al. 1995; Huang-Hellinger et al. 1996). Previously, fMRI had been employed to study the haemodynamic correlates of seizures, relying on visual observation of the patient for interpretation of the BOLD signal changes. Ictal BOLD changes are, however, generally widespread, long lasting and difficult to interpret, particularly without concurrent EEG (Jackson et al. 1994; Detre et al. 1995, 1996; Krings et al. 2000; see Salek-Haddadi et al. 2003 for review).

Analysis of scalp IEDs is not without its problems. Scalp IEDs may reflect propagated activity rather than the source. Furthermore, even when the scalp IEDs are representative of the source or sources, there are no unique solutions to the generator location problem, and such solutions depend upon critical assumptions (such as the number of sources). EEG–fMRI is free from such assumptions and may therefore give a more accurate indication of the source or sources of IEDs.

EEG–fMRI may also help with surgical evaluation, and this chapter will mainly deal with this subject. The assessment of curative resective surgery is aimed at identifying the epileptogenic zone (Rosenow and Luders 2001). This relies upon the convergence of presurgical investigations, including clinical history, seizure semiology, scalp EEG, neuroimaging and neuropsychometry. Discordance between these may lead to a lesser chance of surgical success and the need for further investigation (e.g. further imaging, invasive EEG recordings).

M. C. Walker (✉)
Department of Clinical and Experimental Epilepsy, Institute of Neurology, University College London, Queen Square, London, WC1N 3BG, UK
e-mail: mwalker@ion.ucl.ac.uk

C. Mulert and L. Lemieux (eds.), *EEG– fMRI*
DOI: 10.1007/978-3-540-87919-0_15, © Springer Verlag Berlin Heidelberg 2010

The relative weight that is lent to each of these investigations varies depending on the lobar localisation and the pathogenesis of the epilepsy, and in many instances is either controversial or undetermined. The role of EEG–fMRI in the assessment of people with partial epilepsy remains undecided; there have been studies specifically addressing this issue and these are discussed below. One of the main criticisms that can be levelled at EEG–fMRI (indeed a criticism that can be levelled at other investigations such as magnetoencephalography) is that most studies to date have assessed interictal rather than ictal activity. This raises two questions: what does interictal activity represent, and how does it relate to the epileptogenic zone? We will therefore address the nature of an interictal spike and the relevance of interictal activity to presurgical evaluations before discussing in detail the possible roles of EEG–fMRI.

Up to now, most ictal EEG–fMRI data have been obtained due to the fortuitous occurrence of a seizure or seizures in the course of what was intended to be interictal EEG–fMRI investigations, with the exception of the use of activation procedures in patients with reflex epilepsy. Ictal EEG–fMRI offers the chance to address the main limitation of previous studies into the BOLD changes that occur in conjunction with spontaneous seizures, namely the lack of EEG. However, the technique is limited by the relative rarity and unpredictability of seizures, time constraints and safety considerations due to the confined space of the magnet bore and limited access.

As described in the chapter "Experimental Design and Data Analysis Strategies", regions of BOLD increase or decrease related to events of interest such as epileptiform activity can be identified using EEG-derived linear models of the fMRI time course, in what is effectively a correlation analysis. The main steps in this approach are: EEG event detection and classification; choice of a mathematical representation for the events (e.g. unitary spike, block, etc.); choice of haemodynamic basis set for convolution with the mathematic representation, resulting in an event-related linear model of the event; inclusion of nuisance effects. Individual spikes can be conceived as zero-duration events, at least on the timescale of fMRI, and are therefore usually represented as a mathematical spike with no scope for EEG-derived dynamics to be included in the models of the BOLD time course. However, a number of haemodynamic function basis sets are available for convolution, from the so-called canonical HRF to series of gamma functions, each corresponding to a different set of assumptions and therefore liable to reveal different activation patterns. This is in contrast to (extended) seizures, for which the choice of event mathematical representations is greater (fixed amplitude block, series of spikes, etc.), in addition to the choice of haemodynamic basis sets. Some of these modelling issues will be discussed in greater detail in this chapter.

2
Interictal EEG–fMRI

2.1
What Is an Interictal Spike?

Epileptiform interictal EEG abnormalities include: spikes, which are fast electrographic transients lasting less than 70 ms; and sharp waves, which last 70–120 ms (de Curtis and Avanzini 2001). That these are pathological is supported by their very rare occurrence

(<1%) in healthy individuals (Gregory et al. 1993), and their strong association with epilepsy (Marsan and Zivin 1970). Spikes and sharp waves are often followed by a slow wave lasting hundreds of milliseconds. As discussed below, this slow wave probably represents a period of relative refractoriness. It has been established from concomitant field potential and intracellular recordings that the intracellular correlate of the interictal spike is the paroxysmal depolarising shift (Matsumoto and Marsan 1964), a slow depolarising potential with a high frequency (>200 Hz) burst of action potentials. A number of pathological mechanisms have been proposed to underlie the interictal spike, including the intrinsic burst properties of neurons and the synchronisation of neuronal populations.

The interictal spike is terminated by the activation of hyperpolarising GABA(A) and GABA(B) receptor-mediated currents and calcium-dependent potassium currents (de Curtis and Avanzini 2001; McCormick and Contreras 2001). Therefore, interictal spikes activate hyperpolarising currents, resulting in a postspike refractory period during which neuronal activity is inhibited (de Curtis and Avanzini 2001). The effective activation of these currents by the interictal spike raises the possibility that spikes can be anti-ictogenic. There is evidence that this may be the case, or at least that spikes are intrinsically different from a seizure.

A seizure is not the evolution of spike discharges, but can begin as a distinct high-frequency rhythm. Spike discharges can precede the seizure with progressively less effective after-hyperpolarisations in mesial temporal lobe epilepsy (King and Spencer 1995), but ictal activity remains a distinct phenomenon. Furthermore, increased interictal spiking occurs after the seizure, raising the possibility that this is a compensatory antiepileptic response (de Curtis and Avanzini 2001). Experiments in entorhinal cortex-hippocampal slice preparations have confirmed the antiepileptic potential of spikes. Spike discharges generated in the CA3 region inhibited epileptic activity in the entorhinal cortex, so that sectioning of the Schaffer collaterals led to potentiation of entorhinal cortex seizure activity (Barbarosie and Avoli 1997). This leads to two important conclusions: first, interictal spikes can have an inhibitory effect; second, they can have this effect remote from where the spikes arise.

Since interictal spikes are not a normal characteristic of the brain, they are necessarily indicative of pathology. However, they are not necessarily indicative of the area from which seizures arise. This raises an important question: does all the spiking cortex (in addition to the area in which a seizure arises) have to be removed for a successful surgical outcome; in other words, once the ictogenic area has been removed can the irritative zone generate seizures? If this were so then identifying the full extent of the irritative zone would be critical to directing surgery and to predicting surgical outcome.

It appears that the irritative zone has different implications for different aetiologies and lobar localisations. Furthermore, not all spikes are equal and certain patterns appear to carry greater weight, perhaps being more indicative of cortex that can initiate seizures as well as maintain interictal discharges.

2.2
Interictal Epileptiform Activity in Presurgical Assessment

This relevance of interictal activity depends on lobe and aetiology. The predictive value of IEDs in temporal lobe epilepsy has been the subject of numerous conflicting studies. Nevertheless, a number of conclusions can be drawn about interictal activity and temporal lobe epilepsy. The side that most consistently has interictal spikes has a high chance (>90%) of being the side from which seizures arise (Blume et al. 1993, 2001a). However, in a single recording session, this probability drops to approximately 75% (Blume et al. 2001a). This is similar for scalp, depth and subdural recordings. Reassuringly, the most consistent spikes recorded with subdural electrodes have a >90% chance of arising from the same lobe and >70% chance of arising from the same gyrus as the seizures (Blume et al. 2001a). Although subdural electrodes have a limited coverage, these translate into a high chance that seizures arise ipsilateral to and in the vicinity of interictal spikes. Furthermore, repeated recordings lead to improved specificity. Prominent contralateral interictal activity and/or interictal activity discordant with the ictal onset zone carry a decreased chance of surgical success (Palmer et al. 1999; Schulz et al. 2000).

These results suggest that localising interictal activity in temporal lobe epilepsy may give accurate information on the epileptogenic zone and an indication of prognosis following surgical resection. The data for interictal activity in patients with extratemporal lobe seizures are less promising. This is because of frequent propagation (often to other lobes) and larger irritative and epileptogenic zones. However, MEG studies and source localisation with high-density scalp EEG have revealed that, even in extratemporal studies, there can be a considerable concordance between interictal activity and ictal onset zone (Herrendorf et al. 2000; Stefan et al. 2003). Indeed, it has been suggested that highly localised MEG activity in some instances may obviate the requirement for intracranial EEG recordings.

The use of scalp EEG to identify interictal activity has another consequence. Recent evidence suggests that synchronous or nearly synchronous activation of as much as 10–20 cm^2 of gyral cortex is necessary to give a spike detectable by scalp electrodes (Tao et al. 2007). The immediate conclusion is that any method that relies on scalp EEG activity will only detect activations involving large cortical areas. Alternatively, a positive consequence of this filtering may be the effective selection of more significant and relevant interictal activity.

Therefore, interictal activity commonly overlaps with the seizure onset zone but is often more extensive. Does it reveal cortex beyond the ictal onset zone that needs to be resected in order to obtain a successful surgical outcome? Studies in patients with encephalomalcia suggest that resection of spiking cortex is necessary for a good surgical outcome (Kazemi et al. 1997), while studies of patients with mesial temporal lobe epilepsy are controversial (Schwartz et al. 1997). Certainly removal of the whole area from which discharges arise is unnecessary for surgical success. Indeed, a note of caution needs to be made in the interpretation of many studies in that larger resections are, a priori, likely to be associated with better surgical outcome; the challenge is to remove as little cortex as necessary to have a successful outcome. Certain spikes seem to be of greater importance, such as leading discharges—those that occur on a millisecond basis prior to others (Alarcon et al. 1997). Further, paroxysmal fast and runs of repetitive spikes have greater significance than isolated spikes in cortical dysplasia (Widdess-Walsh et al. 2007). All spikes are therefore not equal.

What implications do these findings have for the application of EEG–fMRI in focal epilepsy?

1. There may be a difference in its utility between temporal and extratemporal lobe epilepsies
2. EEG–fMRI may be of greater localising value in certain aetiologies
3. Scalp EEG–fMRI may be limited to the most significant spikes involving the largest cortical areas
4. The area revealed by EEG–fMRI is likely to be larger than the epileptogenic zone
5. Scalp EEG–fMRI is unlikely to be able to differentiate spikes that are of greatest importance (e.g. leading spikes) because of the temporal resolution of fMRI

These indicate that EEG–fMRI may have utility as an additional presurgical investigation, perhaps to guide intracranial EEG placement. Even in this respect, certain problems remain. Many patients (see below) may not have suitable discharges on scalp EEG and therefore cannot be used in EEG–fMRI studies. In addition, the scalp EEG spikes are likely to represent only a proportion of spikes that are occurring in a region, and since EEG–fMRI in effect compares BOLD signal at the time of scalp spikes with that at the time of no spikes on scalp EEG, then the power of this method may be reduced, resulting in a failure to detect significant BOLD changes. These factors may substantially reduce the impact of EEG–fMRI on presurgical investigation. For this reason, the search for other EEG features (such as focal fast activity or focal slow) or other EEG analyses that may correlate with activity in the epileptogenic zone recorded with intracranial electrodes is now the subject of much research.

2.3
Methodology

2.3.1
Data Acquisition

The technological aspects of EEG–fMRI data acquisitions are discussed in the chapters "EEG Instrumentation and Safety", "EEG Quality: Origin and Reduction of the EEG Cardiac-Related Artefact", "EEG Quality: The Image Acquisition Artefact", "Image Quality Issues" and "Specific Issues Related to EEG–fMRI at $B_0 > 3$ T", and the different data acquisition modes (and data analysis) are discussed in the chapter "Experimental Design and Data Analysis Strategies". Here we will focus on the main methodological aspects of studies on patients with epilepsy. In brief, EEG–fMRI has mainly been performed on conventional MR scanners using BOLD-weighted EPI sequences, with field strengths in the range 1.5–3 T, and using EEG recording equipment specifically designed for EEG–fMRI.[1] So-called "MR-compatible" EEG devices are designed to minimise the electromagnetic interactions between the two data acquisition systems (artefacts in the EEG and images), ensure data synchrony (commonly achieved by recording a scanner

---

[1] Arterial spin labelling EEG–fMRI has also been demonstrated (Stefanovic et al. 2005; Hamandi et al. 2008).

clock-derived signal as one of the EEG or auxiliary channels), record the ECG and mini-mise the additional health risks to the subject.

Patients are generally at rest in the MR scanner. Manipulation of drug levels has been used in some studies to modulate the rate of IED, creating "control" and "active" states with corresponding sets of scans acquired in separate, successive sessions (Seeck et al. 1998). Special attention to mechanical means of head immobilisation is recommended, as patients are more prone to motion than healthy volunteers. Initial EEG–fMRI in epilepsy studies universally utilised "spike- or EEG-triggered fMRI", employing a form of inter-leaved multimodal acquisition, whereby two sets of fMRI datasets were acquired in one session: one set consisting of (single or burst) scans acquired following the detection of an event of interest (e.g. IED) on EEG, and another set of scans acquired following periods of normal background (control state). Spike-triggered fMRI was a way of avoiding the prob-lem of image acquisition artefact, which is caused by the switching magnetic gradients and obscures the EEG. Following technological developments that made it possible to remove or reduce the image acquisition artefact, continuous EEG–fMRI became possible, provid-ing good-quality EEG data throughout the scanning process. This is now the favoured acquisition mode due to its ability to visualise the entire EEG, which may increase sensi-tivity but also has advantages from the point of view of fMRI modelling. For example, in spike-triggered fMRI, scans were acquired roughly from 4 s following an event of interest, based on the assumption that the BOLD change would peak at around 5–6 s postspike; the lack of temporal continuity in the control scan dataset hinders baseline modelling. It also has the advantage of not requiring online identification of spikes.

2.3.2
Data Analysis

The primary aim of EEG–fMRI data analysis is usually the identification of regions of IED-related BOLD change, and the time course of those changes is an important second-ary aim. This is the conventional brain-mapping problem of event-related fMRI, with the difference that the experimental design is totally unknown until after the data have been acquired and the EEG has been reviewed, in contrast to conventional paradigm-driven fMRI studies.

The most commonly used fMRI mapping approach is based on building a general linear model (GLM) of the BOLD time course (see the chapter "Experimental Design and Data Analysis Strategies" for a further explanation of the GLM-based approach to fMRI analy-sis). For data acquired using the spike-triggered scheme, the two sets of scans ("spike" and "control") were simply compared voxel-wise using a t test. For continuous EEG–fMRI, one must attempt to model the entire fMRI time series, which is a greater challenge. In summary, the main steps of the GLM building process to identify areas of interest in epi-lepsy are: (1) identification of events of interest (spikes, runs of spikes, other pathological discharges); (2) classification of the events of interest (grouping according to morphology, field topography); (3) mathematical representation of the events of interest (as "zero-duration/delta function" events, blocks of event runs, etc); (4) choice of a model of the HRF (canonical HRF, inclusion of temporal and dispersion derivatives) for convolution with (3) or another basis set (e.g. Fourier over block). The result is a set of regressors representing the BOLD changes predicted to occur in relation to the IED.

The reliable identification of EEG events of interest requires dedicated review software to reduce or remove pulse-related and image acquisition artefacts (see the chapters "EEG Quality: Origin and Reduction of the EEG Cardiac-Related Artefact" and "EEG Quality: The Image Acquisition Artefact"). EEG event markers are defined in real time and in relation to the fMRI scan series, thanks to scan time markers on the EEG record provided by the scanner–EEG synchronisation mechanism. The resulting event markers form the basis of the modelling of the effects of interest.

The baseline is the other, equally important, side of the statistical comparison that is applied at every brain voxel to reveal BOLD changes linked to the effect or effects of interest (spikes). In EEG terms, the intervals between the marked events of interest are usually considered to constitute the control state. In fact, this "baseline state" is subject to multiple sources of signal variation: physiological (neurological and other) and artefactual (head motion or scanner related). For example, we know from intracranial EEG recordings that the scalp EEG is a very biased and limited representation of physiological or pathological brain activity, reflecting a fundamental limitation of EEG–fMRI. Nonetheless, the effects of confounding factors on the fMRI signal may be added to the model, such as motion and cardiac via the ECG (see Salek-Haddadi et al. 2003).

The parameters (mathematical weight of each regressor) of the resulting GLM are then estimated at each voxel, and can be tested against the null hypothesis (i.e. parameter estimate not significantly different from zero). The z scores for each effect are then mapped across the scanned brain to produce statistical parametric maps (SPM).

An important point to keep in mind is that, given a particular EEG record, one may have a large number of possible GLMs, each effectively corresponding to a different set of questions or hypotheses about the relationship between EEG and BOLD. For example, different EEG observers are likely to identify and classify events differently, and will produce different GLMs. Given a set of EEG events, one may choose to focus on detecting the brain regions for which the spike-related BOLD time course has a fixed shape (e.g. canonical HRF), or to identify brain regions for which the spike-related BOLD time course can have any of a wide variety of shapes (e.g. using the Fourier basis set). The former maximises sensitivity to a specific pattern (the same response is expected irrespective of position), while the latter can be used to both estimate the shape of the time course and identify inter-regional variations in the relationship between event of interest and BOLD signal (i.e. the time course of the BOLD change can vary across the brain).

The principal outputs of fMRI model estimations are statistical maps and time plots of the estimated event-related responses. For example, localisation of the regional BOLD changes is often assessed in relation to the epileptogenic or irritative zones (known or presumed) to provide evidence of validity or potential clinical utility (e.g. as a potential noninvasive adjunct to current localisation techniques). The interpretation of the maps can be facilitated by co-registering them with more anatomically accurate MR images, such as those obtained from T1-weighted volumetric sequences, and the use of atlases (also often based on volumetric sequences or on photographic atlases) for anatomical labelling. However, both methods are prone to error due to differences in the physics of image formation for the two types of sequence, which can result in significant co-registration errors and mislocalisation/labelling (see Gholipour et al. 2007, 2008 for reviews). Concordance of the BOLD maps has been assessed in relation to the presumed or known irritative zone (or epileptogenic zone) at various scales, from lobar (BOLD cluster located in the same lobe) to millimetric (by measurement in Cartesian space or along the cortical surface).

The interpretation of the shape of the BOLD change over time is of interest from two points of view: the assessment of deviations from the "canonical" HRF observed during physiological tasks, and the direction of the epilepsy-related BOLD changes relative to baseline. The first can be addressed by modelling the BOLD changes related to spikes (considered as zero-duration events) using a flexible basis set such as the Fourier expansion (Josephs et al. 1997; also see the chapter "Experimental Design and Data Analysis Strategies"). The first application of continuous EEG–fMRI illustrated the interest in using a flexible modelling approach to plot the spike-related BOLD time course (see Fig. 1). Given the generally biphasic nature of the HRF, with its initial peak followed by an undershoot, assigning a sign to such transient changes is largely a matter of convention. One possibility is to call an "activation" any region that reaches statistical significance for a *t* test over the regressor built by convolution of the canonical (or similar) HRF with the chosen mathematical representation of the event of interest, and a "deactivation" any region for which this is the case for the inverted HRF; for more flexible models of transient changes that do not rely on the canonical HRF, an alternative is to use the sign of the largest deviation from zero over the fitted response's duration.

2.4
Relevance of the Observed BOLD Changes

The observation that local field potentials in the brain correlate with a positive fMRI BOLD signal is important for the interpretation of EEG–fMRI findings in partial epilepsy (Logothetis et al. 2001). Importantly, it was the field potentials and not the single unit spiking (action potential) activity that correlated best with the BOLD signal. Therefore, the generator of BOLD signal correlates well with the generator of the EEG signal, which is also generated by field potentials and not by action potentials. However, EEG and BOLD measure different aspects of brain activity—electrical signal vs. metabolic signal—and these may be generated by different cells. In addition, EEG reflects neuronal synchrony (see the chapters "EEG: Origin and Measurement" and "Locally Measured Neuronal Correlates of Functional MRI Signals"). BOLD activation is therefore likely to represent the source and possibly the propagation of IEDs. Although BOLD activations are often maximal in the spiking temporal lobe, there are often widespread activations in disparate (including contralateral) temporal and extratemporal regions (Kobayashi et al. 2006b). These incongruent activations probably represent the propagation of interictal activity.

IED-related BOLD changes can occur in the form of activation (positive BOLD) and deactivation (negative BOLD). What do BOLD deactivations represent? Local deactivations could represent vascular steal. However, there is evidence that negative BOLD signals correlate with GABA concentrations and relative neuronal inactivity (Shmuel et al. 2006; Northoff et al. 2007), leading to the possibility that negative BOLD can result from cortical inhibition. These propositions are critical for the interpretation of EEG–fMRI in partial

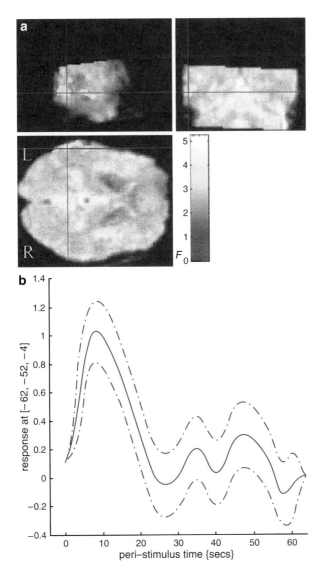

Fig. 1a–b Interictal continuous EEG–fMRI. Fifty-year-old patient with chronic encephalitis of the left hemisphere and intractable partial and secondary generalised seizures. Thirty-seven high-amplitude (>200 μV) stereotyped sharp waves maximal at T3 (left mid-temporal) focal were the most prominent feature. **a** SPM{F} of the spike-related events in the continuous EEG–fMRI experiment projected onto orthogonal slices of the mean EPI, showing activation localisation in the left temporal region. The F contrast was a unit matrix across a 16-term Fourier basis set used to model the event-related change. The crosshair is placed at the global statistical maximum. **b** Estimated time course of IED-related BOLD signal at global maximum (adapted from Lemieux et al. 2001)

epilepsy, because interictal spikes are the result of excitatory synaptic activity but result in both local and more distant inhibition (see above). This would, to some extent, explain the association of IEDs with not only local positive BOLD signals but also local and distant negative BOLD signals. A further explanation of BOLD deactivations associated with IEDs is the possibility that interictal activity may disrupt resting-state brain activity, such as the so-called "default mode network" (Raichle et al. 2001; Gotman et al. 2005; Laufs et al. 2006b, 2007). In either case, BOLD deactivations are more likely to be imprecise and discordant than BOLD activations. This is largely borne out by studies in patients with partial epilepsy. In a relatively unselected population of patients with partial epilepsy (Salek-Haddadi et al. 2006), positive BOLD responses were more likely to be concordant with electroclinical localisation, although negative BOLD signal did provide additional information. In this study, BOLD signal activations/deactivations were classified as concordant, concordant plus (in which the maximum BOLD change was concordant but other activated areas were discordant), or discordant (Salek-Haddadi et al. 2006). Spike-associated BOLD changes were observed in 23 patients: activations were concordant in ten patients, concordant plus in five, discordant in two, while deactivations were concordant in one patient, concordant plus in two patients, and discordant in seven (Salek-Haddadi et al. 2006). A further study in only eight patients reached a similar conclusion (Liu et al. 2008). Nevertheless, a recent study (Benar et al. 2006) found that the negative BOLD responses may represent EEG activity measured using intracranial EEG, and, in some instances, may provide concordant information.

There is therefore considerable evidence that EEG–fMRI activations can be concordant with electroclinical localisation and are more likely to be concordant than deactivations. BOLD activations are also likely to overlap with or be adjacent to intracranial lesions (Krakow et al. 1999; Al-Asmi et al. 2003; Salek-Haddadi et al. 2006).

2.5
Clinical Utility

For an assessment of clinical utility, three further questions need to be addressed: (1) what is the yield of EEG–fMRI in unselected patients undergoing presurgical assessment? (2) How closely does EEG–fMRI correlate with intracranial investigation? (3) What is the added value of EEG–fMRI in presurgical assessment?

Unfortunately, none of these questions has yet been adequately addressed. In the only study that addressed replicability in focal epilepsy (Krakow et al. 1999), six out of ten patients had activations that were confirmed on a subsequent scan. The largest "unselected" group of patients with focal epilepsy was 63 patients (25 males), four of whom were excluded (mainly due to excessive head movement). These patients were, however, included in this study only if they had frequent interictal discharges (spikes, polyspikes, sharp waves) on a recent EEG. Examination of other studies reveals that a similar criterion was used (Lazeyras et al. 2000; Al-Asmi et al. 2003; Kobayashi et al. 2006b) or sometimes that even more stringent criteria were used (Krakow et al. 1999). Even with this criterion in this study, 25 of the patients (42%) had no IEDs. Of the remaining 34, 11 had no change in BOLD signal. Therefore out of the original 63 patients, EEG–fMRI revealed activations/deactivations in 23 (37%). This is comparable to other studies, such as a study of 38 patients with intractable partial epilepsy in which only 31 studies from 48 could be analysed, mainly because of a lack of IEDs, and there was a significant fMRI activation in only 12 (25% of all studies, and 39% of those that could be analysed). Therefore, even when frequent interictal discharges are present on a previous EEG, there is a significant chance that no further information will be revealed by EEG–fMRI. A number of studies have analysed the features of IEDs associated with a BOLD signal change; these are: frequent epileptiform discharges, runs of epileptiform discharges, higher amplitude discharges and discharges with similar morphology (Krakow et al. 1999; Al-Asmi et al. 2003; Kobayashi et al. 2006b; Salek-Haddadi et al. 2006). Continuous fMRI has enabled post hoc analysis rather than manual triggering and so increases the yield (Al-Asmi et al. 2003), and the yield may be better at 3 T rather than 1.5 T (Federico et al. 2005). Since one of the main problems is the lack of IEDs, then it is important to be more inclusive (i.e. less rigorous) of possible interictal EEG abnormalities or to use a method that relies less on correlation with scalp EEG such as independent component analysis (ICA) of the fMRI data (Rodionov et al. 2007). Another approach is to analyse other scalp EEG activity such as focal slow, which has been shown in a small number of patients to have a strong concordance with site of lesion and intracranial EEG investigation (Federico et al. 2005; Laufs et al. 2006a). The tendency of expert observers to exclude discharges that are not clearly epileptiform, as encountered in clinical practice, may also limit the technique's sensitivity. The detection of more subtle IEDs using a more integrative analysis of the EEG and fMRI may provide an avenue for improvement (Liston et al. 2006). This has been used with some success, but is an area that requires further research.

The other question is whether the canonical HRF is the best model for IED-related changes or whether deviant, noncanonical BOLD signal changes yield useful additional information; systematic investigation of this issue suggests that in adults, noncanonical changes are relatively rare and likely to be discordant, and are therefore likely to decrease the specificity of the method (Lemieux et al. 2008; see also Salek-Haddadi et al. 2006). This is line with the observation that the yield of EEG–fMRI (i.e. proportion of cases in whom IEDs are captured that show significant activations) has not drastically increased following the transition from spike-triggered (with its assumption of a canonical spike-related response) at roughly 50–60% to continuous EEG–fMRI (capable of capturing a much greater number of events and greater modelling capability) at roughly 60–70%, although no satisfactory comparison exists. Although the use of multiple haemodynamic response functions in fMRI analysis may increase the yield to 80% (Kobayashi et al. 2006b), this may also be at the expense of specificity, and further studies are required. It is important to note that deviations from the canonical response have not been subjected to the same scrutiny for normal stimuli in healthy subjects as it has been in epilepsy. Therefore, the specificity of deviant responses to epilepsy is unknown.

A critical issue is the degree of concordance of intracranial EEG with scalp EEG–fMRI. Two potential problems when addressing this issue are: the limited coverage by intracranial EEG, and the fact that the fMRI BOLD (at 1.5 T) originates mainly from relatively large veins that drain the neuronally activated area (Lai et al. 1993), resulting in a discrepancy between signal location and active cortex. Notwithstanding this, studies suggest a significant concordance between intracerebral EEG and BOLD signal (Lazeyras et al. 2000; Al-Asmi et al. 2003). In the largest series to date (five patients) (Benar et al. 2006), it was observed that at least one contact of intracranial EEG was active that was sampled near a region of EEG-associated BOLD signal change.

Does EEG–fMRI give added value? A study comparing EEG–fMRI with scalp EEG source localisation has demonstrated a good degree of concordance at the lobar level (Lemieux et al. 2001). A study of five patients compared scalp EEG source localisation, EEG–fMRI and intracranial EEG (Benar et al. 2006). EEG–fMRI compared favourably against EEG source localisation. Within an error of 20 mm, the percentage matches between BOLD activations and intracranial EEG were better than those between EEG source localisation and intracranial EEG. Importantly, BOLD and EEG source localisation identified distinct areas of intracranial EEG activity (Benar et al. 2006). This study did not consider surgical outcome or concordance with ictal intracranial recordings, but it indicates that EEG–fMRI and EEG source localisation can give distinct information.

An alternative approach to determining added value is to consider patients who have been turned down for surgery. A study of 29 patients rejected for surgery because of an inability to localise a single source with EEG were selected for EEG–fMRI study (Zijlmans et al. 2007). All of these patients were noted to have frequent IEDs (>10 in 40 min) on a previous EEG. Of these 29 patients, a significant BOLD response was observed in 15. Eight patients had a BOLD signal that was topographically related to interictal discharges. For four patients (14%), there was felt to be enough information to proceed to intracranial studies. Two had intracranial studies and in both there was concordance between BOLD activation and ictal onset zone, but only one was operated on because of the proximity of the seizure onset zone to eloquent cortex in the other patient. The operated patient had a significant improvement (Engel grade II), but was not rendered seizure free.

In addition to directing the placement of intracranial electrodes, or possibly in the future removing the need for intracranial electrodes, another aspect of added value is if the EEG–fMRI is able to improve the prediction of surgical success. This is relatively unexplored.

2.6
The Influence of Lesions

It is likely that different lesions will have different effects on the BOLD signal generated by IEDs. This question has not been systematically studied, and there are only small case series. An important consideration is EEG–fMRI in malformations of cortical development, as these (in particular focal cortical dysplasia) comprise a significant proportion of MRI-negative cases (McGonigal et al. 2007). From a large study of patients with partial epilepsy, four of eight patients with malformations of cortical development had concordant activations (the other four had no activations) (Salek-Haddadi et al. 2006). This concordance has been confirmed in a further study using 3 T MRI in six patients (Federico et al. 2005). In all subjects there was a detectable BOLD signal change, and in four of six (67%) subjects there was a precise concordance of the BOLD activation with the location of the malformation of cortical development. The other two patients did not have lesional change that could be explained by lack of sensitivity (too few spikes), an epileptogenic zone distant from the area of observable malformation, or ongoing epileptiform discharges that were not detected on scalp EEG and so would contaminate the control fMRI periods (Federico et al. 2005). An additional observation is that only part of the lesion showed significant BOLD change, perhaps due to a more restricted irritative zone or a lack of statistical power. Also, there were distant activations.

In an investigation of 14 patients with either nodular or band heterotopia out of 26 studies, 23 were analysed and 22 had a significant BOLD change (Kobayashi et al. 2006c). 67% of the nodular heterotopia group activations and 100% of the band heterotopia group activations were in the heterotopia and/or surrounding cortex. Deactivations were also associated with the heterotopia but less robustly.

Polymicrogyria is a widespread abnormality associated with epilepsy. Evidence from intracranial EEG investigation and experimental work suggests that the epileptogenic region can be outside the predominant structural abnormality. An EEG–fMRI study revealed significant BOLD changes in 89% of the studies with 61.5% (8/13) of the maximal activations involving the lesion (Kobayashi et al. 2005).

These studies suggest that malformations of cortical development can be the main source of epileptiform activity, that such activity is detectable by EEG–fMRI, and that it may be associated with BOLD activations more than deactivations. This holds promise for the analysis of patients with apparently normal structural imaging.

What about other lesions? It would be important to consider vascular lesions because of potential problems. The problem with areas into which there has been bleeding or in which there is blood is that there may be considerable BOLD signal loss. It is therefore not surprising that five patients with cavernoma and EEG–fMRI signal change showed no responses within the lesion or its immediate periphery (Kobayashi et al. 2007). Reassuringly, two patients had perilesional BOLD changes, but the others had distant activations. This raises the distinct prospect that vascular lesions may be less suitable for EEG–fMRI studies.

3
Ictal EEG–fMRI

As mentioned previously, due to the practical difficulties and risks associated with acquiring MR scans during seizures, ictal EEG–fMRI has had a much lesser impact than interictal EEG–fMRI. Up to now, there are only four case reports and three small group studies of 43 patients (Di Bonaventura et al. 2006b), nine patients (Salek-Haddadi et al. 2008) and eight patients (Tyvaert et al. 2008) that are available in the published literature. Nonetheless, ictal EEG–fMRI may play an important role in epilepsy research in future, as it provides the opportunity to explore haemodynamic and electrophysiological changes taking place during a seizure, which is the defining event of epilepsy and central to the clinical evaluation of patients with drug-resistant epilepsy.

Ictal is derived from the Latin word *ictus*, which is used to describe a sudden neurologic event like stroke or an epileptic seizure (Sykes 1982; Blume et al. 2001b). Ictal is used to describe anything pertaining to epileptic seizures that is a manifestation of excessive and/ or hypersynchronous, self-limited activity of neurons in the brain (Blume et al. 2001b).

In the following, we discuss the limitations and review the clinical applications of ictal EEG–fMRI in patients with focal epilepsy.

3.1
Limitations of Ictal EEG–fMRI

Certain methodological and procedural factors have core importance in ictal EEG–fMRI, limiting its applicability, and they deserve careful consideration at this stage of the discussion.

3.1.1
Unpredictable Nature of Seizures

Due to the difficulty of predicting the occurrence and the relative rarity of spontaneous seizures, ictal EEG–fMRI has been reported in patients with either frequent or inducible seizures only, or as fortuitous occurrences of spontaneous seizures in studies of interictal activity, thereby severely limiting the practical utility of ictal EEG–fMRI. Daily absence seizures, pseudo absence seizures, tonic and atonic seizures (Di Bonaventura et al. 2006b), focal electrographic seizures (Kobayashi et al. 2006a; Salek-haddadi et al. 2002; Tyvaert et al. 2008), partial seizures with minimal motion (Di Bonaventura et al. 2006a, b; Tyvaert et al. 2008) and inducible seizures of reading epilepsy (Salek-Haddadi et al. 2008) have been investigated so far. Moreover, it is not always possible to record ictal events in all selected patients; e.g. only six out of nine (Salek-Haddadi et al. 2008) and 16 out of 43 patients (Di Bonaventura et al. 2006b) had ictal events. While the likelihood of recording seizures generally increases with acquisition time, this is limited to roughly 90–120 min by resource and patient comfort considerations.

3.1.2
Seizure-Related Motion

Seizure-related motion is a fundamental feature affecting the image quality and leads to false-positive or false-negative results in EEG–fMRI (Hajnal et al. 1994; Lund et al. 2005; Lemieux et al. 2007). Thus, by selecting cases in whom stereotypical seizures have less motion, an effort has been made to minimise this problem. In addition, vacuum cushions significantly reduce motion-related noise on the EEG and fMRI (Benar et al. 2003; Lemieux et al. 2007). After acquisition, fMRI scans can be corrected for motion by slice-timing correction, realignment, spatial smoothing, and later by incorporation of the estimated rigid body realignment parameters (Fig. 2) as confounding covariates in the design matrix to remove any residual artefacts (Salek-Haddadi et al. 2008; Tyvaert et al. 2008). Another approach to counteracting the signal changes, secondary to motion events during image acquisition, is scan nulling, where additional regressors for each motion event are modelled in the design matrix. Scan nulling reduces the effect of motion significantly (Lemieux et al. 2007). Seizure-related motion also affects EEG quality (see Fig. 2).

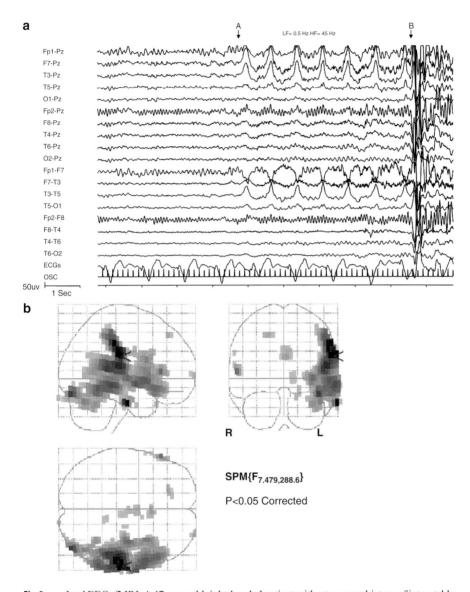

Fig. 2a–c Ictal EEG–fMRI. A 47-year-old right-handed patient with a two-year history of intractable generalised tonic-clonic seizures. An electrographic seizure started approximately 3 min into the acquisition, with focal rhythmic delta activity emerging abruptly and being unilaterally maximum over the F7/T3 electrodes (see Fig 1); it lasted for the next 15 s prior to evolving into a localised (F7/T3) 5 Hz theta rhythm and decaying slowly over the next 26 s. Brief EEG motion artefact was evident 5 s into the seizure. **a** EEG segment showing seizure onset (point *A*) and motion artefact on EEG (point *B*). **b** SPM showing seizure-related BOLD activation result of F test across 16-term Fourier basis set; cluster is shown on spatially normalised "glass brain". *Red arrowhead* shows global statistical maximum. **c** Regional ictal BOLD signal change (*green*, maximum change in cluster; *blue*, estimated change averaged over whole cluster; *red*, fitted sine function) in relation to motion as assessed by an fMRI time series realignment process (*red, green, blue*, X, Y and Z translations, and the corresponding rotations below). Note the negative BOLD signal prior to seizure onset (adapted from Salek-Haddadi et al. 2002)

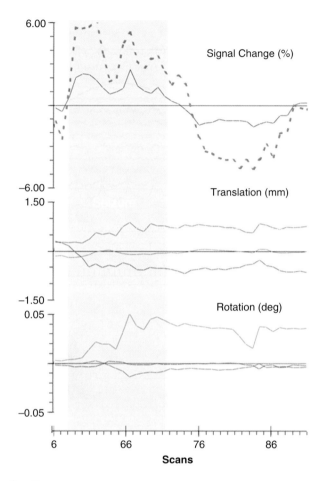

Fig. 2a–c (continued)

3.2
Detection of Ictal Activity

In some instances, ictal EEG activity is easy to differentiate from interictal EEG activity (Fig. 2; Kobayashi et al. 2006a; Salek-haddadi et al. 2002). However, this is often the exception, and even in these instances seizure onset may precede scalp EEG ictal activity. Various other methods can be employed to detect clinical seizures, such as button pressing by the patient (Salek-Haddadi et al. 2008), observing and identifying clinical changes inside the scanner similar to typical clinical seizure (Di Bonaventura et al. 2006b;Tyvaert et al. 2008) or following a verbal signal from the patient (Di Bonaventura et al. 2006b). Although subject to uncertainty and imprecision, when precise synchronisation with the EEG recording is unavailable, these time markers can be used as a basis for modelling the associated BOLD changes.

3.3
General Linear Model Building

As for interictal studies the usual data preprocessing and modelling steps are commonly applied to the ictal fMRI time series; a high-pass filter is applied to the data and design matrix, according to the noise characteristics of the scanner and the inclusion of autoregressive models to estimate the intrinsic temporal autocorrelation structure of the data. However, modelling the effects of interest linked to ictal activity is a priori a much more challenging task than for interictal activity for a number of reasons: the long durations of the events of interest give scope for yet-unknown patterns of signal change, affecting the choice of a mathematical representation for the events of interest and haemodynamic basis set; the potentially greater degree of interevent variability makes it more difficult to classify and group events; the possibility of pathological activity not reflected on scalp EEG or linked to behavioural changes (baseline problem); the potential for greater head and body motion. In addition, any interictal activity should be incorporated into the model.

Different EEG patterns have been used so far in various studies for modelling purposes, which include slow-wave discharges (Salek-Haddadi et al. 2008), sharp rhythmic activity, sharp fast activity, rhythmic bilateral discharges (Tyvaert et al. 2008), slow waves (Di Bonaventura et al. 2006b), spikes, polyspikes and spike wave discharges (Salek-Haddadi et al. 2002, 2003, 2008; Tyvaert et al. 2008).

In Salek-Haddadi et al. (2002), a single 45-s duration ictal event was modelled with a Fourier basis set spanning the entire event, thereby allowing for an almost arbitrary BOLD signal time course at any given location. In a study of patients with reading epilepsy, events (spikes and onset of ictal activity) identified on EEG and represented as stick functions were convolved with a canonical haemodynamic response function and its first temporal derivative (Salek-Haddadi et al. 2008). In Tyvaert et al. (2008), ictal events were modelled taking into account event duration and convolved with four haemodynamic response functions.

The inclusion of regressors to account for motion-related fMRI signal effects and close examination of the temporal relationship between motion and signal change are generally advisable, and case selection based on a maximum allowable degree of motion is also possible, although the choice of a specific threshold value is problematic.

3.4
Application of Ictal EEG–fMRI

Despite the issues highlighted above, EEG–fMRI has been successful in revealing interesting patterns of BOLD signal change related to ictal events captured on scalp EEG in a small number of cases.

3.4.1
Localisation Potential of Ictal EEG–fMRI

Ictal EEG–fMRI has shown the potential to localise the epileptogenic zone. The first case report showed a region of significant BOLD change concordant with the electrographic focus (Salek-Haddadi et al. 2002). The use of a flexible basis set revealed BOLD time-course variations across the activated region, and a suggestion of change prior to the EEG onset, but their pathological significance is unclear due to the level of inter-regional variability observed in healthy subjects (Aguirre et al. 1998). The large amplitude of the BOLD activation was deemed consistent with the levels of blood flow changes commonly observed using PET and SPECT (Salek-Haddadi et al. 2002).

In a study of malformations of cortical development (Tyvaert et al. 2008), and in a case study of Rasmussen encephalitis (Di Bonaventura et al. 2006a), ictal EEG–fMRI results were consistent with the electroclinically determined epileptogenic zone and intracranial recordings where available. Based on this small, highly selected sample, it appears that BOLD changes linked to ictal events are of stronger amplitude and are therefore possibly more likely to be detected than those linked to interictal activity, particularly in cases where the scalp EEG is a good representation of the overall ictal activity.

3.4.2
Mechanism of Epilepsy

In reading epilepsy (Salek-Haddadi et al. 2008), ictal EEG–fMRI revealed activations in cortical and subcortical areas, concordant with EEG changes. This observation points towards the early recruitment of subcortical structures, which may propagate and synchronise cortical activity. This has provided further evidence for a corticosubcortical network in seizure generation.

Tyvaert et al. studied patients with different types of malformations of cortical development, often demonstrating different BOLD patterns for ictal and interictal activity in lesions, overlying cortex and distant areas (Tyvaert et al. 2008; see Fig. 3). BOLD responses were found to be significantly greater for ictal compared to interictal activity. Studies in patients with focal cortical dysplasia demonstrated BOLD activations involving the lesion during both interictal and ictal recording. In contrast, patients with band heterotopias had BOLD activations with interictal epileptic activity involving the lesion and areas distant to the lesion, whereas ictal BOLD increases involved the lesion only. Similarly, patients with nodular heterotopia also showed some discordance between BOLD changes with ictal and interictal epileptic activity; ictal activity originated in the overlying cortex, whereas spike-related BOLD changes were congruent with the nodular heterotopia and distant cortex (Tyvaert et al. 2008). The significance of these observations remains to be assessed.

4
Conclusions

EEG–fMRI, with its capacity to reveal 3D, whole-brain maps of haemodynamic changes related to pathological EEG patterns, is a unique tool for the study of epilepsy. While the technique's yield—comparable to that of MEG—remains limited, and studies to date have

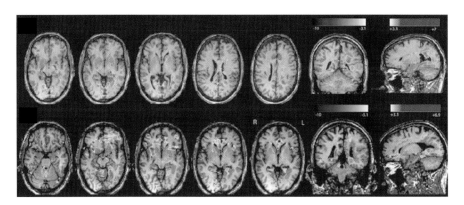

Fig. 3 BOLD maps of interictal and ictal activity in patient with malformation of cortical development (adapted from Tyvaert et al. 2008). *Upper*: Interictal increase of BOLD signal involving nodular heterotopia (in right occipitotemporal region) during right posterior temporoparietal spikes; *lower*: ictal activations involving overlying cortex only

been limited to selected cases, it has provided new localising information and revealed previously unseen brain networks in a large proportion of the patients studied, which now number in the hundreds. The combination of fMRI with EEG allows the application of powerful hypothesis-driven fMRI analysis techniques to reveal haemodynamic changes specifically correlated with pathological EEG patterns such as IED. However, this means that this approach to EEG–fMRI also suffers from some of the limitations of EEG, in particular its limited sensitivity, which can result in a poor baseline against which postulated BOLD changes can be assessed. The application of more sophisticated EEG analysis techniques and the use of EEG markers of the epileptogenic zone other than clear IEDs (such as focal slow or fast activity) may lead to more objective and reliable GLMs. Efforts are being made to both improve our understanding of the relationship between epileptiform discharges and BOLD signals, with the ultimate aim of improving sensitivity, and to find other ways of recognising BOLD patterns of epileptic activity.

References

Aguirre GK, Zarahn E, & D'esposito M (1998), "The variability of human, BOLD hemodynamic responses", Neuroimage. 8. 4. 360–369

Al-Asmi A, Benar CG, Gross DW, Khani YA, Andermann F, Pike B, Dubeau F, Gotman J (2003) fMRI activation in continuous and spike-triggered EEG–fMRI studies of epileptic spikes. Epilepsia 44:1328–1339

Alarcon G, Garcia Seoane JJ, Binnie CD, Martin Miguel MC, Juler J, Polkey CE, Elwes RD, Ortiz Blasco JM (1997) Origin and propagation of interictal discharges in the acute electrocorticogram. Implications for pathophysiology and surgical treatment of temporal lobe epilepsy. Brain 120 (Pt 12):2259–2282

Barbarosie M, Avoli M (1997) CA3-driven hippocampal-entorhinal loop controls rather than sustains in vitro limbic seizures. J Neurosci 17:9308–9314

Benar C, Aghakhani Y, Wang Y, Izenberg A, Al-Asmi A, Dubeau F, & Gotman J (2003), "Quality of EEG in simultaneous EEG-fMRI for epilepsy", Clin.Neurophysiol. 114. 3. 569–580

Benar CG, Grova C, Kobayashi E, Bagshaw AP, Aghakhani Y, Dubeau F, Gotman J (2006) EEG–fMRI of epileptic spikes: concordance with EEG source localization and intracranial EEG. Neuroimage 30:1161–1170

Blume WT, Borghesi JL, Lemieux JF (1993) Interictal indices of temporal seizure origin. Ann Neurol 34:703–709

Blume WT, Holloway GM, Wiebe S (2001a) Temporal epileptogenesis: Localizing value of scalp and subdural interictal and ictal EEG data. Epilepsia 42:508–514

Blume WT, Luders HO, Mizrahi E, Tassinari C, van Emde BW, Engel J Jr (2001b) Glossary of descriptive terminology for ictal semiology: report of the ILAE task force on classification and terminology. Epilepsia 42(9):1212–1218

Detre JA, Alsop DC, Aguirre GK, & Sperling MR (1996), "Coupling of cortical and thalamic ictal activity in human partial epilepsy: demonstration by functional magnetic resonance imaging", Epilepsia. 37. 7. 657–661

Detre JA, Sirven JI, Alsop DC, O'Connor MJ, & French JA (1995), "Localization of subclinical ictal activity by functional magnetic resonance imaging: correlation with invasive monitoring", Ann.Neurol. 38. 4. 618–624

de Curtis M, Avanzini G (2001) Interictal spikes in focal epileptogenesis. Prog Neurobiol 63: 541–567

Di Bonaventura BC, Carnfi M, Vaudano AE, Pantano P, Garreffa G, Le PE, Maraviglia B, Bozzao L, Manfredi M, Prencipe M, Giallonardo AT (2006a) Ictal hemodynamic changes in late-onset Rasmussen encephalitis. Ann Neurol 59(2):432–433

Di Bonaventura BC, Vaudano AE, Carni M, Pantano P, Nucciarelli V, Garreffa G, Maraviglia B, Prencipe M, Bozzao L, Manfredi M, Giallonardo AT (2006b) EEG/fMRI study of ictal and interictal epileptic activity: Methodological issues and future perspectives in clinical practice. Epilepsia 47(Suppl 5):52–58

Federico P, Archer JS, Abbott DF, Jackson GD (2005) Cortical/subcortical BOLD changes associated with epileptic discharges: an EEG–fMRI study at 3 T. Neurology 64:1125–1130

Gholipour A, Kehtarnavaz N, Briggs R, Devous M, & Gopinath K (2007), "Brain functional localization: a survey of image registration techniques", IEEE Trans.Med.Imaging. 26. 4. 427–451

Gholipour A, Kehtarnavaz N, Briggs RW, Gopinath KS, Ringe W, Whittemore A, Cheshkov S, & Bakhadirov K (2008a), "Validation of non-rigid registration between functional and anatomical magnetic resonance brain images", IEEE Trans.Biomed.Eng. 55. 2 Pt 1. 563–571

Gholipour A, Kehtarnavaz N, Gopinath K, Briggs R, & Panahi I (2008b), "Average field map image template for Echo-Planar image analysis", Conf.Proc.IEEE Eng Med.Biol.Soc. 2008. 94–97

Gotman J, Grova C, Bagshaw A, Kobayashi E, Aghakhani Y, Dubeau F (2005) Generalized epileptic discharges show thalamocortical activation and suspension of the default state of the brain. Proc Natl Acad Sci USA 102(42):15236–15240

Gregory RP, Oates T, Merry RT (1993) Electroencephalogram epileptiform abnormalities in candidates for aircrew training. Electroencephalogr Clin Neurophysiol 86:75–77

Hajnal JV, Myers R, Oatridge A, Schwieso JE, Young IR, & Bydder GM (1994), "Artifacts due to stimulus correlated motion in functional imaging of the brain", Magn Reson.Med. 31. 3. 283–291

Hamandi K, Powell HW, Laufs H, Symms MR, Barker GJ, Parker GJ, Lemieux L, & Duncan JS (2008), "Combined EEG-fMRI and tractography to visualise propagation of epileptic activity", J. Neurol.Neurosurg.Psychiatry. 79. 5. 594–597

Herrendorf G, Steinhoff BJ, Kolle R, Baudewig J, Waberski TD, Buchner H, Paulus W (2000) Dipole-source analysis in a realistic head model in patients with focal epilepsy. Epilepsia 41:71–80

Hill RA, Chiappa KH, Huang-Hellinger F, & Jenkins BG (1995), "EEG during MR imaging: differentiation of movement artifact from paroxysmal cortical activity", Neurology. 45. 10: 1942–1943

Huang-Hellinger F, Hans C, McCormack G, Cohen M, Kwong KK, Sutton JP, Savoy RL, Weisskoff RM, Davis TL, Baker JR, Belliveau JW, Rosen BR (1995), "Simultaneous functional magnetic resonance imaging and electrophysiological recording", Hum Brain Mapp. 3:13–23

Ives JR, Warach S, Schmitt F, Edelman RR, & Schomer DL (1993), "Monitoring the patient's EEG during echo planar MRI", Electroencephalogr.Clin.Neurophysiol. 87. 6. 417–420

Jackson GD, Connelly A, Cross JH, Gordon I, & Gadian DG (1994), "Functional magnetic resonance imaging of focal seizures", Neurology. 44. 5. 850–856

Josephs O, Turner R, Friston K (1997), "Event-related fMRI", Hum Brain Mapp. 5: 243–248

Kazemi NJ, So EL, Mosewich RK, O'Brien TJ, Cascino GD, Trenerry MR, Sharbrough FW (1997) Resection of frontal encephalomalacias for intractable epilepsy: Outcome and prognostic factors. Epilepsia 38:670–677

King D, Spencer S (1995) Invasive electroencephalography in mesial temporal lobe epilepsy. J Clin Neurophysiol 12:32–45

Kobayashi E, Hawco CS, Grova C, Dubeau F, Gotman J (2006a) Widespread and intense BOLD changes during brief focal electrographic seizures. Neurology 66(7):1049–1055

Kobayashi E, Bagshaw AP, Benar CG, Aghakhani Y, Andermann F, Dubeau F, Gotman J (2006b) Temporal and extratemporal BOLD responses to temporal lobe interictal spikes. Epilepsia 47:343–354

Kobayashi E, Bagshaw AP, Gotman J, Dubeau F (2007) Metabolic correlates of epileptic spikes in cerebral cavernous angiomas. Epilepsy Res 73:98–103

Kobayashi E, Bagshaw AP, Grova C, Gotman J, Dubeau F (2006c) Grey matter heterotopia: what EEG–fMRI can tell us about epileptogenicity of neuronal migration disorders. Brain 129:366–374

Kobayashi E, Bagshaw AP, Jansen A, Andermann F, Andermann E, Gotman J, Dubeau F (2005) Intrinsic epileptogenicity in polymicrogyric cortex suggested by EEG–fMRI BOLD responses. Neurology 64:1263–1266

Kobayashi E, Hawco CS, Grova C, Dubeau F, Gotman J (2006d) Widespread and intense BOLD changes during brief focal electrographic seizures. Neurology 66:1049–1055

Krakow K, Woermann FG, Symms MR, Allen PJ, Lemieux L, Barker GJ, Duncan JS, Fish DR (1999) EEG-triggered functional MRI of interictal epileptiform activity in patients with partial seizures. Brain 122(Pt 9):1679–1688

Krings T, Topper R, Reinges MH, Foltys H, Spetzger U, Chiappa KH, Gilsbach JM, & Thron A (2000), "Hemodynamic changes in simple partial epilepsy: a functional MRI study", Neurology. 54. 2. 524–527

Lai S, Hopkins AL, Haacke EM, Li D, Wasserman BA, Buckley P, Friedman L, Meltzer H, Hedera P, & Friedland R (1993), "Identification of vascular structures as a major source of signal contrast in high resolution 2D and 3D functional activation imaging of the motor cortex at 1.5T: preliminary results", Magn Reson.Med. 30. 3. 387–392

Laufs H, Hamandi K, Salek-Haddadi A, Kleinschmidt AK, Duncan JS, Lemieux L (2007) Temporal lobe interictal epileptic discharges affect cerebral activity in "default mode" brain regions. Hum Brain Mapp 28:1023–1032

Laufs H, Hamandi K, Walker MC, Scott C, Smith S, Duncan JS, Lemieux L (2006a) EEG–fMRI mapping of asymmetrical delta activity in a patient with refractory epilepsy is concordant with the epileptogenic region determined by intracranial EEG. Magn Reson Imaging 24:367–371

Laufs H, Lengler U, Hamandi K, Kleinschmidt A, Krakow K (2006b) Linking generalized spike-and-wave discharges and resting state brain activity by using EEG/fMRI in a patient with absence seizures. Epilepsia 47:444–448

Lazeyras F, Blanke O, Zimine I, Delavelle J, Perrig SH, Seeck M (2000) MRI, (1)H-MRS, and functional MRI during and after prolonged nonconvulsive seizure activity. Neurology 55: 1677–1682

Lemieux L, Salek-haddadi A, Josephs O, Allen P, Toms N, Scott C, Krakow K, Turner R, & Fish DR (2001), "Event-related fMRI with simultaneous and continuous EEG: description of the method and initial case report", Neuroimage. 14. 3. 780–787

Lemieux L, Salek-haddadi A, Lund TE, Laufs H, Carmichael D (2007) Modelling large motion events in fMRI studies of patients with epilepsy. Magn Reson Imaging 25(6):894–901

Lemieux L, Laufs H, Carmichael D, Paul JS, Walker MC, Duncan JS (2008) Noncanonical spike-related BOLD responses in focal epilepsy. Hum Brain Mapp 29:329–345

Liu Y, Yang T, Yang X, Liu I, Liao W, Chen H, Zhou D (2008) EEG–fMRI study of the interictal epileptic activity in patients with partial epilepsy. J Neurol Sci 268(1–2):117–123

Liston AD, De Munck JC, Hamandi K, Laufs H, Ossenblok P, Duncan JS, & Lemieux L (2006), "Analysis of EEG-fMRI data in focal epilepsy based on automated spike classification and Signal Space Projection", Neuroimage. 31. 3. 1015–1024

Logothetis NK, Pauls J, Augath M, Trinath T, Oeltermann A (2001) Neurophysiological investigation of the basis of the fMRI signal. Nature 412:150–157

Lund TE, Norgaard MD, Rostrup E, Rowe JB, & Paulson OB (2005), "Motion or activity: their role in intra- and inter-subject variation in fMRI", Neuroimage. 26. 3. 960–964

Marsan CA, Zivin LS (1970) Factors related to the occurrence of typical paroxysmal abnormalities in the EEG records of epileptic patients. Epilepsia 11:361–381

Matsumoto H, Marsan CA (1964) Cortical cellular phenomena in experimental epilepsy: interictal manifestations. Exp Neurol 9:286–304

McCormick DA, Contreras D (2001) On the cellular and network bases of epileptic seizures. Annu Rev Physiol 63:815–846

McGonigal A, Bartolomei F, Regis J, Guye M, Gavaret M, Trebuchon-Da Fonseca A, Dufour H, Figarella-Branger D, Girard N, Peragut JC, Chauvel P (2007) Stereoelectroencephalography in presurgical assessment of MRI-negative epilepsy. Brain 130:3169–3183

Northoff G, Walter M, Schulte RF, Beck J, Dydak U, Henning A, Boeker H, Grimm S, Boesiger P (2007) GABA concentrations in the human anterior cingulate cortex predict negative BOLD responses in fMRI. Nat Neurosci 10:1515–1517

Palmer CA, Geyer JD, Keating JM, Gilliam F, Kuzniecky RI, Morawetz RB, Bebin EM (1999) Rasmussen's encephalitis with concomitant cortical dysplasia: the role of GluR3. Epilepsia 40: 242–247

Raichle ME, MacLeod AM, Snyder AZ, Powers WJ, Gusnard DA, Shulman GL (2001) A default mode of brain function. Proc Natl Acad Sci USA 98:676–682

Rodionov R, De Martino F, Laufs H, Carmichael DW, Formisano E, Walker M, Duncan JS, Lemieux L (2007) Independent component analysis of interictal fMRI in focal epilepsy: Comparison with general linear model-based EEG-correlated fMRI. Neuroimage 38:488–500

Rosenow F, Luders H (2001) Presurgical evaluation of epilepsy. Brain 124:1683–1700

Salek-Haddadi A, Diehl B, Hamandi K, Merschhemke M, Liston A, Friston K, Duncan JS, Fish DR, Lemieux L (2006) Hemodynamic correlates of epileptiform discharges: An EEG–fMRI study of 63 patients with focal epilepsy. Brain Res 1088:148–166

Salek-haddadi A, Lemieux L, Merschhemke M, Friston KJ, Duncan JS, Fish DR (2003) Functional magnetic resonance imaging of human absence seizures. Ann Neurol 53(5):663–667

Salek-haddadi A, Mayer T, Hamandi K, Symms M, Josephs O, Fluegel D, Woermann F, Richardson MP, Noppeney U, Wolf P, Koepp MJ (2008) Imaging seizure activity: a combined EEG/EMG–fMRI study in reading epilepsy. Epilepsia 50(2):256–264

Salek-haddadi A, Merschhemke M, Lemieux L, Fish DR (2002) Simultaneous EEG-correlated ictal fMRI. Neuroimage 16(1):32–40

Seeck M, Lazeyras F, Michel CM, Blanke O, Gericke CA, Ives J, Delavelle J, Golay X, Haenggeli CA, de TN, & Landis T (1998), "Non-invasive epileptic focus localization using EEG-triggered functional MRI and electromagnetic tomography", Electroencephalogr.Clin.Neurophysiol. 106. 6. 508–512

Schulz R, Luders HO, Hoppe M, Tuxhorn I, May T, Ebner A (2000) Interictal EEG and ictal scalp EEG propagation are highly predictive of surgical outcome in mesial temporal lobe epilepsy. Epilepsia 41:564–570

Schwartz TH, Bazil CW, Walczak TS, Chan S, Pedley TA, Goodman RR (1997) The predictive value of intraoperative electrocorticography in resections for limbic epilepsy associated with mesial temporal sclerosis. Neurosurgery 40:302–309; discussion 309–311

Shmuel A, Augath M, Oeltermann A, Logothetis NK (2006) Negative functional MRI response correlates with decreases in neuronal activity in monkey visual area V1. Nat Neurosci 9: 569–577

Stefan H, Hummel C, Scheler G, Genow A, Druschky K, Tilz C, Kaltenhauser M, Hopfengartner R, Buchfelder M, Romstock J (2003) Magnetic brain source imaging of focal epileptic activity: A synopsis of 455 cases. Brain 126:2396–2405

Stefanovic B, Warnking JM, Kobayashi E, Bagshaw AP, Hawco C, Dubeau F, Gotman J, & Pike GB (2005), "Hemodynamic and metabolic responses to activation, deactivation and epileptic discharges", Neuroimage. 28. 1. 205–215

Sykes JB (ed) (1982) The concise Oxford dictionary, 7th edn. Clarendon, Oxford

Tao JX, Baldwin M, Hawes-Ebersole S, Ebersole JS (2007) Cortical substrates of scalp EEG epileptiform discharges. J Clin Neurophysiol 24:96–100

Tyvaert L, Hawco C, Kobayashi E, LeVan P, Dubeau F, Gotman J (2008) Different structures involved during ictal and interictal epileptic activity in malformations of cortical development: an EEG–fMRI study. Brain 131(Pt 8):2042–2060

Widdess-Walsh P, Jeha L, Nair D, Kotagal P, Bingaman W, Najm I (2007) Subdural electrode analysis in focal cortical dysplasia: predictors of surgical outcome. Neurology 69:660–667

Zijlmans M, Huiskamp G, Hersevoort M, Seppenwoolde JH, van Huffelen AC, & Leijten FS (2007), "EEG–fMRI in the preoperative work-up for epilepsy surgery", Brain. 130. Pt 9. 2343–2353

EEG–fMRI in Idiopathic Generalised Epilepsy (Adults)

16

Patrick Carney and Graeme Jackson

1
Idiopathic Generalised Epilepsy

1.1
Definition and Classification

At the highest level, epilepsy syndromes are classified as being either focal or generalised (Commission on Classification and Terminology of the International League Against Epilepsy 1981, 1989).

Focal epilepsies appear to arise from a localised part of the brain and then spread (Commission on Classification and Terminology of the International League Against Epilepsy 1989). They are usually identified by pinpointing the onset of seizures from a specific location, and there will often be a focal structural abnormality. A more challenging problem for imaging is understanding the structures involved in idiopathic generalised epilepsy (IGE), which does not have identifiable lesions and appears to arise bilaterally and symmetrically throughout the brain (Blumenfeld 2005; Commission on Classification and Terminology of the International League Against Epilepsy 1989).

IGE is a syndrome that occurs in otherwise neurologically normal individuals who have generalised seizure types, and a characteristic ictal or interictal EEG showing generalised spike and wave (GSW) discharges (Nordli 2005). IGE is common and accounts for approximately 20% of epilepsy diagnoses (Jallon and Latour 2005). IGE is classified into subsyndromes on the basis of age of onset and predominant seizure type. The three major seizure types seen in IGE are absence seizures (AS), myoclonus and generalised tonic-clonic seizures (GTCS) (Jallon and Latour 2005).

GTCS are the most recognisable of the generalised seizures. They are prolonged and have characteristic motor activity. AS, on the other hand, are brief (rarely lasting more than 20s), and involve a loss of attention with subtle or no associated movement. Myoclonus is a brief event (usually less than 1 s), and involves a single jerk of axial muscles without loss

P. Carney (✉)
Brain Research Institute, Austin Health, Florey Neuroscience Institutes, University of Melbourne, Melbourne, Australia

C. Mulert and L. Lemieux (eds.), *EEG– fMRI*
DOI: 10.1007/978-3-540-87919-0_16, © Springer Verlag Berlin Heidelberg 2010

of consciousness (Commission on Classification and Terminology of the International League Against Epilepsy 1981).

Using a combination of these seizure types and the age at seizure onset, IGE is subclassified into the following groups according to the Commission on Classification and Terminology of the International League Against Epilepsy (1989):

- Childhood absence epilepsy (CAE)
- Juvenile absence epilepsy (Tae et al. 2006)
- Juvenile myoclonic epilepsy (JME)
- Epilepsy with GTCS

The extent to which subsyndrome classification identifies true physiological differences between the disorders in people with "IGE" is, however, uncertain (Luders et al. 2006).

1.2
The EEG in Idiopathic Generalised Epilepsy

The EEG signature of IGE is GSW. These discharges are typically 3–4 Hz, and consist of surface negative slow waves that alternate with surface negative spikes. Spikes are high amplitude, are usually single or double, and are seen bilaterally over a broad field, but tend to be maximal in the frontal midline region (Blumenfeld 2005). However, there is some variability in the morphology of the GSW that appears to relate to the underlying IGE subsyndrome. Faster spike and wave discharges and polyspike components are more typical of JME. GSW discharges are also seen ictally (Blumenfeld 2005).

2
Mechanisms of Generalised Spike and Wave in Idiopathic Generalised Epilepsy

The pattern of GSW seen on EEG requires the synchronous firing of neurons in a large area of cortex. In 1968 Pierre Gloor published the generalised corticoreticular theory of generalised discharges (Gloor 1968). GSW, he proposed, arose from interactions between ascending inputs from the thalamus and a diffusely hyperexcitable cortex. This framework has underpinned much of the research into how GSW might arise.

The physiological role of thalamocortical networks in the maintenance of the sleep–wake cycle, awareness and cognition is well established (Kostopoulos 2000; Pinault and O'Brien 2005; Steriade 2005). The possibility that aberrations of these normal physiological oscillations lead to GSW has been studied extensively by Steriade (2005, 2006) and Steriade and Amzica (2003). This has led to the popular theory that the underlying network substrate for generalised discharges, particularly in AS, are the networks involved in sleep and wakefulness. This view comes from both clinical observation and animal models of sleep and generalised discharges (Kostopoulos 2000; Steriade and Amzica 2003).

More recently, however, data from animal studies—especially from rat models of AS—have suggested a cortical generator in the sensorimotor cortex for the development of the SW discharge in AS (Pinault and O'Brien 2005; Meeren et al. 2002). In this model, oscillations of thalamocortical circuits tend to involve the sensorimotor cortex and do not resemble sleep spindles as closely (Pinault and O'Brien 2005). There is little question that thalamocortical networks underpin the generation of GSW; however, whether there is a focal generator and the pathways that underlie this generation are unclear.

EEG–fMRI offers a new way to assess the applicability of theories developed in animal models to human epilepsy. As discussed in the chapter "BOLD Response and EEG Gamma Oscillations", several studies have looked at the application of EEG–fMRI to existing animal models of spontaneous and induced GSW (Nersesyan et al. 2004; Tenney et al. 2003, 2004). These studies have found positive BOLD signal in the thalamus, predominantly ventral, and in the cortex, particularly parietal sensory cortex. Negative BOLD response is not prominent in these models. These studies would support the emerging view that focal cortical areas may be important for the generation of spike and wave.

3
EEG–fMRI in Human IGE

3.1
Early EEG–fMRI Studies

The first publications on EEG–fMRI used event-triggered recordings to avoid the image acquisition artefact on EEG (see the chapters "EEG Instrumentation and Safety" and "EEG Quality: The Image Acquisition Artefact"). This required continuous observation of the EEG, and when a discharge was seen, EPI images were acquired with a time lag of 2–3 s between the onset of interictal activity and the initiation of scanning (Krakow et al. 1999; Archer et al. 2003).

Using this approach, Archer et al. (2003) suggested that IGE was associated with prominent BOLD decreases in the posterior midline structures, referred to as the REST (random episodic silent thinking) (Mazoyer et al. 2001) network,[1] as well as diffuse cortical activations (Fig. 1). The patients had AS persisting into adult life and frequent interictal epileptiform abnormalities. Thalamic involvement was not seen in these patients. The technique, originating from the Queens Square group, of continuously and simultaneously acquiring EEG and MRI data was a major advance (Lemieux et al. 2001) and enabled the study of an IGE patient with AS (Salek-Haddadi et al. 2003). This clearly demonstrated that the thalamus can be strongly activated in AS.

EEG–fMRI is currently carried out in a variety of centres using various commercial and in-house technologies that can offer high-quality artefact removal for EEGs recorded in an operating scanner. While this has led to a substantial improvement in the accuracy and reliability of the identification of epileptiform activity in the MRI scanner, artefacts can still easily be misinterpreted as epileptiform activity. Careful scrutiny and a high degree of skill are required to make sure that epileptiform activity is not left in the background or that movement artefacts of various types are not included in the analysis.

---

[1]Otherwise referred to as the default mode network (DMN).

a – fMRI deactivation:

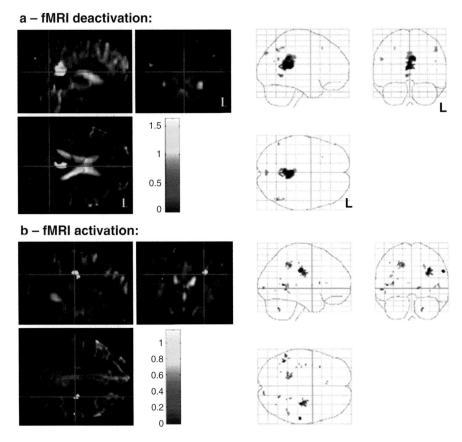

b – fMRI activation:

Fig. 1a–b Group analysis (conjunction analysis of five subjects) of spike and wave-associated "deactivation" (**a**) and activation (**b**) from Archer et al. (2003). On the *left*, results have been overlaid onto averaged, normalised EPI of subject D, and thresholded at $P < 0.001$ uncorrected. *Blue lines* represent the slice planes of the orthogonal images, with t scores indicated in the colour scale. On the *right*, results are displayed projected onto the "glass brain". Spike and wave-associated activation and particularly deactivation are relatively circumscribed, consistent with a common effect across subjects. Note that, for all figures, the radiological convention for orientation has been used (left is as indicated on the images)

3.2
Overview of EEG–fMRI Data

3.2.1
EEG–fMRI and Patient Selection

There has been a bias towards selecting patients with high rates of interictal activity to enhance the power of the analysis in EEG–fMRI studies, possibly with the aim of demonstrating an effect (significant epilepsy-related BOLD change), particularly in early studies. The largest cohort of patients with IGE studied using EEG–fMRI was reported by the Queen Square group (Hamandi et al. 2006). They investigated a series of 46 patients who were

Table 1 Demographic details of the patients in the study by Hamandi et al. (2006)

	JAE	JME	CAE	IGE-GTCS
Patients	14	9	3	6
Mean age	30	34	32	32
Number of drugs	0–4	1–4	0–1	0–3
Frequency of GSW	2.5–4	2–5	3–4	2–4

a. JAE

b. JME

c. IGE-GTCS

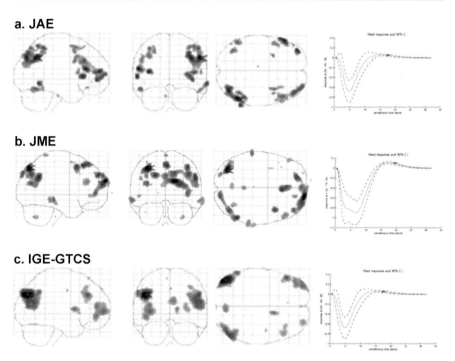

Fig. 2a–c Examples of mean intensity projections from single-subject SPM analyses showing cortical signal change with GSW involving symmetrical bifrontal, biparietal, posterior cingulate/precuneus in three patients with different diagnostic syndromes. **a** JAE; **b** JME; **c** IGE-GTCS (Hamandi et al. 2006)

consecutively studied and classified according to the 1989 ILAE Commission on Classification (Commission on Classification and Terminology of the International League Against Epilepsy 1989). Thirty-two patients were classified as having IGE, whilst the remaining patients were classified as having symptomatic generalised epilepsy (SGE). Table 1 outlines the features of these IGE subtypes. The youngest patients in this study were 18 years of age, while the oldest patient was a 53-year-old man with a diagnosis of CAE. Twenty of the patients were on two or more agents to control their seizures although, in many cases, they were still having frequent seizures and displayed prominent interictal activity.

Given the small numbers overall, a comparison of IGE subsyndromes was not possible, although representative examples of the different subgroups are shown in Fig. 2. The authors noted a significant degree of intersubject variability. They did not explore the extent to which the intersubject variability and indeed the identified networks are a phenomenon of EEG–fMRI, medication, or IGE subtype.

The largest series of patients with IGE from the Montreal group involved 15 patients who were selected on the basis of active interictal GSW (Aghakhani et al. 2004). Patients were again classified according the ILAE criteria. Seven patients were classified as having JAE, four with CAE, one patient had JME, while the remainder had GTCS alone. Patients ranged in age from 18 to 66; all but one were being treated with anticonvulsants, while ten continued to have seizures despite treatment with one or more medications. Five of the patients were receiving carbamazepine alone or in combination with other anticonvulsants, which may exacerbate epilepsy in patients with IGE, particularly AS. Patients had either spike or polyspike waves of 2.5–4 Hz.

Labate et al. (2005) published the results for a patient with a typical case of CAE not on medications. A robust thalamic response was clearly demonstrated. Similar patterns of activation and deactivation have been seen amongst all of the major groups performing EEG–fMRI (Hamandi et al. 2006; Labate et al. 2005; Gotman et al. 2005). While there is commonality between some findings, there is also considerable variability within and between groups. Only small numbers of typical patients have been studied. The variability may reflect the influence of clinical factors, particularly the need to select intractable, perhaps atypical, patients with a high frequency of interictal discharges.

The study by Hamandi et al. employing simultaneous EEG and interleaved BOLD and arterial spin labelling (ASL) fMRI to measure cerebral blood flow (CBF) in four patients found that GSW-related BOLD increases and decreases consistently reflect increases and decreases in CBF, respectively (Hamandi et al. 2008; Carmichael et al. 2008).

3.2.2
BOLD Signal Change in the Thalamus

Given the apparently central role of the thalamus in generalised spike wave events, we would expect robust positive BOLD response (PBR). However, thalamic signal change has not been seen consistently, particularly in the two largest case series to date. Hamandi et al. (2006) demonstrated thalamic signal changes in less than 50% of patients. Their group analysis demonstrated PBR in the thalamus on the right only (Fig. 2). Thalamic signal change was seen in twelve of the 15 subjects in the series from Montreal (Aghakhani et al. 2004). Thalamic involvement was most common in anterior regions. The use of a random effects linear model to group studies Gotman et al. (2005) showed significant bilateral and symmetrical PBR in the thalamus (Fig. 3). The reasons for this failure to demonstrate thalamic activity in all cases of IGE could be biological or technical leading to insufficient signal-to-noise.

3.2.3
Factors Influencing Thalamic BOLD Changes

Technical: MRI Field Strength

The above studies were performed at 1.5 T. The Melbourne experience at higher magnetic field strength (3 T) is of common bilateral and symmetrical PBR involving the thalamus

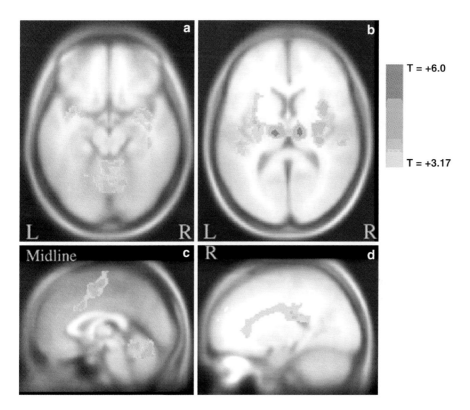

Fig. 3a–d   Significant positive BOLD response (PBR) observed from the group analysis of 15 IGE patients obtained by using the haemodynamic response function (HRF) peaking at 5 s (**a–c**) and at 7 s (**d**), corrected $P < 0.05$ for spatial extent. Functional data are superimposed on the average brain template of the Montreal Neurological Institute. **a** Axial view showing activation in the cerebellum and inferior part of the insula cortex. **b** Axial view showing the PBR involving the thalami and insular cortex. **c** Sagittal interhemispheric view showing activation along a wide band of mesial frontal cortex and within the cerebellum. **d** Sagittal view of the right hemisphere 2 cm away from the midline showing activation within the ventricles. This activation was bilateral and followed the ventricles until the trigone (Gotman et al. 2005)

(Labate 2005 and unpublished data; see Fig. 4). Laufs et al. (2006) repeated EEG–fMRI on an adult with frequent AS at 1.5 and 3 T and found thalamic PBR only at the higher field strength. In a further study comparing four subjects, a patient with SGE and atypical AS was also seen to have thalamic PBR only at 3 T, although this was not the case for other subjects with IGE (Hamandi et al. 2008). High-MRI field strength may improve the resolution of thalamic change during GSW.

Technical/Biology Interaction: HRF Time Course

The standard (or canonical) haemodynamic response function (HRF) with peak amplitude at 5–6 s post event onset (Glover 1999; Friston et al.) has been commonly used to model

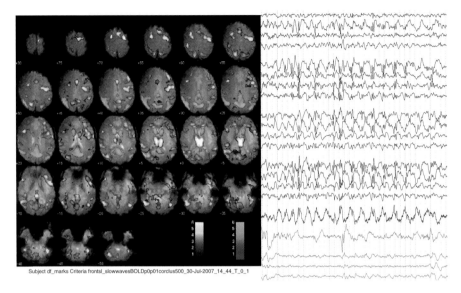

Fig. 4 18-year-old male with CAE. The image on the *left* shows *t*-score maps for PBR (*red-yellow* colour scale) and negative BOLD response (*blue/green* colour scale). Highest *t* scores are seen in the thalamus (positive) and posterior midline structures (negative). The image on the *left* shows the typical EEG appearance of the patient's generalised discharge recorded in the MRI scanner

the BOLD signal change associated with GSW. The Montreal Group have looked at changes to the timing of the HRF and found thalamic changes been best seen using the standard HRF (Aghakhani et al. 2004; Gotman et al. 2005). Moeller et al. (2008) studied the time course of the BOLD response in a cohort of young patients with IGE and found that when event onset was shifted 3–6 s prior to the onset of GSW, PBR in the thalamus was seen consistently in all patients and tended to localise to the mesial thalamus. It may be that analysis strategies that allow for intersubject variations in BOLD time course will reveal reproducible thalamic BOLD signal increases in all patients.

Biological: Absence Seizures Are Different

The IGE subsyndrome or EEG event type may be important factors in relation to the areas that are revealed to be involved using EEG–fMRI. Published studies, as well as our unpublished experience, suggest a robust thalamic BOLD change is more likely to be seen in patients with AS. In Hamandi et al. (2006), positive bilateral BOLD response occurred predominantly in patients who had frequent AS regardless of IGE subsyndrome. Patients with SGE with atypical AS appear to have particularly robust thalamic involvement. In Aghakani et al. (2004) and Gotman et al. (2005), 12 of the 15 patients studied had absence epilepsy with bilateral PBR predominating and a clear PBR seen in the thalamus bilaterally. AS are often frequent and cause prolonged bursts of spike wave (Sadleir et al. 2006). It is not known whether the thalamic activation reflects the prolonged nature of AS or a difference in the nature of these events. In one study (Aghakhani et al. 2004), no significant difference was seen between short and long discharges in a small group of patients studied.

Robust data at high field may show the thalamus to be an integral part of the network when the discharges are spike and wave in form.

Cortical BOLD Signal

As seen in Archer's initial spike-triggered study, Hamandi et al. (2006) also demonstrated significant variability in cortical signal. Although predominantly bilateral, both PBR and NBR are seen. The parietal areas involving the supramarginal gyrus and posterior cingulate and the angular gyrus commonly show NBR. In Halmadi's study, significant areas of frontal NBR involved the inferior and superior frontal gyri and inferior, middle and superior gyri. Similarly, left–right differences in these areas are variable. Figure 5 shows the group analysis, with NBR in green predominating in bilateral cortical areas.

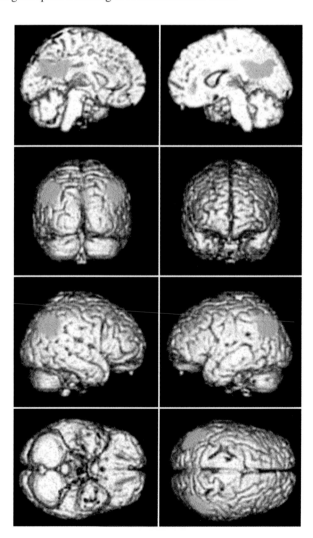

Fig. 5 SPM overlaid onto canonical brain of positive HRF (*red*) and negative HRF (Greenberg et al. 1992) (uncorrected $P < 0.001$), illustrating the thalamic and cortical distribution of BOLD changes to GSW in the IGE group analysis. This shows bilateral parietal (46, −51, 32), (−44, −62, 34) and posterior cingulate/precuneus (6, −48, 17) deactivation and thalamic activation (12, −11, 4); we suspect the activation around the ventricles is due to modelled changes in CSF pulsation as a result of the widespread haemodynamic changes occurring during GSW (Hamandi et al. 2006)

A similar pattern of bilateral cortical involvement was seen in the Montreal series (Aghakhani et al. 2004). Patterns could be divided into diffuse involvement, where all cortical areas were connected, and multiregional involvement. Cortical signal change also varied according to its anterior vs. posterior predominance. PBR in the cortex had an earlier-peaking HRF than the NBR, which peaked at 7–9s (Fig. 6).

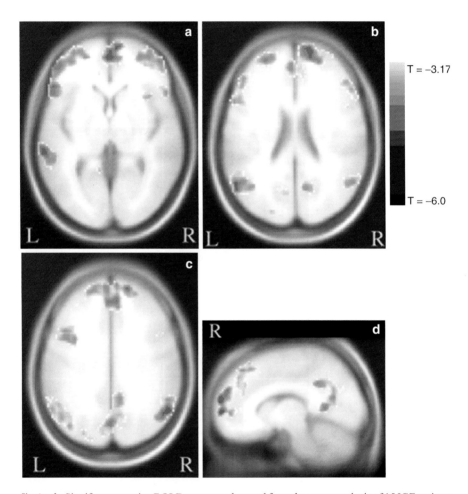

Fig. 6a–d Significant negative BOLD response observed from the group analysis of 15 IGE patients obtained using HRF peaking at 9 s, corrected $P < 0.05$ for spatial extent. **a** Axial view showing bilateral deactivations in mesial and lateral anterior frontal areas (cluster 10) and in the left posterior temporal area (cluster 13). **b** Axial view 1 cm higher than **a** and showing deactivations in frontal regions (cluster 10), in parietal areas (clusters 11 and 12), and in the posterior cingulate gyrus (cluster 11). **c** Axial view 2 cm above **b** and showing the same frontal and parietal clusters. **d** Sagittal view of the right hemisphere 1 cm away from the midline and showing a deactivation within the mesial prefrontal area (cluster 10) and the posterior cingulate gyrus (cluster 11) (Gotman et al. 2005)

Negative Cortical BOLD Response and the REST Network

Negative BOLD responses in areas of association cortex have been described in numerous EEG–fMRI studies in IGE and reflect a consistent pattern of involvement that appears to involve reduction in activity in the brain's resting-state network. These task-induced decreases in regional brain function have been identified in a number of different functional imaging paradigms using fMRI and PET (Damoiseaux et al. 2006; Raichle et al. 2001). These paradigms, as in EEG–fMRI, compare a specific task to a non-task period, which is generally called rest, but which involves its own degree of mental activity. The mental rest period involves internalised cognitive activity, including random thoughts and free associations of ideas, memories, visual and auditory information (Mazoyer et al. 2001; Andreasen et al. 1995). Furthermore, this is integrated with physiological information such as body position and sensation.

EEG–fMRI papers in IGE have been particularly interested in the relationship between activation and rest and its influence on the NBR. In all paradigms used in the three main centres using continuous EEG–fMRI, patients have been instructed to rest comfortably, usually with eyes closed, and not to perform any particular task for long periods of time while EPI data are continuously acquired. This long rest period is then compared to periods of GSW. It is believed that the appearance of relative deactivations in cortical areas during GSW may actually reflect cessation of the REST mode of the resting brain caused by the GSW (Gotman et al. 2005; Laufs et al. 2006). The fact that NBR responses appear to occur later than PBR may reflect that the REST mode is switched off following the onset of increased thalamocortical activity during a generalised discharge (Gotman et al. 2005). A possible interpretation is that GSW, whether during an AS (where awareness is clearly impaired) or during interictal activity (where it is difficult to assess awareness), may lead to cessation of normal REST network conscious activity.

Positive Cortical BOLD; Implications for Epilepsy Networks

Greater variability exists in the published literature in relation to areas of PBR during EEG–fMRI in IGE patients. Given the theoretical pathways involved in the generation of GSW activity, we would hypothesise activation of the thalamus linked to variable regions of activation in the cortex leading to PBR in these regions. These expected phenomena are not seen consistently across studies.

Hamandi et al. (2006) found that the primary cortices were rarely involved in the PBR. Aghakhani et al. (2004) found two basic patterns of PBR in IGE subjects. The first, a multiregional pattern, involved separate cortical regions with usually a bilateral and symmetric distribution. The alternative pattern involved a more diffuse pattern of bilateral symmetric involvement, with the cortical regions linked. Our findings at the BRI have similarly identified these patterns (Fig. 7). At this stage, however, it remains difficult to identify what underlies these differences or to ascribe clinical phenomena that may underpin these changes.

Studies in GAERS and WAG/Rij rats have demonstrated focal changes in the sensorimotor cortex during AS during both electrophysiological studies (Pinault and O'Brien 2005)

Fig. 7 Eight-year-old with absence seizures showing bilateral rolandic activation on the cortical surface image

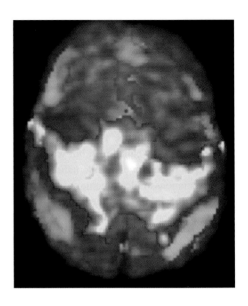

and EEG–fMRI studies (Nersesyan et al. 2004; Tenney et al. 2003, 2004). Focal cortical PBR in the sensorimotor cortex has also been noted in patients with IGE studied by us, raising the possibility that EEG–fMRI may help to further explore this hypothesis in humans.

What Structures Are Involved Outside of the Thalamocortical Network?

Areas of the brain outside of the cortex and thalamus have not been consistently identified. Cerebellar PBR has been noted (Gotman et al. 2005), while our experience at BRI and those reported in other publications (Hamandi et al. 2006) have shown frequent involvement of the caudate nucleus with bilateral and symmetrical NBR. Otherwise, extrapyramidal motor involvement has not been identified in most published EEG–fMRI literature.

4
Structures and Networks: Future Directions for EEG–fMRI in IGE

EEG–fMRI is a noninvasive tool that provides spatial information about brain haemodynamics (particularly blood flow) during generalised spike-wave discharge. Well-developed animal models have shown that intact thalamocortical networks are crucial to the generation of GSW. EEG–fMRI studies of IGE have confirmed the role of thalamus and cortex in the human disease phenotype.

However, there is variability in the findings for BOLD response to IGE discharges that may be due to selection of atypical cases, and variation in analytical methods with the awareness that the timing of the BOLD response may not be linked to the interictal discharge in the way that a cognitive or motor event is. Variability in the power of the analysis in individual case studies is also a difficult problem to deal with given the variable frequency of epileptiform events. Alternatively, or as well, there may be biological differences in individual cases.

To progress further and define the biology underlying generalised discharges, homogeneous phenotypes need to be studied with optimised analytical methods, and the effects of drugs need to be considered.

Patient cohorts in EEG–fMRI typically reflect the severe end of the IGE spectrum, with treatment-refractory seizures and multiple medications. Important issues include: what contributes to the variability in these phenotypes, and how does the underlying epilepsy network itself contribute to seizure frequency and pharmacoresistance? The effect of medications on EEG patterns may also be important. It is difficult to use the BOLD response as a tool to understand the epilepsy networks in IGE when we are dealing with a heterogeneous population with clinical factors that potentially influence the biology of the generation of spike and wave. We expect that attention to cohort selection and homogeneous and "typical" cohorts may provide consistent results.

Recent studies in children have highlighted the value of "purer" cohorts of patients with IGE to help gain greater insight into the role of phenotypic factors in the activation maps generated by EEG–fMRI (Moeller et al. 2008a, b; see the chapter "EEG–fMRI in Children with Epilepsy"). It appears that the thalamic, posterior parietal, caudate and possibly brainstem structures are a necessary component of the generation of generalised spike wave and AS. What remains to be clarified is whether variable areas of frontal and temporal cortical BOLD reflect differences in the mechanism of generation of GSW, and whether this has phenotypic and clinical implications. Furthermore, as we develop new techniques to understand the interplay of fluctuations in the BOLD signal over time, we may become more be able to identify the roles of the various structures identified by BOLD imaging in generating GSW.

5
Conclusion

Spike-and-wave-related PBR in the thalamus and NBR distributed in the REST network areas are seen consistently across studies, while other phenomena, including PBR in cortical areas, are less consistent. PBR in the thalamus accords with the view that the thalamus plays a central role in the generation of spike wave. NBR in the REST network may reflect GSW-related interruption of usual conscious cortical processing.

EEG–fMRI has already contributed to our understanding of the underlying effects of GSW on cortical function. The reproducible pattern of rest network deactivation supports a role of GSW in altering conscious awareness. The contribution of the spatial information of the imaging at the time of the epileptiform discharge provides us with a remarkable new tool to investigate the areas of the brain that are involved in seizures. It enables us to explore the interaction of subcortical structures with the cortex, and to explore the timing of neuronal events in the brain that underlie the hypersynchronisation that is the hallmark of epileptic activity.

Acknowledgements We thank Dr Danny Flanagan and Dr David Abbott for developing the analytical methodology and data analysis.

References

Aghakhani Y, Bagshaw AP, Benar CG, et al. (2004) fMRI activation during spike and wave discharges in idiopathic generalized epilepsy. Brain 127:1127–1144

Andreasen NC, O'Leary DS, Cizadlo T, et al. (1995) Remembering the past: two facets of episodic memory explored with positron emission tomography. Am J Psychiatry 152:1576–1585

Archer JS, Abbott DF, Waites AB, Jackson GD (2003) fMRI "deactivation" of the posterior cingulate during generalized spike and wave. Neuroimage 20:1915–1922

Avoli M, Rogawski MA, Avanzini G (2001) Generalized epileptic disorders: an update. Epilepsia 42:445–457

Blumenfeld H (2005) Cellular and network mechanisms of spike-wave seizures. Epilepsia 46(Suppl 9):21–33

Carmichael DW, Hamandi K, Laufs H, Duncan JS, Thomas DL, Lemieux L (2008) An investigation of the relationship between BOLD and perfusion signal changes during epileptic generalised spike wave activity. Magn Reson Imaging 26(7):870–873

Commission on Classification and Terminology of the International League Against Epilepsy (1981) Proposal for revised clinical and electroencephalographic classification of epileptic seizures. Epilepsia 22:489–501

Commission on Classification and Terminology of the International League Against Epilepsy (1989) Proposal for revised classification of epilepsies and epileptic syndromes. Epilepsia 30:389–399

Damoiseaux JS, Rombouts SA, Barkhof F, et al. (2006) Consistent resting-state networks across healthy subjects. Proc Natl Acad Sci USA 103:13848–13853

Gloor P (1968) Generalized cortico-reticular epilepsies. Some considerations on the pathophysiology of generalized bilaterally synchronous spike and wave discharge. Epilepsia 9:249–263

Glover GH (1999) Deconvolution of impulse response in event-related BOLD fMRI. Neuroimage 9:416–429

Gotman J, Grova C, Bagshaw A, et al. (2005) Generalized epileptic discharges show thalamocortical activation and suspension of the default state of the brain. Proc Natl Acad Sci USA 102:15236–15240

Greenberg DA, Durner M, Delgado-Escueta AV, et al. (1992) Evidence for multiple gene loci in the expression of the common generalized epilepsies. Neurology 42:56–62

Hamandi K, Laufs H, Noth U, et al. (2008) BOLD and perfusion changes during epileptic generalised spike wave activity. Neuroimage 39:608–618

Hamandi K, Salek-Haddadi A, Laufs H, et al. (2006) EEG–fMRI of idiopathic and secondarily generalized epilepsies. Neuroimage 31:1700–1710

Jallon P, Latour P (2005) Epidemiology of idiopathic generalized epilepsies. Epilepsia 46(Suppl 9):10–14

Kostopoulos GK (2000) Spike-and-wave discharges of absence seizures as a transformation of sleep spindles: the continuing development of a hypothesis. Clin Neurophysiol 111(Suppl 2):S27–S38

Krakow K, Woermann FG, Symms MR, et al. (1999) EEG-triggered functional MRI of interictal epileptiform activity in patients with partial seizures. Brain. 1999;122(Pt 9):1679–1688

Labate A, Briellmann RS, Abbott DF, et al. (2005) Typical childhood absence seizures are associated with thalamic activation. Epileptic Disord 7:373–377

Laufs H, Lengler U, Hamandi K, et al. (2006) Linking generalized spike-and-wave discharges and resting state brain activity by using EEG/fMRI in a patient with absence seizures. Epilepsia 47:444–448

Lemieux L, Salek-Haddadi A, Josephs O, et al. (2001) Event-related fMRI with simultaneous and continuous EEG: description of the method and initial case report. Neuroimage 14:780–787

Luders HO, Acharya J, Alexopoulos A, et al. (2006) Are epilepsy classifications based on epileptic syndromes and seizure types outdated? Epileptic Disord 8:81–85

Mazoyer B, Zago L, Mellet E, et al. (2001) Cortical networks for working memory and executive functions sustain the conscious resting state in man. Brain Res Bull 54:287–298

Meeren HK, Pijn JP, Van Luijtelaar EL, et al. (2002) Cortical focus drives widespread corticothalamic networks during spontaneous absence seizures in rats. J Neurosci 22:1480–1495

Moeller F, Siebner HR, Wolff S, et al. (2008a) Changes in activity of striato-thalamo-cortical network precede generalized spike wave discharges. Neuroimage 39:1839–1849

Moeller F, Siebner HR, Wolff S, et al. (2008b) Simultaneous EEG–fMRI in drug-naive children with newly diagnosed absence epilepsy. Epilepsia 49:1510–1519

Nersesyan H, Hyder F, Rothman DL, Blumenfeld H (2004) Dynamic fMRI and EEG recordings during spike-wave seizures and generalized tonic-clonic seizures in WAG/Rij rats. J Cereb Blood Flow Metab 24:589–599

Nordli DR Jr (2005) Idiopathic generalized epilepsies recognized by the International League Against Epilepsy. Epilepsia 46(Suppl 9):48–56

Pinault D, O'Brien TJ (2005) Cellular and network mechanisms of genetically-determined absence seizures. Thalamus Relat Syst 3:181–203

Raichle ME, MacLeod AM, Snyder AZ, et al. (2001) A default mode of brain function. Proc Natl Acad Sci USA 98:676–682

Sadleir LG, Farrell K, Smith S, et al. (2006) Electroclinical features of absence seizures in childhood absence epilepsy. Neurology 67:413–418

Salek-Haddadi A, Lemieux L, Merschhemke M, et al. (2003) Functional magnetic resonance imaging of human absence seizures. Ann Neurol 53:663–667

Steriade M (2005) Sleep, epilepsy and thalamic reticular inhibitory neurons. Trends Neurosci 28:317–324

Steriade M (2006) Neuronal substrates of spike-wave seizures and hypsarrhythmia in corticothalamic systems. Adv Neurol 97:149–154

Steriade M, Amzica F (2003) Sleep oscillations developing into seizures in corticothalamic systems. Epilepsia 44(Suppl 12):9–20

Tae WS, Hong SB, Joo EY, et al. (2006) Structural brain abnormalities in juvenile myoclonic epilepsy patients: volumetry and voxel-based morphometry. Korean J Radiol 7:162–172

Tenney JR, Duong TQ, King JA, et al. (2003) Corticothalamic modulation during absence seizures in rats: a functional MRI assessment. Epilepsia 44:1133–1140

Tenney JR, Marshall PC, King JA, Ferris CF (2004) fMRI of generalized absence status epilepticus in conscious marmoset monkeys reveals corticothalamic activation. Epilepsia 45:1240–1247

Michael Siniatchkin and Francois Dubeau

Abbreviations

BECTS   Benign epilepsy with centrotemporal spikes
BOLD   Blood oxygenation level dependent
EEG   Electroencephalography
fMRI   Functional magnetic resonance imaging
HRF   Haemodynamic response function

1
EEG–fMRI in Children with Epilepsy

Childhood epilepsies differ from adult epilepsies in aetiology, pathogenesis, seizure semiology, electroencephalography (EEG) patterns, and prognosis (Roger et al. 2005). The immature brain is more prone to developing seizures, and epileptic discharges are more frequent and less localised in children than in adults (Holmes 1997). The clinical manifestations are also age-correlated and can vary within a patient throughout the maturation process (Ben-Ari 2006). Some epileptic syndromes are seen only in infants or children, such as the West syndrome and severe myoclonic epilepsy of infancy, idiopathic occipital epilepsies and benign epilepsy with centrotemporal spikes (Roger et al. 2005). Most of our understanding of the networks involved in the generation and propagation of epileptic activity in the immature brain derives from animal models, rather than from the study of human epilepsies.

The combination of EEG and fMRI, which permits the study of the haemodynamic correlates of spontaneous brain activity such as interictal epileptiform discharges (IED), provides a unique opportunity to investigate epileptogenic networks in vivo in patients with

M. Siniatchkin (✉)
University Hospital of Pediatric Neurology, Christian-Albrechts-University of Kiel, Scjwanenweg 20,
24105 Kiel, Germany
e-mail: m.siniatchkin@pedneuro.uni-kiel.de

C. Mulert and L. Lemieux (eds.), *EEG– fMRI*
DOI: 10.1007/978-3-540-87919-0_17, © Springer Verlag Berlin Heidelberg 2010

epilepsy (see the chapters "EEG–fMRI in Adults with Focal Epilepsy" and "EEG–fMRI in Idiopathic Generalised Epilepsy (Adults)", as well as Gotman et al. 2006; Laufs and Duncan 2007). It is a noninvasive technique that can be applied serially or longitudinally to children of all ages, and it is one that could provide essential information on the maturation process and on developmental changes due to epilepsy. However, the use of EEG–fMRI in the paediatric population is associated with a host of methodological issues regarding data acquisition and analysis.

2
Methodological Issues Specific to Paediatric EEG–fMRI Studies

2.1
Patient Selection and Scanning

One of the most challenging aspects of performing fMRI in children is obtaining sufficient cooperation from them so that adequate data can be collected. There are two main aspects to this issue: first, anxiety must be minimised so that the child will agree to enter the scanner and remain for the entirety of the exam; second, it is necessary to ensure that the child stays motionless throughout the entire study (20–30 min on average). In some recent studies, sedation has been used for children undergoing EEG–fMRI (Jacobs et al. 2007, 2008a, b; Moeller et al. 2008b), especially in very young children and children with developmental delay. For unsedated children, who are usually older and do not have an intellectual handicap, anxiety can be reduced if a relative or someone familiar to the child is present in the MR room during data acquisition; if EEG–fMRI is simulated first and the child is trained for the test; and, finally, if external stimulation (video and audio tapes) is used as early as possible before the test to distract the child (Rosenberg et al. ; Gaillard et al. 2001; Poldrack et al. 2002). Relaxation techniques may help in some cases (Quirk et al. 1989).

Even well-prepared or sedated children are subject to motion (head and body movements) during the acquisition time. For instance, to reduce the effect of head motion on EEG–fMRI results, algorithms are used to improve the quality and sensitivity of fMRI analysis (Friston et al. 1996; Lemieux et al. 2007). Despite these difficulties, a survey of the literature reveals that EEG–fMRI studies have been conducted successfully in approximately 140 children with epilepsy to date. In our experience, so far, the recordings have been well tolerated and good-quality fMRI data have been obtained (see below).

2.2
Modelling IED-Related BOLD Changes in Children: Variability and Developmental Changes

The haemodynamic response function (HRF) for external stimuli is known to change over the course of normal development, most notably during infancy (Richter and Richter 2003; Schapiro et al. 2004). Whereas acoustic and visual stimulation results in positive blood oxygenation level dependent (BOLD) responses (activations) in adults, several studies have reported negative BOLD responses (deactivations) to the same sensory stimulation in infants (for review Poldrack et al. 2002). Despite a great deal of variability, there is a general pattern of BOLD responses at different stages of development. Up to eight weeks, a significant proportion of children shows no BOLD changes. Older infants and children demonstrate negative BOLD responses in most cases until the age of three years (Morita et al. 2000; Yamada et al. 2000; Martin et al. 1999). In children older than three years, the positive BOLD response dominates and persists throughout maturation.

The term "HRF" designates the BOLD time course in response to a brief stimulus, and in the field of EEG–fMRI applied to epilepsy, HRF commonly refers to the BOLD change associated with brief discharges such as focal spikes. The effects of epilepsy and brain maturation on the shape of the HRF(amplitude, polarity and latency) are not well characterised. Jacobs et al. (2007) recently underlined the impact of age on IED-related BOLD changes, and demonstrated that children with focal lesional epilepsy show deactivations more frequently than activations in the irritative zone compared to adults with the same type of epilepsy. In another study, the same group (Jacobs et al. 2008b) analysed the latency of the IED-related positive and negative BOLD changes using a Fourier basis set (see the chapter "Experimental Design and Data Analysis Strategies") in 37 children with focal epilepsy (age range: 3 months to 18 years). The peak time of the positive BOLD changes in the youngest children (0–2 years) was significantly longer (mean: 7.74 s) than in the other older age groups. Moreover, the negative BOLD changes peaked later than HRF for positive BOLD responses in all age groups. The influence of age on the HRF in children may be explained by a different vascular response to neural activity compared to adults, by a higher synaptic density and increased rates of synaptogenesis resulting in a higher energy demand in the cortex of infants and young children, or by an increased venous capacitance effect that is usually found in the paediatric age group (Chugani 1998; Meek et al. 1998).

Changes in brain state (vigilance, drowsiness and sleep), the effect of anaesthetics or sedative drugs and the effect of the antiepileptic medication itself probably modulate the BOLD signal and hence influence the fMRI results. For instance, more negative BOLD responses are observed if children are sedated during the EEG–fMRI studies (Altman and Bernal 2001; Bell et al. 2005; Born et al. 1998; Moehring et al. 2008). Whatever the mechanism and explanation, the choice of basis set for fMRI modelling may be particularly important in paediatric studies, with possible implications for the technique's yield (Jacobs et al. 2007).

3
Results of EEG–fMRI Studies in Paediatric Epilepsy

3.1
Idiopathic Focal Epilepsies

Initial applications of EEG–fMRI in children were carried out in cases with benign focal epilepsies. Benign focal epilepsies represent a group of epileptic disorders that are related to well-localised focal EEG patterns (very suitable for assessing correspondence between EEG and fMRI results), are rarely seen in children with an intellectual handicap, and are only present during childhood because they are associated with a specific developmental state of the brain (Dalla Bernardina et al. 2005). Seizures in benign epilepsy with centrotemporal spikes (BECTS) typically begin with parasthesiae and jerking in the mouth, face and hand, usually with a preserved level of consciousness, thus supporting their origin in the inferior central sulcus. Children with BECTS also often show neuropsychological abnormalities such as attention deficit and abnormal executive functions.

Archer et al. (2003) were the first to report on spike-triggered fMRI performed in a 12-year-old girl with BECTS and using a 3 T MR scanner. Unilateral focal activation was seen in the left sensorimotor cortex ($p < 0.001$, uncorrected) near the face area following left rolandic spikes. Interestingly, they also described fMRI deactivation in the medial frontal region, adjacent to the cingulate sulcus ($p = 0.004$, corrected), a location consistent with areas involved in attention and concentration, which may provide a link with the aforementioned neuro psychological deficits.

In more extensive studies, Boor et al. (2003, 2007) found similar results. The authors first investigated seven children (range, 5–12 years) with BECTS using a 1.5 T MR scanner and analysed data using an event-related study design. The fMRI results demonstrated spike-correlated activation in the perisylvian central region in three of five patients with sufficient spikes for fMRI analysis (sensorimotor cortex, face and hand area, $p < 0.05$ corrected in all patients). In a second study in 11 children (range, 5–12 years) also with BECTS, they (Boor et al. 2007) compared the results of the spike-correlated fMRI analysis (1.5 T scanner) with results of multiple source analysis. BOLD activations, consistent with the locations of the initial central dipoles, were found in four of seven patients with sufficient spike activity during scanning ($p < 0.05$, corrected). There were additional large areas of BOLD activations in three of these patients, extending into the Sylvian fissure and the insula. These were identified as propagated activity by multiple source analysis. This study was able to discriminate the spike onset zone from propagated epileptiform source activity using the spatial resolution of the EEG–fMRI technique and the temporal resolution of the multiple source analysis (Fig. 1). The sensitivity of the EEG–fMRI

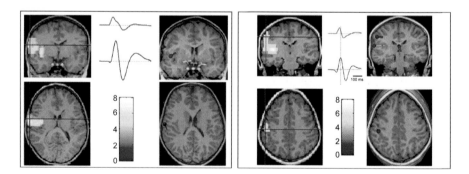

Fig. 1 Examples of two patients with benign epilepsy with centrotemporal spikes (Boor et al. 2007). For each patient, the *left* picture shows results from an event-related EEG–fMRI study. Only significant activations (FWE corrected, $p < 0.05$) are presented. The *right* picture demonstrates the localisation of equivalent current dipoles (calculated with BESA@) for generators of epileptic activity (*red*) and propagated activity (*blue*). Note the good concordance between dipole localisation and activation in the centrotemporal region in both patients. The figure illustrates how the combination of EEG source imaging and fMRI may disclose the physiological significance of activated brain regions and separate areas of initiation and propagation of epileptic activity

technique was, however, relatively low in both studies: 57 and 60% of the patients with identifiable spikes during scanning showed significant spike-correlated activations, respectively. This relatively low sensitivity (even in subjects that were sleeping) may be explained by the use of a low magnetic field MR scanner, no artefact correction (EEG was analysed during the periods between the gradient artefacts), or by a suboptimal model of the HRF. The authors did not test for the occurrence of BOLD decreases.

Lengler et al. (2007) used EEG–fMRI in a heterogeneous group of ten children (range, 4–16 years, with different clinical diagnoses and sedation: 3/7 patients fell asleep during EEG–fMRI scanning). In the seven patients in whom IEDs were recorded during the EEG–fMRI session, positive or negative BOLD signal changes were found in perisylvian, central, premotor and prefrontal regions (one child with additional bilateral occipital activation), confirming similar results to those in the previous studies (Archer et al. 2003; Boor et al. 2003) in children with BECTS. However, the areas of deactivation did not show any consistent pattern of distribution. The authors used two liberal statistical threshold values ($p < 0.001$ or $p < 0.05$ uncorrected).

Siniatchkin and colleagues (2007a) investigated seven children (range, 6–8 years) with benign centrotemporal spikes (three with BECTS) with a 3 T MR scanner. Using a new EEG pulse artefact correction method and automated spike detection system, significant activations were observed in the central and sensorimotor areas in 6/7 patients ($p < 0.05$, corrected), representing an increase in EEG–fMRI sensitivity.

Leal et al. (2006, 2007), in two EEG–fMRI studies of four children with different types of occipital lobe epilepsy (OLE)—two with a Gastaut type of benign OLE, one with idiopathic photosensitive OLE and one with Panayiotopoulos syndrome, showed that the IED-related BOLD signal changes (mostly increases) map to different cortical occipital and parietal areas in the different OLE syndromes. They suggested that EEG–fMRI provided a more satisfactory mapping of the irritative zone than those obtained from EEG source analysis. They were able to improve the electroclinical correlation for their subjects, and they concluded that EEG–fMRI is a powerful method for studying OLEs, and possibly by extension other benign idiopathic epilepsies of childhood.

3.2
Symptomatic and Cryptogenic Focal Epilepsies

An important motivation for performing EEG–fMRI studies in epilepsy is to use this method to map the epileptogenic and irritative zones for surgical purposes. In adults, attempts have been made to reveal the epileptogenic zone using EEG–fMRI within a preoperative work-up for epilepsy surgery in a selected group of patients (Zijlmans et al. 2007). EEG–fMRI studies in lesional pharmacoresistant epilepsies are of particular interest, especially from a clinical point of view. However, before the method finds a place in the clinical routine, validation studies demonstrating correspondence between lesions and BOLD signal changes are needed (Al-Asmi et al. 2003; Salek-Haddadi et al. 2006). It can be hypothesised that different lesions may cause activations of different epileptogenic networks, which will be specifically displayed by EEG–fMRI (Kobayashi et al. 2005, 2007). Also, the EEG–fMRI method may be a useful tool for studying and understanding lesional, perilesional and remote regions (Kobayashi et al. 2006a, b). Very few studies have been performed in children because a great number of children with lesional or cryptogenic pharmacoresistant epilepsies have a severe developmental delay and often need sedation to undergo fMRI. In view of the lack of evidence of a clinical benefit resulting from EEG–fMRI, investigations of children under sedation may represent an additional problem from an ethical point of view. So far, three studies have been done in children with lesional epilepsies, and these have clearly demonstrated the feasibility and the potential of this method in clinical practice.

De Tiege et al. (2007) presented, for the first time in a paediatric population, the results from EEG–fMRI studies in six children (range, 8–15 years) with symptomatic (one with focal dysplasia, two with cortical atrophy, and one with polymicrogyria and periventricular occipital grey matter heterotopia) and cryptogenic (two patients), pharmacoresistant focal epilepsy. The EEG–fMRI investigations were part of the presurgical evaluation program, and the authors wished to evaluate its usefulness in localising the epileptogenic zone. MRI acquisitions were carried out in a 1.5 T scanner for 18 min without sedation. BOLD changes were revealed in all cases: four demonstrated significant activations only, one child showed activation and deactivation, and the remaining one presented with a widespread deactivation. In four children (66%), activations colocalised with the presumed location of the epileptic focus, and in a fifth, colocalisation was seen for both activation

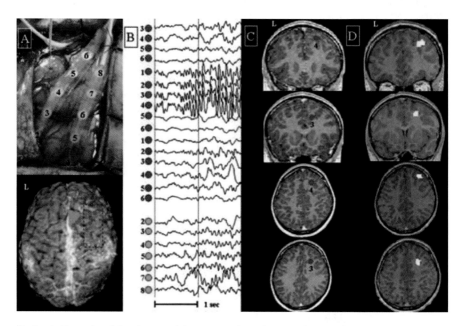

Fig. 2a–d Example of the close spatial correspondence between intracranial EEG recordings and EEG–fMRI activations in a child suffering from focal epilepsy. **a** Surface positions of three subdural strips (*green, blue,* and *violet circles*) and depth electrodes (*red circle*) relative to the brain lesion (focal cortical dysplasia in *green*). **b** A sample from the intracranial recording that shows that seizures started at contacts 1–4 of the depth electrodes (*red circle*). **c** Locations of contacts 3 and 4 of the depth electrode (*red circle*) involved in seizure onset on coronal and axial brain scans. **d** Colocalised activations found with EEG–fMRI (reproduced from De Tiege et al. 2007 with permission)

and deactivation. Moreover, EEG–fMRI was found to colocalise with either invasive EEG monitoring (one patient, Fig. 2), with a brain lesion (two patients), or with ictal SPECT (two patients), suggesting a potential role of this method in noninvasively mapping the haemodynamic changes associated with epileptic activity in children.

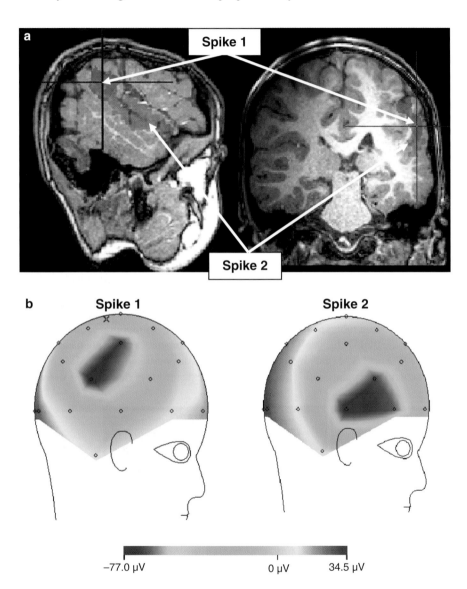

Fig. 3a–b   EEG–fMRI results. **a** Results for an eight-year-old boy with a right-hemispheric extended perisylvian polymicrogyria and focal seizures. **b** The patient exhibited two types of interictal epileptiform discharges (*Spike 1* and *Spike 2*) in the right centroparietal and right temporal areas. Note the good correspondence between bioelectrical activity (**b**) and cortical deactivation. (**a**) In this patient, and as in many other cases, the locations of the negative BOLD response were consistent with those of the lesion and epileptiform discharges (reproduced from Jacobs et al. 2007 with permission)

In a more extensive study, Jacobs et al. (2007) analysed 13 children (age range 5–17 years) with pharmacoresistant lesional focal epilepsy (four with polymicrogyria, eight with gliosis and atrophy as a result of ischaemic insults, intracranial haemorrhages or head trauma, and one with multiple cavernomas) who underwent a 20-min EEG–fMRI acquisition using a 3 T MR scanner under sedation-induced sleep (chloral hydrate or chlorpro-tixen). Because most of these children had multifocal epileptiform activity, a total of 25 spike types were analysed using individual HRFs (see Sect. 2.2). In 84% of the studies, BOLD responses were localised in the lesion or presumed irritative zone. Activation cor-responding to the lesion was seen in 20% and deactivation in 52% of the studies. In the area of spike generation, activation was found in 48% of studies and deactivation in 36%. This study first confirmed that, despite the necessarily short recording times (20 min or less) utilised, EEG–fMRI can provide localising information in sedated children using a high-field 3 T scanner. Second, and in contrast to studies in adults (Kobayashi et al. 2005; Salek-Haddadi et al. 2006), deactivations in the lesion and the irritative zone were more common than activations (Fig. 3). The differences observed in the study of De Tiege et al. (2007) can be explained, at least in part, by the fact that scans were performed without sedation. The impact of age, sleep and sedation on the BOLD response clearly need to be analysed further, and future studies should focus on the significance of deactivation with respect to the epileptogenic network.

In another study by Jacobs et al. (2008b;), five children (mean age: 5.2 ± 5.1 years) with tuberous sclerosis complex (TSC) and pharmacoresistant focal epilepsy were studied in a 3 T MR scanner. Thirteen different types of IED were analysed. A BOLD response was found in at least one tuber localised in the lobe responsible for spike generation and the presumed seizure onset zone (according to EEG video telemetry) in all patients. In four patients, the same tubers were involved in the generation of topographically different spikes and the BOLD changes were always multifocal, sometimes involving tubers distant from the IED field. The study by Jacobs et al. (2008b) demonstrated an extended epilepto-genic network in patients with TSC that was more extended than the networks described

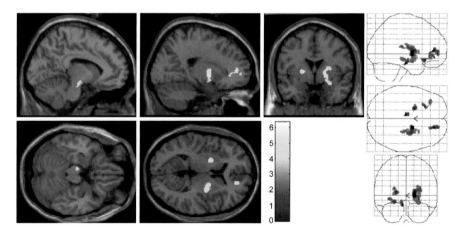

Fig. 4 Results of group analysis in children with West syndrome (reproduced from Siniatchkin et al. 2007b with permission). High-voltage slow-wave activity within the hypsarrhythmia was associated with BOLD signal increases in brain voxels representing putamen and brain stem

in PET and SPECT studies (Chugani et al. 1998). It was, however, possible to identify specifically active epileptogenic tubers. EEG–fMRI may provide a noninvasive way to identify surgical targets in patients with multiple lesions.

3.3
Epileptic Encephalopathies

West syndrome is a prototype of severe epileptic encephalopathies of infancy, consisting of tonic spasms, psychomotor developmental delay and the characteristic electroencephalographic pattern of hypsarrhythmia. The EEG features are characterised in most cases by a multifocal spike and sharp wave activity, synchronous or asynchronous high-voltage slow-wave activity, and attenuation of the background EEG (Dulac 2001; Hrachovy and Frost 2003). The long-term outcome of infantile spasms is usually poor, and the mechanisms involved in the generation of hypsarrhythmia are poorly understood.

In order to study the involvement and specificity of cortical and subcortical structures in the generation of multifocal interictal spikes and high-amplitude slow-wave activity in hypsarrhythmia, Siniatchkin et al. (2007b) investigated eight infants (mean age: 7.62 ± 2.87 months; range: 4–12 months) with West syndrome and hypsarrhythmia and compared them with a group of eight children (mean age: 20.7 ± 12.5 months; range: 4–38 months) suffering from pharmacoresistant focal epilepsy using combined EEG and fMRI recordings in a 3 T MR scanner (the children were all sedated). Haemodynamic changes related to epileptiform discharges and high-voltage slow-wave activity were analysed separately. This study showed that, in West syndrome, interictal spikes were associated with positive BOLD changes in the cerebral cortex (especially in occipital areas), comparable to the cortical activations found in the group of children with focal epilepsy. High-amplitude slow-wave activity in hypsarrhythmia was commonly associated with BOLD signal changes in brainstem and putamen (Fig. 4), with frequent involvement of the thalamus and different cortical areas. No association was found between slowing of the EEG and the BOLD signal in children with focal epilepsy. Metabolic changes in cortex, putamen and brainstem associated with West syndrome have been demonstrated in numerous PET studies (Chugani et al. 1992; Chiron et al. 1993; Metsähonkala et al. 2002). In this disorder, EEG–fMRI was able to reveal differences between the neuronal networks responsible for the generation of epileptiform discharges and for the slow-wave activity for the first time. Finally, this study demonstrated the feasibility of applying the EEG–fMRI method in infants and very young children, meaning that this technique is potentially useful for studying other types of infantile or paediatric encephalopathy with or without epileptic activity.

De Tiege et al. (2007) used EEG–fMRI in a 9.5-year-old girl who developed cognitive and behavioural regression in association with epilepsy with continuous spikes and waves during sleep, in order to assess potential pathophysiological links between epileptic activity and development regression. Runs of intense bilaterally synchronous epileptic discharges were found to be associated with BOLD activations in the right frontal, parietal and temporal cortices, possibly indicating the source of epileptic activity, and with deactivations in the lateral and medial frontoparietal cortices, posterior cingulate gyrus and cerebellum. The authors proposed that those areas of deactivation reflect the interference of the epileptic activity with normal brain function, explaining the neuropsychological deterioration. These areas of deactivation also corresponded well to the "default mode network" (DMN) of the brain (Laureys et al. 2004; Raichle and Mintun 2006). Previous EEG–fMRI studies have suggested that the deactivation in DMN associated with epileptiform activity may represent a disturbance in the cognitive network underlying consciousness processing resulting from IED (Aghakhani et al. 2004; Gotman et al. 2005; Hamandi et al. 2006; Laufs et al. 2006). The study by De Tiege et al. (2007) is a good example of how the EEG–fMRI technique can be used to investigate the functional consequences of epilepsy.

3.4
Idiopathic Generalised Epilepsies

Labate et al. (2005) presented results from an EEG–fMRI study of an untreated seven-year-old girl with new-onset idiopathic generalised epilepsy (IGE), frequent absence seizures and eyelid myoclonia. Bursts of 3-Hz spike wave and polyspike-wave epileptiform discharges registered in a 3 T MR scanner were associated with prominent, bilateral activation in the thalamus ($p < 0.05$, corrected), and less pronounced areas of cortical activation and deactivation. These results were replicated and extended by Moeller et al. (2008a), who demonstrated significant bilateral activation in thalamus and bilateral deactivation (negative BOLD signal changes) in frontal and parietal cortex as well as precuneus in six untreated children (range, 5–9 years) with typical 3/s absence seizures using a 3 T MR scanner ($p < 0.05$, corrected). A random-effect group analysis confirmed a common pattern of thalamic BOLD increase and cortical decreases (the latter resembling the DMN) and deactivation of the caudate nucleus bilaterally. These few observations of absence seizures in children extend the findings on generalised spike wave paroxysms performed in adults with IGE (see the chapter "EEG–fMRI in Idiopathic Generalised Epilepsy (Adults)" and Aghakhani et al. 2004; Gotman et al. 2005; Hamandi et al. 2006; Laufs et al. 2006). These preliminary data seem to suggest that the age of subjects and antiepileptic medication (all of the studies in adults have been done in treated patients and often with drug-resistant IGE) do not influence the haemodynamic and metabolic responses during spike-and-wave activity, and thus possibly reflect stable and typical neuronal networks.

However, the morphology of generalised paroxysms seems to be related to different patterns of activation. Moeller et al. (2008b) demonstrated that, in six children with short generalised polyspike-and-wave paroxysms (PSWs), the neuronal network consisting of thalamic activation and deactivation in cortex and caudate nucleus may be observed several seconds (on average 6 s) before the onset of the discharges on scalp EEG—the early thalamic activation is followed by a cortical deactivation and then by a deactivation in the caudate nucleus; and that the PSWs seen on surface EEG occur only at the end of the activation of the described thalamocortical network. On the other hand, typical 3 Hz absence seizures do not show this temporal activation pattern (Fig. 5); instead, the thalamocortical network is active only at the onset of the seizure (Moeller et al. 2008a). Since children from both studies (Moeller et al. 2008a, b) shared diagnoses (both patients with PSW and 3 Hz generalised paroxysms have had absence seizures), 3 Hz and PSW showed different activation patterns in the same patient (Fig. 5), and some children in the study of Moeller et al. (2008b) were sedated and were asleep throughout the recording and some were not,

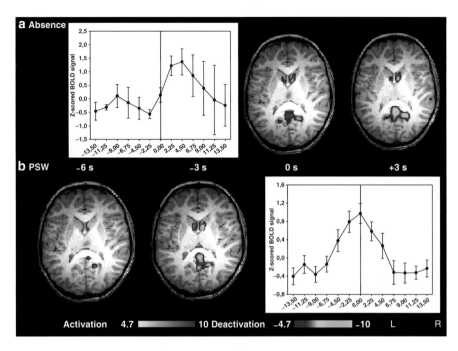

Fig. 5a–b Involvement of the typical neuronal network (thalamic activation and deactivation in precuneus, frontoparietal cortex and caudate nucleus) associated with generalised epileptiform discharges in an eight-year-old boy with juvenile absence epilepsy. This patient presented with both 3/s absence seizures (**a**) and generalised irregular polyspike-wave paroxysms (PSWs) (**b**). The figure represents BOLD change patterns at 3 and 6 s prior to epileptiform discharges (−3 and −6), at the beginning of the discharge (0) and 3 s after the discharge (3). The diagram demonstrates the time course of the normalised BOLD signal extracted from the voxel in the thalamus with the maximal *t* value (for a more detailed description, see Moeller et al. 2008b). The *x*-axis shows the time (s) around the beginning of a generalised paroxysm (point 0). Note that with the 3/s spike-and-wave discharge, the change in the BOLD signal in the striatothalamocortical network occurs at the beginning of the discharge (**a**). In contrast, this network already shows changes 6 s before PSWs are seen in the surface EEG (**b**).

Advanced methods of spike detection and advances in fMRI modelling may increase the sensitivity of EEG–fMRI studies in the paediatric population. Changes in the neurovascular coupling and haemodynamics related to brain maturation require further investigation. The effects of sleep, sedation and antiepileptic medication remain to be investigated more systematically in larger groups of patients, as their impact on the sensitivity of EEG–fMRI and the localisation of BOLD responses remains unknown.

The combination of EEG and fMRI should help to study brain function in a variety of epileptic syndromes, providing more insight into the state of the brain during epileptic activity. Finally, the clinical value of EEG–fMRI has to be validated. EEG–fMRI maps must be compared with data from established investigations, including intracranial EEG recordings, other methods of functional neuroimaging (PET, SPECT), and EEG source analysis. One major problem is to determine whether BOLD signal changes represent areas of initial epileptic activity or areas of propagation. Ultimately, informative results will come from comparisons with epilepsy surgery outcome studies.

References

Aghakhani Y, Bagshaw AP, Benar CG, Hawco C, Andermann F, Dubeau F, Gotman J (2004) fMRI activation during spike and wave discharges in idiopathic generalized epilepsy. Brain 127:11271144

Al-Asmi A, Benar CG, Gross DW, Aghakhani Y, Andermann F, Pike B, Dubeau F, Gotman J (2003) fMRI activation in continuous and spike-triggered EEG–fMRI studies of epileptic spikes. Epilepsia 44:1328–1339

Altman NR, Bernal B (2001) Brain activation in sedated children: auditory and visual functional MR imaging. Radiology 221:56–63

Archer JS, Briellman RS, Abbott DF, Syngeniotis A, Wellard RM, Jackson GD (2003) Benign epilepsy with centro-temporal spikes: spike triggered fMRI shows somato-sensory cortex activity. Epilepsia 44:200–204

Bell EC, Willson MC, Wilman AH, Dave S, Silverstone PH (2005) Differential effects of chronic lithium and valproate on brain activation in healthy volunteers. Hum Psychopharmacol 20: 415–424

Ben-Ari Y (2006) Basic developmental rules and their implication for epilepsy in the immature brain. Epileptic Disord 8:91–102

Boor R, Jacobs J, Bauermann T, Scherg M, Boor S, Vucurevic G, Kutschke G, Stoeter P (2007) Combined spike-related functional MRI and multiple source analysis in the non-invasive spike localization of benign rolandic epilepsy. Clin Neurophysiol 118 (4):901–909

Boor S, Vucurevic G, Pfleiderer C, Stoeter P, Kutschke G, Boor R. (2003). EEG-related functional MRI in benign childhood epilepsy with centrotemporal spikes. Epilepsia 44:688–692

Born P, Leth H, Miranda MJ, Rostrup E, Stensgaard A, Peitersen B, Larsson HB, Lou HC (1998) Visual activation in infants and young children studied by functional magnetic resonance imaging. Pediatr Res 44:578–583

Chiron C, Dulac O, Bulteau C, Nuttin C, Depas G, Raynaud C, Syrota A (1993) Study of regional cerebral blood flow in west syndrome. Epilepsia 34:707–715

Chugani DC, Chugani HT, Muzik O, Shah JR, Shah AK, Canady A, Mangner TJ, Chakraborty PK (1998) Imaging epileptogenic tubers in children with tuberous sclerosis complex using alpha-[11C]methyl-L-tryptophan positron emission tomography. Ann Neurol 44:858–866

Chugani HT (1998) A critical period of brain development: studies of cerebral glucose utilization with PET. Prev Med 27:184–188

Chugani HT, Shewmon DA, Sankar R (1992) Infantile spasms: II. Lenticular nuclei and brain stem activation on positron emission tomography. Ann Neurol 31:212–219

Dalla Bernardina B, Sgro V, Fejerman N (2005) Epilepsy with centro-temporal spikes and related syndomes. In: Roger J, Bureau M, Dravet C, Genton P, Tassinari CA, Wolf P (eds) Epileptic syndromes in infancy, childhood and adolescence. John Libbey Eurotext, Montrouge, pp 203–226

De Tiege X, Laufs H, Boyd SG, Harkness W, Allen PJ, Clark CA, Connelly A, Cross JH (2007) EEG–fMRI in children with pharmacoresistant focal epilepsy. Epilepsia 48:385–389

Dulac O (2001) What is West syndrome? Brain Dev 23: 447–452

Friston KJ, Williams S, Howard R (1996) Movement-related effects in fMRI time-series. Magn Res Med 35:346–355

Gaillard WD, Grandin CB, Xu B (2001) Developmental aspects of pediatric fMRI: considerations for image acquisition, analysis, and interpretation. Neuroimage 13:239–249

Gotman J, Grova C, Bagshaw A, Kobayashi E, Aghakhani Y, Dubeau, F (2005) Generalized epileptic discharges show thalamocortical activation and suspension of the default state of the brain. Proc Natl Acad Sci USA 102:15236–15240

Gotman J, Kobayashi E, Bagshaw AP, Benar CG, Dubeau F (2006) Combining EEG and fMRI: a multimodal tool for epilepsy research. J Magn Reson Imaging 23:906–920

Hamandi K, Salek-Haddadi A, Laufs H, Liston A, Friston K, Fish DR, Duncan JS, Lemieux L (2006) EEG–fMRI of idiopathic and secondary generalized epilepsies. Neuroimage 31:1700–1710

Holmes GL (1997) Epilepsy in the developing brain: lessons from the laboratory and clinic. Epilepsia 38:12–30

Hrachovy RA, Frost JD (2003) Infantile epileptic encephalopathy with hypsarrhythmia (infantile spasms/west syndrome). J Clin Neurophysiol 20:408–425

Jacobs J, Hawco C, Kobayashi E, Boor R, LeVan P, Stephani U, Siniatchkin M, Gotman J (2008a) Variability of the hemodynamic response function with age in children with epilepsy. Neuroimage 40:601–614

Jacobs J, Kobayashi E, Boor R, Muhle H, Wolff S, Hawco C, Dubeau F, Jansen O, Stephani U, Gotman J, Siniatchkin M (2007) Hemodynamic responses to interictal epileptiform discharges in children with symptomatic epilepsy. Epilepsia 48:2068–2078

Jacobs J, Rohr A, Moeller F, Boor R, Kobayashi E, Stephani U, Gotman J, Siniatchkin M (2008b) Evaluation of epileptogenic networks in children with tuberous sclerosis complex using EEG–fMRI. Epilepsia 49:816–825

Kobayashi E, Bagshaw AP, Benar CG, Aghakhani Y, Andermann F, Dubeau F, Gotman J (2006a) Temporal and extratemporal BOLD responses to temporal lobe interictal spikes. Epilepsia 47:343–354

Kobayashi E, Bagshaw AP, Gotman J, Dubeau F (2007) Metabolic correlates of epileptic spikes in cerebral cavernous angiomas. Epilepsy Res 73:98–103

Kobayashi E, Bagshaw AP, Grova C, Gotman J, Dubeau F (2006b) Grey matter heterotopia: what EEG–fMRI can tell us about epileptogenicity of neuronal migration disorders. Brain 129:366–374

Kobayashi E, Bagshaw AP, Jansen A, Andermann F, Andermann E, Gotman J, Dubeau F (2005) Intrinsic epileptogenicity in polymicrogyric cortex suggested by EEG–fMRI BOLD responses. Neurology 12:1263–1266

Labate A, Briellmann RS, Abbott DF, Waites AB, Jackson GD (2005) Typical childhood absence seizures are associated with thalamic activation. Epileptic Disord 7:373–377

Laufs H, Duncan JS (2007) Electroencephalography/functional MRI in human epilepsy: what it currently can and cannot. Curr Opin Neurol 20:417–423

Laufs H, Lengler U, Hamandi K, Kleinschmidt A, Krakow K (2006) Linking generalized spike-and-wave discharges and resting state brain activity by using EEG/fMRI in a patient with absence seizures. Epilepsia 47:444–448

Laureys S, Owen AM, Schiff ND (2004) Brain function in coma, vegetative state, and related disorders. Lancet Neurol 3:537–546

Leal A, Dias A, Vieira JP, Secca M, Jordao C (2006) The BOLD effect of interictal spike activity in childhood occipital lobe epilepsy. Epilepsy 47:1536–1542

Leal A, Nunes S, Martins A, Secca M, Jordao C (2007) Brain mapping of epileptic activity in a case of idiopathic occipital lobe epilepsy (panayiotopoulos syndrome). Epilepsia 48:1179–1183

Lemieux L, Salek-Haddadi A, Lund TE, Laufs H, Carmichael D (2007) Modelling large motion events in fMRI studies of patients with epilepsy. Magn Reson Imaging 25:894–901

Lengler U, Kafadar I, Neubauer BA, Krakow K (2007) fMRI correlates of interictal epileptic activity in patients with idiopathic benign focal epilepsy of childhood. A simultaneous EEG-functional MRI study. Epilepsy Res 75:29–38

Martin E, Joeri P, Loenneker T, Ekatodramis D, Vitacco D, Henning J, Marcar VL (1999) Visual processing in infants and children studied using functional MRI. Pediatr Res 46:135–140

Meek JH, Firbank M, Elwell CE, Atkinson J, Braddick O, Wyatt JS (1998) Regional hemodynamic responses to visual stimulation in awake infants. Pediatr Res 43:840–843

Metsähonkala L, Gaily E, Rantala H, Salmi E, Valanne L, Aarimaa T, Liukkonen E, Holopainen I, Granström ML, Erkinjuntti M, Grönroos T, Sillanpaa M (2002) Focal and global cortical hypometabolism in patients with newly diagnosed infantile spasms. Neurology 58:1646–1651

Moehring J, Moeller F, Jacobs J, Siebner H, Wolff S, Jansen O, Stephani U, Siniatchkin M. (2008) The influence of sleep on BOLD response in children with epilepsy. Neurosci Lett 443:61–66

Moeller F, Siebner H, Wolff S, Muhle H, Boor R, Granert O, Jansen O, Stephani U, Siniatchkin M (2008a) EEG–fMRI in children with untreated childhood absence epilepsy. Epilepsia 49:1510–1519

Moeller F, Siebner H, Wolff S, Muhle H, Boor R, Granert O, Jansen O, Stephani U, Siniatchkin M (2008b) Changes in activity of striato-thalamo-cortical network precede generalized spike wave discharges. NeuroImage 39:1839–1849

Morita T, Kochiyama T, Yamada H, Konishi Y, Yonekura Y, Matsumura M, Sadato N (2000) Difference in the metabolic response to photic stimulation of the lateral geniculate nucleus and the primary visual cortex of infants: a fMRI study. Neurosci Res 38:63–70

Poldrack RA, Pare-Blagoev EJ, Grant PE (2002) Pediatric functional magnetic resonance imaging: progress and challenges. Top Magn Reson Imaging 13:61–70

Quirk ME, Letendre AJ, Ciottone RA, Langley JF (1989) Evaluation of three psychologic interventions to reduce anxiety during MR imaging. Radiology 173:759–762

Raichle ME, Mintun MA (2006) Brain work and brain imaging. Annu Rev Neurosci 29:449–476

Richter W, Richter M (2003) The shape of the fMRI BOLD response in children and adults changes systematically with age. NeuroImage 20:1122–1131

Roger J, Bureau M, Dravet C, Genton P, Tassinari CA, Wolf P (2005) Epileptic syndromes in infancy, childhood and adolescence. John Libbey Eurotext, Montrouge

Rosenberg DR, Sweeney JA, Gillen JS (1997) Magnetic resonance imaging of children without sedation: preparation with simulation. J Am Acad Child Adolesc Psychiatry 36:853–859

Salek-Haddadi A, Diehl B, Hamandi K, Merschhemke M, Liston A, Friston K, Duncan JS, Fish DR, Lemieux L (2006) Hemodynamic correlates of epileptiform discharges: an EEG–fMRI study of 63 patients with focal epilepsy. Brain Res 1088:148–166

Schapiro MB, Schmithorst VJ, Wilke M, Byars AW, Strawsburg RH, Holland SK (2004) BOLD fMRI signal increases with age in selected brain regions in children. Neuroreport 15:2575–2578

Siniatchkin M, Moeller F, Jacobs J, Stephani U, Boor R, Wolff S, Jansen O, Siebner H, Scherg M (2007a) Spatial filters and automated spike detection based on brain topographies improve sensitivity of EEG–fMRI studies in focal epilepsy. Neuroimage 37:834–843

Siniatchkin M, van Baalen A, Jacobs J, Moeller F, Moehring J, Boor R, Wolff S, Jansen O, Stephani U (2007b) Different neuronal networks are associated with spikes and slow activity in hypsarrhythmia. Epilepsia 48:2312–2321

Yamada H, Sadato N, Konishi Y, Muramoto S, Kimura K, Tanaka M, Yonekura Y, Ishii Y, Ithoh H (2000) A milestone for normal development of the infantile brain detected by functional MRI. Neurology 55:218–223

Zijlmans M, Huiskamp G, Hersevoort M, Seppenwoolde JH, van Huffelen AC, Leijten FSS (2007) EEG–fMRI in the preoperative work-up for epilepsy surgery. Brain 130:2343–2353

Activation Studies

Combining EEG and fMRI in Pain Research   **18**

G.D. Iannetti and A. Mouraux

1
Introduction

In 1976, Carmon et al. showed, for the first time, that radiant heat pulses generated by a CO_2 laser stimulator could, when directed to the skin, elicit brain potentials in the ongoing human electroencephalogram (EEG). Such laser pulses were later demonstrated to activate $A\delta$ and C skin nociceptors in a *selective* and *synchronous* fashion (see Plaghki and Mouraux 2003 for a review). Since this first report, numerous studies have relied on laser-evoked brain potentials (LEPs) to assess the function of nociceptive somatosensory pathways and to gain insight into the neural processes that underlie the perception of pain. In the late 1980s, a number of studies used multichannel EEG recordings to examine the topographical distribution of LEPs (Treede et al. 1988) and model their underlying neural sources, and thus started to identify the different brain areas activated by nociceptive somatosensory input (Bromm and Chen 1995; Tarkka and Treede 1993). A consistent finding across these studies is that LEPs are well explained by the combination of a midline source (usually assigned to the anterior part of the cingulate cortex, ACC), and a pair of bilateral opercular sources (usually assigned to secondary somatosensory cortex, i.e. SII, and/or insular cortex). In some studies (Tarkka and Treede 1993) an additional parietal source was added to the model and assigned to the primary somatosensory cortex (SI) contralateral to the stimulated side (see Garcia-Larrea et al. 2003 for a review).

These early findings were later corroborated by a large number of studies using magnetoencephalography (MEG; Ploner et al. 2002), direct intracranial recording of local field potentials (Frot and Mauguiere 2003), and neuroimaging methods that sample neural activity indirectly by measuring stimulus-evoked changes in regional cerebral blood flow (PET and fMRI; Davis et al. 1998; Peyron et al. 1999). Several meta-analyses have

G. D. Iannetti (✉)
Department of Physiology, Anatomy and Genetics, University of Oxford, South Parks Road, Oxford, OX1 3QX, UK
e-mail: giandomenico.iannetti@dpag.ox.ac.uk

C. Mulert and L. Lemieux (eds.), *EEG–fMRI*   **365**
DOI: 10.1007/978-3-540-87919-0_18, © Springer Verlag Berlin Heidelberg 2010

reviewed the existing data on EEG, MEG, PET and fMRI responses to nociceptive stimulation (Apkarian et al. 2005; Garcia-Larrea et al. 2003; Peyron et al. 1999), and have confirmed the existence of a common set of brain regions responding to nociceptive stimuli, including bilateral thalamus, bilateral SII, bilateral insula, ACC, prefrontal cortex and, less consistently, contralateral SI cortex. A number of investigators have hypothesised that this network of brain areas, usually referred to as the "pain matrix" (Melzack 1999), reflects brain activities that are specifically involved in the processing of nociceptive input, and thus that it may constitute a "cerebral signature for pain" (Tracey and Mantyh 2007).

However, to date, the actual functional significance of brain responses elicited by nociceptive stimuli remains largely unknown. As a matter of fact, clear experimental evidence in support of the notion that these brain responses reflect truly nociceptive-specific brain processes is lacking. On the contrary, there is accumulating evidence suggesting that these responses are very indirectly related to pain perception. For example, when nociceptive laser stimuli are presented at short and constant interstimulus intervals (ISI) (thus increasing the temporal expectancy of the stimulus, and hence reducing its saliency), a clear dissociation between the magnitude of LEPs and the magnitude of perceived pain can be observed (Iannetti et al. 2008). Similarly, when brain responses to nociceptive stimuli are compared directly to the brain responses elicited by stimuli belonging to other sensory modalities (Kunde and Treede 1993; Lui et al. 2008; Mouraux and Iannetti 2009), results show that the elicited responses are strikingly similar, and thus that the greater part of the brain responses to nociceptive stimuli may actually reflect multimodal brain processes (i.e. brain processes that are elicited by sensory stimuli regardless of sensory modality).

One reason for the poor understanding of the functional significance of nociceptive-related EEG and fMRI brain responses is represented by the limited spatial resolution of EEG and the limited temporal resolution of fMRI. These intrinsic limitations make it difficult to tease out physiologically distinct brain activities contributing to the measured responses, as these appear lumped in space when sampled with EEG and lumped in time when sampled with fMRI. Therefore, because EEG signals contain the temporal information that is missing in fMRI signals, and because fMRI signals contain the spatial resolution that is missing in EEG signals (i.e. both methods provide complementary spatiotemporal information), the scientific community has shown an increasing interest in the simultaneous recording of EEG and fMRI responses. Here, we will show that combining EEG and fMRI is not sufficient to sample neural activity with the temporal resolution of EEG and the spatial resolution of fMRI. Nevertheless, we will also show that, when methods are used to analyse the recorded signals at the single-trial level, combining these two neuroimaging methods can lead to novel physiological information about the cortical processing of nociceptive input.

In the following sections we will (1) examine the general issues related to the simultaneous collection of EEG and fMRI responses to nociceptive stimuli, (2) examine the practical issues related to the simultaneous collection of EEG and fMRI responses to nociceptive stimuli, (3) review the studies that have attempted to combine such recordings, and (4) illustrate, with some novel results, how single-trial estimation of EEG data can drive the analysis of fMRI data and thus provide novel physiological information.

2
Combining EEG and fMRI in Pain Research: General Issues

The spatial and temporal resolution of a given functional neuroimaging technique is defined as its ability to distinguish two distinct events in space and time, respectively.

As discussed in the chapter "EEG: Origin and Measurement", scalp EEG detects changes in electric potentials that are generated mainly by the summation of slow postsynaptic activity occurring in regularly oriented cortical neurons, thus providing a direct measure of spontaneous and stimulus-evoked neuronal activity on a millisecond timescale (Speckmann and Elger 1999). However, because the skin, skull and meningeal layers interposed between the brain and the recording electrodes distort and exert a spatial low-pass filtering on neuronal electrical currents, the recorded scalp signals have a spatial resolution on the order of centimetres, thus preventing discrimination between distinct but spatially neighbouring neural sources of activity (Nunez and Srinivasan 2006). This issue is particularly relevant when considering nociceptive-related LEPs, which are thought to arise mostly from nonsuperficial brain structures like the operculoinsular cortex and the cingulate cortex, meaning that the recorded signal is particularly affected by volume conduction.

In contrast, blood oxygen level dependent (BOLD) fMRI samples neural activity indirectly, by detecting changes in blood oxygenation that are linked, but not equivalent, to changes in neuronal activity; see also the chapter "Locally Measured Neuronal Correlates of Functional MRI Signals" (Kwong et al. 1992; Ogawa et al. 1992). It is often stated that fMRI, unlike EEG, has an excellent spatial resolution (in the order of millimeters). However, it is important to mention that the actual spatial resolution of BOLD–fMRI is compromised by the fact that the haemodynamic response to neural activity is not necessarily restricted to the locus of this neural activity, a notion that has been described previously as "watering the entire garden for the sake of one thirsty flower" (Malonek and Grinvald 1996). Furthermore, when performing analyses at the group level, inter-subject spatial registration requires the warping of single subject data, a procedure that can lead to distortions and even displacements of activity between neighbouring cerebral lobes (Ozcan et al. 2005). The temporal resolution of fMRI is limited by the variable delay between the onset of neural activity and the subsequent haemodynamic response, as well as by the long-lasting nature of this haemodynamic response (both on the order of several seconds (Menon and Goodyear 2001)). Furthermore, the temporal profile of the haemodynamic response may vary across subjects and brain regions (Lee et al. 1995; Robson et al. 1998). Consequently, the temporal resolution of BOLD–fMRI is very low, making it extremely difficult to unravel neural processes separated in time by less than a few seconds.

When considering these physiological properties, it becomes apparent that achieving optimal spatiotemporal resolution by exploiting the higher temporal resolution of EEG and the higher spatial resolution of BOLD–fMRI is not obvious. As a matter of fact, almost all studies that have collected EEG and fMRI data simultaneously have not succeeded in achieving this goal. The fundamental reason for this is that *EEG and fMRI do not necessarily sample the same neural activity.*

The lack of correspondence between neural activity sampled by EEG and fMRI is particularly striking when comparing EEG and fMRI responses elicited by sensory stimuli.

Sensory event-related potentials (ERPs) are short-lasting EEG responses that are mainly related to transient changes in the peripheral sensory input. Sensory ERPs only reflect the fraction of stimulus-triggered brain activity that is (1) synchronous enough to summate into a measurable scalp potential, (2) spatially organised into an "open-field" configuration, and (3) time-locked and phase-locked to the onset of the stimulus (Regan 1989). For example, (1) the neural activity triggered by a slowly rising thermal stimulus will not yield a measurable ERP because the neural activity it elicits is not synchronous enough; (2) the neural activity originating from a "closed field" structure such as a subcortical nucleus will not yield a measurable ERP because the electrical fields generated by each neuron cancel each other; and (3) the neural activity consisting of stimulus-triggered modulations of the magnitude of ongoing EEG oscillations (i.e. event-related synchronisation, ERS, and event-related desynchronisation, ERD) will not yield a measurable ERP because these oscillations are not phase locked to the onset of the stimulus. In contrast, the BOLD–fMRI signal is relatively independent of the synchronicity of the afferent volley, the spatial configuration of the underlying source, and most importantly, it integrates stimulus-triggered neural activity over a much longer timescale.

This mismatch between the neural activity sampled by ERPs and the neural activity sampled by fMRI can mislead the interpretation of combined ERP and fMRI recordings, even if the data are not collected in the same experimental session. For example, an approach that is commonly used to combine ERP and fMRI data is to exploit the spatial resolution of fMRI in order to better define the neural generators of scalp ERPs (Christmann et al. 2002; Mulert et al. 2004). Indeed, the problem of estimating the location and extent of electrical sources contributing to a given scalp ERP signal (i.e. the EEG inverse problem; Nunez and Srinivasan 2006) is fundamentally ill-posed, as this scalp ERP can be explained by an infinite number of source configurations. Therefore, in order to obtain a unique solution, constraints must be imposed on the model (Michel et al. 2004). With this aim, a number of investigators have used the location of stimulus-induced BOLD–fMRI responses as a "functional constraint" (fMRI-constrained ERP source localisation (Christmann et al. 2002; Mulert et al. 2004)). However, it is important to take into account that only a fraction of the stimulus-triggered neural activity contributes to the scalp ERP, and that this fraction constitutes only a subset of the longer-lasting neural activities subserving the BOLD–fMRI response. Therefore, although fMRI-constrained ERP source localisation can certainly improve the solution of the inverse problem by constraining the placement of dipolar sources to brain areas that are metabolically active, it can produce false-positive results by allowing the misplacement of dipolar sources in brain regions that are metabolically active but do not contribute to the ERP response. This crucial aspect of EEG and fMRI data fusion remains the subject of investigation.

When considering nociceptive somatosensory input, the fact that the BOLD–fMRI signal integrates neural activity over a long timescale is likely to generate a particularly significant mismatch between nociceptive-related neural activity that is sampled by EEG and fMRI. The perceptual correlate of a single strong nociceptive stimulus is long-lasting and multidimensional. Besides its sensory-discriminative dimension, it also encompasses motivational and emotional dimensions. Because ERPs almost exclusively reflect transient changes in neural activity, they probably capture only the initial part of the long-lasting neural response related to the perception of pain. In contrast, because fMRI data integrates neural responses over a long timescale, they probably more closely reflect the neural activity related to the perception as a whole.

The contributions of different populations of peripheral nociceptive afferents to the recorded brain response are likely to further increase the mismatch between the neural activity sampled by EEG and fMRI. This is due to the fact that nociceptive stimuli activate two different types of peripheral skin nociceptors: small myelinated Aδ and unmyelinated C nociceptors. While the activation of Aδ nociceptors results in sharp, short-lasting "prick-ing" sensations, the activation of C nociceptors conveys dull, long-lasting "burning" or "aching" sensations that spread well beyond the spatial limits of the stimulus. For this rea-son, brief and intense laser stimuli elicit a typical dual sensation of "first" (Aδ-related) and "second" (C-related) pain (Lewis and Ponchin 1937). Yet, For reasons that are still debated (e.g. Mouraux and Iannetti 2008), LEPs only reflects brain responses related to the activa-tion of Aδ nociceptors (Mouraux et al. 2004). This leads to the possibility of an important mismatch between the brain activity underlying LEPs (which is strictly related to the acti-vation of Aδ nociceptors, and thus to the perception of "first pain") and the brain activity underlying the BOLD–fMRI response (which integrates neural activity on a longer time scale, and may thus reflect a combination of brain activity related to the activation of both Aδ and C nociceptors).

For all of these reasons, before addressing the problem of *how* EEG and fMRI responses to nociceptive stimulation can be concomitantly recorded, it is crucial to discuss *why* this should be done, and in which instances it may yield physiological information that is unob-tainable using data collected in two separate experimental sessions. As discussed in the chap-ter "EEG Instrumentation and Safety", sampling EEG and fMRI data in a truly simultaneous fashion is a technically challenging task. The experimental setup is complex, and issues related to subject safety and quality of collected data must be addressed using dedicated EEG hard-ware (Lemieux et al. 1997). Magnetic susceptibility effects and radiofrequency interactions associated with EEG electrodes and wires cause signal dropouts and geometric distortions on MR images (Bonmassar et al. 2001). Degradation of image signal-to-noise ratio due to electromagnetic noise emitted by the EEG recording headbox has also been described (Krakow et al. 2000). Most importantly, the collected EEG data are contaminated by severe MR-induced artefacts. These consist mainly of "pulse" artefacts caused by cardiac pulse-related move-ments and blood flow effects within the scanner's static magnetic field, and "imaging" artefacts caused by radiofrequency and gradient switching during image acquisition. Pulse artefacts are regular, have a relatively low amplitude, and occur even when MR images are not being acquired. In contrast, imaging artefacts are large and obscure the EEG completely (Allen et al. 2000). The reduction of these artefacts, although feasible, is a complex and time-demanding procedure (Niazy et al. 2005). In addition, the increased subject discomfort related to combining the EEG setup with the constraints of the MR environment reduces the possi-ble duration of the experimental session, and thus limits the complexity of the experimental design. For all of these reasons, repeating the same experimental paradigm in two separate experimental sessions, is, in most cases, a more rewarding strategy (Iannetti et al. 2005a).

Nevertheless, as detailed more extensively in the chapter "Principles of Multimodal Functional Imaging and Data Integration" the simultaneous recording of EEG and fMRI unleashes its potential in two particular circumstances: (1) when the neural activity under investigation displays a certain level of *unpredictability*, and (2) when the experimental design introduces important *time-dependent effects* such as habituation, learning, or between-session variability in the effect of a given pharmacological compound.

Outside the field of pain research, typical examples of such circumstances are studies examining ictal and interictal activities in epileptic patients (Hamandi et al. 2008), sleep stages (Wehrle et al. 2007), and spontaneous fluctuations of ongoing EEG rhythms (Laufs et al. 2003). Also, combining EEG and fMRI within a single recording session may be useful when examining the time-dependent effect of drugs on the processing of sensory input and, in particular, the effect of anaesthetic agents on the processing of nociceptive input (Rogers et al. 2004). Lastly, when studies focus on brain responses that are strongly dependent on cognitive variables such as the focus of selective attention or the general level of arousal, the peculiar attentional context and the additional sensory stimulation inherent to a working MR scanner can introduce important, non-task-related differences when comparing data collected in separate sessions.

In the field of pain research (see also Sect. 5), the intrinsic variability of the brain responses to nociceptive stimulation introduces a degree of unpredictability that makes the simultaneous and *continuous* acquisition of EEG and fMRI data the only possible approach to assessing physiologically meaningful between-trial variations of EEG and BOLD–fMRI brain responses, and examining their relationship with behavioural measures (e.g. intensity of pain perception, reaction-time latency). In addition, the simultaneous (but not necessarily continuous) acquisition of EEG and fMRI data can be important in the evaluation of drug effects, when a significant within-subject, between-session variation in the response to the drug (e.g. the potential development of tolerance to opioids) is expected.

3
Combining EEG and fMRI in Pain Research: Practical Issues

3.1
Selectivity of the Nociceptive Input in EEG–fMRI Studies

Noxious heat stimuli are most frequently used in EEG and fMRI studies of nociception, because they selectively activate nociceptive-specific transduction mechanisms in afferents located in the superficial layers of the skin (Julius and Basbaum 2001). If the temperature of the skin is raised above the thermal activation threshold of Aδ ($\sim$46°C) and C nociceptors ($\sim$40°C) (Treede et al. 1995), the stimulus will be transduced into a nociceptive afferent volley. Noxious heat can be delivered using either thermal conduction (contact thermodes) or thermal radiation (infrared lasers). Alternative methods to activate Aδ and C skin nociceptors include high-intensity mechanical (Slugg et al. 2004) and electrical stimulation (Naka and Kakigi 1998). However, both methods present issues related to the lack of selectivity of the elicited somatosensory afferent volley.

Whatever the techniques used to sample neural activity, it is important to ascertain that the brain responses elicited by the nociceptive stimulus are truly related to the processing of nociceptive input (and not to the processing of another type of sensory input). For this reason, heat nociceptive stimulation is preferred to electrical or mechanical noxious stimulation, as the latter concomitantly activate low-threshold mechanoreceptors and corresponding Aβ fibres (for a discussion on this topic see Baumgartner et al. 2005; Plaghki and Mouraux 2003). For the same reason, radiant heat stimulation is preferred to contact heat stimulation, as contact thermodes unavoidably activate non-nociceptive Aβ-fibre afferents, both tonically (because the contact of the thermode with the skin results in the activation of slowly adapting non-nociceptive mechanoreceptors) and phasically (because changing the location of the thermode from trial to trial results in the activation of fast-adapting non-nociceptive mechanoreceptors; Greffrath et al. 2007). Because the activation of Aβ-fibre afferents induced by contact thermodes is not strictly synchronous with the onset of the thermal stimulus, and because the averaging procedures used to reveal ERPs cancels out signal changes that are not strictly time locked to the stimulus onset, its contribution to contact heat-evoked potentials may be considered negligible (CHEPs; Chen et al. 2001). In contrast, when contact thermodes are used to elicit BOLD–fMRI brain responses, the contribution from both tonic and phasic non-nociceptive Aβ-fibre input is likely to become significant, because the BOLD signal integrates neural activity over a much longer timescale (see also Sect. 2 and the chapter "The Basics of Functional Magnetic Resonance Imaging"), and it has been shown that even long-lasting tonic stimuli may elicit a significant "sustained" BOLD response (Bandettini et al. 1997).

Another advantage of radiant over conductive heat is that infrared laser stimulators heat the skin much faster (up to 10,000°C/s; Plaghki and Mouraux 2003) than contact thermodes (up to 70°C/s for thermodes specifically designed for the recording of ERPs; Baumgartner et al. 2005). Therefore, because nociceptors are activated much more synchronously (quasi-simultaneously) by laser stimuli than by contact heat stimuli, laser stimuli elicit ERPs more reliably than contact thermodes (Baumgartner et al. 2005; Iannetti et al. 2006; see also Sect. 2).

Lastly, the recent reintroduction of intra-epidermal needle electrodes as a method to selectively activate nociceptive fibres should be mentioned. This method was originally proposed by Bromm and Meier (1984), and was subsequently refined by Inui et al. (2002). A thin (diameter: 0.5 mm) needle anode is inserted into the epidermal layer of the skin, where the free nerve endings of Aδ and C fibres lie. The anode is surrounded by a circular cathode. In this configuration, the current flows tangentially to the skin surface and, if the current is kept low, it will activate intra-epidermal nociceptors directly and selectively. The actual selectivity of the method still requires further validation, but if confirmed, this technique could become a valid alternative to infrared laser stimulation for providing selective nociceptive stimuli in the MR environment, not only because it is easy to implement (the stimulus is generated using conventional electrical stimulators), but also because the direct activation of nociceptive fibres generates an extremely synchronous afferent volley.

3.2
Delivery of Nociceptive Stimuli in the EEG–fMRI Environment

When performing pain-related EEG–fMRI studies, an important issue to consider is that the equipment involved in the delivery of the nociceptive stimulus must be "compatible" with the strong magnetic field of the MR scanner, as it must function normally and any additional health risk for the subject and investigators must be assessed. Short-wavelength laser pulses (e.g. Nd:YAP lasers: λ = 1.34 µm) can be easily transmitted through inexpensive optical fibres. Recently, optical fibres capable of transmitting longer-wavelength CO_2 pulses (λ = 10.6 µm) have also been made available, but they are much more expensive (Plaghki and Mouraux 2003). Using such fibres, laser stimuli can be delivered inside the scanner room whilst keeping the laser source outside. A number of contact thermodes have been developed to deliver noxious heat within the MR environment (Wise et al. 2002). Furthermore, both transcutaneous and intra-epidermal electrical stimuli are easily delivered in the MR scanner room, provided that safety measures related to the presence of electric currents are considered. Finally, several laboratories (e.g. Lui et al. 2008) have built custom pneumatically driven devices to deliver noxious mechanical stimuli inside the MR scanner room.

Taking these different factors into consideration, it appears that noxious heat pulses generated by infrared laser stimulators constitute, at present, the best method of producing nociceptive sensory input for the concurrent recording of EEG and fMRI because they (1) are entirely selective for nociceptors, (2) elicit a nociceptive afferent volley that is synchronous enough to elicit reliable ERPs, and (3) can be delivered safely inside the scanner using optical fibres.

3.3
Experimental Design

Interleaved vs. continuous EEG–fMRI acquisition. As discussed in the chapter "EEG Instrumentation and Safety", the main source of contamination of the EEG by MR-related artefacts is represented by the gradient switching that occurs during image acquisition. For this reason, several studies aiming at recording ERPs and fMRI within the same experimental session rely on an *interleaved* experimental design. In such a design, the introduction of short pauses in the acquisition of MR images (e.g. 3 s of image acquisition alternated with 3 s without image acquisition) allows the recording of segments of EEG data unaffected by the imaging artefact. However, interleaving EEG and fMRI acquisition has important practical and theoretical limitations, mainly represented by inefficient sampling of the neural activity and the consequent haemodynamic response, and by a reduction in the flexibility of the stimulus presentation paradigm (Garreffa et al. 2004; Nebel et al. 2005). Furthermore, the data can be affected by pulse-related artefacts on the EEG that are also correlated with the stimulus or task (see the chapter "EEG Quality: Origin and Reduction of the EEG Cardiac-Related Artefact"). The alternative is to acquire EEG and fMRI data simultaneously and *continuously* using an event-related experimental design, and then rely on offline signal-processing methods to remove the contaminating artefacts (Niazy et al. 2005).

Interstimulus interval. The rate of stimulus presentation can affect the magnitude of EEG responses elicited by nociceptive stimuli very significantly. When the ISI is kept constant across trials, it has been shown that the shorter the ISI, the smaller the recorded EEG response (Raij et al. 2003; Truini et al. 2004). For this reason, some investigators have recommended the use of an ISI of more than 4 s (Raij et al. 2003). However, it has been also shown that when the ISI is randomised across trials, thus making the occurrence of the nociceptive stimulus *unpredictable*, the magnitude of the EEG response is unaffected by stimulus repetition, even at ISIs as short as 280 ms (Mouraux et al. 2004; Mouraux and Iannetti 2008a). Consequently, if fMRI and EEG responses to nociceptive stimulation are sampled in an interleaved manner, it is crucial to present the nociceptive stimuli using the same ISI and stimulation paradigm, or else the functional significance of the brain responses sampled using EEG and fMRI may be very different. To date, the relationship between ISI parameters and the magnitude of nociceptive-evoked fMRI responses has not been explicitly studied.

Number of stimuli. Another practical issue to consider when designing the experiment is the number of nociceptive stimuli required to elicit reliable EEG and fMRI responses. Most studies recording ERPs elicited by nociceptive stimulation average a total of 20–40 stimuli (Treede et al. 2003). When using an event-related design, a similar number of stimuli are usually used to assess fMRI responses to nociceptive stimulation. The magnitude of EEG responses to nociceptive stimuli can vary greatly as a function of the parameters of the nociceptive stimulus and the stimulated body district. For example, fast-rising nociceptive stimuli yield a more synchronous afferent volley, thus providing a stronger spatiotemporal summation at central synapses that enhances the intensity of perceived pain and increases the magnitude of measured brain responses (Iannetti et al. 2004). Similarly, and because of the shorter conduction distance and the higher density of skin nociceptors, nociceptive stimuli delivered to a proximal body district (e.g. the trigeminal territory) yield brain responses of significantly shorter latency and larger amplitude than nociceptive stimuli delivered to a distal body district (e.g. the foot) (Truini et al. 2005).

Displacement of the stimuli. To avoid nociceptor fatigue or sensitisation, and to allow passive cooling of the skin, the laser beam must be moved slightly after each stimulus (Treede et al. 2003). This is usually achieved by manually displacing the laser beam inside the scanner room. However, although common in fMRI studies, this approach is far from being optimal, because (1) it is necessary to provide the experimenter with some form of cue about when the beam has to be displaced, thus making the procedure prone to mistakes, and (2) it makes it difficult to define the exact location of stimulated spots. For these reasons, the development of computer-controlled MR-compatible devices to displace the laser beam automatically would be desirable, particularly when the time interval between two consecutive stimuli is short (Lee et al. 2009).

4
Studies Combining EEG and fMRI in Pain Research

To date, only two studies have simultaneously collected EEG and BOLD–fMRI responses to nociceptive stimulation (Christmann et al. 2007; Iannetti et al. 2005a).

Iannetti et al. (2005a) demonstrated for the first time the feasibility of recording reliable laser-evoked EEG and fMRI responses in a truly simultaneous and continuous fashion (i.e. using a single and *continuous* acquisition of EEG and fMRI data). They showed that the

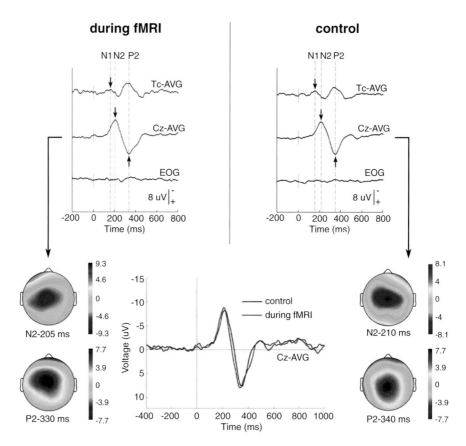

Fig. 1 Comparison between the grand-average waveforms (data from seven subjects) and scalp topographies of laser-evoked brain potentials (LEPs) recorded during simultaneous and continuous fMRI at 3 T (*left panel*) and LEPs recorded in a control session outside the scanner room (*right panel*). The same recording equipment and experimental paradigm were used in both sessions. LEPs were elicited by stimulation (Nd:YAP laser) of the right hand dorsum. Negativity is plotted upwards. Recordings from the vertex (Cz) and the temporal electrode contralateral to the stimulated side (Tc) are computed against average reference (AVG). Electro-oculogram (EOG) was recorded to monitor eye blinks. *Arrows* indicate early N1 and late N2–P2 components. Scalp topographies are shown at N2 and P2 peak latencies. Note the similarity between the latencies, amplitudes and scalp topographies of N2 and P2 waves obtained in the fMRI and in the control session (*lower panel*). Reproduced from Iannetti et al. (2005a)

latency, the amplitude, and the scalp distribution of LEPs recorded during fMRI acquisition are not significantly different from the latency, the amplitude, and the scalp distribution of LEPs recorded outside the MR scanner (Fig. 1). This finding has two important implications. First, because of the observed similarities, it indicates that, in most experimental designs, multimodal integration of LEP and fMRI results can be carried out using data collected in separate, single-modality experiments unless one is interested in studying individual trials.

Second, because it shows that reliable LEPs can be recorded during a truly simultaneous collection of fMRI data, it demonstrates the possibility of performing EEG-driven analysis of fMRI data in pain research (see Sect. 5).

Christmann et al. (2007) recorded EEG and fMRI responses elicited by the electrical transcutaneous stimulation of the right thumb, and observed a good concordance between the strength and the location of the fMRI response and the modelled sources contributing to the ERP. However, the use of high-intensity electrical stimuli is not selective for nociceptive afferents. Furthermore, the comparison of of averaged EEG (equivalent dipoles) and BOLD responses over partially overlapping sets of neuronal events does not represent an optimal exploitation of the simultaneously acquired data, namely the analysis of individual trials.

In summary, neither the study of Iannetti et al. (2005a) nor that of Christmann et al. (2007) provide novel physiological information that could not have been obtained by recording EEG and fMRI pain-related responses in two separate experimental sessions.

5
Future Directions: EEG-Driven Analysis of fMRI BOLD Responses to Nociceptive Stimulation

Whatever the neuroimaging modality, the magnitude of the activity elicited by the selective stimulation of nociceptive afferents displays a significant amount of trial-to-trial variability (Iannetti et al. 2005b; Purves and Boyd 1993). Most often, because this variability is spontaneous (i.e. cannot be explained by identified experimental factors), it is discarded as physiologically meaningless noise. However, one person's noise is another's signal, so to speak, and both the peripheral and central sources of this variability could contain information that is physiologically relevant. Two peripheral factors contribute particularly to the variability of brain responses to nociceptive stimuli, namely the different number of afferents stimulated from trial to trial, and the significant variance in the conduction velocity of primary nociceptive afferents (Treede et al. 1998). Furthermore, an increasing number of studies have shown that a great part of the variability of any given brain response results from dynamic fluctuations of the ongoing cortical activity (Arieli et al. 1996), possibly related to fluctuations of vigilance, expectation and attentional focus, or changes in task strategy. Therefore, exploring the trial-to-trial variability of EEG and fMRI brain responses, as well as exploring its relationship with behavioural variables (e.g. intensity of perception, reaction-time latency), may provide important insights into the functional significance of the different processes that underlie these brain responses.

In the following section, we will show how the trial-to-trial variability of EEG responses can be used to drive the analysis of simultaneously recorded fMRI responses, and thereby establish relationships between temporally distinct peaks of the EEG response and spatially distinct clusters of the fMRI–BOLD response (Fig. 2). We will (1) examine different methods that are used to estimate the magnitude of stimulus-evoked EEG responses at the level of single trials, and (2) illustrate how these different methods can be used to drive the analysis of simultaneously acquired fMRI data.

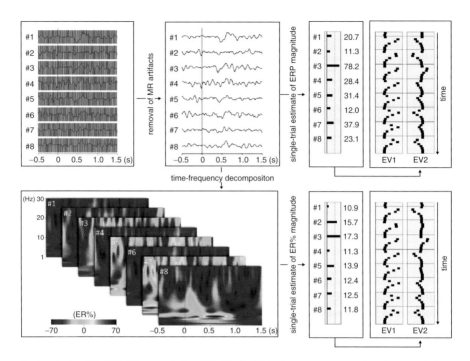

Fig. 2 Single-trial EEG-driven analysis of BOLD–fMRI brain responses to nociceptive stimulation. EEG and fMRI data are recorded simultaneously and continuously. The peristimulus EEG recordings (−0.5 to +1.0 s relative to stimulus onset) are contaminated with severe MR-related artefacts. These artefacts are efficiently removed using a method based on a principal component analysis (PCA) (Niazy et al. 2005). Once MR-related artefacts have been removed, different approaches can be used to quantify, within each single epoch, the magnitude of both phase-locked (i.e. event-related potentials, ERPs; see also Fig. 3) and non-phase-locked (i.e. event-related synchronisation and event-related desynchronisation, ERS and ERD; see also Fig. 4) EEG responses (Mouraux and Iannetti,2008b). Single-trial estimates of the magnitude of laser-evoked EEG responses are consequently used as regressors in the general linear model analysis of fMRI time series to identify voxels whose BOLD signal time courses correlate with the trial-to-trial variability of laser-evoked EEG responses. Two regressors are used for each single-subject analysis, one representing the mean amplitude of the EEG response (*EV1*), the other representing the trial-to-trial variability of the EEG response (*EV2*)

5.1
Single-Trial Estimation of the Magnitude of Stimulus-Evoked EEG Responses

A simple way to obtain a single-trial estimate of the magnitude of stimulus-evoked EEG responses consists of visually identifying and measuring a defined peak of activity within each single EEG epoch. This approach has been shown to be reasonably effective for nociceptive ERPs, as these are of particularly large amplitude (Iannetti et al. 2005b; Purves and Boyd 1993). However, it has three important limitations: (1) it is prone to the introduction of involuntary biases by the observer, (2) it leads to an overestimation of response magnitude, since some single-trial estimates are likely to reflect the spurious detection of uncorrelated noise resembling the searched-for visual template, and (3) the obtained results are difficult to replicate, as they are observer dependent.

Recently, Mayhew et al. (2006) showed that a multiple linear regression approach can be used to obtain an unbiased and accurate estimate of the latency and amplitude of single-trial nociceptive ERPs. In this method, a basis set of regressors and their temporal derivatives are obtained from the average ERP waveform. This basis set is then regressed against each single EEG epoch, thus providing a quantitative measure of the latencies and amplitudes of the different peaks of the ERP waveform (Fig. 3B).

However, ERPs reflect only a fraction of the EEG response to a given stimulus. Indeed, the stimulus also triggers transient increases (event-related synchronisation, ERS) and decreases (event-related desynchronisation, ERD) of the power of ongoing EEG oscillations. Identifying ERS and ERD requires estimating the average time-varying power of EEG oscillations. This can be obtained by performing a joint time–frequency decomposition of EEG epochs using, for example, the continuous wavelet transform (see Fig. 4). ERS and ERD are subsequently identified by averaging time–frequency maps across trials. To estimate the magnitude of ERS and ERD at the level of single trials, time-frequency regions of interest can be defined and used to mask the activity within each single trial. Importantly, this approach has the potential to identify nociceptive-related EEG responses that correlate more closely with fMRI responses, because a number of studies have suggested that the BOLD–fMRI signal could, at least in other sensory modalities, be more tightly related to the occurrence of longer-lasting ERD and ERS.

5.2
Correlation Between EEG and fMRI Responses at Single-Trial Level

The analytical steps necessary for the extraction of physiologically relevant information embedded in the trial-to-trial variability of simultaneously acquired EEG and fMRI brain responses to nociceptive stimulation are outlined in Fig. 2. After the removal of the pulse and imaging artefacts (Niazy et al. 2005), EEG signals are filtered and segmented into peri-stimulus epochs. A continuous wavelet transform can be used to build a time–frequency matrix expressing single-trial signal amplitude as a function of time and frequency. A single-trial estimate of EEG response magnitude is then obtained either from the original signal in the time domain (e.g. the amplitude of the N2 and P2 peaks at the vertex, estimated using a multiple linear regression approach; see Fig. 3B) or in the time–frequency domain (e.g. the percent increase or decrease of oscillation amplitude corresponding to a focus of event-related synchronisation or desynchronisation, estimated within a defined time–frequency region of interest; see Fig. 4B). These single-trial estimates of the magnitude of the EEG response are used to build a function of the predicted haemodynamic response, which is finally included as an additional regressor in the GLM used to analyse the fMRI time series. This method allows the identification of voxels whose BOLD signal time course correlates with the trial-to-trial variability of the measured EEG response. The same approach can be used to correlate the trial-to-trial variability of laser-evoked EEG responses with the fMRI–BOLD signal decomposed into a set of spatially independent maps and time courses using a spatial probabilistic independent component analysis (PICA; Beckmann and Smith 2004).

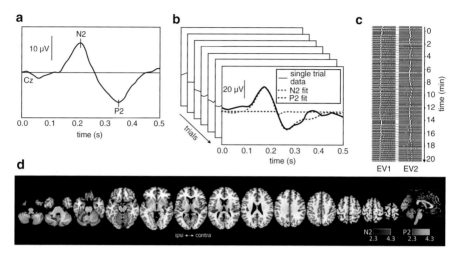

Fig. 3a–d Correlation between the trial-to-trial variability of LEPs and the simultaneously recorded BOLD–fMRI signal. EEG and fMRI responses to nociceptive laser stimuli were recorded simultaneously and continuously in five subjects. For each subject, 60 laser stimuli were applied to the left hand dorsum, and 60 laser stimuli to the right hand dorsum. **a** shows the LEP waveform obtained by averaging peristimulus EEG epochs across trials (electrode Cz vs. nose reference, data from one representative subject). The response is characterised by a negative deflection (N2) followed by a positive deflection (P2). The average LEP waveform was used to create a set of four regressors formed by the N2 waveform, the P2 waveform, and their temporal derivatives (Mayhew et al. 2006). A multiple linear regression of the basis set of the four regressors against each single EEG epoch was used to model each single-trial ERP, and thus obtain an estimate of the amplitude and latency of N2 and P2 peaks in each single trial (**b**). The *black* waveform corresponds to a single representative EEG epoch. The *red* and *blue* dashed waveforms correspond to the automated fittings of the N2 and P2 deflections. The single-trial estimates of N2 and P2 amplitudes were subsequently used to create regressors and thereby investigate the correlation between the trial-to-trial variability of the N2 and P2 EEG peaks and the simultaneously and continuously recorded BOLD signal, using two separate single-subject analyses (one for each peak). For each analysis, two regressors were used (**c**). The first (*EV1*) represented the average amplitude of the peak of interest. The second (*EV2*) represented the trial-to-trial variability of the peak of interest. (**d**) shows the results obtained at group level (the hemisphere ipsilateral to the stimulated side is shown on the *left*). Voxels whose BOLD signal time courses were significantly correlated with the trial-to-trial variability of the N2 EEG peak are shown in *red*, while voxels whose time course was significantly correlated with the trial-to-trial variability of the P2 EEG peak are shown in *green*. Analysis was done using a mixed effects analysis and cluster-based thresholding ($z > 2.3$, $p < 0.05$). Note how the variability of the N2 peak correlates with the BOLD signal time course of voxels located in the ipsilateral and contralateral posterior insula. Also note how the variabilities of both the N2 and P2 peaks correlate with the BOLD signal time course of voxels located in the vicinity of the hand area of the contralateral primary somatosensory cortex.

PICA decomposes the fMRI data into a linear combination of independent spatiotemporal components (ICs), each hypothesised to reflect independent physical or physiological sources of BOLD signal change (Fig. 5). The approach has the advantage of allowing the correlation of the single-trial variability of EEG responses to physiologically relevant independent patterns of BOLD–fMRI activity (see also Bagshaw and Warbrick 2007). Finally,

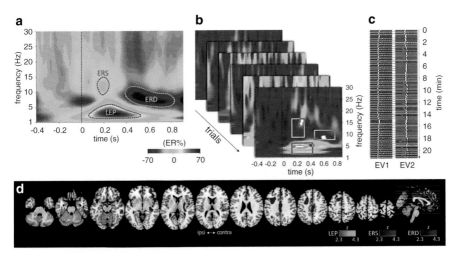

Fig. 4a–d Correlation between the trial-to-trial variability of laser-evoked EEG responses identified in the time–frequency domain and the simultaneously recorded BOLD–fMRI signal. EEG and fMRI responses to nociceptive laser stimuli were recorded simultaneously and continuously in five subjects. For each subject, 60 laser stimuli were applied to the left hand dorsum, and 60 laser stimuli to the right hand dorsum. A time–frequency decomposition of each single EEG epoch (electrode Cz vs. nose reference) was performed using the continuous wavelet transform to generate a map of EEG oscillation power as a function of time and frequency. The maps are expressed as the percentage of change (ER%) relative to a prestimulus reference interval (−400 to −100 ms). Across-trial averaging of these maps (**a**) reveals both phase-locked LEPs and non-phase-locked laser-induced modulations of the power of ongoing EEG oscillations (*ERS* and *ERD*). Three time–frequency regions of interest (ROIs) were defined, centred around the locations of the three main foci of activity. (ROI-LEP: 150–450 ms and 1–5 Hz; ROI-ERS: 150–300 ms and 8–17 Hz; ROI-ERD: 500–800 ms and 8–12 Hz.) Within each ROI, the mean of the 10% of pixels displaying the greatest increase (ROI-LEP and ROI-ERS) or decrease (ROI-ERD) in amplitude was calculated for each single EEG epoch (**b**). Single-trial estimates of LEP, ERS, and ERD magnitude were subsequently used to create regressors and thereby investigate the correlation between the trial-to-trial variability of each of the three laser-evoked EEG responses and the simultaneously recorded BOLD signal, using three separate single-subject analyses. For each analysis, two regressors were used (**c**). The first (*EV1*) represented the average amplitude of the EEG response. The second (*EV2*) represented the trial-to-trial variability of the EEG response. (**d**) shows the results obtained at the group level (the hemisphere ipsilateral to the stimulated side is shown on the *left*). Voxels whose BOLD signal time courses were significantly correlated with the trial-to-trial variability of ROI-LEP, ROI-ERS, and ROI-ERD are shown respectively in *green*, *red* and *blue*. Analysis was done using a mixed effects analysis and cluster-based thresholding ($z > 2.3$, $p < 0.05$)

the same approach can be applied to the exploration of single-trial information that is not derived from the EEG, such as the energy of the eliciting sensory stimulus or the intensity of the perceived sensation (see Fig. 6; Niazy 2006).

Acknowledgments   G.D. Iannetti is University Research Fellow of The Royal Society. A. Mouraux is a Marie-Curie Postdoctoral Research Fellow and a "Chargé de Recherché" of the Belgian National Fund for Scientific Research.

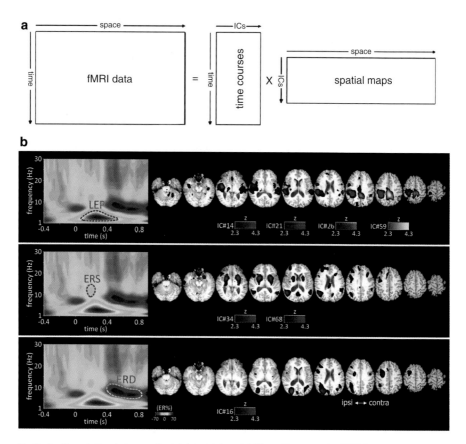

Fig. 5a–b Correlation between the trial-to-trial variability of laser-evoked EEG responses and the BOLD–fMRI signal decomposed into a set of spatially-independent maps and time courses using a spatial probabilistic independent component analysis (PICA; Beckmann and Smith 2004). EEG and fMRI responses to nociceptive laser stimuli were recorded simultaneously and continuously in five subjects. For each subject, 60 laser stimuli were applied to the left hand dorsum, and 60 laser stimuli to the right hand dorsum. PICA was used to decompose the fMRI data into a linear combination of independent spatiotemporal components (ICs), each reflecting an independent physical or physiological source of BOLD signal change (**a**). A time–frequency decomposition of EEG epochs (electrode Cz vs. nose reference) was used to obtain single-trial estimates of phase-locked (LEP) and non-phase-locked (ERS and ERD) EEG responses (see Fig. 4 for details). These single-trial estimates were subsequently used to create regressors and thereby investigate the correlation between the trial-to-trial variability of each of these three laser-evoked EEG responses and the time course of each IC. (**b**) shows the results obtained in one representative subject. The spatial maps of ICs whose time courses were significantly ($p < 0.01$) correlated with the trial-to-trial variability of the LEP response, the ERS response and the ERD response are shown in the *upper*, *middle* and *lower rows*, respectively. Note how the variability of the LEP response (**b**, *top row*) correlates with the temporal profile of ICs located in the contralateral insular cortex (*purple*), secondary somatosensory cortex (*blue*), and in the hand area of the primary somatosensory cortex (*red*), while the ERS response (**b**, *middle row*) correlates with the temporal profile of ICs located in the deep insular cortex bilaterally. In contrast, the variability of the ERD response (**b**, *bottom row*) correlates with the temporal profile of ICs located in posterior brain regions (*red*)

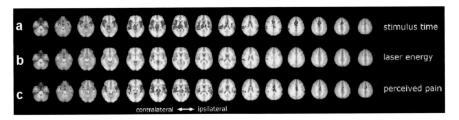

Fig. 6a–b   Single-trial analysis of laser-evoked BOLD–fMRI responses. The *top row* (**a**) displays the mean laser-evoked fMRI responses modelled using only the temporal information of stimulus onset, while the *middle* and the *bottom rows* display the correlation between the trial-to-trial variability of the energy of laser stimulation (**b**), the intensity of perceived pain (**c**), and the BOLD–fMRI signal (group-level results obtained from a total of seven subjects). For each subject, 60 laser stimuli of three different energies (20 stimuli for each energy) were applied to the left hand dorsum. After each stimulus, the subjects were asked to rate the elicited sensation on a numerical scale (ranging from 0 to 10, where 0 was "no pain" and 10 "pain as bad as it could be"). Note how the magnitude of the fMRI response in the contralateral operculoinsular region more closely reflects the intensity of the nociceptive somatosensory input. Note also how the bulk of the fMRI response to laser stimulation is more closely related to the perceived magnitude of pain than to the applied stimulus energy, suggesting that these responses are more related to the intensity of the perceived sensation than to the intensity of the incoming nociceptive afferent volley. Analysis was done using a mixed effects analysis and cluster-based thresholding ($z > 1.6$, $p < 0.05$). Data from Iannetti and Niazy (Niazy 2006)

References

Allen PJ, Josephs O, Turner R (2000) A method for removing imaging artefact from continuous EEG recorded during functional MRI. Neuroimage 12:230–9

Apkarian AV, Bushnell MC, Treede RD, Zubieta JK (2005) Human brain mechanisms of pain perception and regulation in health and disease. Eur J Pain 9:463–84

Arieli A, Sterkin A, Grinvald A, Aertsen A (1996) Dynamics of ongoing activity: explanation of the large variability in evoked cortical responses. Science 273:1868–71

Bagshaw AP, Warbrick T (2007) Single trial variability of EEG and fMRI responses to visual stimuli. Neuroimage 38:280–92

Bandettini PA, Kwong KK, Davis TL, Tootell RB, Wong EC, Fox PT, et al. (1997) Characterization of cerebral blood oxygenation and flow changes during prolonged brain activation. Hum Brain Mapp 5:93–109

Baumgartner U, Cruccu G, Iannetti GD, Treede RD (2005) Laser guns and hot plates. Pain 116:1–3

Beckmann CF, Smith SM (2004) Probabilistic independent component analysis for functional magnetic resonance imaging. IEEE Trans Med Imaging 23:137–52

Bonmassar G, Hadjikhani N, Ives JR, Hinton D, Belliveau JW (2001) Influence of EEG electrodes on the BOLD fMRI signal. Hum Brain Mapp 14:108–115

Bromm B, Chen AC (1995) Brain electrical source analysis of laser evoked potentials in response to painful trigeminal nerve stimulation. Electroencephalogr Clin Neurophysiol 95:14–26

Bromm B, Meier W (1984) The intracutaneous stimulus: a new pain model for algesimetric studies. Methods Find Exp Clin Pharmacol 6:405–10

Carmon A, Mor J, Goldberg J (1976) Evoked cerebral responses to noxious thermal stimuli in humans. Exp Brain Res 25:103–7

Chen AC, Niddam DM, Arendt-Nielsen L (2001) Contact heat evoked potentials as a valid means to study nociceptive pathways in human subjects. Neurosci Lett 316:79–82

Christmann C, Koeppe C, Braus DF, Ruf M, Flor H (2007) A simultaneous EEG–fMRI study of painful electric stimulation. Neuroimage 34:1428–37

Christmann C, Ruf M, Braus DF, Flor H (2002) Simultaneous electroencephalography and functional magnetic resonance imaging of primary and secondary somatosensory cortex in humans after electrical stimulation. Neurosci Lett 333:69–73

Davis KD, Kwan CL, Crawley AP, Mikulis DJ (1998) Event-related fMRI of pain: entering a new era in imaging pain. Neuroreport 9:3019–23

Frot M, Mauguiere F (2003) Dual representation of pain in the operculo-insular cortex in humans. Brain 126:438–50

Garcia-Larrea L, Frot M, Valeriani M (2003) Brain generators of laser-evoked potentials: from dipoles to functional significance. Neurophysiol Clin 33:279–92

Garreffa G, Bianciardi M, Hagberg GE, Macaluso E, Marciani MG, Maraviglia B, et al. (2004) Simultaneous EEG–fMRI acquisition: how far is it from being a standardized technique? Magn Reson Imaging 22:1445–55

Greffrath W, Baumgartner U, Treede RD (2007) Peripheral and central components of habituation of heat pain perception and evoked potentials in humans. Pain 132:301–11

Hamandi K, Laufs H, Noth U, Carmichael DW, Duncan JS, Lemieux L (2008) BOLD and perfusion changes during epileptic generalised spike wave activity. Neuroimage 39:608–18

Iannetti GD, Hughes NP, Lee MC, Mouraux A (2008) The determinants of laser-evoked EEG responses: pain perception or stimulus saliency? J Neurophysiol 100:815–28

Iannetti GD, Leandri M, Truini A, Zambreanu L, Cruccu G, Tracey I (2004) Adelta nociceptor response to laser stimuli: selective effect of stimulus duration on skin temperature, brain potentials and pain perception. Clin Neurophysiol 115:2629–37

Iannetti GD, Niazy RK, Wise RG, Jezzard P, Brooks JC, Zambreanu L, et al. (2005a) Simultaneous recording of laser-evoked brain potentials and continuous, high-field functional magnetic resonance imaging in humans. Neuroimage 28:708–19

Iannetti GD, Zambreanu L, Cruccu G, Tracey I (2005b) Operculoinsular cortex encodes pain intensity at the earliest stages of cortical processing as indicated by amplitude of laser-evoked potentials in humans. Neuroscience 131:199–208

Iannetti GD, Zambreanu L, Tracey I (2006) Similar nociceptive afferents mediate psychophysical and electrophysiological responses to heat stimulation of glabrous and hairy skin in humans. J Physiol 577:235–48

Inui K, Tran TD, Hoshiyama M, Kakigi R (2002) Preferential stimulation of Adelta fibers by intra-epidermal needle electrode in humans. Pain 96:247–52

Julius D, Basbaum AI (2001) Molecular mechanisms of nociception. Nature 413:203–10

Krakow K, Allen PJ, Symms MR, Lemieux L, Josephs O, Fish DR (2000) EEG recording during fMRI experiments: image quality. Hum Brain Mapp 10:10–15

Kunde V, Treede RD (1993) Topography of middle-latency somatosensory evoked potentials following painful laser stimuli and non-painful electrical stimuli. Electroencephalogr Clin Neurophysiol 88:280–9

Kwong KK, Belliveau JW, Chesler DA, Goldberg IE, Weisskoff RM, Poncelet BP, et al. (1992) Dynamic magnetic resonance imaging of human brain activity during primary sensory stimulation. Proc Natl Acad Sci USA 89:5675–9

Laufs H, Krakow K, Sterzer P, Eger E, Beyerle A, Salek-Haddadi A, et al. (2003) Electroencephalographic signatures of attentional and cognitive default modes in spontaneous brain activity fluctuations at rest. Proc Natl Acad Sci USA 100:11053–8

Lee AT, Glover GH, Meyer CH (1995) Discrimination of large venous vessels in time-course spiral blood-oxygen-level-dependent magnetic-resonance functional neuroimaging. Magn Reson Med 33:745–54

Lee MC, Mouraux A, Iannetti GD. Characterizing the cortical activity through which pain emerges from nociception. J Neurosci. 2009 Jun 17;29(24):7909–16

Lemieux L, Allen PJ, Franconi F, Symms MR, Fish DR (1997) Recording of EEG during fMRI experiments: patient safety. Magn Reson Med 38:943–52

Lewis T, Ponchin EE (1937) The double pain response of the human skin to a single stimulus. Clin Sci 3:67–76

Lui F, Duzzi D, Corradini M, Serafini M, Baraldi P, Porro CA (2008) Touch or pain? Spatio-temporal patterns of cortical fMRI activity following brief mechanical stimuli. Pain 138(2):362–74

Malonek D, Grinvald A (1996) Interactions between electrical activity and cortical microcirculation revealed by imaging spectroscopy: implications for functional brain mapping. Science 272:551–4

Mayhew SD, Iannetti GD, Woolrich MW, Wise RG (2006) Automated single-trial measurement of amplitude and latency of laser-evoked potentials (LEPs) using multiple linear regression. Clin Neurophysiol 117:1331–44

Melzack R (1999) From the gate to the neuromatrix. Pain (Suppl) 6:S121–6

Menon RS, Goodyear BG (2001) Spatial and temporal resolution in fMRI. In: Jezzard P, Matthews PM, Smith SM (eds) Functional MRI: an introduction to methods. Oxford University Press, Oxford, pp 145–58

Michel CM, Murray MM, Lantz G, Gonzalez S, Spinelli L, Grave De Peralta R (2004) EEG source imaging. Clin Neurophysiol 115:2195–222

Mouraux A, Guerit JM, Plaghki L (2004) Refractoriness cannot explain why C-fiber laser-evoked brain potentials are recorded only if concomitant Adelta-fiber activation is avoided. Pain 112:16–26

Mouraux A, Iannetti GD (2008a) A review of the evidence against the "first come first served" hypothesis. Comment on Truini et al. [Pain 2007;131:43–7]. Pain 136:219–21; author reply 222–3

Mouraux A, Iannetti GD. Across-trial averaging of event-related EEG responses and beypnd. Magn Reson Imaging. 2008 Sep; 26 (7) : 1041–54. Review.

Mouraux and Iannetti 2009 ("Nociceptive laser-evoked brain potentials do not reflect nociceptive-specific neural activity. J Neurophysiol. 2009 Jun; 101 (6) : 3258–69. Epub 2009 Apr 1)

Mulert C, Jager L, Schmitt R, Bussfeld P, Pogarell O, Moller HJ, et al. (2004) Integration of fMRI and simultaneous EEG: towards a comprehensive understanding of localization and time-course of brain activity in target detection. Neuroimage 22:83–94

Naka D, Kakigi R (1998) Simple and novel method for measuring conduction velocity of A delta fibers in humans. J Clin Neurophysiol 15:150–3

Nebel K, Stude P, Wiese H, Muller B, de Greiff A, Forsting M, et al. (2005) Sparse imaging and continuous event-related fMRI in the visual domain: a systematic comparison. Hum Brain Mapp 24:130–43

Niazy RK (2006) Simultaneous electroencephalography and functional MRI: methods and applications (doctoral dissertation). University of Oxford, Oxford

Niazy RK, Beckmann CF, Iannetti GD, Brady JM, Smith SM (2005) Removal of FMRI environment artefacts from EEG data using optimal basis sets. Neuroimage 28:720–37

Nunez PL, Srinivasan R (2006) Electric fields of the brain. The neurophysics of EEG. Oxford University Press, New York

Ogawa S, Tank DW, Menon R, Ellermann JM, Kim SG, Merkle H, et al. (1992) Intrinsic signal changes accompanying sensory stimulation: functional brain mapping with magnetic resonance imaging. Proc Natl Acad Sci U S A 89:5951–5

Ozcan M, Baumgartner U, Vucurevic G, Stoeter P, Treede RD (2005) Spatial resolution of fMRI in the human parasylvian cortex: comparison of somatosensory and auditory activation. Neuroimage 25:877–87

Peyron R, Garcia-Larrea L, Gregoire MC, Costes N, Convers P, Lavenne F, et al. (1999) Haemodynamic brain responses to acute pain in humans: sensory and attentional networks. Brain 122 (Pt 9):1765–80

Plaghki L, Mouraux A (2003) How do we selectively activate skin nociceptors with a high power infrared laser? Physiology and biophysics of laser stimulation. Neurophysiol Clin 33:269–77

Ploner M, Gross J, Timmermann L, Schnitzler A (2002) Cortical representation of first and second pain sensation in humans. Proc Natl Acad Sci USA 99:12444–8

Purves AM, Boyd SG (1993) Time-shifted averaging for laser evoked potentials. Electroencephalogr Clin Neurophysiol 88:118–22

Raij TT, Vartiainen NV, Jousmaki V, Hari R (2003) Effects of interstimulus interval on cortical responses to painful laser stimulation. J Clin Neurophysiol 20:73–9

Regan D (1989) Human brain electrophysiology. Evoked potentials and evoked magnetic fields in science and medicine. Elsevier, New York

Robson MD, Dorosz JL, Gore JC (1998) Measurements of the temporal fMRI response of the human auditory cortex to trains of tones. Neuroimage 7:185–98

Rogers R, Wise RG, Painter DJ, Longe SE, Tracey I (2004) An investigation to dissociate the analgesic and anesthetic properties of ketamine using functional magnetic resonance imaging. Anesthesiology 100:292–301

Slugg RM, Campbell JN, Meyer RA (2004) The population response of A- and C-fiber nociceptors in monkey encodes high-intensity mechanical stimuli. J Neurosci 24:4649–56

Speckmann E, Elger C (1999) Introduction to the neurophysiological basis of the EEG and DC potentials. In: Niedermeyer E, Lopes Da Silva F (eds) Electroencephalography: basic principles, clinical applications, and related fields. Lippincott, Williams & Wilkins, Baltimore, pp 15–27

Tarkka IM, Treede RD (1993) Equivalent electrical source analysis of pain-related somatosensory evoked potentials elicited by a CO_2 laser. J Clin Neurophysiol 10:513–9

Tracey I, Mantyh PW (2007) The cerebral signature for pain perception and its modulation. Neuron 55:377–91

Treede RD, Kief S, Holzer T, Bromm B (1998) Late somatosensory evoked cerebral potentials in response to cutaneous heat stimuli. Electroencephalogr Clin Neurophysiol 70:429–41

Treede RD, Lorenz J, Baumgartner U (2003) Clinical usefulness of laser-evoked potentials. Neurophysiol Clin 33:303–14

Treede RD, Meyer RA, Campbell JN (1998) Myelinated mechanically insensitive afferents from monkey hairy skin: heat-response properties. J Neurophysiol 80:1082–93

Treede RD, Meyer RA, Raja SN, Campbell JN (1995) Evidence for two different heat transduction mechanisms in nociceptive primary afferents innervating monkey skin. J Physiol 483(Pt 3): 747–58

Truini A, Galeotti F, Romaniello A, Virtuoso M, Iannetti GD, Cruccu G (2005) Laser-evoked potentials: normative values. Clin Neurophysiol 116:821–6

Truini A, Rossi P, Galeotti F, Romaniello A, Virtuoso M, De Lena C, et al. (2004) Excitability of the Adelta nociceptive pathways as assessed by the recovery cycle of laser evoked potentials in humans. Exp Brain Res 155:120–3

Wehrle R, Kaufmann C, Wetter TC, Holsboer F, Auer DP, Pollmacher T, et al. (2007) Functional microstates within human REM sleep: first evidence from fMRI of a thalamocortical network specific for phasic REM periods. Eur J Neurosci 25:863–71

Wise RG, Rogers R, Painter D, Bantick S, Ploghaus A, Williams P, et al. (2002) Combining fMRI with a pharmacokinetic model to determine which brain areas activated by painful stimulation are specifically modulated by remifentanil. Neuroimage 16:999–1014

Mouraux A, Iannetti GD. Across-trial averaging of event-related EEG responses and beyond. Magn Reson Imaging. 2008 Sep;26(7):1041-54. Review.

Simultaneous EEG and fMRI of the Human Auditory System

19

Christoph S. Herrmann, Andre Brechmann, and Henning Scheich

1
Introduction

While attempting to examine the physiological correlates of human cognitive functions, neuroscientists are restricted to noninvasive measures when dealing with healthy subjects. Correlates of cognitive brain processes are present in electromagnetic fields and haemodynamic responses that can be recorded with electroencephalography (EEG) and functional magnetic resonance imaging (fMRI), respectively. While EEG offers a temporal resolution on the millisecond timescale, intracranial sources of activity must be inferred from extracranial recordings—a phenomenon referred to as the inverse problem. fMRI offers spatial resolution on the millimetre scale but suffers from a suboptimal temporal resolution, since the blood oxygen level dependent (BOLD) signal is an indirect haemodynamic consequence of electrical brain activity.

Combining EEG and fMRI is an approach that promises to integrate the good temporal resolution of EEG with the good spatial resolution of fMRI (for recent reviews, see Debener et al. 2006; Herrmann and Debener (2007); Menon and Crottaz-Herbette 2005). However, it should be noted that some authors have questioned the implicit assumption that both measures pick up more or less the same neural activity. A number of studies have demonstrated that EEG and BOLD responses do not reflect identical neural activity, resulting in the notion of EEG signals without fMRI correlates, and vice versa (Ritter and Villringer 2006).

EEG and fMRI setups are both complicated technical environments that require sophisticated hard- and software as well as skilled personnel for operation. Thus, even slight disturbances such as a nearby electromechanical device in EEG or metal parts inside the MR scanner can result in severe artefacts and corrupted signal quality. Therefore, the recording of EEG signals inside the MR scanner certainly compromises EEG signal quality (e.g. Warbrick and Bagshaw 2008) and can also affect the quality of MR images (e.g. Mullinger et al. 2008).

C. S. Herrmann (✉)
Department of Biological Psychology, Otto-von-Guericke University, PO box 4120, 39016 Magdeburg, Germany
e-mail: christoph.herrmann@ovgu.de

C. Mulert and L. Lemieux (eds.), *EEG–fMRI*
DOI: 10.1007/978-3-540-87919-0_19, © Springer Verlag Berlin Heidelberg 2010

Two types of artefacts obscure EEG data when recording inside an MR scanner. The first is the so-called cardioballistic artefact. This refers to the cardiac cycle and its amplitude scales in proportion to the magnetic field strength (Debener et al. 2008). It is commonly agreed that the cardioballistic artefact is related to the pulsatile movement of the head and/or the pulsatile movement of EEG electrodes. It is therefore also referred to as the pulse artefact. EEG electrodes and EEG leads are conductive, and the movement of conductive material in a static magnetic field induces a current that is picked up by the EEG. Numerous articles deal with this artefact and offer effective mechanisms to correct it (e.g. Bonmassar et al. 2002; Debener et al. 2007; Ellingson et al. 2004; Niazy et al. 2005).

The second type of artefact is caused by MRI gradient switching and radiofrequency (RF) pulses and is referred to as gradient artefact (GA). This artefact is limited to the time required to acquire the images. For many purposes, the GA can be avoided through the interleaved data recording of EEG and fMRI (see the section on sparse sampling below). However, even in the case of temporally overlapping EEG recording and acquisition of MR slices, the artefact can be corrected by adequate software algorithms (e.g. Allen et al. 2000; Felblinger et al. 1999; Ritter et al. 2007; Sijbersa et al. 2000).

Despite the feasibility and elegance of simultaneously recording EEG and BOLD responses, and the potential insights to be gained by this method, it should be noted that many research questions do not require such a technically challenging approach. Whenever it is sufficient to have subjects perform a task twice, it is much more convenient to perform the two types of recordings separately. In many cases, one of the two measurements may suffice to answer relevant research questions.

2
Specifics of Auditory Recordings

The scanner environment is especially unsuitable for auditory experiments requiring a number of special hardware and software solutions. There are at least three problems specific to auditory experiments, which are addressed in subsequent sections:

- The static magnetic field interferes with auditory equipment
- The transient magnetic fields generate noise that interferes with auditory perception
- The scanner noise generates a BOLD response that needs to be distinguished from the auditory response to the acoustic stimuli

Further details of problems with auditory experiments inside MR scanners are discussed in valuable review articles (McJury and Shellock 2000; Moelker and Pattynama 2003; Palmer et al. 2006).

2.1
Interference of the Static Magnetic Field

To begin with, there is a strong magnetic field that precludes the use of standard auditory equipment such as headphones. The static magnetic fields of commercially available scanners currently range from 1 to 7 T. Ferromagnetic devices cannot be brought into the scanner since they would be attracted by the magnet, potentially resulting in accidents. Thus, standard headphones with metallic leads cannot be operated inside a scanner. In addition, the transient magnetic fields used for slice selection and readout would induce currents in metallic leads that, in turn, would produce undesirable sounds in the headphones. A preliminary but suboptimal solution has been the design of air-pressure devices, such as those already used in magnetoencephalography (MEG). Unfortunately, these devices sometimes show problems such as asymmetric levels. Meanwhile, a number of special sound delivery devices have been designed that can cope with the hostile conditions and are sufficiently precise for auditory experiments (Baumgart et al. 1998; Palmer et al. 1998).

2.2
Interference of Transient Magnetic Fields

More importantly, the sound created by the scanner interferes with the perception of auditory stimuli. The flow of electric currents induces a magnetic field surrounding the conductor. If the conductor lies within a magnetic field, a force acts upon the conductor, the so-called Lorentz force. This is the case for the gradient coil of an MR scanner that generates the transient magnetic fields for slice selection and readout. The Lorentz force deforms the gradient coils. This deformation spreads to the surrounding air, generating a noise similar to when the membrane of a loudspeaker is being moved (Mansfield et al. 1998). This scanner noise relates to the field strength of the scanner (Price et al. 2001) and usually exceeds 100 dB SPL (sound pressure level), requiring protection for the subjects' ears using earplugs and/or appropriate headphones to avoid damage to the hearing system.

However, even after significant suppression, the remaining noise still interferes with auditory perception. It has been demonstrated that the noise from the MR scanner's echo planar imaging (EPI) sequences results in significant changes in a subjects' auditory MEG responses during an auditory experiment (Herrmann et al. 2000), and similar findings have been obtained for event-related potentials (ERP) (Novitski et al. 2001, 2003). Thus, specific suitable experimental paradigms must be designed for recording inside a MR scanner. Two suggestions for such a design are given below.

2.3
BOLD Response to Scanner Noise

Another problem for auditory fMRI experiments is the fact that the scanner noise results in a BOLD response. Bandettini et al. (1998) contrasted images that were taken after a scanning period with others that were preceded by silence. The results showed an activation of the primary auditory cortex due to the scanner noise. It was subsequently shown using an auditory discrimination task that when the MR scanner noise was present (due to slice acquisition) it was modulating the BOLD response in auditory cortex (Shah et al. 1999). By investigating the time course of the scanner noise activating the auditory cortices, Hall et al. (2000) were able to demonstrate that primary and secondary auditory cortex showed peaks 4–5 s after stimulus onset that decayed after a further 5–8 s. This time course indicates that noise contamination in auditory designs can be substantially reduced by using long repetition times of about 9–13 s.

It should be noted that scanner noise also poses a problem for non-auditory experiments. For example, BOLD responses in the visual cortex have been reported to decrease by 50% during the presence of scanner noise (Cho et al. 1998).

2.4
Sparse Sampling

A potential solution to the problem of scanner noise could be to present stimuli during silent periods of the scanning protocol, as suggested by Hall et al. (2000). The noise is only audible when the scanner is actually scanning a volume of the brain. However, the scanning procedure does not need to be continuous; it can be performed intermittently in order to allow silent periods for stimulation. Since the BOLD response lags the electrical brain response by about 6 s, there is the possibility of presenting an auditory stimulus in silence. The lagging BOLD response for the same trial is recorded subsequent to generating the described noise. This approach was initially developed for auditory fMRI acquisition. However, it also offers the possibility of recording the EEG response during silence, and hence in the absence of gradient artefacts. This procedure is illustrated in Fig. 1 and has been called sparse sampling (Hall et al. 1999) or clustered acquisition (Edmister et al. 1999).

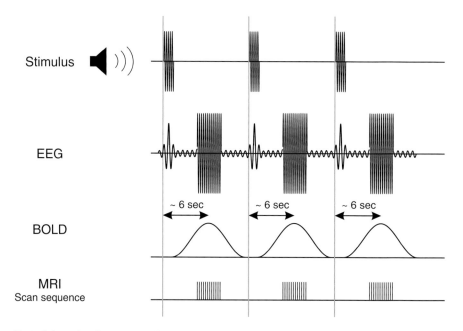

Fig. 1 Schematic of sparse sampling. The MRI scan sequence is not continuous but sparse (*bottom trace*). This allows the presentation of auditory stimuli in silence (*top trace*), i.e. interleaved with the MR scanner noise. In addition, this provides the opportunity to record the EEG response (e.g. an ERP) while there are no scanner artefacts in the EEG. The lagging BOLD response to the same stimuli can then be recorded after a few seconds, creating noise and EEG artefacts. However, these are not as disturbing as if they were simultaneous to the presentation of auditory stimuli and EEG recording

Sparse sampling has been repeatedly applied in auditory experiments, revealing numerous phenomena of the auditory cortex (Gaab et al. 2003; Müller et al. 2003; Tanaka et al. 2000; Zaehle et al. 2004).

Conventional sparse sampling results in a lack of temporal information on the BOLD signal, because one volume is scanned after each stimulus presentation. It has been proposed that the stimulus presentation time should be jittered with respect to the time at which image acquisition begins (Belin et al.1999). Enhanced temporal resolution is also offered by a new interleaved imaging protocol (Schwarzbauer et al. 2006). In addition, a new clustered version of sparse sampling provides better statistical results than conventional sparse sampling (Zaehle et al. 2007).

2.5
Silent fMRI Acquisition

A different solution to the problem of scanner noise interfering with auditory experiments lies in suppressing the noise in the first place. As described above, the noise stems from the transient magnetic fields—the so-called gradients—and gets louder along with a stronger transient (Moelker et al. 2003). On the one hand, this poses a problem due to the constantly increasing field strengths of MR scanners. On the other hand, it offers a handle on how to tackle the problem. The noise is generated by the Lorentz forces due to gradient currents. Hennel et al. (1999) used this knowledge to suggest an approach for reducing scanner noise. They used sinusoidal instead of rectangular gradient slopes, reducing the number of harmonics in the spectrum, and a longer gradient duration, thus reducing the steepness of the gradient. This resulted in a reduction in scanner noise by 40 dBA for spin-echo and gradient-echo pulse sequences whose harmonics are audible (the fundamental gradient frequencies below 100 Hz are barely audible). However, it was not as successful for faster EPI or FLASH (fast low-angle shot) sequences, which have a fundamental gradient frequency that is already in the audible range and so suppression of the harmonics is not as effective. Another approach is to use simultaneous multislice excitation (SIMEX) sequences that acquire multiple slices with one multifrequency RF pulse, resulting in fewer pulses per scan (Loenneker et al. 2001). While the SIMEX sequences were applied as a block design, Yang et al. (2000) carried out an event-related silent sequence, revealing a 54% signal increase as compared to a conventional technique, and suggesting tonotopic maps within Heschl's gyrus. Amaro et al. (2002) compared conventional and silent acquisition protocols as well as a block design and an event-related design, demonstrating that the silent event-related design yielded maximal BOLD responses to a single auditory cue. Low-noise FLASH sequences were applied to demonstrate central functions of the auditory system, such as sound-level dependence (Brechmann et al. 2002).

2.6
Adjusting Auditory Stimulus Frequencies

The sound produced by the scanner is like a complex tone (cf. Fig. 2). A typical EPI sequence has a spectral peak at the switching periodicity of the magnetic transients, plus harmonics and subharmonics that lie within the frequency range of 500–5,000 Hz (Hedeen

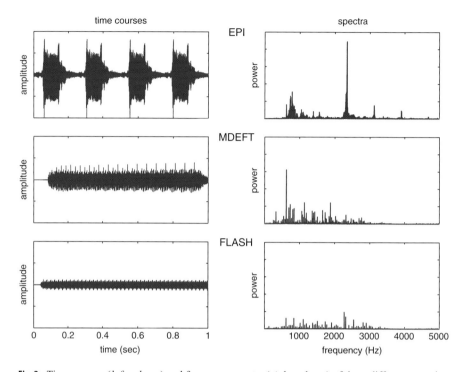

Fig. 2 Time courses (*left column*) and frequency spectra (*right column*) of three different scanning protocols. Echo planar imaging (EPI) has a sharp peak in the audible frequency range. MDEFT (modified driven-equilibrium Fourier tomography) has a lower cut-off frequency and reduced power. Low-noise FLASH is the quietest of the three sequences

and Edelstein 1997; Counter et al. 2000). Unfortunately, this is also the frequency range of human speech and of many auditory stimuli. Thus, the scanner noise could selectively influence the stimuli that fall within the same frequency range through a process called masking (Brosch et al. 1999). Novitski et al. (2006) were able to demonstrate this effect by recording MEG in a pitch change detection task and comparing a silent background to simulated scanner noise. The authors were able to show that the amplitude of the mismatch negativity (MMN) reflecting the automatic detection of the pitch change is only affected by scanner noise when it overlaps spectrally with the auditory stimulus. This is a potential explanation of findings by Le et al. (2001), who discovered that the perception of sine tones was reduced when they overlapped spectrally with scanner noise.

Importantly, these results offer another approach to auditory fMRI experiments. MR sequences could be designed in such a way as not to overlap with the auditory stimuli in an experiment. However, this method is probably only feasible in research environments where MR physicists are capable of programming their own sequences. In a clinical setting, another approach is more promising. The scanner noise of the available scanning sequences can easily be recorded on a digital sound recorder. Please note that special caution must be applied to ensure that ferromagnetic devices are not brought close to the scanner! A Fourier transform can be used to analyse the frequency spectrum of the scanner noise, and stimuli can be designed to lie outside the main peaks of the spectrum.

This method seems especially appropriate when the design of the experiment excludes the possibility of applying sparse sampling. This would, for example, be the case when trying to implement n-back working memory tasks with fixed latencies (e.g. Brechmann et al. 2007), or when investigating auditory streaming that requires a certain amount of time to build up (e.g. Micheyl et al. 2007).

3
Simultaneous EEG and fMRI in Auditory Experiments

In order to avoid the abovementioned obstacles to recording EEG inside a MRI scanner, a number of early studies have recorded EEG and BOLD responses from the same subjects in two separate EEG and fMRI recording sessions.

Menon et al. (1997) analysed P3, an ERP, in response to rare target stimuli in order to investigate processes of auditory target detection. They were able to demonstrate that the dipole locations of the inverse solution for P3 coincided with the maximum BOLD activations within the temporoparietal cortex. Subsequently, a second group analysed P3a, an ERP response to novel auditory stimuli, and found foci in the superior temporal gyrus (Opitz et al. 1999). Later that same year, a third group analysed P3 in response to auditory as well as visual targets and was able to describe a whole network of brain regions involved in target processing (Linden et al. 1999). This research led to the method of "fMRI-constrained source modelling" for EEG as well as MEG (Fujimaki et al. 2002). Numerous studies have applied similar approaches in auditory experiments (e.g. Doeller et al. 2003; Opitz et al. 2002; Crottaz-Herbette and Menon 2006).

A further important method involves carrying out parametric studies separately in EEG and fMRI, and then correlating the EEG and BOLD responses in order to find out which of them co-varies with respect to the same parameter. This approach has been applied by Horovitz et al. (2002) in an auditory oddball paradigm, and it revealed that the BOLD response in some brain regions (e.g. supramarginal gyrus and right medial frontal gyrus) co-varies with P3 amplitude, while other regions (ACC) are activated by targets but show no signs of co-variation.

One point of criticism in relation to separate recording protocols is that it appears to be impossible to control whether a subject performs in exactly the same manner in both experiments (Debener et al. 2006). For separate recordings, it seems necessary to test for order of session effects. In numerous psychophysiological studies, these tests have revealed significant differences depending on whether subjects performed an experiment for the first time or repeated a known experimental paradigm in a second session. This is easily conceivable for paradigms explicitly investigating learning and memory processes. One should note that even the most basic perceptual and cognitive operations can also show signs of adaptation over time, so that temporal aspects of sessions or the order of trials should be taken into account. A further criticism is that even minor changes in an experimental setup can result in significant changes in the subjects' behavioural and physiological responses. For example, changing a subject from a seated upright position, as is common in EEG recordings, into a supine position, which is necessary for fMRI scanners, may influence physiological responses and behaviour.

In order to overcome the problems of separate recordings, EEG and BOLD responses have been recorded simultaneously. The first such study of the auditory system applied the abovementioned approach of correlating the parametric variation of an ERP component with the BOLD response in a simultaneous recording (Liebenthal et al. 2003). The authors were able to identify brain regions where the BOLD response co-varied with the strength of the MMN. Subsequently, another group set out to investigate P3 during target processing, revealing an enhancement for targets concurrent with increased BOLD activity in the temporoparietal junction, frontal areas, and the insula (Mulert et al. 2004). Scarff et al. (2004) have used simultaneous recordings of EEG and BOLD responses in order to compare the anatomical locations of the N1 generators. Source reconstruction of ERP data revealed dipole locations in the superior temporal gyrus that coincided with the centre of gravity of the BOLD responses. However, the authors also reported some differences between ERP dipoles and BOLD activity in terms of asymmetry and the inferior–superior axis of the brain. Otzenberger et al. (2005) further extended previous findings by showing that different P3 components such as target P3 and novelty P3 could be discriminated in a simultaneous recording, a finding that has recently been replicated (Strobel et al. 2008). Another study investigated the influence of task difficulty on MMN amplitude and fMRI activation (Sabri et al. 2006). The authors were able to show that the superior temporal gyrus and sulcus were more strongly activated in the difficult auditory task. By combining a current source density reconstruction of ERP data and simultaneously recorded BOLD responses, Mulert et al. (2005) were able to demonstrate that both measures revealed a dependence upon the sound level of auditory stimuli. Recently, Debener et al. (2007) showed how three different methods of artefact removal in simultaneous recordings differentially affect both auditory N1 amplitude and signal-to-noise ratio (SNR).

Lately, a very important aspect of simultaneous recordings has been addressed: the analysis of single-trial data. Due to the parallel acquisition of EEG and BOLD responses, parameters of the two measurements can be correlated across single trials, potentially leading to a better understanding of the coupling of the two (Debener et al. 2006). It has been convincingly demonstrated that the amplitude of ERP components varies systematically over time, reflecting cognitive processes, and that this variation can be used to identify those brain regions where the BOLD contrast shows the same variation (Eichele et al. 2005). In a similar way, Benar et al. (2007) were able to demonstrate that the amplitude of P3 correlated positively with BOLD activity in the ACC, which is believed to reflect attentional processes. In addition, a negative correlation of P3 latency with BOLD activity in medial frontal regions probably reflects processes of action planning or performance monitoring, since P3 latency was also negatively correlated with subjects' reaction times.

4
Low-Noise fMRI Sequences for Simultaneous Experiments

In a recent experiment, we conducted a simultaneous recording where functional imaging was performed by adapting a conventional FLASH sequence using long gradient-ramp rise times (2,500 μs). This reduced the scanner noise to a quasi-continuous sound of 54 dB

SPL peak amplitude (Thaerig et al. 2008). The MRI measurement was performed on a 3 T head scanner (Bruker MEDSPEC 30/60). Four slices of 8 mm thickness oriented parallel to the Sylvian fissure were collected, covering the superior temporal plane in both hemispheres. The low-noise imaging protocol applied was introduced by Scheich et al. (1998). The volume acquisition time was 10.5 s. Breaks of 200 ms were inserted to improve gradient artefact detection during analysis. EEG was recorded simultaneously with a BrainAmp MR+ in a block-design fashion.

The observed AEPs show the typical, expected morphology (cf. Fig. 3): a P1 was followed by an N1 and a P2. The strongest N1 as well as P2 responses were observed at frontocentral electrodes. The peak-to-peak amplitude of the N1–P2 complex was enhanced for 80 dB HL stimulation (13.5 ± 2.1 µV) compared to 60 dB HL (10.6 ± 1.8 µV; $T(5) = 4.35, p < 0.01$). Thus, we were able to replicate the level dependency that had already been demonstrated in numerous EEG studies outside the scanner (Beagley and Knight 1967; Rapin et al. 1966). In addition, our approach of using low-noise sequences proved useful for simultaneously recording EEG during an auditory fMRI experiment.

However, due to the long duration of the acquisition of a single volume (10.5 s), many volumes were contaminated by movement artefacts enhanced by the metallic electrodes. Thus, half of the participants had to be excluded from further analysis. For the remaining

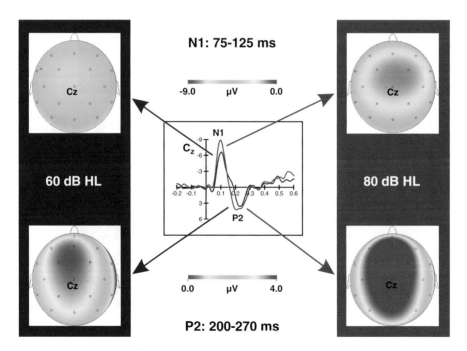

Fig. 3 Auditory event-related potentials recorded simultaneously with the BOLD response during MR scanning. The N1 component of the ERP shows the typical dependence upon sound level, i.e. larger amplitudes for higher sound pressure (80 dB HL) compared to 60 dB HL. Topographic maps reveal the strong resemblance of ERPs recorded outside the scanner (adapted from Thäerig et al. 2008)

three participants for whom the data could be analysed, BOLD responses were found in predefined regions of interest in the auditory cortex. Figure 4 displays the BOLD activations of those three single subjects in response to 60 dB HL and 80 dB HL FM tones. BOLD responses covered auditory areas TA, T1, T2, and T3 (Brechmann and Scheich 2005), which included Heschl's gyrus and planum temporale. On a descriptive level, BOLD responses were enhanced for 80 dB HL vs. 60 dB HL stimulation. This was the case for both the number of voxels and the amplitude of the BOLD signal. The BOLD effect was pronounced over the right hemisphere.

Our fMRI findings are compatible with the notion that the BOLD signal captures the stimulus-evoked auditory processes more reliably when recorded via low-noise sequences. This was also suggested by fMRI experiments that either used low-noise or EPI sequences to study sound level dependence. Jäncke et al. (1998) used EPI sequences and only found increases in the number of activated voxels, while Brechmann et al. (2002) found increases in both signal amplitude and the number of activated voxels when using low-noise sequences.

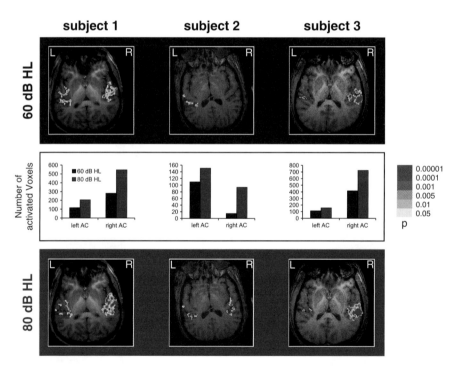

Fig. 4 The fMRI activation of the auditory cortex in response to 60 dB HL (*top row*) and 80 dB HL (*bottom row*) FM tones in three individual subjects. The amplitude of the BOLD signal is enhanced in response to 80 dB HL tones. *Middle row*: The number of activated voxels in the auditory region of interest demonstrated an enhancement in 80 dB (*red*) vs. 60 dB (*blue*) tones (adapted from Thäerig et al. 2008)

5
Conclusions

In this chapter, we have discussed the problems of simultaneously recording EEG and BOLD responses in auditory experiments, and we introduced potential solutions. Because sparse sampling avoids both the interfering noise from the scanner and the gradient arte-fact in EEG, it represents a good option for auditory experiments. Due to the fact that the scanner noise can mask even subsequent auditory stimuli, it seems advantageous to design auditory stimuli in such a way as not to overlap spectrally with the scanner noise. Our own data found silent scanning sequences to be well suited for EEG analysis. However, fMRI data had to be excluded from half of the subjects due to strong movement artefacts during the long acquisition time required for one volume scan (10.5 s). A combination of silent sequences using intermediate acquisition times with sparse sampling to avoid gradient artefacts will probably offer better results still.

References

Allen PJ, Josephs O, Turner R (2000) A method for removing imaging artifact from continuous EEG recorded during functional MRI. Neuroimage 12(2):230–239

Amaro E Jr, Williams SC, Shergill SS, Fu CH, MacSweeney M, Picchioni MM, Brammer MJ, McGuire PK (2002) Acoustic noise and functional magnetic resonance imaging: current strate-gies and future prospects. J Magn Reson Imaging 16(5):497–510

Bandettini PA, Jesmanowicz A, Van Kylen J, Birn RM, Hyde JS (1998) Functional MRI of brain activation induced by scanner acoustic noise. Magn Reson Med 39(3):410–416

Baumgart F, Kaulisch T, Tempelmann C, Gaschler-Markefski B, Tegeler C, Schindler F, Stiller D, Scheich H (1998) Electrodynamic headphones and woofers for application in magnetic reso-nance imaging scanners. Med Phys 25(10):2068–2070

Beagley HA, Knight JJ (1967) Changes in auditory evoked response with intensity. J Laryngol Otol 81(8):861–873

Belin P, Zatorre RJ, Hoge R, Evans AC, Pike B (1999) Event-related fMRI of the auditory cortex. Neuroimage 10(4):417–429

Bénar CG, Schön D, Grimault S, Nazarian B, Burle B, Roth M, Badier JM, Marquis P, Liegeois-Chauvel C, Anton JL (2007) Single-trial analysis of oddball event-related potentials in simul-taneous EEG–fMRI. Hum Brain Mapp 28(7):602–613

Bonmassar G, Purdon PL, Jääskeläinen IP, Chiappa K, Solo V, Brown EN, Belliveau JW (2002) Motion and ballistocardiogram artifact removal for interleaved recording of EEG and EPs dur-ing MRI. Neuroimage 16(4):1127–1141

Brechmann A, Baumgart F, Scheich H (2002) Sound-level-dependent representation of frequency modulations in human auditory cortex: a low-noise fMRI study. J Neurophysiol 87(1):423–433

Brechmann A, Gaschler-Markefski B, Sohr M, Yoneda K, Kaulisch T, Scheich H (2007) Working memory specific activity in auditory cortex: potential correlates of sequential processing and maintenance. Cereb Cortex 17(11):2544–2552

Brechmann A, Scheich H (2005) Hemispheric shifts of sound representation in auditory cortex with conceptual listening. Cereb Cortex 15(5):578–587

Brosch M, Schulz A, Scheich H (1999) Processing of sound sequences in macaque auditory cortex: response enhancement. J Neurophysiol 82(3):1542–1559

Cho ZH, Chung SC, Lim DW, Wong EK (1998) Effects of the acoustic noise of the gradient systems on fMRI: a study on auditory, motor, and visual cortices. Magn Reson Med 39(2):331–335

Counter SA, Olofsson A, Borg E, Bjelke B, Häggström A, Grahn HF (2000) Analysis of magnetic resonance imaging acoustic noise generated by a 4.7 T experimental system. Acta Otolaryngol 120(6):739–743

Crottaz-Herbette S, Menon V (2006) Where and when the anterior cingulate cortex modulates attentional response: combined fMRI and ERP evidence. J Cogn Neurosci 18(5):766–780

Debener S, Mullinger KJ, Niazy RK, Bowtell RW (2008) Properties of the ballistocardiogram artefact as revealed by EEG recordings at 1.5, 3 and 7 T static magnetic field strength. Int J Psychophysiol 67(3):189–199

Debener S, Strobel A, Sorger B, Peters J, Kranczioch C, Engel AK, Goebel R (2007) Improved quality of auditory event-related potentials recorded simultaneously with 3-T fMRI: removal of the ballistocardiogram artefact. Neuroimage 34(2):587–597

Debener S, Ullsperger M, Siegel M, Engel AK (2006) Single-trial EEG–fMRI reveals the dynamics of cognitive function. Trends Cogn Sci 10(12):558–563

Doeller CF, Opitz B, Mecklinger A, Krick C, Reith W, Schröger E (2003) Prefrontal cortex involvement in preattentive auditory deviance detection: neuroimaging and electrophysiological evidence. Neuroimage 20(2):1270–1282

Edmister WB, Talavage TM, Ledden PJ, Weisskoff RM (1999) Improved auditory cortex imaging using clustered volume acquisitions. Hum Brain Mapp 7(2):89–97

Eichele T, Specht K, Moosmann M, Jongsma ML, Quiroga RQ, Nordby H, Hugdahl K (2005) Assessing the spatiotemporal evolution of neuronal activation with single-trial event-related potentials and functional MRI. Proc Natl Acad Sci USA 102(49):17798–17803

Ellingson ML, Liebenthal E, Spanaki MV, Prieto TE, Binder JR, Ropella KM (2004) Ballistocardiogram artifact reduction in the simultaneous acquisition of auditory ERPS and fMRI. Neuroimage 22(4):1534–1542

Felblinger J, Slotboom J, Kreis R, Jung B, Boesch C (1999) Restoration of electrophysiological signals distorted by inductive effects of magnetic field gradients during MR sequences. Magn Reson Med 41(4):715–721

Fujimaki N, Hayakawa T, Nielsen M, Knösche TR, Miyauchi S (2002) An fMRI-constrained MEG source analysis with procedures for dividing and grouping activation. Neuroimage 17(1):324–343

Gaab N, Gaser C, Zaehle T, Jancke L, Schlaug G (2003) Functional anatomy of pitch memory-an fMRI study with sparse temporal sampling. Neuroimage 19(4):1417–1426

Hall DA, Haggard MP, Akeroyd MA, Palmer AR, Summerfield AQ, Elliott MR, Gurney EM, Bowtell RW (1999) "Sparse" temporal sampling in auditory fMRI. Hum Brain Mapp 7(3):213–223

Hall DA, Summerfield AQ, Gonçalves MS, Foster JR, Palmer AR, Bowtell RW (2000) Time-course of the auditory BOLD response to scanner noise. Magn Reson Med 43(4):601–606

Hedeen RA, Edelstein WA (1997) Characterization and prediction of gradient acoustic noise in MR imagers. Magn Reson Med 37(1):7–10

Hennel F, Girard F, Loenneker T (1999) "Silent" MRI with soft gradient pulses. Magn Reson Med 42(1):6–10

Herrmann CS, Oertel U, Wang Y, Maess B, Friederici AD (2000) Noise affects auditory and linguistic processing differently: an MEG study. Neuroreport 11(2):227–229

Herrmann CS, Debener S (2007) Simultaneous recording of EEG and BOLD responses: a historical perspective. Int J Psychophysiol 67(3):161–168.

Horovitz SG, Skudlarski P, Gore JC (2002) Correlations and dissociations between BOLD signal and P300 amplitude in an auditory oddball task: a parametric approach to combining fMRI and ERP. Magn Reson Imaging 20(4):319–325

Jäncke L, Shah NJ, Posse S, Grosse-Ryuken M, Müller-Gärtner HW (1998) Intensity coding of auditory stimuli: an fMRI study. Neuropsychologia 3 (9):875–883

Le TH, Patel S, Roberts TP (2001) Functional MRI of human auditory cortex using block and event-related designs. Magn Reson Med 45(2):254–260

Liebenthal E, Ellingson ML, Spanaki MV, Prieto TE, Ropella KM, Binder JR (2003) Simultaneous ERP and fMRI of the auditory cortex in a passive oddball paradigm. Neuroimage 19(4): 1395–1404

Linden DE, Prvulovic D, Formisano E, Völlinger M, Zanella FE, Goebel R, Dierks T (1999) The functional neuroanatomy of target detection: an fMRI study of visual and auditory oddball tasks. Cereb Cortex 9(8):815–823

Loenneker T, Hennel F, Ludwig U, Hennig J (2001) Silent BOLD imaging. MAGMA 13(2):76–81

Mansfield P, Glover PM, Beaumont J (1998) Sound generation in gradient coil structures for MRI. Magn Reson Med 39(4):539–550

McJury M, Shellock FG (2000) Auditory noise associated with MR procedures: a review. J Magn Reson Imaging 12(1):37–45

Menon V, Crottaz-Herbette S (2005) Combined EEG and fMRI studies of human brain function. Int Rev Neurobiol 66:291–321

Menon V, Ford JM, Lim KO, Glover GH, Pfefferbaum A (1997) Combined event-related fMRI and EEG evidence for temporal-parietal cortex activation during target detection. Neuroreport 8(14):3029–3037.

Micheyl C, Carlyon RP, Gutschalk A, Melcher JR, Oxenham AJ, Rauschecker JP, Tian B, Courtenay Wilson E (2007) The role of auditory cortex in the formation of auditory streams. Hear Res 229(1–2):116–131

Moelker A, Pattynama PM (2003) Acoustic noise concerns in functional magnetic resonance imaging. Hum Brain Mapp 20(3):123–141

Moelker A, Wielopolski PA, Pattynama PM (2003) Relationship between magnetic field strength and magnetic-resonance-related acoustic noise levels. MAGMA 16(1):52–55

Mulert C, Jäger L, Propp S, Karch S, Störmann S, Pogarell O, Möller HJ, Juckel G, Hegerl U (2005) Sound level dependence of the primary auditory cortex: Simultaneous measurement with 61-channel EEG and fMRI. Neuroimage 28(1):49–58

Mulert C, Jäger L, Schmitt R, Bussfeld P, Pogarell O, Möller HJ, Juckel G, Hegerl U (2004) Integration of fMRI and simultaneous EEG: towards a comprehensive understanding of localization and time-course of brain activity in target detection. Neuroimage 22(1):83–94

Müller BW, Stude P, Nebel K, Wiese H, Ladd ME, Forsting M, Jueptner M (2003) Sparse imaging of the auditory oddball task with functional MRI. Neuroreport 14(12):1597–1601

Mullinger K, Debener S, Coxon R, Bowtell R (2008) Effects of simultaneous EEG recording on MRI data quality at 1.5, 3 and 7 Tesla. Int J Psychophysiol 67(3):178–188

Niazy RK, Beckmann CF, Iannetti GD, Brady JM, Smith SM (2005) Removal of FMRI environment artifacts from EEG data using optimal basis sets. Neuroimage 28(3):720–737

Novitski N, Alho K, Korzyukov O, Carlson S, Martinkauppi S, Escera C, Rinne T, Aronen HJ, Näätänen R (2001) Effects of acoustic gradient noise from functional magnetic resonance imaging on auditory processing as reflected by event-related brain potentials. Neuroimage 14(1 Pt 1):244–251

Novitski N, Anourova I, Martinkauppi S, Aronen HJ, Näätänen R, Carlson S (2003) Effects of noise from functional magnetic resonance imaging on auditory event-related potentials in working memory task. Neuroimage 20(2):1320–1328

Novitski N, Maess B, Tervaniemi M (2006) Frequency specific impairment of automatic pitch change detection by fMRI acoustic noise: An MEG study. J Neurosci Methods 155(1): 149–159

Opitz B, Mecklinger A, Friederici AD, von Cramon DY (1999) The functional neuroanatomy of novelty processing: integrating ERP and fMRI results. Cereb Cortex 9(4):379–391

Opitz B, Rinne T, Mecklinger A, von Cramon DY, Schröger E (2002) Differential contribution of frontal and temporal cortices to auditory change detection: fMRI and ERP results. Neuroimage 15(1):167–174

Otzenberger H, Gounot D, Foucher JR (2005) P300 recordings during event-related fMRI: a feasibility study. Cogn Brain Res 23(2-3):306–315.

Palmer AR, Bullock D, Chambers J (1998) A high output high quality sound system for use in auditory fMRI. Neuroiamge 7:S359

Palmer AR, Chambers J, Hall DA (2006) New fMRI methods for hearing and speech. Acoust Sci Tech 27(3):125–133

Price DL, De Wilde JP, Papadaki AM, Curran JS, Kitney RI (2001) Investigation of acoustic noise on 15 MRI scanners from 0.2 T to 3 T. J Magn Reson Imaging 13(2):288–293

Rapin I, Schimmel H, Tourk LM, Krasnegor NA, Pollak C (1966) Evoked responses to clicks and tones of varying intensity in waking adults. Electroencephalogr Clin Neurophysiol 21(4): 335–344

Ritter P, Becker R, Graefe C, Villringer A (2007) Evaluating gradient artifact correction of EEG data acquired simultaneously with fMRI. Magn Reson Imaging 25(6):923–932

Ritter P, Villringer A (2006) Simultaneous EEG–fMRI. Neurosci Biobehav Rev 30(6):823–838

Sabri M, Liebenthal E, Waldron EJ, Medler DA, Binder JR (2006) Attentional modulation in the detection of irrelevant deviance: a simultaneous ERP/fMRI study. J Cogn Neurosci 18(5): 689–700

Scarff CJ, Reynolds A, Goodyear BG, Ponton CW, Dort JC, Eggermont JJ (2004) Simultaneous 3-T fMRI and high-density recording of human auditory evoked potentials. Neuroimage 23(3): 1129–1142

Scheich H, Baumgart F, Gaschler-Markefski B, Tegeler C, Tempelmann C, Heinze HJ, Schindler F, Stiller D (1998) Functional magnetic resonance imaging of a human auditory cortex area involved in foreground–background decomposition. Eur J Neurosci 10(2):803–809

Schwarzbauer C, Davis MH, Rodd JM, Johnsrude I (2006) Interleaved silent steady state (ISSS) imaging: A new sparse imaging method applied to auditory fMRI. Neuroimage 29(3):774–782

Shah NJ, Jäncke L, Grosse-Ruyken ML, Müller-Gärtner HW (1999) Influence of acoustic masking noise in fMRI of the auditory cortex during phonetic discrimination. J Magn Reson Imaging 9(1):19–25

Sijbersa J, Van Audekerke J, Verhoye M, Van der Linden A, Van Dyck D (2000) Reduction of ECG and gradient related artifacts in simultaneously recorded human EEG/MRI data. Magn Reson Imaging 18(7):881–886

Strobel A, Debener S, Sorger B, Peters JC, Kranczioch C, Hoechstetter K, Engel AK, Brocke B, Goebel R (2008) Novelty and target processing during an auditory novelty oddball: a simultaneous event-related potential and functional magnetic resonance imaging study. Neuroimage 40(2):869–883.

Tanaka H, Fujita N, Watanabe Y, Hirabuki N, Takanashi M, Oshiro Y, Nakamura H (2000) Effects of stimulus rate on the auditory cortex using fMRI with "sparse" temporal sampling. Neuroreport 11(9):2045–2049

Thaerig S, Behne N, Schadow J, Lenz D, Scheich H, Brechmann A, Herrmann CS (2008) Sound level dependence of auditory evoked potentials: simultaneous EEG recording and low-noise fMRI. Int J Psychophysiol 67(3):235–241

Warbrick T, Bagshaw AP (2008) Scanning strategies for simultaneous EEG–fMRI evoked potential studies at 3 T. Int J Psychophysiol 67(3):169–177

Yang Y, Engelien A, Engelien W, Xu S, Stern E, Silbersweig DA (2000) A silent event-related functional MRI technique for brain activation studies without interference of scanner acoustic noise. Magn Reson Med 43(2):185–190

Zaehle T, Schmidt CF, Meyer M, Baumann S, Baltes C, Boesiger P, Jancke L (2007) Comparison of "silent" clustered and sparse temporal fMRI acquisitions in tonal and speech perception tasks. Neuroimage 37(4):1195–1204

Zaehle T, Wüstenberg T, Meyer M, Jäncke L (2004) Evidence for rapid auditory perception as the foundation of speech processing: a sparse temporal sampling fMRI study. Eur J Neurosci 20(9):2447–2456

Visual System

20

Robert Becker, Petra Ritter, and Arno Villringer

1
Simultaneous EEG–fMRI of the Visual System: Signal Quality

Combining both EEG and fMRI is still a challenging task. A large number of studies on the feasibility of EEG–fMRI for the visual system have been performed because it is an accessible and well-described system.

A general question when performing EEG–fMRI experiments is whether typical neural patterns of the visual system as measured by EEG, such as alpha rhythm or visual evoked potentials (VEPs), are modified by the strong static magnetic field inside the MR environment. Despite two studies reporting changed evoked potentials during exposure to the strong magnetic field of the MR environment (Bunkrad et al. 1989; Sammer et al. 2005), most other studies have reported typical evoked potentials (EPs) within the magnetic field, although without systematic comparison to non-MR EPs. Typical configurations have been shown for VEPs (Bonmassar et al. 1999; Kruggel et al. 2000; Muri et al. 1998; Negishi et al. 2004; Comi et al. 2005; Becker et al. 2005, see also Fig. 1) and for visual oddball P300 potentials (Otzenberger et al. 2005; Negishi et al. 2004). The recording of VEPs at high MR B_0 fields (4.7 T) was demonstrated for monkeys (Schmid et al. 2006). EEG source localisation was also shown to be feasible for EEG data from inside the MR tomograph by Bonmassar et al. (2001) and Im et al. (2006). Depending on whether EPs were recorded in an interleaved manner (i.e. during nonacquisition intervals of the MR sequence) or continuously, the data had to be corrected for either the ballistocardiogram (BCG) or for both BCG and MR imaging artefacts.

Another question is whether the imaging of metabolic responses is impaired by the EEG equipment inside the MR environment. Lazeyras et al. (2001) found that functional imaging during visual stimulation yielded similar activations for fMRI with simultaneous EEG acquisition and for fMRI acquisition alone.

R. Becker (✉)
Department of Neurology, Charité Universitätsmedizin, Charitéplatz 1, 10117 Berlin, Germany
e-mail: robert.becker@charite.de

C. Mulert and L. Lemieux (eds.), *EEG– fMRI*
DOI: 10.1007/978-3-540-87919-0_20, © Springer Verlag Berlin Heidelberg 2010

Fig. 1 The effect of MR gradient artefact removal on the average VEP for one subject (*bottom right*). Accompanying slices (*top row and bottom left*) show the corresponding fMRI activations (from Becker et al. 2005)

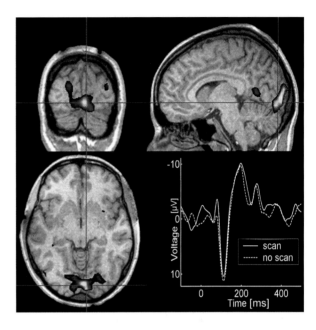

In general, it can be stated that average VEPs can be recorded reliably in the scanner using conventional artefact removal techniques. Depending on the magnetic field strength, single-trial analysis or the analysis of nonaveraged data may be hampered by BCG residuals. Because it is a complex signal that varies in both time and space, it may not always be completely removable (Debener et al. 2007).

2
fMRI-Informed EEG of the Visual System

With the aid of EEG it is possible to analyse temporally highly resolved dynamics of evoked responses during visual stimulation. However, due to the inverse problem, an exact and unconstrained localisation of these evoked responses is not possible (Helmholtz 1853). Since the visual areas in humans are densely clustered at the occipital pole, and an increasing number of generators may be concurrently active with subsequent stages of processing, the differentiation of neural sources by EEG source localisation in the visual system is additionally intricate (Vanni et al. 2004). Thus, the motivation for using EEG–fMRI for this purpose is to benefit from the high spatial resolution of fMRI and improve the localisation of visual evoked responses in the visual system. In this section, we focus on EEG–fMRI that performs source localisation constrained by or compared to fMRI. Strictly evaluated, unconstrained EEG dipole modelling with fMRI does not fall into this category of fMRI-informed EEG, but it is included to maintain topical integrity.

2.1
Localising Visual Evoked Potentials

In a typical pattern-onset stimulation, the first component (called C1, with a peak latency of around 60–100 ms) is commonly believed to be generated by striate cortex. However, the origin of the following component, P1 (peaking around 100–130 ms), is more uncertain, and possibly reflects extrastriate generators as well as generators within primary visual areas (Di Russo et al. 2002). Thus, one motivation for fMRI-informed EEG is to shed more light on the question of generator sites for EP components. The idea behind fMRI-informed EEG is to constrain the location of the dipole by identifying regions that exhibit significantly increased BOLD activity (e.g. caused by visual stimulation) while keeping the orientation and strength of the dipole flexible for further dipole fitting (also called "seeding"). An unconstrained EEG–fMRI study by Di Russo et al. (2002) showed a promising substantial overlap between activated fMRI sites and EEG dipoles. Also, Bonmassar et al. (2001), who performed unconstrained and fMRI-constrained source localisation over the entire EP window during a checkerboard pattern reversal task, found that the sources were consistently located in the calcarine sulcus with a more focal distribution in the fMRI-constrained localisation approach, along with a slightly lower dipole power than in the unconstrained analysis.

An EEG–fMRI study by Di Russo et al. (2002) used unconstrained EEG dipole modelling to localise sources of early visual evoked components, tracing the pathway from the primary visual cortex (earliest component, C1) via extrastriate areas (P1/posterior N1 component) to higher-cognitive areas, such as in the parietal lobe (anterior N1). Dipoles were fitted sequentially, according to the peak latencies of observed components. The comparison with fMRI activations for the same experimental setup yielded generally good agreement between activated fMRI sites and EEG dipoles. However, they also stated that localising generators for components later than C1/P1 becomes an increasingly difficult task, because the number of putative temporally and spatially overlapping generators accumulates in subsequent processing stages.

In an fMRI-constrained manner, Di Russo et al. (2007) localised generators of steady-state visual evoked potentials (SSVEPS), and reported that the visual areas V1 (primary visual cortex) and V5/MT (middle temporal) were the two major generators that contributed to SSVEPS. Interestingly, two out of the four fMRI activation sites were shown to only marginally contribute to the explained variance of the dipole model when seeded, and were thus discarded. The resulting two-dipole seeded model corresponded well to the unseeded two-dipole model although it explained slightly less variance.

In contrast to the seeding approach used in the aforementioned studies, Vanni et al. (2004) also integrated the orientation of the fMRI-activated cortical areas (using 3D anatomical information from high-resolution structural MRI). The authors noted that high spatial concordance of anatomical and functional MR scans is crucial to this approach because dipole position and orientation may otherwise be distorted, leading to incorrect initial forward models. Orientation is especially susceptible to any misalignment. The goal was to identify the hierarchical cortical processing of visual stimulation. While it was possible to separate visual areas V1, V2 and V3 spatially by fMRI, the fMRI-constrained dipole modelling did not always succeed in assigning each of these areas a distinct dipole. For example, V2 sources were often collapsed together with either V1 or V3 sources.

A tacit assumption that is normally accepted when seeding fMRI-constrained dipoles is that the fMRI activation sites used to constrain the dipole solution are regions that show positive BOLD responses. The rationale for doing so was questioned by Whittingstall et al. (2007), who first performed fMRI-unconstrained source localisation for visual checkerboard stimulation. When comparing results to BOLD fMRI activations they found that the early N75 component dipole localisation reflected the peak positive BOLD response in or near V1, while, in contrast to Di Russo et al. (2002), the P100 (or P1) localisation result yielded a region that also exhibited significant voxels with negative BOLD responses. The authors argued that this negative response, especially when interpreted as an inhibitory process and not mere vascular stealing, may also play an important role in the processing of visual stimuli. However, it is not clear whether the P100 can be regarded as originating from inhibitory processes. Studies in monkeys indicate that, depending on the exact type of stimulation (i.e. flash stimulation or pattern reversal), the simian homologue of the P100 may reflect either at least partially inhibitory processes (i.e. net hyperpolarisation from stellate cells in primary visual cortex) or excitatory processes (i.e. net depolarisation of pyramidal neurons) (Schroeder et al. 1991).

2.2
Visual Attention and Other Cognitive Processes

Localising EP components that reflect attention or other cognitive processes such as target detection with the help of EEG or fMRI is attractive because the underlying neuroanatomy is less well known than it is for processing in primary visual areas. A seminal study on direct neuronal and vascular-metabolic activity associated with attentional effects in the visual system was performed not with EEG–fMRI but with EEG-PET by Heinze et al. (1994). By using separate PET and EEG sessions, they studied the effect of visual selective attention with PET-constrained dipole modelling. They found a close correspondence between unconstrained and PET-constrained EEG dipoles reflecting the effect of visual attention in the P1 EP component. Both the PET activation and the EEG dipole were located in the fusiform gyrus. These results were confirmed by an EEG–fMRI study performed by Mangun et al. (1998) without dipole modelling, which showed that there was a comparable visual spatial attention-related increase in BOLD activity in the posterior fusiform and middle occipital gyri accompanied by a modulated P1 component of the EPs. There was no BOLD modulation of the calcarine sulcus (i.e. in primary visual area V1).

However, there is debate over whether primary visual areas like V1 can also be modulated by top-down mediated attention. Martinez et al. (1999) examined this question with EEG–fMRI and found a divergence between fMRI and EP results. The fMRI results did show a modulation of primary visual cortex activity by attention, whereas the attentional effect in the EP occurred 70 ms after stimulus onset, and corresponding fMRI-unconstrained dipoles indicated that extrastriate region V3 was the putative generator site. In a follow-up study, Di Russo et al. (2003) tried to answer the question of whether the attentional effect in V1, as found by fMRI, could possibly be explained by re-entrant modulatory activity from higher visual areas like V3. They showed that the effect of visual attention did not involve modulation of the early visual evoked component (i.e. C1 around 70 ms, which was shown to be localised in V1). However, they found responses later than the N1 component (150–225 ms range) that were also localised to V1. Since this component also behaved similarly to the early C1 component in terms of reversing polarity upon changing between upper and lower visual field stimulation, the authors argued that there was evidence of an attention-dependent modulation of V1. This would point in a similar direction to the findings of Martinez et al. (1999), with the twist here that the influence of attention in primary visual cortex was paralleled by both the fMRI activations and the late time window EP-dipole sources. Di Russo et al. (2003) used an fMRI "semiconstrained" dipole analysis, which in contrast to a fully seeded model also allowed changes in the initial positions of dipoles, which were defined by significant fMRI activation sites.

Another example of a well-examined cognitive process is the detection of an infrequent target during a (visual) oddball task that elicits the so-called P3 component arising roughly 300–600 ms after the target stimulus. Attempts have been made to localise it via EEG dipole modelling studies, but with inconsistent results (Bledowski et al. 2004). Sometimes this component is divided into P3a and P3b components. While P3a is said to mainly reflect the processing of distractor events, P3b is what is classically referred to as P3 and reflects the detection of novel, infrequent events in general. fMRI studies have shown the involvement of regions like the anterior cingulate cortex (ACC) and the supramarginal gyrus (SMG) (Ardekani et al. 2002). Similar regions were also reported by Linden et al. (1999) for uninformed EEG–fMRI during a visual and auditory oddball task. Bledowski et al. (2004) were interested in separating the P3a and P3b responses. They performed a separate-session three-stimulus visual oddball task (frequent, infrequent distractor and infrequent target) with fMRI-informed source localisation of P3a and P3b responses, and found that a broadly distributed network of sources accounted for the respective P3a and P3b responses. Their approach was to start from a common set of six pairs of fMRI seeds for both target and distractor conditions. Analysis of the time courses of resulting dipole moments indicated that the insula and the precentral sulcus seemed to be contributing more to the P3a component than to the P3b. Crottaz-Herbette and Menon (2006) used a different fMRI-informed EEG localisation approach. By performing a two-stimulus (frequent standard and infrequent target) auditory and visual oddball task, each resulting in a modality-dependent set of fMRI seeds for dipole fitting, they identified the ACC as being the main contributor to the N2b–P3a effect in both sensory modalities. For the visual oddball P3b component, they noted the involvement of inferior parietal areas (this was also reported by Bledowski et al. 2004).

Concerning the different results for generators of the P3 component, it should be said that, with an increasing number of assumed dipoles, dipole fitting often yields highly satisfactory results in terms of explaining the variance of EP waveforms. However, equally efficient solutions may exhibit quite different positions of dipoles. Thus, fMRI constraints are used to constrain the solution space. If the fMRI constraints differ prior to dipole fitting, the positions of the dipoles should also differ.

Apart from the visual oddball studies addressed above, there are also studies focusing on other higher-cognitive processes, like the processing of perceptual illusions or transitions, figure-ground separation, or the construction of objects from incomplete information. An innovative electrophysiological paradigm was used by Appelbaum et al. (2006), who separated the neuronal processes for the figure and background regions of a visual stimulus by "tagging" them with distinct spectral properties; in other words, they were textures characterised by different temporal frequencies. The resulting separate time courses of the figure and background components were subjected to cortical current density (CCD) analysis constrained by fMRI activations. These source reconstructions suggested that the figure region information was routed to the lateral occipital cortex (LOC), but that this was not the case for the processing of background region information.

Schoth et al. (2007) used the rotating Necker cube as a visual stimulus, which, in contrast to other illusionary multistable stimuli, has a predictable transition point between its different modes of perception. In this study, fMRI activations of the rotating Necker cube were used as constraints for current density reconstruction of the VEP related to the arising perceptual transition. It revealed initial processing in Brodmann area 18 and subsequent spreading along the visual dorsal stream.

Concerning the topic of higher-cognitive perceptual processes, Sehatpour et al. (2006) employed EEG–fMRI to identify neural networks that are active during "perceptual closure", which means the filling in of required information for a partially fragmented or distorted visual image in order to actively construct a recognisable object again. The major contributor to perceptual closure, as found by fMRI, was LOC. Without using a priori information from fMRI activations, EEG source analysis of the accompanying Ncl ("negativity related to closure") EP component yielded similar regions within the LOC to those found by fMRI.

Croize et al. (2004) used a combined MEG, EEG and fMRI approach together with unconstrained source localisation to examine visuospatial short-term memory processing. While there was largely good agreement between localised EEG current densities and MEG dipoles with fMRI activation sites, only the MEG covered a memory-encoding component in a late time window (around 400 ms) corresponding to right premotor areas. as observed by fMRI. The authors argued that this may be due to the well-known differential sensitivities of EEG and MEG to either radial or tangential sources, respectively.

Summarising the above studies, it can be said that complementing the EEG dipole models with the associated changes in fMRI activity largely confirmed the results of unconstrained dipole fitting in EEG studies. Also, the use of fMRI-guided dipoles seemed to lead to efficient models in terms of low residual variance. However, a direct comparison of the unconstrained vs. the constrained model approach was not always provided. When it was, the constrained model tended to explain slightly less variance. Some fMRI seeds also had to be discarded due to their inefficiency at explaining the variance of the EP waveform. In our view, findings of nonoverlapping activity are as interesting as findings of overlapping activity, which however appear to be emphasised in published studies.

3
EEG-Informed fMRI of the Visual System

In contrast to the previously described approach of fMRI-informed EEG, the approach of EEG-informed fMRI implies deriving information from the EEG (such as amplitudes of VEPs or spontaneous activity) that can be used to identify regions that exhibit BOLD responses co-varying with the selected parameter. Instead of constraining a dipole solution, it creates a new model of predicted BOLD activity, which can then be tested.

3.1
Spontaneous EEG Oscillations

The posterior alpha rhythm that oscillates around 10 Hz and its connection to the visual system has been known for almost eight decades now (Berger 1929). However, although it is one of the most prominent spontaneous rhythms in the human brain, a clear localisation of its generators has not been achieved. There is also ongoing debate regarding the functional role of the posterior alpha rhythm for visual processing (Makeig et al. 2002; Barry et al. 2000; Becker et al. 2008). Together with the evidence that spontaneous activity resembles activity during stimulation in many respects (Tsodyks et al. 1999), examining spontaneous activity may also contribute significantly to our understanding of event-related processes.

In several combined EEG–fMRI studies, a close relation between the posterior alpha rhythm and fMRI BOLD signal changes was reported (Goldman et al. 2002; Laufs et al. 2003a, b, 2006; Moosmann et al. 2003; Goncalves et al. 2006; de Munck et al. 2007; Feige et al. 2005). In those EEG-informed fMRI studies, the EEG parameter of interest was the amplitude of the alpha rhythm. The envelope of the alpha rhythm convolved with the haemodynamic response function (HRF) was normally used as a predictor for the fMRI signal. Despite the similar approaches used, the (EEG-informed fMRI) results were not completely consistent. Many studies showed a negative correlation between the alpha rhythm amplitude and the BOLD signal in occipital areas, and positive correlations in the thalamus (Goldman et al. 2002; Moosmann et al. 2003; de Munck et al. 2007; Feige et al. 2005, see Fig. 2). This could point to the concept of the alpha rhythm being a gating mechanism for the visual system.

In contrast, some studies (Laufs et al. 2003a, b, 2006; Goncalves et al. 2006) have also reported frontoparietal negative correlations for some subjects, pointing to a more global and modality-independent role of alpha rhythm in vigilance. In this respect, Matsuda et al. (2002) showed that, for a smooth-pursuit eye-movement task, there was a decrease in BOLD activation or even complete abolition of activations in several visual areas during low levels of arousal. Henning et al. (2006) found that the event-related BOLD response to eye closure and opening can change drastically during diminished subject vigilance. This was also reflected in a changed or even inverted alpha-rhythm modulation following eye opening. Interestingly, correlating the alpha power with the BOLD signal did not yield inverse results.

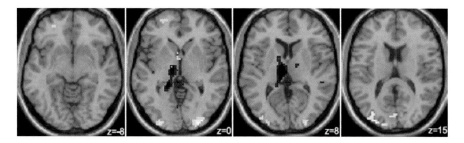

Fig. 2.   Results from a correlation analysis between alpha amplitude and BOLD signal (modified from Moosmann et al. 2003). Group analysis of six subjects, $p < 0.05$ corrected for multiple comparisons. *Yellow*: Significantly negative correlations. *Blue*: Significantly positive correlations

de Munck et al. (2007) were specifically interested in whether the time course of the metabolic correlate of the alpha rhythm follows the temporal assumptions of the HRF. The correlations between the BOLD signal and the alpha-rhythm power in the occipital and parietal regions showed similar lags as previously supposed when using the canonical HRF, while the correlation in the thalamus was less delayed (by several seconds).

In these types of studies, the simultaneous acquisition of EEG and fMRI is crucial. Only when using EEG–fMRI (in this case necessarily acquired simultaneously) it is possible in principle to relate fluctuating EEG activity to concurrent BOLD activity. However, one must always bear in mind that *the* single posterior alpha rhythm may simply not exist (for a discussion of this issue, see Shaw 2003). Further clarification, diversification and classification of spontaneous rhythms will be required to help disentangle the partially inconsistent results. It remains to be clarified how, and to what extent, the alpha rhythm and its associated BOLD signal changes modify task-related activity in the visual system.

Another approach to investigating spontaneous activity with EEG–fMRI was pursued by Mantini et al. (2007), who decomposed BOLD activity into independent clusters reflecting so-called resting-state networks (RSNs) and correlated the BOLD signal in these networks with the EEG spectral activity as averaged across all electrodes, and found distinct correlation patterns for each RSN. This is a promising result for further investigation of the relation between RSNs and EEG rhythms. An extension of this approach would be to

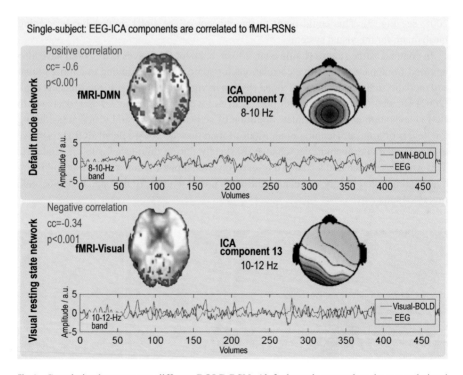

Fig. 3 Correlation between two different BOLD RSNs (default mode network at the *top* and visual component at the *bottom*) and the EEG-ICA components for a single subject (modified from Ritter et al. 2008)

preserve distinct and topographically specific EEG rhythms and examine their relationship to RSN BOLD activity. Results from such an approach are shown in Fig. 3. This shows the topography and time courses of two different RSNs (a visual network and the default mode network; Raichle et al. 2001) and those of two distinct spontaneous EEG components (as identified via independent component analysis, ICA) that correlate maximally with the RSNs. This result demonstrates that spatially and spectrally neighbouring EEG components can exhibit different relationships with different RSNs (Ritter et al. 2008).

3.2
Task-Related EEG Activity

Concerning EEG-informed fMRI studies of task-related activity, so far (2008) no studies have correlated single-trial EEG activity with BOLD, as has been done for other systems (Debener et al. 2005; Benar et al. 2007; Eichele et al. 2005). Existing studies use either parametric information to inform the fMRI procedure at the within-subject level, or they use EEG parameters to perform correlation analysis across subjects.

For example, Horovitz et al. (2004) parametrically varied the noise level in a picture and correlated the resulting effect on the N170 peak EP amplitude with fMRI activations, and identified a highly significant correlation with the fusiform gyrus. The authors concluded that this supports the idea of the fusiform gyrus contributing to the generation of the N170 EP component, since both entities show corresponding effects of experimental manipulation of the noise level.

Rose et al. (2005) focussed on the effect of working memory load on visual processing. They found that it phasically modulates the activity in the LOC (i.e. this region is increasingly activated with higher visibility of objects), with a steeper slope for less working memory load. Separate-session EEG revealed that this phasic modulatory BOLD effect of working memory is paralleled by the EP in a time window at around 170 ms. Assuming a linear relationship between EEG–fMRI measures, it was possible to assign these temporal dynamics to the LOC area. Another approach was employed by Philiastides and Sajda (2007), who used parameters estimated from a previous EEG study to model the BOLD response during different stages of a perceptual decision task in an fMRI experiment, which allowed them to identify distinct cortical networks for each stage.

Other studies used EEG parameters for correlation analyses across subjects to identify the relationship between interhemispheric coherence and involved visual areas. Knyazeva et al. (2006a) showed using EEG-informed fMRI (separate sessions) that visual area V4 was more active during stimulation with iso-oriented gratings than during stimulation with orthogonally oriented gratings. EEG analysis showed that stimulation with iso-oriented gratings was also accompanied by increased interhemispheric coherence of occipital electrodes in the beta band. Additionally, there was a significant correlation of interhemispheric coherence across subjects with visual area V4. The results were taken as evidence for the involvement of this extrastriate site in early perceptual grouping, since iso-oriented gratings obey the Gestalt principles (in this case collinearity and common fate). In another study, Knyazeva et al. (2006b) used different spatial frequencies of stimulation and a similar analysis and experimental approach as that used in the aforementioned study. They showed that, independent of spatial frequency, interhemispheric lower beta-band synchronisation was highly correlated with the activation of ventral extrastriate areas, while synchronisation of the higher beta band corresponded to more dorsal extrastriate areas.

4
Uninformed EEG–fMRI and Other Approaches

Aside from fMRI-informed EEG and EEG-informed fMRI, combined EEG–fMRI studies can also be performed in a mutually "uninformed" way, where each modality is analysed separately. These studies will be discussed in the following section, with the exception of EEG–fMRI studies with unconstrained source localisation, which are actually uninformed but have been already described in the section on fMRI-informed EEG.

4.1
Event-Related Oscillations

Foucher et al. (2003) related EPs and event-related gamma band activity to the BOLD signal and postulated a closer correspondence between BOLD and gamma than between BOLD and the EP response, arguing that non-phase-locked EEG responses should be considered when modelling the haemodynamic response. During a visual oddball task, a weaker P3 component was produced during target than during novel detection, while BOLD activity increased. This was paralleled by a stronger spectral response in the gamma range (32–38 Hz) in EEG.

Another study by Fiebach et al. (2005) also examined effects of event-related gamma band activity during a different task. Using a visual lexical decision task, parallel behaviour between gamma and BOLD was observed: upon the presentation of pseudo-words, BOLD activity in defined areas, gamma band response and phase synchrony between electrodes increased, while these effects were inverted but still parallel upon the presentation of words. Of course, this experimental task differs fundamentally from that above; however, it is still worthwhile discussing such diverging results in the context of a universal relationship between rhythmic activity and BOLD responses.

4.2
Visual Attention and Other Cognitive Processes

Gazzaley et al. (2005) reported top-down modulated magnitude and speed of neural activity as measured with EEG and fMRI. Amplitudes of evoked responses in both EEG and fMRI (neural activity) were modulated by an attentional paradigm showing faces and scenes, respectively. For fMRI, there was higher activity in the parahippocampal place area (PPA) for the remember scenes vs. the ignore scenes condition, and higher activity in the fusiform face area (FFA) for the remember faces vs. the ignore faces condition.

Concerning the EEG results, The EP difference waveform for this contrast also yielded a significant amplitude as well as latency effect for the face-selective N170 component, which had not been reported before. Mangun et al. (1998) showed that there was a visual spatial attention-related increase in BOLD activity in the posterior fusiform and middle occipital gyri accompanied by a modulated P1 component of the ERPs. They did not report on later effects of attention, and in contrast to the aforementioned studies they found no consistent activation of V1.

Muller et al. (2005) used a multistable visual motion paradigm where subjects responded to spontaneous transitions of the perceptual mode of the stimulus. Transitions between different modes were marked by alpha and beta activity decreases and delta increases in the EEG before transition. Regions of increased BOLD activity included right anterior insula, MT and supplementary motor area (SMA), while thalamus and right superior temporal gyrus (STG) showed decreases in BOLD activity.

5
Investigating Neurovascular Coupling in the Visual System by EEG–fMRI

The question of whether a linear coupling between neural activity and BOLD signal can be assumed has occupied investigators since the beginning of fMRI-based research. This assumption is also relevant when employing an EEG-informed fMRI approach, which relies on an appropriate description of BOLD activity by the respective EEG parameters.

In a pioneering study, Logothetis et al. (2001) found a higher correspondence between local field potentials (LFPs) and the BOLD signal than between multiunit activity (MUA) and BOLD. Since the EEG is also said to reflect synchronised synaptic activity rather than action potentials, this is a promising result for "straightforward" EEG–fMRI analysis. However, the idea that there is always a direct linear relationship between the two measures of neural activity, which is basically assumed when correlating EEG parameters with BOLD, is at the very least doubtful, as we will explain below with exemplary studies on the visual system.

Huettel et al. (2004) attempted to link intracranially recorded human visual event-related local field potentials (ER LFPs) and BOLD fMRI in separate sessions by experimentally manipulating stimulus duration. They found a divergence between consistently (nonlinearly) increasing BOLD activity in calcarine and fusiform cortex for longer stimulation, and differing EP responses from these two regions (i.e. an onset-sustained response that was partially dependent on stimulus duration as well as a pure onset response that was independent of stimulus duration). This supports the notion that the BOLD signal integrates information on a longer timescale, which complicates the estimation of the direct neural basis from BOLD measurements. Janz et al. (2001) showed that the adaptation effect for repetitive stimulation from a checkerboard reversal, as seen in the BOLD signal, is not plainly mirrored and cannot be accounted for completely by adaptation effects as observed in the accompanying visual evoked potential. This would speak against a straightforward inference from BOLD to EEG and vice versa, thus demanding adjusted approaches in order to model the haemodynamic response as a consequence of electrophysiological properties.

Wan et al. (2006) also examined the nonlinearity of the visual event-related BOLD and EP responses with concurrent EEG–fMRI by modulating stimulus frequency and contrast. Interestingly, when estimating neuronal efficacy from BOLD rather than using this parameter directly, a comparison of it to mean power of electrical activity (which is nonlinear by nature) resulted in a linear correlation between both indices of neural activity, indicating that the observed nonlinearity may have a neural basis.

Guy et al. (1999) studied EEG and fMRI responses to periodic stimulation. A new measure created by correlating the EEG with the VEP template was created (VEPEG) and compared with the fMRI BOLD signal. Both measures mirrored the fundamental frequency of the stimulus presentation and both of them exhibited a poststimulus negativation, which may point to similar neural processes after stimulus offset. Singh et al. (2003) examined the effect of changing the frequency of a checkerboard flash stimulation on BOLD and EP responses, and found a robust correlation between strength of SSVEPs (amplitudes) and BOLD response activations.

Henning et al. (2005) found a divergence between EEG and fMRI effects when applying different types of visual stimulation, such as pattern reversal, motion onset and motion reversal of a starfield stimulus. While EPs (especially N2 components) were the most enhanced by motion onset, fMRI activation (with its maximum in visual area MT) was largest for motion reversal. They argue that this may be due to both modalities reflecting different processes. In the light of a more complete description of neural activity, it would have been of interest to investigate whether non-phase-locked EEG responses could explain the divergent effects.

In another study, Bucher et al. (2006) examined the effect of maturation (i.e. the transition from adolescence to adulthood) on luminance and motion-related evoked responses in EEG and fMRI. They reported a latency effect of maturation for motion-contrast EPs (N1, around 120–270 ms), which was not, however, mirrored by a change in BOLD responses.

The one single-trial EEG–fMRI study that the authors are aware of (Bagshaw and Warbrick 2007) analyses EEG and fMRI single-trial data from separate sessions. The authors report a robust correlation between the experimentally manipulated latency variabilities of EEG and BOLD single trials, which hints that the observed variability may share a common neural origin. However, further real single-trial studies are required to obtain more direct evidence for that assumption.

In general, more complex biophysical models of the relationship between EEG and fMRI activity are needed to clarify the origins of reported divergent effects. One step in this direction is the forward model of Sotero and Trujillo-Barreto (2008), which was able to reproduce VEPs and concurrent BOLD patterns as well as the spontaneous alpha rhythm with its accompanying typical BOLD activity. A biophysical model that could actually produce the overlaps as well as the observed divergences between EEG and fMRI would be of great value, since this would contribute to a better understanding of the nature of both modalities.

6
Outlook

The following section attempts to sum up what has been achieved so far and at the same time discuss what is still missing. First, we critically examine whether the frequently stated expectation of EEG–fMRI, that of providing both high spatial and temporal resolution of brain activity, has been met with respect to studies of the visual system.

Without restricting ourselves to the visual system, EEG–fMRI experiments yield two kinds of measures: one highly temporally resolved measure from the EEG and one spatially highly resolved signal from the fMRI measurement. What we actually would like to get is one merged signal that has both high spatial and high temporal resolution. However, what we normally obtain is a temporal correlation between BOLD activity and an HRF-convolved EEG time course (EEG-informed fMRI) or a spatial colocalisation between a BOLD cluster and an EEG source (fMRI-informed EEG). These types of temporal or spatial overlaps hint at relevant connections between the two modalities but do not necessarily represent causal relations.

The use of fMRI constraints for EEG source modelling suffers from the problem that fMRI clusters do not always reflect neural activity that contributes to EEG scalp potentials. Thus, it is prone to errors caused by inappropriate modelling of assumed sources of brain activity. Of course, substantial overlap between unconstrained EEG dipoles and fMRI activations has been shown. If we use an appropriate model, we can attribute the temporal dynamics of an EEG dipole to an fMRI cluster.

In EEG-informed fMRI, regions are identified that show a correlation between BOLD activity and a certain EEG parameter. Here, relationships between EEG parameters and BOLD activity other than linear correlations should also be considered. Also, the critical assumption that the chosen EEG parameter indexes neuronal activity may not always be justified (e.g. in the case of BCG contamination of EEG parameters).

Concerning examinations of neurovascular coupling, depending on the examined EEG parameter—EP amplitudes, single-trial activity, spontaneous or event-related oscillatory activity—the characterisation of the EEG-BOLD relationship will vary, which is also reflected in the results of the studies on neurovascular coupling in the visual system discussed above. Even a complete description of all conceivable EEG parameters may not appropriately reflect the neural processes of a certain region, leading to suboptimal modelling of BOLD responses.

Given the option of directly measuring neuronal activity with the help of MRI (sometimes termed "direct" (f)MRI), the concurrent use of EEG would be finally made obsolete, since the MR signal would then provide high temporal and spatial resolution for one and the same measure. The visual system has already been used several times as a starting point for such attempts, but contradictory conclusions have been drawn about its feasibility, since either favourable but indirect results (Bianciardi et al. 2004; Konn et al. 2004) or rather disencouraging results have been obtained when using concurrent EEG for validation (Mandelkow et al. 2007).

Having summarised the results of EEG–fMRI studies in the visual system, in our opinion, the strength of EEG–fMRI is not so much its potential to actually merge both modalities in order to obtain one single measure, as in direct fMRI. Instead, by using simultaneous EEG–fMRI, we are able to observe interactions between these two measures, which may reveal new insights into how, for example, spontaneous rhythms change the way that events are processed.

Acknowledgements The authors would like to thank Daniel Margulies, Matthias Reinacher and Frank Freyer for proofreading the manuscript, and Antje Kraft for helpful discussions. This work was supported by the German Federal Ministry of Education and Research BMBF (Berlin Neuroimaging Center; Bernstein Center for Computational Neuroscience) and the German Research Foundation DFG (Berlin School of Mind and Brain; SFB 618-B4).

References

Appelbaum LG, et al. (2006) Cue-invariant networks for figure and background processing in human visual cortex. J Neurosci 26(45):11695–708

Ardekani BA, et al. (2002) Functional magnetic resonance imaging of brain activity in the visual oddball task. Brain Res Cogn Brain Res 14(3):347–56

Bagshaw AP, Warbrick T. (2007) Single trial variability of EEG and fMRI responses to visual stimuli. Neuroimage 38(2):280–92

Barry RJ, et al. (2000) EEG alpha activity and the ERP to target stimuli in an auditory oddball paradigm. Int J Psychophysiol 39(1):39–50

Becker R, et al. (2005) Visual evoked potentials recovered from fMRI scan periods. Hum Brain Mapp 26(3):221–30

Becker R, et al. (2008) Influence of ongoing alpha rhythm on the visual evoked potential. Neuroimage 39(2):707–16

Benar CG, et al. (2007) Single-trial analysis of oddball event-related potentials in simultaneous EEG–fMRI. Hum Brain Mapp 28(7):602–13

Berger H (1929) Über das Elektrenkephalogram des Menschen. Arch Psychiatr Nervenkr (87):527–570

Bianciardi M, et al. (2004) Combination of BOLD-fMRI and VEP recordings for spin-echo MRI detection of primary magnetic effects caused by neuronal currents. Magn Reson Imaging 22(10):1429–40

Bledowski C, et al. (2004) Localizing P300 generators in visual target and distractor processing: a combined event-related potential and functional magnetic resonance imaging study. J Neurosci 24(42):9353–60

Bonmassar G, et al. (1999) Visual evoked potential (VEP) measured by simultaneous 64-channel EEG and 3T fMRI. Neuroreport 10(9):1893–7

Bonmassar G, et al. (2001) Spatiotemporal brain imaging of visual-evoked activity using interleaved EEG and fMRI recordings. Neuroimage 13(6 Pt 1):1035–43

Bucher K, et al. (2006) Maturation of luminance- and motion-defined form perception beyond adolescence: A combined ERP and fMRI study. Neuroimage 31(4):1625–36

Bunkrad M, et al. (1989) Visual evoked cortical potentials modified by a NMR magnetic field of 0.24 Tesla. Fortschr Ophthalmol 86(6):702–5

Comi E, et al. (2005) Visual evoked potentials may be recorded simultaneously with fMRI scanning: A validation study. Hum Brain Mapp 24(4):291–8

Croize AC, et al. (2004) Dynamics of parietofrontal networks underlying visuospatial short-term memory encoding. Neuroimage 23(3):787–99

Crottaz-Herbette S, Menon V. (2006) Where and when the anterior cingulate cortex modulates attentional response: combined fMRI and ERP evidence. J Cogn Neurosci 18(5):766–80

Debener S, et al. (2005) Trial-by-trial coupling of concurrent electroencephalogram and functional magnetic resonance imaging identifies the dynamics of performance monitoring. J Neurosci 25(50):11730–7

Debener S, et al. (2008) Properties of the ballistocardiogram artefact as revealed by EEG recordings at 1.5, 3 and 7 T static magnetic field strength. Int J Psychophysiol 67(3):189–99

de Munck JC, et al. (2007) The hemodynamic response of the alpha rhythm: An EEG/fMRI study. Neuroimage 35(3):1142–51

Di Russo F, et al. (2002) Cortical sources of the early components of the visual evoked potential. Hum Brain Mapp 15(2):95–111

Di Russo F, et al. (2003) Source analysis of event-related cortical activity during visuo-spatial attention. Cereb Cortex 13(5):486–99

Di Russo F, et al. (2007) Spatiotemporal analysis of the cortical sources of the steady-state visual evoked potential. Hum Brain Mapp 28(4):323–34

Eichele T, et al. (2005) Assessing the spatiotemporal evolution of neuronal activation with single-trial event-related potentials and functional MRI. Proc Natl Acad Sci USA 102(49): 17798–803

Feige B, et al. (2005) Cortical and subcortical correlates of electroencephalographic alpha rhythm modulation. J Neurophysiol 93(5):2864–72

Fiebach CJ, et al. (2005) Neuronal mechanisms of repetition priming in occipitotemporal cortex: spatiotemporal evidence from functional magnetic resonance imaging and electroencephalography. J Neurosci 25(13):3414–22

Foucher JR, et al. (2003) The BOLD response and the gamma oscillations respond differently than evoked potentials: an interleaved EEG–fMRI study. BMC Neurosci 4:22

Gazzaley A, et al. (2005) Top-down enhancement and suppression of the magnitude and speed of neural activity. J Cogn Neurosci 17(3):507–17

Goldman RI, et al. (2002) Simultaneous EEG and fMRI of the alpha rhythm. Neuroreport 13(18):2487–92

Goncalves SI, et al. (2006) Correlating the alpha rhythm to BOLD using simultaneous EEG/fMRI: Inter-subject variability. Neuroimage 30(1):203–13

Guy CN, et al. (1999) fMRI and EEG responses to periodic visual stimulation. Neuroimage 10(2):125–48

Heinze HJ, et al. (1994) Combined spatial and temporal imaging of brain activity during visual selective attention in humans. Nature 372(6506):543–6

Helmholtz H (1853) Über einige Gesetze der Vertheilung elektrischer Ströme in körperlichen Leitern mit Anwendung auf die thierisch-elektrischen Versuche. Annalen der Physik 165(6): 211–33

Henning S, et al. (2005) Simultaneous recordings of visual evoked potentials and BOLD MRI activations in response to visual motion processing. NMR Biomed 18(8):543–52

Henning S, et al. (2006) Task- and EEG-correlated analyses of BOLD MRI responses to eyes opening and closing. Brain Res 1073–1074:359–64

Horovitz SG, et al. (2004) Parametric design and correlational analyses help integrating fMRI and electrophysiological data during face processing. Neuroimage 22(4):1587–95

Huettel SA, et al. (2004) Linking hemodynamic and electrophysiological measures of brain activity: evidence from functional MRI and intracranial field potentials. Cereb Cortex 14(2):165–73

Im CH, et al. (2006) Functional cortical source imaging from simultaneously recorded ERP and fMRI. J Neurosci Methods 157(1):118–23

Janz C, et al. (2001) Coupling of neural activity and BOLD fMRI response: new insights by combination of fMRI and VEP experiments in transition from single events to continuous stimulation. Magn Reson Med 46(3):482–6

Knyazeva MG, et al. (2006a) Imaging of a synchronous neuronal assembly in the human visual brain. Neuroimage 29(2):593–604

Knyazeva MG, et al. (2006b) Interhemispheric integration at different spatial scales: the evidence from EEG coherence and FMRI. J Neurophysiol 96(1):259–75

Konn D, et al. (2004) Initial attempts at directly detecting alpha wave activity in the brain using MRI. Magn Reson Imaging 22(10):1413–27

Kruggel F, et al. (2000) Recording of the event-related potentials during functional MRI at 3.0 Tesla field strength. Magn Reson Med 44(2):277–82

Laufs H, et al. (2003a) EEG-correlated fMRI of human alpha activity. Neuroimage 19(4):1463–76

Laufs H, et al. (2003b) Electroencephalographic signatures of attentional and cognitive default modes in spontaneous brain activity fluctuations at rest. Proc Natl Acad Sci USA 100(19):11053–8

Laufs H, et al. (2006) Where the BOLD signal goes when alpha EEG leaves. Neuroimage 31(4): 1408–18

Lazeyras F, et al. (2001) Functional MRI with simultaneous EEG recording: feasibility and application to motor and visual activation. J Magn Reson Imaging 13(6):943–8

Linden DE, et al. (1999) The functional neuroanatomy of target detection: an fMRI study of visual and auditory oddball tasks. Cereb Cortex 9(8):815–23

Logothetis NK, et al. (2001) Neurophysiological investigation of the basis of the fMRI signal. Nature 412(6843):150–7

Makeig S, et al. (2002) Dynamic brain sources of visual evoked responses. Science 295(5555): 690–4

Mandelkow H, et al. (2007) Heart beats brain: the problem of detecting alpha waves by neuronal current imaging in joint EEG-MRI experiments. Neuroimage 37(1):149–63

Mangun GR, et al. (1998) ERP and fMRI measures of visual spatial selective attention. Hum Brain Mapp 6(5–6):383–9

Mantini D, et al. (2007) Electrophysiological signatures of resting state networks in the human brain. Proc Natl Acad Sci USA 104(32):13170–5

Martinez A, et al. (1999) Involvement of striate and extrastriate visual cortical areas in spatial attention. Nat Neurosci 2(4):364–9

Matsuda T, et al. (2002) Influence of arousal level for functional magnetic resonance imaging (fMRI) study: simultaneous recording of fMRI and electroencephalogram. Psychiatry Clin Neurosci 56(3):289–90

Moosmann M, et al. (2003) Correlates of alpha rhythm in functional magnetic resonance imaging and near infrared spectroscopy. Neuroimage 20(1):145–58

Muller TJ, et al. (2005) The neurophysiological time pattern of illusionary visual perceptual transitions: a simultaneous EEG and fMRI study. Int J Psychophysiol 55(3):299–312

Muri RM, et al. (1998) Recording of electrical brain activity in a magnetic resonance environment: distorting effects of the static magnetic field. Magn Reson Med 39(1):18–22

Negishi M, et al. (2004) Removal of time-varying gradient artifacts from EEG data acquired during continuous fMRI. Clin Neurophysiol 115(9):2181–92

Philiastides MG, Sajda P. (2007) EEG-informed fMRI reveals spatiotemporal characteristics of perceptual decision making. J Neurosci 27(48):13082–91

Raichle ME, et al. (2001) A default mode of brain function. Proc Natl Acad Sci USA 98(2):676–82

Ritter P, et al. (2008) Relation between spatially and spectrally confined EEG rhythms and fMRI resting state networks. In: 14th Ann Meet OHBM, Melbourne, Australia, 15–19 June 2008

Rose M, et al. (2005) The functional and temporal characteristics of top-down modulation in visual selection. Cereb Cortex 15(9):1290–8

Sammer G, et al. (2005) Acquisition of typical EEG waveforms during fMRI: SSVEP, LRP, and frontal theta. Neuroimage 24(4):1012–24

Schmid MC, et al. (2006) Simultaneous EEG and fMRI in the macaque monkey at 4.7 Tesla. Magn Reson Imaging 24(4):335–42

Schoth F, et al. (2007) Cerebral processing of spontaneous reversals of the rotating Necker cube. Neuroreport 18(13):1335–8

Schroeder CE, et al. (1991) Striate cortical contribution to the surface-recorded pattern-reversal VEP in the alert monkey. Vision Res 31(7–8):1143–57

Sehatpour P, et al. (2006) Spatiotemporal dynamics of human object recognition processing: an integrated high-density electrical mapping and functional imaging study of "closure" processes. Neuroimage 29(2):605–18

Shaw JC (2003) More on alpha rhythm characteristics. The brain's alpha rhythms and the mind. Elsevier, Amsterdam, pp 15–32

Singh M, et al. (2003) Correlation between BOLD–fMRI and EEG signal changes in response to visual stimulus frequency in humans. Magn Reson Med 49(1):108–14

Sotero RC, Trujillo-Barreto NJ (2008) Biophysical model for integrating neuronal activity, EEG, fMRI and metabolism. Neuroimage 39(1):290–309

Tsodyks M, et al. (1999) Linking spontaneous activity of single cortical neurons and the underlying functional architecture. Science 286(5446):1943–6

Vanni S, et al. (2004) Sequence of pattern onset responses in the human visual areas: an fMRI constrained VEP source analysis. Neuroimage 21(3):801–17

Wan X, et al. (2006) The neural basis of the hemodynamic response nonlinearity in human primary visual cortex: implications for neurovascular coupling mechanism. Neuroimage 32(2):616–25

Whittingstall K, et al. (2007) Evaluating the spatial relationship of event-related potential and functional MRI sources in the primary visual cortex. Hum Brain Mapp 28(2):134–42

Cognition

Susanne Karch and Christoph Mulert

1
Advantages and Disadvantages of Simultaneous EEG–fMRI Recordings of Cognitive Functions

In cognitive neuroscience, there has been growing interest in the utilisation of simultaneous and combined EEG–fMRI recordings in cognitive paradigms in order to obtain datasets with high spatial and temporal resolution (Debener et al. 2007a; Mulert et al. 2008a). Due to the obvious technical challenges of simultaneous EEG–fMRI, EEG and fMRI data have often been obtained in separate sessions (Bledowski et al. 2004a, b). There are, however, several reasons why simultaneous EEG–fMRI acquisition seems to make sense when investigating cognition. Mental processes don't need to be identical, even if an identical cognitive paradigm is conducted several times. Differences in the participant's mood, vigilance and familiarity with the task, for example, have been shown to be important for cognitive processes as well as for the underlying brain activations (Debener et al. 2006; Matsuda et al. 2002; Menon and Crottaz-Herbette 2005). Often, the same stimuli cannot be used twice, e.g. stimuli used in learning and memory experiments or planning tasks. Simultaneous EEG–fMRI recordings have the advantage of an identical environment, the same stimulation conditions, and the same subject state, e.g. time of day, time spent on the task, level of arousal. In addition, this method appears to be advantageous for studying distinct samples (e.g. children or aged people) in order to avoid multiple sessions involving extended periods of time (Menon and Crottaz-Herbette 2005). Multiple sessions might not be feasible, reliable or practical in clinical studies, e.g. when focussing on the effect of medication on cognitive processes (Menon and Crottaz-Herbette 2005). Additionally, various processing stages of cognitive tasks—e.g. stimulus encoding and evaluation, memory, selection of action and guiding decisions—can be decomposed ("mental chronometry") (Linden 2007; Posner 1978) using EEG and fMRI. In tasks focussing on higher cognitive functions (e.g. executive functions, memory), both

S. Karch (✉)
Functional Brain Imaging Branch, Department of Psychiatry and Psychotherapy of the LMU, Munich, Nussbaumstr. 7, 80336 Munich, Germany
e-mail: susanne.karch@med.uni-muenchen.de

C. Mulert and L. Lemieux (eds.), *EEG–fMRI*
DOI: 10.1007/978-3-540-87919-0_21, © Springer Verlag Berlin Heidelberg 2010

nonspecific processes (e.g. attention, arousal) and specific abilities (e.g. planning, cognitive flexibility, encoding) are required for successful task execution. EEG–fMRI data may be useful for distinguishing neural correlates of specific and nonspecific aspects of cognitive functioning. Furthermore, EEG–fMRI studies allow for the localisation of cognition-related brain structures to be combined with neurophysiological mechanisms, e.g. functional coherence of brain regions.

Some of the disadvantages of simultaneous EEG–fMRI measurements are the reduced signal-to-noise ratio of EEG data obtained in the scanner (Menon and Crottaz-Herbette 2005), and technical problems (e.g. ballistocardiogram artefacts) (Allen et al. 1998; Niazy et al. 2005; see the chapters "EEG Quality: Origin and Reduction of the EEG Cardiac-Related Artefact", "EEG Quality: The Image Acquisition Artefact"). Also, simultaneous EEG–fMRI measurements may be more stressful for participants, due to prolonged sessions or disagreeable circumstances during the acquisition of the data (e.g. the discomfort stemming from the EEG cap, cables, etc.) for instance.

2
Cognitive Functions

2.1
Attention

Attention is the cognitive process of maintaining the mental focus on one or several aspects of the environment (e.g. a specific issue, object or activity) while ignoring other things in order to deal effectively with the information at the attentional focus. Diverse aspects of cognitive functioning are included in this concept, such as the ability to maintain a consistent behavioural response during continuous and repetitive activity (sustained attention) and in the face of distraction or competing stimuli (selective attention). This concept also refers to the capacity for mental flexibility that allows individuals to shift their focus of attention and to alter between tasks with different cognitive requirements (alternating attention) as well as to respond simultaneously to multiple task demands (divided attention) (Sohlberg and Mateer 1989).

The examination of neural responses is crucial for evaluating the functional efficiency of brain functions. In electroencephalographic investigations, attention has frequently been examined using the so-called oddball paradigm, as well as mismatch-associated paradigms. One of the most important aspects of electrophysiological responses is the so-called P300 component, a positive component observed about 300–600 ms after the presentation of a stimulus. The P300 has gained importance in studies of cognition in healthy individuals, and has also proved to be abnormal in many clinical conditions, including aging, schizophrenia, depression, Alzheimer's disease, and psychopathy (Ford et al. 1994; Kawasaki et al. 2004; McCarley et al. 1991; Polich and Corey-Bloom 2005; Polich and Herbst 2000; van der Stelt et al. 2004). For this reason, neural generators of event-related potentials (ERPs) have attracted considerable interest (Bledowski et al. 2004a).

2.1.1
Oddball Paradigm

The *oddball paradigm* has been associated with attention and information processing capacity. During this task, participants detect and respond to infrequent target events embedded in a series of repetitive events (Sutton et al. 1965). The detection of novel, salient information is crucial in order to facilitate the adaptation to a rapidly changing environment (Sokolov 1963). The oddball paradigm entails top-down regulated attention to a stimulus. Sometimes novel stimuli that do not require a behavioural response (deviants) are also presented in this task. The presentation of deviants enables the ongoing focused attention to be broken and the attention to be attracted (Bledowski et al. 2004a).

Aberrant electrophysiological responses associated with rare, task-relevant stimuli have been reported about 300–500 ms after the presentation of the task, especially in frontocentral and parietal brain regions (P3/P300). This ERP is thought to reflect the mental processes underlying the allocation of attentional resources to an incoming stimulus and its evaluation, as well as decision making and memory updating (Calhoun et al. 2006). There are two components of the P300: P3a and P3b. P3a has a more frontal distribution and is thought to be associated with an orienting response (Friedman et al. 2001). Variations related to the P3b appear a little later and primarily have a parietal distribution. The P3b is associated with context updating, context disclosure, event categorisation and processing capacity (Donchin and Coles 1988; Kok 2001).

Halgren and colleagues used intracranial recordings to identify P3-related neural generators (Halgren et al. 1998). The results supported the view that P3a is primarily related to paralimbic areas as well as frontal, parietal and cingulate brain regions. The integration of context information (P3b) engaged frontotemporal cortices, association cortices, and the hippocampus. Brain responses to oddball tasks have been extensively studied using fMRI (e.g. Horovitz et al. 2002; Kiehl et al. 2005b; Linden et al. 1999; McCarthy et al. 1997; Menon et al. 1997). It is assumed that oddball paradigms elicit activations in a widespread cortical network, including the anterior temporal gyrus, the inferior and superior parietal lobes, anterior and posterior cingulate cortex, the thalamus, and lateral frontal brain regions. Some studies have found a rightward lateralisation in frontal, temporal and parietal regions (Kiehl et al. 2005a; Stevens et al. 2005). There is evidence that some brain activities are related to specific task modalities. For example, the activity of the postcentral gyrus in the button press condition was thought to reflect the somatosensory component of the motor response (Linden et al. 1999). By contrast, the angular gyrus and intraparietal region were exclusively activated when subjects counted rare events (Linden et al. 1999). Modality-independent activations (e.g. within the frontal operculum and the insular cortex as well as the parietal and frontal lobes) are said to form a network for saliency detection (Linden et al. 1999).

In order to improve the understanding of target-associated brain activity, a precise localisation of the generators of P3 was aimed for in several studies. Menon and colleagues (1997) ranked among the first to combine EEG and fMRI analysis; however, the data were obtained in separate sessions. Spatiotemporal modelling of event-related potentials based on dipole locations derived from the event-related brain activation provided evidence that the temporoparietal cortex is the main generator of the P300. These brain regions were activated in the interval 285–610 ms following the onset of the target stimulus. The authors concluded that the supramarginal gyrus is critically involved in generating a prominent brain signal in the postprocessing of salient stimuli for evaluation, categorisation, response and decision making (Menon et al. 1997).

A different approach was the comparison of fMRI findings with those of an independent localisation of event-related potentials using low-resolution electromagnetic tomography (LORETA) (Mulert et al. 2004). In this study, ERPs and fMRI data were acquired at the same time as the participants performed an auditory oddball paradigm. The comparison of the centres of gravity of BOLD responses with the current source density derived from LORETA analysis revealed highly concordant responses in the temporoparietal junction, the supplementary motor area (SMA)/anterior cingulate cortex (ACC), the insula, and the middle frontal gyrus. However, fMRI activations of the motor cortex were not represented in the P300 potential. Concerning the time course of brain responses, the activation seemed to start in the temporal lobe and the temporoparietal junction, and the last activity was observed in the frontal and supplementary motor cortex (Mulert et al. 2004).

Bledowski and colleagues intended to distinguish neuroanatomical correlates related to generators of the P3a component, which is mainly evoked by distractor events, from those of P3b, which has been associated with the detection of rare events in general (targets and distractors) (Bledowski et al. 2004a, b), using EEG and fMRI acquired in separate sessions. Results of a visual oddball paradigm with three different conditions (frequent, rare, distractor) revealed that targets elicited a posterior P3b; distractor stimuli were followed by a frontocentral P3a ERP. Both conditions produced BOLD responses in the temporoparietal junction and the right prefrontal gyrus. Furthermore, target processing led to bilateral perisylvian responses, whereas the frontal eye fields, bilateral superior parietal cortices, and left prefrontal cortex contributed to distractor processing (Bledowski et al. 2004a). An fMRI-based EEG model was designed to directly relate the data sets: fMRI-constrained seeding points were located in the prefrontal cortex, precentral sulcus, inferior parietal lobe, posterior parietal cortex, inferior temporal cortex, anterior insula, right superior temporal sulcus, as well as the cingulate gyrus. The results revealed that all sources had contributed to the target and distractor condition. However, distinct neural processes seemed to be related to the processing of targets and distractors: frontal areas and the insula contributed mainly to P3a, which was compatible with a more anterior distribution on the scalp. By contrast, P3b was mainly produced by higher visual and supramodal association areas (e.g. parietal and inferior temporal areas) (Bledowski et al. 2004b). Altogether, the results confirmed previous reports about a supramodal target detection system (Linden et al. 1999). Beyond this, some task-specific subsystems associated with P3a and P3b components seemed to exist (Bledowski et al. 2004a; b).

Furthermore, it was suggested that a separation of brain regions according to their diverse response properties is possible (Horovitz et al. 2002). A parametric design was used in which the probability of infrequent stimuli was modulated. Combined EEG–fMRI analyses revealed probability-induced changes in P3 amplitudes related to fMRI responses of the supramarginal gyri, the thalamus, the insula and the right medial frontal gyrus. Other brain regions, such as the ACC, showed reliable activations during the oddball task but responses were not modulated according to the P3 amplitude.

The study of Crottaz-Herbette and colleagues (2006) was especially concerned with the influence of the ACC in attentional control. A simple auditory and visual oddball task was used to examine if, and to what extent, early attentional effects were influenced by top-down processes from the ACC. The importance of the ACC in attentional control has been

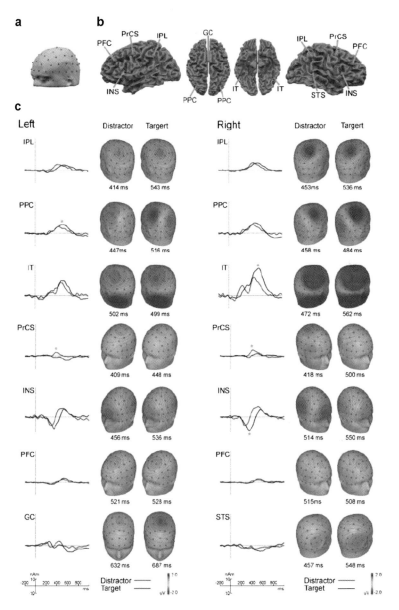

Fig. 1a–c Combined EEG and fMRI study using a novelty paradigm; dipoles were seated in BOLD clusters. Source activity in target and distractor condition. **a** Surface of a standard head (MNI template) with a standard 81-electrode configuration. **b** Position of the regional sources on a surface reconstruction of the MNI template brain. **c** Source activity waves and topographical maps of scalp voltage in the main current flow direction of each regional source for the target and distractor conditions. * indicates significant differences between regional source peak amplitudes in the target and distractor conditions; *PFC*, prefrontal cortex; *INS*, anterior insula; *PrCS*, precentral sulcus; *IPL*, inferior parietal lobe; *GC*, cingulate gyrus; *PPC*, posterior parietal cortex; *IT*, inferior temporal sulcus; *STS*, superior temporal sulcus. (Bledowski et al. 2004b; copyright 2004 Society for Neuroscience)

demonstrated before, for example in tasks requiring selective attention or the inhibition of prepotent responses (Botvinick et al. 2001; Bush et al. 2000; Carter et al. 1999; Gehring and Knight 2000; Milham and Banich 2005). As expected, the presentation of infrequent stimuli led to significantly greater responses in the ACC, as well as enhanced contributions from the SMA, inferior parietal cortex, basal ganglia, cerebellum, and left premotor cortex. Modality-specific variations were produced, especially in the primary sensory cortices; for example, the visual oddball paradigm was associated with greater BOLD responses in the lingual and fusiform gyri, the middle and inferior occipital gyri, temporoparietal regions, and the cerebellum (Crottaz-Herbette and Menon 2006). Although attention-related activation of the ACC was similar in both modalities, its connectivity was remarkably dependent on its modality: the auditory task produced an enhanced effective connectivity between the ACC and Heschl's gyrus, the left middle and superior temporal gyri, the left and right precentral and postcentral gyri, the supramarginal gyrus, the caudate, the thalamus, and the cerebellum. During the visual oddball task, the ACC showed an increased connectivity with the striate cortex, the precuneus/cuneus, and the posterior cingulate gyrus. ERP recordings confirmed that oddball tasks elicit prominent frontocentral and central N2 and P3a signals. The fMRI-constrained dipole modelling showed that the ACC is the major generator of the N2b-P3a components of the ERP. Summarised, the functional MRI results of the study suggest a top-down attentional modulation of early sensory processing by the ACC. The authors concluded that these results provide evidence for a model of attentional control based on dynamic bottom-up and top-down interactions between the ACC and primary sensory regions (Crottaz-Herbette and Menon 2006).

Calhoun and colleagues performed a spatial independent component analysis (ICA) of the haemodynamic change data and a temporal ICA of the ERPs in order to derive a spatiotemporal decomposition. The results provided evidence for initial auditory processing and corresponding preparatory motor activity. These initial activations were followed by N2-related activations in association areas and motor execution regions. The early P3a was associated with enhanced neural responses of thalamic regions and posterior superior parietal lobe areas, as well as decreases in orbitofrontal brain regions. However, the late P3b showed associations with posterior temporal and temporoparietal lobe regions, in addition to lateral prefrontal areas (Calhoun et al. 2006).

The effect of trial-by-trial variability on neurofunctional parameters, for instance due to variations in the experimental design or variations in arousal, has been explored in other similar studies (Benar et al. 2007; Debener et al. 2007a; Eichele et al. 2005). Trial-by-trial variability has been reported for both EEG (Effern et al. 2000; Jung et al. 2001) and fMRI (Duann et al. 2002; Kruggel and von Cramon 1999). In simultaneous EEG–fMRI experiments, information about changes in the event-related EEG activity of each trial was used as a parameter for fMRI analysis. Eichele and colleagues (2005) distinguished three independent stages during oddball processing. The main sources of early ERP components (P2; ~170 ms) were located in temporal and frontal lobes. The authors suggested that P2 indicates matching processes between sensory input and a neuronal representation of stimuli selected for further processing. Later, electrophysiological responses (N2) were related to the anterior frontomedian cortex and parahippocampal regions, and appeared to be linked with the detection of a mismatch and memory processes, rather than attentional processes (Eichele et al. 2005). The most extensive variations were related to the P300 about 320 ms after stimulus presentation. As expected, BOLD responses were found in frontal, temporal, and parietal brain regions, especially in the right hemisphere. Similar changes have been associated with a mechanism elicited when a memory representation of the recent stimulus context is updated, as opposed to the detection of deviancy (Eichele et al. 2005) (Fig. 2).

Furthermore, there was some evidence for a relation between P3 latency and cognitive functions as well as BOLD responses (Benar et al. 2007): single-trial P3 latency clearly correlated with the reaction time. Significant fMRI activations for the modulation by P300 amplitude and latency were obtained at both the single-subject level and the group level, indicating a link between evoked potentials and fMRI signals: P300 parameters seemed to be associated with fMRI activations in the anterior medial frontal region, the parietal-occipital junction, and the anterior medial frontal region. However, a large variability in the patterns of activations across subjects was observed. Whether the modulation of the ERP reflected a modulation of neural activity visible in the fMRI, or both EEG and fMRI signals were jointly modulated by the same factors (e.g. the level of attention) was not clear (Benar et al. 2007).

In summary, the feasibility of tracking single-trial variations in both the amplitude and the latency of an EEG wave during fMRI scanning was proved. The use of simultaneous EEG–fMRI can be seen as a bridge between the well-established field of evoked cognitive

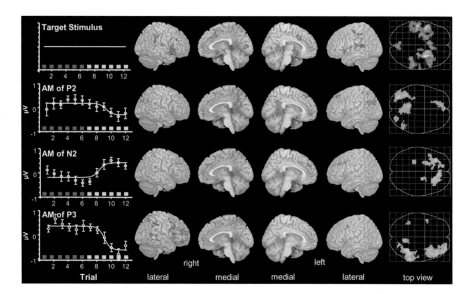

Fig. 2 Simultaneous EEG–fMRI experiment using an oddball paradigm. Amplitude modulation (AM)-correlated fMRI results. Rendered views and maximum-intensity projections of the general target-related activation, and positive (*red*) and negative (*blue*) correlations with the respective AM. Each correlation shows for each voxel the maximum t value from the four electrodes (Fz, FC1, FC2, Cz). The average AM (empty circles ± SEM) and the fitted sigmoid curves are shown to the left of each rendering of the AM-correlated fMRI. *Top row*, target-related activation, $p < 0.05$ (FWE), cluster size >10; *second row*, P2 (170 ms); *third row*, N2 (200 ms); and *fourth row*, P3 (320 ms). All AM-related activations were thresholded at $p < 0.001$ (uncorrected), cluster extent threshold $p < 0.01$. (Eichele et al. 2005; copyright 2005 National Academy of Sciences, USA)

potentials and the fast-growing field of fMRI studies; the study contributes to this goal by linking the fluctuations of the features of a well-known ERP component to the fMRI signal. It also permits the extraction of new information from evoked activity with a very high spatial resolution (Benar et al. 2007).

2.1.2
Mismatch Negativity

The mismatch negativity reflects the registration of differences between an actual presented stimulus and the representation of stimuli in memory (Näätänen and Winkler 1999). The mismatch detection has been associated with preattentive change detection and is considered to be more or less automatic. Mismatch-generating processes have often been associated with the initiation of an involuntary switch to information outside the focus of attention (Giard et al. 1990; Schroger and Wolff 1996). In a sequence of frequently repeated standard stimuli, infrequent auditory stimuli are rarely interspersed during mismatch experiments. In contrast to oddball paradigms, no behavioural response is required. The mismatch negativity is linked to the mismatch between sensory input from a deviant stimulus and neural correlates of sensory information, representing the features of repeatedly presented standard stimuli (Näätänen and Winkler 1999).

Electrophysiologically, mismatch leads to a negative deflection, the so-called mismatch negativity (MMN), which peaks roughly between 100 and 250 ms after deviance onset (Näätänen et al. 1978). The MMN is commonly calculated by subtracting the ERP elicited from the standard information from the ERP produced by the deviant stimulus. The MMN is often followed by a P3a component announcing a switch of attention (Knight 1996). Others concluded that the P3 probably indicates an involuntary switch of attention to salient or novel events; it is elicited when the characteristic of the current stimulus is differs significantly from the preceding stimulus (Katayama and Polich 1998). Imaging studies (Mathiak et al. 2002; Opitz et al. 1999) as well as intracranial recordings (Javitt et al. 1992; Kropotov et al. 1995) provided evidence that the main MMN generators are located in the left and right transverse temporal gyri and the STG. Frontal brain regions are thought to be involved to; e.g. the inferior frontal gyrus (IFG) (Downar et al. 2002; Opitz et al. 2002). Frontal brain regions seemed to be activated at a later stage than temporal regions, and contributed to the switch of attention in response to changes in auditory stimulation (Rinne et al. 2000). Downar and colleagues (2000) assumed that the IFG could be relevant for the evaluation of the potential importance of the stimuli presented.

Using EEG and fMRI responses, Opitz and colleagues (2002) examined the influence of the degree of variation of deviants from standard stimuli on neural parameters. Thus, deviants of three different pitches were presented with an infrequent change of either small, medium or large magnitude. Significant BOLD activations were observed during the presentation of medium and large deviants in the STG and in the opercular part of the right IFG. Temporal lobe activations were more pronounced for large than for medium deviants, whereas the reverse was true for the IFG. Small deviants failed to produce any reliable response during fMRI; however, an MMN was produced in the EEG environment, indicating that they could only be detected during silence. Haemodynamic changes in the STG correlated with the change-related ERP signal between 90 and 120 ms (early MMN), while the IFG response correlated with the MMN in a late time window (140–170 ms). The authors concluded that the right fronto-opercular cortex is part of the neural network generating the MMN and could be attributed to an involuntary amplification or contrast enhancement mechanism (Opitz et al. 2002). The prefrontal cortex might be associated with change detection, but at a later time than temporal regions (Opitz et al. 2002; Rinne et al. 2000).

Liebenthal and colleagues (2003) conducted a simultaneous EEG–fMRI experiment, also using small and large deviants. The ERP analysis revealed MMNs recorded in both large and small deviant conditions, especially in frontal sites. The correlation analysis between MMN amplitudes in Fz and BOLD responses showed that an increased negativity was linked with enhanced responses in the right STG bordering the superior temporal sulcus and in the right posterior superior temporal plane. Additionally, smaller peaks were found in the right posterior STG, Heschl's gyri, the left planum temporale, and the left STG. Altogether, the authors concluded that the results for MMN generators on the superior temporal plane are consistent with dipole analysis and magnetoencephalographic recordings (Giard et al. 1990; Opitz et al. 2002). In addition, generators in each temporal region were hypothesised: one generator near the primary auditory areas on the superior temporal plane is thought to be the first to respond, and probably corresponds to the N1 component. The later generator is believed to be located more anteriorly and laterally, and seems to be associated with the MMN (Liebenthal et al. 2003). The results of the study support the idea that frequency deviancy detection is linked with generators in the right lateral part of the STG. However, a confident differentiation of N1- and MMN-associated brain responses and BOLD activation related to the P3a component was not possible. This study focussed mainly on the feasibility of simultaneous EEG–fMRI measurements for mismatch detection: basically, the results rely on the validation of MMN-associated generators.

The functional roles of various brain regions during mismatch processing were addressed in a study using infrequent deviants with variations in the dimensions of pitch and space (Doeller et al. 2003). A dipole analysis constrained by fMRI was used to compare the ERP and fMRI measurements, which were acquired in separate sessions. The results of dipole analysis confirmed the assumption of two separate MMN components: early MMN amplitude and activity of the STG increased with pitch deviance. However, the right IFG and the late MMN amplitude showed an inverted u-shaped pattern; most pronounced were the BOLD responses where the dissimilarity was moderately pronounced. The right prefrontal cortex seemed to be relevant for auditory pitch discrimination, especially when the differentiability of pitch deviants and standards is low. The authors concluded that these prefrontal mechanisms are probably associated with a top-down modulation of the deviance detection system in the STG (Doeller et al. 2003).

Apart from the magnitude of deviance, the modulation of attention may also matter in mismatch detection. Sabri and colleagues (2006) accomplished a simultaneous EEG–fMRI experiment in which the difficulty of the primary task was modulated. The results demonstrated an enhanced deviant-induced MMN in the easy task compared to the difficult task, whereas the N1 and P3a components were smaller. The frontocentral negativity varied in the temporal dimension between conditions. In the difficult task, the negativity was observed 60–110 ms after the stimulus presentation, indicating a link to the N1 component. In addition, a strong positivity was observed 210–340 ms after the stimulus. In the easy task, the significant negativity instead seemed to be associated with the MMN and was observed 110–170 ms after stimulus presentation. Thus, the underlying electrophysiological processes may be discriminative. Apart from frontal regions, passive deviancy detection, as reflected by the MMN, was connected with activations in the dorsal part of the STG; and involuntary shifting of attention, as reflected by P3a, was observed in the dorsal and ventral parts of the superior temporal cortex, respectively. The authors suggested that the dorsal STG regions were primarily affected by the passive detection of mismatch between the memory influenced by standard tones and the incoming deviant, whereas the ventral region appeared to be modulated by involuntary shifts of attention to task-irrelevant auditory features (Sabri et al. 2006).

Presumably, mismatch detection can be associated with haemodynamic responses of superior temporal as well as frontal brain regions. EEG–fMRI studies have provided evidence for a functional dissociation of these regions, and have yielded further insight into the chronology of brain responses. Another factor that may have an influence on mismatch detection is the focus of attention; this was investigated in a further study.

2.1.3
Preparatory Attention

Most classical studies of preparatory attention are based on the contingent negative variation (CNV) ERP. This negative potential is generated in the interval preceding the stimulus that needs further processing (Gomez et al. 2006). It is suggested that CNV is an index of cortical arousal during anticipatory attention, preparation, motivation, and information processing (Nagai et al. 2004; Tecce 1972). Neurophysiological theories suggest that the CNV reflects a subthreshold activation of the cortex, preparing it to process the next stimulus and response (Rockstroh et al. 1982) as well as to integrate cognitive and motor components (Nagai et al. 2004). The CNV can be induced when a warning stimulus is presented before the target stimulus during a reaction time task. There are several dissociable components of the CNV. The early phase of the CNV, maximal at midline electrodes, encompasses an orienting response. Later variations of the CNV, maximal at the vertex, instead reflect motor preparation. Neuroimaging studies have shown contributions from primary motor cortex, ACC, SMA, frontoparietal regions and subcortical centres (Gomez et al. 2007, 2003; Ioannides et al. 1994).

In a simultaneous EEG–fMRI study, increased BOLD responses in the thalamus, somatomotor cortex, midcingulate, SMA, and insular cortices during the period of CNV generation were demonstrated (Nagai et al. 2004). Additionally, single-trial analysis indicated that the thalamic, anterior cingulate and supplementary motor activity was modulated by the amplitude of the CNV. Thus, thalamocortical interactions appeared to regulate the CNV amplitude (Nagai et al. 2004) (Fig. 3).

2.2
Executive Functions

There are numerous definitions of the concept of executive functions as well as possible subcomponents (e.g. Baddeley and Hitch 1974; Banich 2004; Norman and Shallice

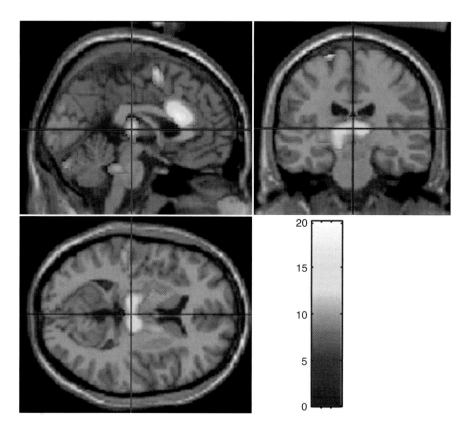

Fig. 3 Brain regions modulated by CNV amplitude. In five subjects, CNV was recorded simultaneously with the acquisition of fMRI data. For these subjects, a fixed-effect analysis was used to determine the correlation of regional brain activity with trial-by-trial changes in measured CNV amplitude (derived from the integral over 3.5 s of baseline-corrected EEG data). F tests of regions were significantly related to activity ($p < 0.05$, corrected), and highlighted bilateral thalamus, ACC/SMA, pons, and cerebellum. The distribution of this activity is plotted on orthogonal sections of a template brain, illustrating the location of thalamic involvement extending into basal ganglia. (Reprinted from Nagai et al. 2004; copyright 2004, with permission from Elsevier)

1986). Executive functioning describes a set of cognitive abilities that control and regulate other abilities and behaviours necessary for goal-directed behaviour. Various abilities are included, such as the ability to initiate and stop actions, to monitor and evaluate performance in relation to goals, to flexibly change and revise plans and behaviour as needed, and to solve problems (Jurado and Rosselli 2007; Lezak 1983). They are necessary for appropriate, socially responsible and effectively self-serving behaviour (Lezak 1983).

Neuroimaging research has shown that executive functioning is mediated by the prefrontal lobes of the cerebral cortex. However, different executive functions are associated with different regions of the frontal lobe (Braver et al. 2001; Carlson et al. 1998; D'Esposito et al. 1998; Stuss and Levine 2002; Watanabe et al. 2002). Also, a wide cerebral network that includes temporal, parietal and subcortical structures and thalamic pathways is activated (e.g. Lewis et al. 2004; Watanabe et al. 2002). Along with the broad heterogeneity of executive functions, various experimental paradigms and tests have been used to acquire these processes.

2.2.1
Cognitive Flexibility

Cognitive flexibility comprises the ability to shift the attention from one perceptual parameter to another. The ability to flexibly adapt mental activity and behaviour according to upcoming environmental requirements is crucial for successful behaviour. Flexible responses can be investigated when using the *Wisconsin Card Sorting Test (WCST)* for example (Grant and Berg 1948). This test comprises a fairly easy task (rearranging cards with simple symbols according to various criteria, e.g. colour). However, no instructions are given on how to complete the task. Only feedback provided after each match enables the subject to acquire the correct rule of classification.

ERP studies revealed a posterior P3b wave associated with the performance of WCST-like tasks (Barcelo et al. 2000). Electrophysiological responses seemed to be modulated along with various aspects of task execution, such as the maintenance of the task compared with shifting to a newly relevant dimension (Barcelo et al. 1997). Furthermore, stimulus presentation elicited an enhanced synchronisation between prefrontal, temporal and posterior association cortex, comprising different frequency ranges (Gonzalez-Hernandez et al. 2002). Functional neuroimaging studies verified the influence of frontal lobes (e.g. Konishi et al. 2002; Lie et al. 2006) as well as temporal and parietal regions (Lie et al. 2006) during the performance of the WCST. So far, there have been no combined or simultaneous EEG–fMRI studies addressing cognitive flexibility and set-shifting abilities. Still, the functional segregation of neural responses related to task components like set shifting, working memory, inhibitory control or feedback was attempted in several fMRI studies (e.g. Konishi et al. 1999; Lie et al. 2006; Monchi et al. 2001). Rule changing in WCST-like tests seemed to be followed by responses in the inferior prefrontal area (Konishi et al. 1999), whereas positive and negative feedback led to increased activation in the dorsolateral prefrontal cortex (DLPFC) (Monchi et al. 2001). Beyond that, negative feedback indicating the need for a mental shift produced an enhanced contribution from a cortical basal ganglia loop (ventrolateral prefrontal cortex, caudate nucleus, thalamus) (Monchi et al. 2001).

2.2.2
Verbal Fluency

Verbal fluency tests require people to generate words in a certain period of time according to semantic or phonematic (e.g. words starting with a certain letter) criteria. The ease of word generation is assessed. Frontal brain regions, especially the DLPFC and the ACC

(Jahanshahi et al. 2000; Phelps et al. 1997), the inferior part of the prefrontal cortex (Paulesu et al. 1997; Phelps et al. 1997), as well as the thalamus (Paulesu et al. 1997) and the superior parietal cortex (Jahanshahi et al. 2000), are of some importance for these tasks. So far, none of the fMRI studies have combined their results with electrophysiological information.

2.2.3
Performance Monitoring

The control and dynamic adjustment of behaviour within changing environmental require-ments are important aspects of performance monitoring. Performance monitoring involves the detection of errors as well as the subsequent adjustment of behaviour, reinforcing adap-tive behaviour (Holroyd et al. 2002).

Erroneous actions, in particular, are highly informative for adjusting future behaviour (Ridderinkhof et al. 2004). Studies of error processing indicated that erroneous responses were associated with negativity at frontocentral midline sites that peaked about 100 ms after an error was made, known as negativity associated with errors (Ne) or error-related negativity (ERN) (Falkenstein et al. 1991; Gehring et al. 1993). Initially the ERN/Ne was interpreted in the context of the *error-monitoring system*: the ERN/Ne was meant to reflect the detection of errors or an attempt to inhibit errors (Gehring et al. 1993; Scheffers and Coles 2000; Scheffers et al. 1996). The ERN/Ne was also interpreted in the context of the *conflict-monitoring system*, where it is essential for the detection of a high degree of response competition and the recruitment of top-down control from the DLPFC, which is again important for improving task performance and reducing conflict (Botvinick et al. 2001; Carter et al. 1998; Cohen et al. 2000).

Imaging studies revealed a contribution from the ACC to error processing and response conflict (Braver et al. 2001; Carter et al. 1998; Ullsperger and von Cramon 2001). There is disagreement regarding the precise location within the ACC. Some studies have reported a contribution from the caudal ACC during response conflict and the activation of the rostral ACC along with error processing (Braver et al. 2001; Kiehl et al. 2000); other stud-ies have reported conflict and error-related brain activations in the caudal ACC (Carter et al. 1998; Menon et al. 2001a, b). Frontomedian areas also appear to be associated with error-induced behavioural changes: greater posterror slowing was associated with increased BOLD responses in frontomedian areas (Garavan et al. 2002). Apart from medial frontal areas, the DLPFC, the (pre)SMA (Kiehl et al. 2000; Menon et al. 2001a, b), and the basal ganglia (Holroyd and Coles 2002) contribute to the modulation of the ERN/Ne.

Combined EEG–fMRI analyses of a *Go/NoGo paradigm* were used to further distin-guish error and conflict-related brain responses (Mathalon et al. 2003). For this purpose, unsuccessful response inhibitions (errors/false alarms) and successful nogo trials (con-flict/correct rejections) were analysed. The results showed the expected ERN/Ne during error trials, especially at Cz, as well as a nogo-related N2. Rostral, caudal, and motor ACC were activated during both conditions. However, responses were more pronounced during the nogo trials compared to error trials, and a tight coupling between inhibition- and error-related brain responses could be demonstrated. The correlation of EEG and fMRI data revealed that error and conflict monitoring (at least partially) recruit the same brain regions, e.g. caudal ACC. These results were consistent with the idea of medial frontal lobe monitoring in error and conflict monitoring. In addition, both processes engage distinct neural circuitry. Error-specific responses were also shown in the rostral ACC, as well as BA 10 and posterior cingulate. Conflict monitoring also recruited the DLPFC and inferior parietal lobule. Thus, error monitoring and conflict monitoring may be dissociable, being subserved by overlapping and distinct ACC regions (Mathalon et al. 2003) (Fig. 4).

Another study used a speeded *flanker task* to analyse neural correlates of ERN and posterror slowing (Debener et al. 2005). During this task, participants were instructed to respond according to the direction of an arrow that was presented on a screen. The arrow was flanked by further arrows pointing in the same (compatible trials) or the opposite direction (incompatible trials). A profound ERN was shown in frontocentral sites, especially for the incongruent error trials. Further analysis showed an association between high single-trial amplitudes and short reaction times for the incompatible errors, whereas incompatible correct trials were related to a small negativity. In addition, the ERN was systematically associated with ensuing behavioural adjustment: higher ERN amplitudes were related to longer reaction times in posterror trials. Single-trial amplitudes also covaried with enhanced BOLD responses in the rostral cingulate zone. Therefore, these results supported the view that the rostral cingulate zone is one source of the ERN and seems to be involved in controlling subsequent adjustment (Debener et al. 2005; Ridderinkhof et al. 2004; Ullsperger and von Cramon 2004).

Performance monitoring also includes the anticipation and inhibition of behavioural responses. *Response anticipation* was assessed by comparing responses after a cue was given to prepare vs. a cue indicating relaxation; *response conflict* was examined by comparing incongruent and congruent trials (Fan et al. 2007). As expected, response anticipation facilitated response execution: the responses were faster when a warning signal was presented before the actual target. In addition, response anticipation was associated with altered electrophysiological responses, especially in midline electrodes (CNV), as well as enhanced cue-associated fMRI activations encompassing a distributed right-lateralised thalamocorticostriatal network and brain areas significant in executive control. A power spectrum analysis of the pretarget period revealed a greater anticipation-related gamma power and decreased responses in theta, alpha and beta bands, especially in frontal brain regions and the superior parietal lobe. The authors assumed that the increased gamma band activity and decreased alpha band activity in regions associated with attention, sensory processing and motor preparation support the assumption that the PFC exerts top-down control of task-relevant brain regions in response anticipation. Response conflict during uncued trials also led to an enhanced contribution of brain regions linked to executive control. Neural responses were enhanced compared to the response anticipation task (cued trials). In summary, common regions of a dorsal frontoparietal network and the ACC seemed to be engaged in the flexible control of a wide range of executive processes. Response anticipation modulated overall activity in the executive control network but did not interact with response conflict processing (Fan et al. 2007) (Fig. 5).

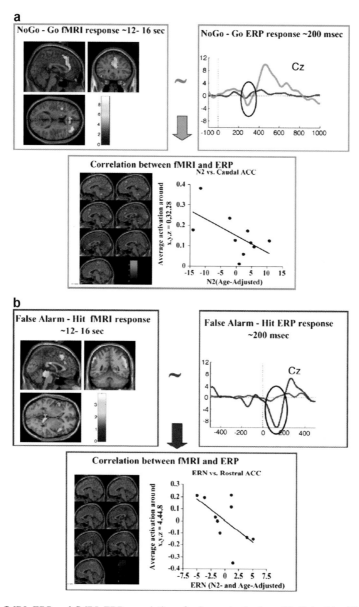

Fig. 4 **a** fMRI, ERP and fMRI–ERP correlations for [correct rejections (NoGo) – hits (Go)] comparisons. Three-planar view for fMRI ($p < 0.001$, uncorrected) (*upper left*); ERPs superimposed on correct rejections and hits from Cz (*upper right*); fMRI and ERP correlations ($p < 0.05$, uncorrected) focussing on the ACC (*lower left*); scatter plot showing that subjects with larger age-adjusted N2 scores have greater caudal ACC activation (*lower right*). **b** fMRI, ERP and fMRI–ERP correlations for [false alarms (NoGo) – hits (Go)] comparisons. Three-planar view for fMRI ($p < 0.05$, uncorrected) (*upper left*); ERPs superimposed on false alarms and hits from Cz (*upper right*); fMRI and ERP correlations ($p < 0.05$, uncorrected) focussing on the ACC (*lower left*); scatter plot showing that subjects with larger age-adjusted N2 scores have greater rostral ACC activation (*lower right*). (Reprint from Mathalon et al. 2003; copyright 2003, with permission from Elsevier)

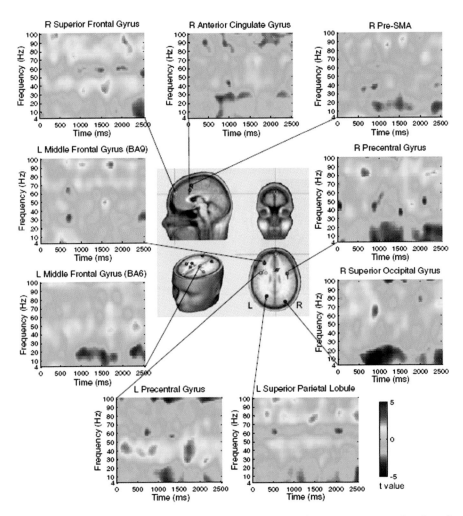

Fig. 5 Power change difference diagrams for the ready minus relax cue contrast as a function of time–frequency, and the dipoles from ERP data. The *centre panel* shows the dipole locations. The *small balls and bars* represent the locations and orientations of the dipoles, respectively. The right superior frontal gyrus shows greater gamma (>30 Hz) power maintained over the cue-target interval, whereas the right superior occipital gyrus shows a power decrease in the theta (4–8 Hz), alpha (8–12 Hz), and beta (12–30 Hz) bands. The cue onset is at 0 ms, and the target onset is at 2,500 ms (Fan et al. 2007; copyright 2007, Society for Neuroscience)

2.2.4
Decision Making

The influence of mental effort on decision-making processes was examined in a simultaneous EEG–fMRI experiment with a forced choice reaction task: the subjects were instructed to accomplish this task under both high- and low-effort conditions (Mulert et al. 2008b).

Mental effort significantly affected the N1 potential but did not show any influence on the P300 potential. In the high-effort condition, single-trial coupling of EEG with fMRI demonstrated N1-related BOLD activity in the ACC and auditory cortex. Upon comparing the N1-specific activity of the high-effort condition and the control condition (passive listening), significant activation was only found in the ACC. Hence, it is suggested that early ACC activation is important in effort-related decision making (Mulert et al. 2008b).

2.2.5
Behavioural Inhibition

The ability to inhibit responses that are inappropriate in the current context is crucial for interactions in the social context (Logan et al. 1984; Shallice 1988). Inhibition capacity can be assessed with *Go/NoGo* tasks for example. Go/NoGo tasks require the subjects to respond to one type of stimulus, representing response execution processes, and to withhold a response to another stimulus.

Electrophysiologically, the response inhibition process seems to be associated with a negative deflection that reaches a frontocentral maximum about 200 ms after the presentation of the respective stimuli (N2) (Falkenstein et al. 1999). More recently, it has been speculated that N2 reflects response conflict rather than inhibitory control (Donkers and van Boxtel 2004; Nieuwenhuis et al. 2003). There is some evidence that the nogo-P3, a positive-going peak observed approximately 300–600 ms after stimulus, is related to response inhibition (Kamarajan et al. 2005; Bekker et al. 2004; Bruin et al. 2001; Pfefferbaum et al. 1985). Inhibition-related haemodynamic responses included the ACC (Braver et al. 2001; Casey et al. 1997; Durston et al. 2002; Liddle et al. 2001), middle and inferior cingulate cortex, anterior insula (Braver et al. 2001; Konishi et al. 1999; Watanabe et al. 2002), (pre)SMA (Garavan et al. 2002; Ullsperger and von Cramon 2001), and parietal brain regions (Garavan et al. 2002; Watanabe et al. 2002). BOLD reactivity was usually stronger in the right hemisphere than the left hemisphere (Garavan et al. 1999; Kelly et al. 2004; Konishi et al. 1999).

Deficits in response inhibition capacities (Go/NoGo paradigm) and associated brain responses (ERPs, fMRI) have been studied, for example, in schizophrenic patients (Ford et al. 2004). In this study, the percentage of false-alarms errors was lower and the percentage of omission errors was higher in patients with schizophrenia than in the control group. P300 amplitudes and fMRI activations associated with go trials differed from those associated with nogo trials less in patients than controls: go-related activations were increased, nogo-associated variations decreased in patients compared to the control group. Enhanced inhibition-related haemodynamic responses in controls compared to schizophrenic patients were shown in a network of brain regions, including medial and lateral frontal regions, the precuneus, the inferior parietal lobe, the gyrus postcentralis, the STG, and the insula. Altogether, these results indicated that go responses were more arduous and deliberate for patients with schizophrenia than for healthy subjects, whereas response inhibition was easier. The combined evaluation of ERPs and BOLD responses revealed a positive association of P300 amplitudes with BOLD responses in the ACC, DLPFC, inferior parietal lobe, and caudate nucleus in healthy subjects. In patients, there was a modest correlation between parietocentral nogo-P3 and ACC activations. Overall, the evaluation of behavioural data, ERPs and fMRI results indicated that healthy subjects set up prepotent response biases during go trials. The effort expended to overcome this tendency during inhibition is reflected in the nogo-P3 amplitude as well as the recruitment of neural structures associated with executive control. Patients with schizophrenia, however, did not show strong response biases; instead, they simply experienced conflict. Furthermore, the DLPFC, the inferior parietal lobe and the striatum did not contribute significantly to task execution in patients (Ford et al. 2004).

The combination of EEG and fMRI helped to generate a hypothesis about different cognitive strategies of psychiatric populations, and neural structures recruited to implement them (Ford et al. 2004).

Response inhibition capacity in alcohol-dependent patients was examined in a simultaneous EEG–fMRI study using an auditory Go/NoGo task (Karch et al. 2007). The results showed that self-rated anxiety considerably influenced cognitive functions and their neural correlates in alcohol-dependent patients: patients with high self-rated anxiety showed significantly elevated activations during response inhibition, especially in the middle/superior frontal gyrus and the right IFG compared to patients with low ratings on these scales. In addition, enhanced activations were shown in temporoparietal brain regions. The integration of EEG and fMRI data produced a positive correlation between P300 amplitudes at frontocentral locations and medial frontal, insular as well as right temporoparietal BOLD responses in healthy subjects. In patients, associations between ERPs and haemodynamic responses were less clear: patients with small anxiety ratings showed positive relations between the insula and frontocentral P300 amplitudes. Contrary to the control subjects, there was no association with medial frontal and temporoparietal regions. Patients with increased anxiety scores, however, revealed correlations between enhanced P300 latencies in FCz and right frontal and inferior parietal activations. Altogether, these results provided evidence that alcohol-dependent patients and healthy subjects recruit different brain regions during behavioural inhibition. In addition, comorbid symptoms of trait anxiety considerably influenced the pattern of brain functions related to cognitive functions in alcohol-dependent subjects (Karch et al. 2007).

2.2.6
Working Memory

Working memory (WM) refers to processes used for temporarily storing and manipulating information (Baddeley 1992). Baddeley and Hitch proposed a WM model based on the assumption of three basic components (*central executive, phonological loop, visuospatial sketchpad*) (Baddeley and Hitch 1974). According to their model, information is stored by silently rehearsing sounds or words in a continuous loop (*phonological loop*). The *visuospatial sketchpad* is engaged when performing visual or spatial tasks. The *central executive* is responsible for the supervision of information integration and for coordinating both systems. Later on, the concept was extended by adding the *episodic buffer*. This buffer is meant to contain images integrating phonological, visual and spatial information, and possibly information not covered in other systems (e.g. semantic information, musical information) (Baddeley 1992). The component is episodic because it is assumed to bind information into a unitary episodic representation.

The DLPFC, the IFG, the ACC and temporoparietal brain regions are suggested to account for WM processes (D'Esposito et al. 2000; Rypma and D'Esposito 1999; Veltman et al. 2003). Within parietal regions, there seems to be a distinction between a ventral pathway for object processing and a dorsal pathway for spatial processing (Cabeza and Nyberg 2000). The phonological store is thought to consist of left parietal activations, whereas the rehearsal process consists of left prefrontal activations (Paulesu et al. 1993).

Bledowski and colleagues (2006) conducted a WM task to further analyse the *mental chronometry* of WM retrieval on the basis of an fMRI-constrained source analysis in order to distinguish various subprocesses of WM abilities. The results indicated early BOLD activations within the inferior temporal cortex associated with the electrophysiological N1 and P3a component, which were followed by responses of the posterior parietal cortex. Late responses were also observed in the ventrolateral prefrontal cortex as well as the medial frontal and premotor areas. The authors proposed that these neural responses might reflect various cognitive stages during task processing, such as perceptual evaluation (inferotemporal), storage buffer operations (posterior parietal cortex), active retrieval (ventrolateral prefrontal cortex), and action selection (medial frontal and premotor cortex) (Bledowski et al. 2006).

Executive dysfunction and deficits in working memory are common in various psychiatric diseases, e.g. schizophrenia (Catafau et al. 1994; Goldman-Rakic 1994; Weinberger et al. 1986). Functional MRI studies focussing on WM tasks in schizophrenic patients found abnormal activations, especially in the PFC (Callicott et al. 2003; Johnson et al. 2006; Manoach et al. 2000; Tan et al. 2005). A combined EEG–fMRI study was designed to distinguish the effect of early perceptual stages from later, memory-related operations on the WM capacities of schizophrenic patients (Haenschel et al. 2007). The WM load was varied parametrically in this study by presenting one, two or three objects during the encoding condition. After a short delay, participants were asked to judge whether or not the stimulus currently presented was part of the initial sample. Perceptual and cognitive stages of WM performance were separated using ERP analysis. The results suggested that early aspects, indicated by the P1 amplitude, and late aspects of encoding and retrieval, represented by P370 amplitude, were abnormal in schizophrenic patients: the P1 and P370 amplitudes were reduced in patients compared to healthy controls. Furthermore, unlike healthy subjects, patients did not show a gradual increase in P1 with increasing task demands. In patients, the P1 reduction was mirrored by reduced activation of visual areas. Altogether, the findings showed the relevance of early sensory deficits for higher-level cognitive dysfunctions in schizophrenia (Haenschel et al. 2007).

Several aspects of executive functioning, such as verbal fluency and cognitive flexibility, have not been addressed in EEG–fMRI studies so far. Functional dissociations of brain regions connected with flexible responses to task demands have been examined in functional MRI studies independent of EEG recordings. Regarding behavioural inhibition and decision making, EEG–fMRI studies have been conducted to further distinguish neural correlates of different aspects of cognition, for example conflict-related and error-related tasks as well as response anticipation and response conflict. In addition, various processing stages of WM retrieval were decomposed (mental chronometry) using combined

EEG–fMRI measurements. Furthermore, the brain activities of healthy subjects were compared to those associated with deficient executive processes in psychiatric patients; these studies provided evidence for distinct patterns of neural responses.

2.3
Memory

There are three main stages in the formation and retrieval of memory:

(1) *Encoding*: processing and combining received information
(2) *Storage* of encoded information
(3) *Retrieval:* calling back stored information

Irrespective of these criteria, memory processes can be classified according to the amount of information being processed, the duration of storage and the kind of information being stored. The *sensory memory* stores impressions of sensory information (e.g. pictures or smells) for the initial 200–500 ms after its presentation. Some of the information in the sensory memory is transferred to the *short-term memory*. The information in the short-term memory can be recalled for several seconds up to 1 min. Much larger quantities of information can be stored in the *long-term memory*, and the information is potentially stored for an unlimited time period. The memory processes can be enhanced via rehearsal. In contrast to the sensory and the short-term memory, the information in the long-term memory is stored semantically. Long-term memory can be divided into the *declarative* and the *procedural memory* (Anderson 1976). The declarative memory contains information that is explicitly stored and retrieved, for example contact-independent facts (*semantic memory*) or personal memories such as emotions and personal associations (*episodic memory*). The procedural memory, however, primarily contains cognitive and motor skills that were formed primarily via repetition and without explicit learning.

Medial temporal lobes are assumed to reliably contribute to memory processes (Cabeza and Nyberg 2000; Yancey and Phelps 2001). In order to examine *encoding processes*, neural activity is measured while subjects learn a series of stimuli. Memory processes are determined by comparing the neural activation in response to items that were later remembered with the neural activation in response to items that were later forgotten. Neurobiological responses during effective encoding and the formation of new declarative memories have been observed in medial temporal lobe structures, including the hippocampus and surrounding parahippocampal cortices (Brewer et al. 1998; Ofen et al. 2007; Otten et al. 2002). The *storage of information* appears to be related to a network of cortical brain regions, e.g. association cortices. *Retrieval processes* seem to be associated with enhanced responses of the prefrontal cortex and temporal regions (Cabeza and Nyberg 2000; de Zubicaray et al. 2007; Habib and Nyberg 2008; Henson 2005), intraparietal sulcus and precuneus (Henson et al. 2005), and the parietal cortex (de Zubicaray et al. 2007; Heun et al. 2004).

Iidaka and colleagues (2006) aimed to disentangle the conscious recollection of information from familiarity-based judgments using fMRI and ERP. To achieve this, an old/new recognition task was designed. In addition, the level of processing was modulated in order to test whether retrieval activity in the cortical and subcortical structures was affected by the depth of processing during memory encoding. During the encoding phase of the experiment, pictures were presented to the left or right of a fixation cross; in the deep-encoding condition, the subjects judged whether the picture was manmade or natural; in the shallow-encoding condition, the subjects judged whether the object was presented on the left or the right side of the screen. The recognition task consisted of target items (hits; i.e. shown during the encoding task) and new objects (i.e. not shown during the encoding task). In addition, some new items were presented repeatedly (repetitions). The subjects were asked to judge whether the picture presented was old or new.

The findings of the study were consistent with those of former studies supposing a frontoparietal involvement during retrieval success. In addition, the study demonstrated that parietal activity associated with retrieval success produced by deeply encoded items was greater than that produced by shallowly encoded items. However, functional discrepancies appeared: the correct recognition of items presented during the encoding task led to enhanced prefrontal activity compared to the repetition condition; instead, the ventral part of the precentral gyrus was activated. A comparison of correct recognitions (hits) with repetitions revealed that left prefrontal regions were more activate during the hit condition. The authors concluded that this indicated that left prefrontal cortex activation was primarily associated with the conscious and successful recognition of old items. In contrast, the right inferior parietal area was more likely to be related to familiarity-based judgement than to recollection-based judgement. Connectivity analysis indicated that retrieval success is modulated by the functional connectivity in the left hemisphere. ERP and independent component analysis showed that the repetition of items is presumably associated with an earlier rise in parietal activity rather than with other items (Iidaka et al. 2006).

Altogether, these studies demonstrated the possibility of distinguishing BOLD responses associated with different aspects of task execution and related to a differential temporal architecture using EEG–fMRI integration.

3
Limitations and Outlook

Current EEG–fMRI studies focussing on cognitive processes have provided further information, for example about the localisation of various aspects of cognitive processing and ERP components. Various methods have been used, such as a comparison of BOLD responses and the localisation of ERPs based on LORETA analysis (Mulert et al. 2004), fMRI-constrained dipole models (Bledowski et al. 2004b; Crottaz-Herbette and Menon 2006) and single-trial analysis (Debener et al. 2005; Eichele et al. 2005; Mulert et al. 2008b). Single-trial analysis was also used to investigate how aspects like habituation influence task execution. Determining the influence of arousal and the default mode of cognitive functioning may represent important aspects of other EEG–fMRI assessments; for instance, the question of whether and to what extent the default mode of brain activity, as represented by BOLD fMRI, accounts for event-related trial-by-trial fluctuations (Debener et al. 2006).

Working memory studies revealed a chronological dissociation of prefrontal and parietal brain regions, suggesting parallel as well as serial retrieval processes (Bledowski et al. 2006). In addition, a functional dissociation of various aspects of cognitive functioning was attempted in several studies: partial overlapping and distinct brain regions were related to error processing and conflict monitoring (Mathalon et al. 2003) as well as response conflict and response anticipation (Fan et al. 2007). Furthermore, associations of BOLD responses with oscillations in various frequency bands were assessed (Meltzer et al. 2007; Sammer et al. 2007).

So far, the number of simultaneous EEG–fMRI studies focussing on the examination of cognitive processes has been limited: combined evaluations of electrophysiological and haemodynamic information, sometimes acquired through diverse samples, still form the majority. The conclusions that could drawn from these studies are limited because some of the main advantages of simultaneous studies are not achieved; for example, the parameters are not acquired under the same conditions, probably resulting in differences regarding factors that potentially influence cognitive abilities like motivation, learning, habituation and arousal.

Most of the simultaneous and combined EEG–fMRI studies that are investigating cognitive abilities are focussing on attention processes. Investigations dealing with other aspects of cognitive functioning, such as executive functions and memory processes, are rare. One reason for this might be the fact that neurobiological aspects of attention take centre stage in electrophysiological studies. These attention-related electrophysiological studies (e.g. the so-called oddball paradigm and studies of mismatch negativity) form the basis of many EEG–fMRI measurements. Methodological difficulties may be the reason why some cognitive functions have only rarely been analysed. Memory processes, for example, fundamentally rely on subcortical brain functions, e.g. the hippocampus. By contrast, the EEG is particularly sensitive to postsynaptic potentials that are generated in superficial layers of the cortex. The electrical activity of deep structures contributes far less to the EEG signal. Thus, memory-related functional changes in deep brain structures cannot be recorded reliably with electroencephalography. Another reason for the limited number of studies focussing on cognitive functions other than attention may be that executive functions, for example, comprise a number of different components; various tasks are used to acquire these processes. Functional results often vary significantly between tasks; even small variations between task demands can produce clear functional differences. Another problem arises through the examination of planning processes and the management of new problems: problems cease to be novel after the first administration of the test, meaning that they cannot be determined reliably using methods which depend on the iterative presentation of similar tasks (e.g. functional MRI, ERPs) (Burgess 1997; Denckla 1996). Lezak (1983) assumed that examining goal setting, structuring and decision making is a difficult task in the highly structured context of a study. In addition, due to the high complexity of executive tasks, basic nonexecutive processes like attention, memory and motor skills may be triggered during task execution (Burgess 1997), various subprocesses are likely, and similar behaviours can have quite different causes (Jurado and Rosselli 2007).

Due to the limited number of studies regarding cognitive functions other than attention, this overview is one-sided. Various aspects of cognitive functioning are not accounted for considering their significance in cognitive psychology and research. The content of this chapter was strongly determined by the number of EEG–fMRI studies presented in the literature thus far. Often, only some aspects of a cognitive domain were accounted for during these studies.

Despite several difficulties to be considered when evaluating executive functions, examining these processes could be a particularly interesting task: interactions between primary sensory areas, unimodal and multimodal association cortices and prefrontal regions, as well as between various parts of the prefrontal cortex are assumed to be of some importance in executive functioning. EEG–fMRI could contribute to the functional dissociation of these processes and their underlying brain responses. The assignment of subprocesses of cognitive functioning to various brain regions can be investigated using temporal information ("mental chronometry"). In addition, new information can be compared with that stored in memory, and interactions between various sensoric and cognitive subprocesses (e.g. encoding) as well as response preparation can be explored (Fig. 6).

Another promising approach is the implementation of EEG–fMRI studies for the evaluation of neuropsychiatric diseases. Apart from structural deficits, the functional disintegration of various brain structures and functions is thought to provide the main neurobiological

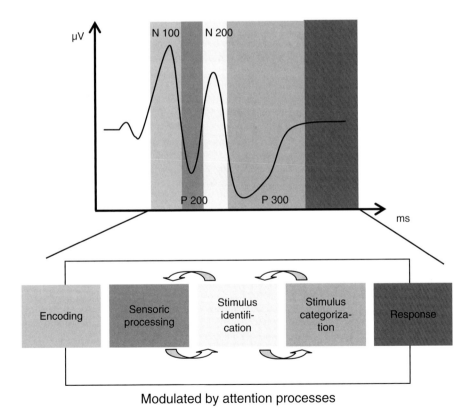

Fig. 6   Exogenous event-related potential in response to auditory information (adapted from Birbaumer and Schmidt 1991)

basis for these diseases. These deficits in brain functions and functional interactions could be evaluated using EEG–fMRI studies and could contribute considerably to a further understanding of neurobiological aspects of these diseases. However, such examinations of neurologic and psychiatric patients as well as children have their limitations: EEG–fMRI investigations tend to be more stressful than single EEG and functional MRI recordings. Furthermore, the recordings are more time consuming; for example, the time required is significantly influenced by the number of electrodes. Due to the extraordinary technical complexity involved, the practicability of incorporating such examinations into the daily clinical routine is limited. As a consequence, only three studies with psychiatric patients have been published so far. However, the relevance of this approach was demonstrated, for example, in a study by Haenschel and colleagues (2007). Their results indicated that working memory deficits of schizophrenic patients were not solely the consequence of dysfunction in prefrontal brain regions. It is more likely that early visual deficits contributed to these deficits.

References

Allen PJ, Polizzi G, Krakow K, Fish DR, Lemieux L (1998) Identification of EEG events in the MR scanner: the problem of pulse artifact and a method for its subtraction. Neuroimage 8(3):229–39

Anderson JR (1976) Language, memory and thought. Erlbaum, Hilldale

Baddeley A (1992) Working memory. Science 255(5044):556–9

Baddeley AD, Hitch GJ (1974) Working memory. In: Bower GA (ed) The psychology of learning and motivation. Academic, New York

Banich MT (2004) Cognitive neuroscience and neuropsychology. Houghton Mifflin, Boston

Barcelo F, Munoz-Cespedes JM, Pozo MA, Rubia FJ (2000) Attentional set shifting modulates the target P3b response in the Wisconsin Card Sorting Test. Neuropsychologia 38(10):1342–55

Barcelo F, Sanz M, Molina V, Rubia FJ (1997) The Wisconsin Card Sorting Test and the assessment of frontal function: a validation study with event-related potentials. Neuropsychologia 35(4):399–408

Bekker EM, Kenemans JL, Verbaten MN (2004) Electrophysiological correlates of attention, inhibition, sensitivity and bias in a continuous performance task. Clin Neurophysiol 115(9):2001–13

Benar CG, Schon D, Grimault S, Nazarian B, Burle B, Roth M, Badier JM, Marquis P, Liegeois-Chauvel C, Anton JL (2007) Single-trial analysis of oddball event-related potentials in simultaneous EEG–fMRI. Hum Brain Mapp 28(7):602–13

Birbaumer N, Schmidt RF (1991) Biologische Psychologie. Springer, Berlin

Bledowski C, Cohen Kadosh K, Wibral M, Rahm B, Bittner RA, Hoechstetter K, Scherg M, Maurer K, Goebel R, Linden DE (2006) Mental chronometry of working memory retrieval: A combined functional magnetic resonance imaging and event-related potentials approach. J Neurosci 26(3):821–9

Bledowski C, Prvulovic D, Goebel R, Zanella FE, Linden DE (2004a) Attentional systems in target and distractor processing: A combined ERP and fMRI study. Neuroimage 22(2):530–40

Bledowski C, Prvulovic D, Hoechstetter K, Scherg M, Wibral M, Goebel R, Linden DE (2004b) Localizing P300 generators in visual target and distractor processing: a combined event-related potential and functional magnetic resonance imaging study. J Neurosci 24(42):9353–60

Botvinick MM, Braver TS, Barch DM, Carter CS, Cohen JD (2001) Conflict monitoring and cognitive control. Psychol Rev 108(3):624–52

Braver TS, Barch DM, Gray JR, Molfese DL, Snyder A (2001) Anterior cingulate cortex and response conflict: effects of frequency, inhibition and errors. Cereb Cortex 11(9):825–36

Brewer JB, Zhao Z, Desmond JE, Glover GH, Gabrieli JD (1998) Making memories: brain activity that predicts how well visual experience will be remembered. Science 281(5380):1185–7

Bruin KJ, Wijers AA, van Staveren AS (2001) Response priming in a go/nogo task: do we have to explain the go/nogo N2 effect in terms of response activation instead of inhibition? Clin Neurophysiol 112(9):1660–71

Burgess P (1997) Theory and methodology in executive function research. In: Rabbitt P (ed) Methodology of frontal executive function. Psychology, Hove

Bush G, Luu P, Posner MI (2000) Cognitive and emotional influences in anterior cingulate cortex. Trends Cogn Sci 4(6):215–22

Cabeza R, Nyberg L (2000) Imaging cognition II: an empirical review of 275 PET and fMRI studies. J Cogn Neurosci 12(1):1–47

Calhoun VD, Adali T, Pearlson GD, Kiehl KA (2006) Neuronal chronometry of target detection: fusion of hemodynamic and event-related potential data. Neuroimage 30(2):544–53

Callicott JH, Mattay VS, Verchinski BA, Marenco S, Egan MF, Weinberger DR (2003) Complexity of prefrontal cortical dysfunction in schizophrenia: more than up or down. Am J Psychiatry 160(12):2209–15

Carlson S, Martinkauppi S, Rama P, Salli E, Korvenoja A, Aronen HJ (1998) Distribution of cortical activation during visuospatial n-back tasks as revealed by functional magnetic resonance imaging. Cereb Cortex 8(8):743–52

Carter CS, Botvinick MM, Cohen JD (1999) The contribution of the anterior cingulate cortex to executive processes in cognition. Rev Neurosci 10(1):49–57

Carter CS, Braver TS, Barch DM, Botvinick MM, Noll D, Cohen JD (1998) Anterior cingulate cortex, error detection, and the online monitoring of performance. Science 280(5364):747–9

Casey BJ, Castellanos FX, Giedd JN, Marsh WL, Hamburger SD, Schubert AB, Vauss YC, Vaituzis AC, Dickstein DP, Sarfatti SE, Rapoport JL (1997) Implication of right frontostriatal circuitry in response inhibition and attention-deficit/hyperactivity disorder. J Am Acad Child Adolesc Psychiatry 36(3):374–83

Catafau AM, Parellada E, Lomena FJ, Bernardo M, Pavia J, Ros D, Setoain J, Gonzalez-Monclus E (1994) Prefrontal and temporal blood flow in schizophrenia: Resting and activation technetium-99m-HMPAO SPECT patterns in young neuroleptic-naive patients with acute disease. J Nucl Med 35(6):935–41

Cohen JD, Botvinick M, Carter CS (2000) Anterior cingulate and prefrontal cortex: who's in control? Nat Neurosci 3(5):421–3

Crottaz-Herbette S, Menon V (2006) Where and when the anterior cingulate cortex modulates attentional response: combined fMRI and ERP evidence. J Cogn Neurosci 18(5):766–80

Debener S, Strobel A, Sorger B, Peters J, Kranczioch C, Engel AK, Goebel R (2007a) Improved quality of auditory event-related potentials recorded simultaneously with 3-T fMRI: removal of the ballistocardiogram artefact. Neuroimage 34(2):587–97

Debener S, Ullsperger M, Siegel M, Engel AK (2006) Single-trial EEG–fMRI reveals the dynamics of cognitive function. Trends Cogn Sci 10(12):558–63

Debener S, Ullsperger M, Siegel M, Fiehler K, von Cramon DY, Engel AK (2005) Trial-by-trial coupling of concurrent electroencephalogram and functional magnetic resonance imaging identifies the dynamics of performance monitoring. J Neurosci 25(50):11730–7

Denckla MBA (1996) Theory and model of executive function: a neuropsychological perspective. In: Lyon G, Krasnegor N (eds) Attention, memory, and executive function. Paul Brooks, Baltimore

D'Esposito M, Aguirre GK, Zarahn E, Ballard D, Shin RK, Lease J (1998) Functional MRI studies of spatial and nonspatial working memory. Brain Res Cogn Brain Res 7(1):1–13

D'Esposito M, Postle BR, Rypma B (2000) Prefrontal cortical contributions to working memory: Evidence from event-related fMRI studies. Exp Brain Res 133(1):3–11 de Zubicaray G, McMahon K, Eastburn M, Pringle AJ, Lorenz L, Humphreys MS (2007) Support for an auto-associative model of spoken cued recall: evidence from fMRI. Neuropsychologia 45(4):824–35

Doeller CF, Opitz B, Mecklinger A, Krick C, Reith W, Schroger E (2003) Prefrontal cortex involvement in preattentive auditory deviance detection: neuroimaging and electrophysiological evidence. Neuroimage 20(2):1270–82

Donchin E, Coles MGH (1988) Is the P300 component a manifestation of context updating? Behav Brain Sci 11:355–72

Donkers FC, van Boxtel GJ (2004) The N2 in go/no-go tasks reflects conflict monitoring not response inhibition. Brain Cogn 56(2):165–76

Downar J, Crawley AP, Mikulis DJ, Davis KD (2000) A multimodal cortical network for the detection of changes in the sensory environment. Nat Neurosci 3(3):277–83

Downar J, Crawley AP, Mikulis DJ, Davis KD (2002) A cortical network sensitive to stimulus salience in a neutral behavioral context across multiple sensory modalities. J Neurophysiol 87(1):615–20

Duann JR, Jung TP, Kuo WJ, Yeh TC, Makeig S, Hsieh JC, Sejnowski TJ (2002) Single-trial variability in event-related BOLD signals. Neuroimage 15(4):823–35

Durston S, Thomas KM, Worden MS, Yang Y, Casey BJ (2002) The effect of preceding context on inhibition: an event-related fMRI study. Neuroimage 16(2):449–53

Effern A, Lehnertz K, Fernandez G, Grunwald T, David P, Elger CE (2000) Single trial analysis of event related potentials: non-linear de-noising with wavelets. Clin Neurophysiol 111(12):2255–63

Eichele T, Specht K, Moosmann M, Jongsma ML, Quiroga RQ, Nordby H, Hugdahl K (2005) Assessing the spatiotemporal evolution of neuronal activation with single-trial event-related potentials and functional MRI. Proc Natl Acad Sci USA 102(49):17798–803

Falkenstein M, Hohnsbein J, Hoormann J, Blanke L (1991) Effects of crossmodal divided attention on late ERP components. II. Error processing in choice reaction tasks. Electroencephalogr Clin Neurophysiol 78(6):447–55

Falkenstein M, Hoormann J, Hohnsbein J (1999) ERP components in Go/Nogo tasks and their relation to inhibition. Acta Psychol (Amst) 101(2–3):267–91

Fan J, Kolster R, Ghajar J, Suh M, Knight RT, Sarkar R, McCandliss BD (2007) Response anticipation and response conflict: an event-related potential and functional magnetic resonance imaging study. J Neurosci 27(9):2272–82

Ford JM, Gray M, Whitfield SL, Turken AU, Glover G, Faustman WO, Mathalon DH (2004) Acquiring and inhibiting prepotent responses in schizophrenia: event-related brain potentials and functional magnetic resonance imaging. Arch Gen Psychiatry 61(2):119–29

Ford JM, White P, Lim KO, Pfefferbaum A (1994) Schizophrenics have fewer and smaller P300s: a single-trial analysis. Biol Psychiatry 35(2):96–103

Friedman D, Cycowicz YM, Gaeta H (2001) The novelty P3: an event-related brain potential (ERP) sign of the brain's evaluation of novelty. Neurosci Biobehav Rev 25(4):355–73

Garavan H, Ross TJ, Murphy K, Roche RA, Stein EA (2002) Dissociable executive functions in the dynamic control of behavior: inhibition, error detection, and correction. Neuroimage 17(4):1820–9

Garavan H, Ross TJ, Stein EA (1999) Right hemispheric dominance of inhibitory control: an event-related functional MRI study. Proc Natl Acad Sci USA 96(14):8301–6

Gehring WJ, Goss B, Coles MG, Meyer DE, Donchin E (1993) A neural system for error detection and compensation. Psychol Sci 4:385–90

Gehring WJ, Knight RT (2000) Prefrontal-cingulate interactions in action monitoring. Nat Neurosci 3(5):516–20

Giard MH, Perrin F, Pernier J, Bouchet P (1990) Brain generators implicated in the processing of auditory stimulus deviance: a topographic event-related potential study. Psychophysiology 27(6):627–40

Goldman-Rakic PS (1994) Working memory dysfunction in schizophrenia. J Neuropsychiatry Clin Neurosci 6(4):348–57

Gomez CM, Flores A, Ledesma A (2007) Fronto-parietal networks activation during the contingent negative variation period. Brain Res Bull 73(1–3):40–7

Gomez CM, Marco J, Grau C (2003) Preparatory visuo-motor cortical network of the contingent negative variation estimated by current density. Neuroimage 20(1):216–24

Gomez CM, Marco-Pallares J, Grau C (2006) Location of brain rhythms and their modulation by preparatory attention estimated by current density. Brain Res 1107(1):151–60

Gonzalez-Hernandez JA, Pita-Alcorta C, Cedeno I, Bosch-Bayard J, Galan-Garcia L, Scherbaum WA, Figueredo-Rodriguez P (2002) Wisconsin Card Sorting Test synchronizes the prefrontal, temporal and posterior association cortex in different frequency ranges and extensions. Hum Brain Mapp 17(1):37–47

Grant DA, Berg EA (1948) A behavioral analysis of degree of reinforcement and ease of shifting to new responses in a Weigl-type card-sorting problem. J Exp Psychol 38:404–11

Habib R, Nyberg L (2008) Neural correlates of availability and accessibility in memory. Cereb Cortex 18(7):1720–6

Haenschel C, Bittner RA, Haertling F, Rotarska-Jagiela A, Maurer K, Singer W, Linden DE (2007) Contribution of impaired early-stage visual processing to working memory dysfunction in adolescents with schizophrenia: a study with event-related potentials and functional magnetic resonance imaging. Arch Gen Psychiatry 64(11):1229–40

Halgren E, Marinkovic K, Chauvel P (1998) Generators of the late cognitive potentials in auditory and visual oddball tasks. Electroencephalogr Clin Neurophysiol 106(2):156–64

Henson R (2005) A mini-review of fMRI studies of human medial temporal lobe activity associated with recognition memory. Q J Exp Psychol B 58(3–4):340–60

Henson RN, Hornberger M, Rugg MD (2005) Further dissociating the processes involved in recognition memory: an FMRI study. J Cogn Neurosci 17(7):1058–73

Heun R, Jessen F, Klose U, Erb M, Granath DO, Grodd W (2004) Response-related fMRI of veridical and false recognition of words. Eur Psychiatry 19(1):42–52

Holroyd CB, Coles MG (2002) The neural basis of human error processing: reinforcement learning, dopamine, and the error-related negativity. Psychol Rev 109(4):679–709

Holroyd CB, Coles MG, Nieuwenhuis S (2002) Medial prefrontal cortex and error potentials. Science 296(5573):1610–1; author reply 1610–1

Horovitz SG, Skudlarski P, Gore JC (2002) Correlations and dissociations between BOLD signal and P300 amplitude in an auditory oddball task: a parametric approach to combining fMRI and ERP. Magn Reson Imaging 20(4):319–25

Iidaka T, Matsumoto A, Nogawa J, Yamamoto Y, Sadato N (2006) Frontoparietal network involved in successful retrieval from episodic memory. Spatial and temporal analyses using fMRI and ERP. Cereb Cortex 16(9):1349–60

Ioannides AA, Fenwick PB, Lumsden J, Liu MJ, Bamidis PD, Squires KC, Lawson D, Fenton GW (1994) Activation sequence of discrete brain areas during cognitive processes: results from magnetic field tomography. Electroencephalogr Clin Neurophysiol 91(5):399–402

Jahanshahi M, Dirnberger G, Fuller R, Frith CD (2000) The role of the dorsolateral prefrontal cortex in random number generation: a study with positron emission tomography. Neuroimage 12(6):713–25

Javitt DC, Schroeder CE, Steinschneider M, Arezzo JC, Vaughan HG Jr (1992) Demonstration of mismatch negativity in the monkey. Electroencephalogr Clin Neurophysiol 83(1):87–90

Johnson MR, Morris NA, Astur RS, Calhoun VD, Mathalon DH, Kiehl KA, Pearlson GD (2006) A functional magnetic resonance imaging study of working memory abnormalities in schizophrenia. Biol Psychiatry 60(1):11–21

Jung TP, Makeig S, Westerfield M, Townsend J, Courchesne E, Sejnowski TJ (2001) Analysis and visualization of single-trial event-related potentials. Hum Brain Mapp 14(3):166–85

Jurado MB, Rosselli M (2007) The elusive nature of executive functions: a review of our current understanding. Neuropsychol Rev 17(3):213–33

Kamarajan C, Porjesz B, Jones KA, Choi K, Chorlian DB, Padmanabhapillai A, Rangaswamy M, Stimus AT, Begleiter H (2005) Alcoholism is a disinhibitory disorder: neurophysiological evidence from a Go/No-Go task. Biol Psychol 69(3):353–73

Karch S, Jager L, Karamatskos E, Graz C, Stammel A, Flatz W, Lutz J, Holtschmidt-Taschner B, Genius J, Leicht G, Pogarell O, Born C, Moller HJ, Hegerl U, Reiser M, Soyka M, Mulert C (2007) Influence of trait anxiety on inhibitory control in alcohol-dependent patients: Simultaneous acquisition of ERPs and BOLD responses. J Psychiatr Res 42(9):734–45

Katayama J, Polich J (1998) Stimulus context determines P3a and P3b. Psychophysiology 35(1):23–33

Kawasaki T, Tanaka S, Wang J, Hokama H, Hiramatsu K (2004) Abnormalities of P300 cortical current density in unmedicated depressed patients revealed by LORETA analysis of event-related potentials. Psychiatry Clin Neurosci 58(1):68–75

Kelly AM, Hester R, Murphy K, Javitt DC, Foxe JJ, Garavan H (2004) Prefrontal-subcortical dissociations underlying inhibitory control revealed by event-related fMRI. Eur J Neurosci 19(11):3105–12

Kiehl KA, Liddle PF, Hopfinger JB (2000) Error processing and the rostral anterior cingulate: an event-related fMRI study. Psychophysiology 37(2):216–23

Kiehl KA, Stevens MC, Celone K, Kurtz M, Krystal JH (2005a) Abnormal hemodynamics in schizophrenia during an auditory oddball task. Biol Psychiatry 57(9):1029–40

Kiehl KA, Stevens MC, Laurens KR, Pearlson G, Calhoun VD, Liddle PF (2005b) An adaptive reflexive processing model of neurocognitive function: supporting evidence from a large scale (n = 100) fMRI study of an auditory oddball task. Neuroimage 25(3):899–915

Knight R (1996) Contribution of human hippocampal region to novelty detection. Nature 383(6597):256–9

Kok A (2001) On the utility of P3 amplitude as a measure of processing capacity. Psychophysiology 38(3):557–77

Konishi S, Hayashi T, Uchida I, Kikyo H, Takahashi E, Miyashita Y (2002) Hemispheric asymmetry in human lateral prefrontal cortex during cognitive set shifting. Proc Natl Acad Sci USA 99(11):7803–8

Konishi S, Nakajima K, Uchida I, Kikyo H, Kameyama M, Miyashita Y (1999) Common inhibitory mechanism in human inferior prefrontal cortex revealed by event-related functional MRI. Brain 122 (Pt 5):981–91

Kropotov JD, Naatnen R, Sevostianov AV, Alho K, Reinikainen K, Kropotova OV (1995) Mismatch negativity to auditory stimulus change recorded directly from the human temporal cortex. Psychophysiology 32(4):418–22

Kruggel F, von Cramon DY (1999) Modeling the hemodynamic response in single-trial functional MRI experiments. Magn Reson Med 42(4):787–97

Lewis SJ, Dove A, Robbins TW, Barker RA, Owen AM (2004) Striatal contributions to working memory: a functional magnetic resonance imaging study in humans. Eur J Neurosci 19(3):755–60

Lezak MD (1983) Neuropsychological assessment. Wiley, New York

Liddle PF, Kiehl KA, Smith AM (2001) Event-related fMRI study of response inhibition. Hum Brain Mapp 12(2):100–9

Lie CH, Specht K, Marshall JC, Fink GR (2006) Using fMRI to decompose the neural processes underlying the Wisconsin Card Sorting Test. Neuroimage 30(3):1038–49

Liebenthal E, Ellingson ML, Spanaki MV, Prieto TE, Ropella KM, Binder JR (2003) Simultaneous ERP and fMRI of the auditory cortex in a passive oddball paradigm. Neuroimage 19(4):1395–404

Linden DE, Prvulovic D, Formisano E, Vollinger M, Zanella FE, Goebel R, Dierks T (1999) The functional neuroanatomy of target detection: an fMRI study of visual and auditory oddball tasks. Cereb Cortex 9(8):815–23

Linden DEJ (2007) What, when, where in the brain? Exploring mental chronometry with brain imaging and electrophysiology. Rev Neurosci 18(2):159–71

Logan GD, Cowan WB, Davis KA (1984) On the ability to inhibit simple and choice reaction time responses: a model and a method. J Exp Psychol Hum Percept Perform 10(2):276–91

Manoach DS, Gollub RL, Benson ES, Searl MM, Goff DC, Halpern E, Saper CB, Rauch SL (2000) Schizophrenic subjects show aberrant fMRI activation of dorsolateral prefrontal cortex and basal ganglia during working memory performance. Biol Psychiatry 48(2):99–109

Mathalon DH, Whitfield SL, Ford JM (2003) Anatomy of an error: ERP and fMRI. Biol Psychol 64(1–2):119–41

Mathiak K, Rapp A, Kircher TT, Grodd W, Hertrich I, Weiskopf N, Lutzenberger W, Ackermann H (2002) Mismatch responses to randomized gradient switching noise as reflected by fMRI and whole-head magnetoencephalography. Hum Brain Mapp 16(3):190–5

Matsuda T, Matsuura M, Ohkubo T, Ohkubo H, Atsumi Y, Tamaki M, Takahashi K, Matsushima E, Kojima T (2002) Influence of arousal level for functional magnetic resonance imaging (fMRI) study: simultaneous recording of fMRI and electroencephalogram. Psychiatry Clin Neurosci 56(3):289–90

McCarley RW, Faux SF, Shenton ME, Nestor PG, Holinger DP (1991) Is there P300 asymmetry in schizophrenia? Arch Gen Psychiatry 48(4):380–3

McCarthy G, Luby M, Gore J, Goldman-Rakic P (1997) Infrequent events transiently activate human prefrontal and parietal cortex as measured by functional MRI. J Neurophysiol 77(3):1630–4

Meltzer JA, Negishi M, Mayes LC, Constable RT (2007) Individual differences in EEG theta and alpha dynamics during working memory correlate with fMRI responses across subjects. Clin Neurophysiol 118(11):2419–36

Menon V, Adleman NE, White CD, Glover GH, Reiss AL (2001a) Error-related brain activation during a Go/NoGo response inhibition task. Hum Brain Mapp 12(3):131–43

Menon V, Anagnoson RT, Mathalon DH, Glover GH, Pfefferbaum A (2001b) Functional neuroanatomy of auditory working memory in schizophrenia: relation to positive and negative symptoms. Neuroimage 13(3):433–46

Menon V, Crottaz-Herbette S (2005) Combined EEG and fMRI studies of human brain function. Int Rev Neurobiol 66:291–321

Menon V, Ford JM, Lim KO, Glover GH, Pfefferbaum A (1997) Combined event-related fMRI and EEG evidence for temporal-parietal cortex activation during target detection. Neuroreport 8(14):3029–37

Milham MP, Banich MT (2005) Anterior cingulate cortex: an fMRI analysis of conflict specificity and functional differentiation. Hum Brain Mapp 25(3):328–35

Monchi O, Petrides M, Petre V, Worsley K, Dagher A (2001) Wisconsin Card Sorting revisited: distinct neural circuits participating in different stages of the task identified by event-related functional magnetic resonance imaging. J Neurosci 21(19):7733–41

Mulert C, Jager L, Schmitt R, Bussfeld P, Pogarell O, Moller HJ, Juckel G, Hegerl U (2004) Integration of fMRI and simultaneous EEG: Towards a comprehensive understanding of localization and time-course of brain activity in target detection. Neuroimage 22(1):83–94

Mulert C, Pogarell O, Hegerl U (2008a) Simultaneous EEG–fMRI: perspectives in psychiatry. Clin EEG Neurosci 39(2):61–4

Mulert C, Seifert CL, Leicht G, Kirsch V, Ertl M, Karch S, Moosmann M, Lutz J, Moller HJ, Hegerl U, Pogarell O, Jager L (2008b) Single-trial coupling of EEG and fMRI reveals the involvement of early anterior cingulate cortex activation in effortful decision making. Neuroimage 42:158–68

Näätänen R, Gaillard AW, Mantysalo S (1978) Early selective-attention effect on evoked potential reinterpreted. Acta Psychol (Amst) 42(4):313–29

Näätänen R, Winkler I (1999) The concept of auditory stimulus representation in cognitive neuroscience. Psychol Bull 125(6):826–59

Nagai Y, Critchley HD, Featherstone E, Fenwick PB, Trimble MR, Dolan RJ (2004) Brain activity relating to the contingent negative variation: an fMRI investigation. Neuroimage 21(4):1232–41

Niazy RK, Beckmann CF, Iannetti GD, Brady JM, Smith SM (2005) Removal of FMRI environment artifacts from EEG data using optimal basis sets. Neuroimage 28(3):720–37

Nieuwenhuis S, Yeung N, van den Wildenberg W, Ridderinkhof KR (2003) Electrophysiological correlates of anterior cingulate function in a go/no-go task: effects of response conflict and trial type frequency. Cogn Affect Behav Neurosci 3(1):17–26

Norman DA, Shallice T (1986) Attention to action: willed and automatic control of behavior. In: Davidson RJ, Schwartz GE, Shapiro D (eds) Consciousness and self-regulation, vol 4. Plenum, New York

Ofen N, Kao YC, Sokol-Hessner P, Kim H, Whitfield-Gabrieli S, Gabrieli JD (2007) Development of the declarative memory system in the human brain. Nat Neurosci 10(9):1198–205

Opitz B, Mecklinger A, Friederici AD, von Cramon DY (1999) The functional neuroanatomy of novelty processing: integrating ERP and fMRI results. Cereb Cortex 9(4):379–91

Opitz B, Rinne T, Mecklinger A, von Cramon DY, Schroger E (2002) Differential contribution of frontal and temporal cortices to auditory change detection: fMRI and ERP results. Neuroimage 15(1):167–74

Otten LJ, Henson RN, Rugg MD (2002) State-related and item-related neural correlates of successful memory encoding. Nat Neurosci 5(12):1339–44

Paulesu E, Frith CD, Frackowiak RS (1993) The neural correlates of the verbal component of working memory. Nature 362(6418):342–5

Paulesu E, Goldacre B, Scifo P, Cappa SF, Gilardi MC, Castiglioni I, Perani D, Fazio F (1997) Functional heterogeneity of left inferior frontal cortex as revealed by fMRI. Neuroreport 8(8):2011–7

Pfefferbaum A, Ford JM, Weller BJ, Kopell BS (1985) ERPs to response production and inhibition. Electroencephalogr Clin Neurophysiol 60(5):423–34

Phelps EA, Hyder F, Blamire AM, Shulman RG (1997) FMRI of the prefrontal cortex during overt verbal fluency. Neuroreport 8(2):561–5

Polich J, Corey-Bloom J (2005) Alzheimer's disease and P300: review and evaluation of task and modality. Curr Alzheimer Res 2(5):515–25

Polich J, Herbst KL (2000) P300 as a clinical assay: rationale, evaluation, and findings. Int J Psychophysiol 38(1):3–19

Posner MI (1978) Chronometric explorations of mind. Oxford University Press, New York

Ridderinkhof KR, Ullsperger M, Crone EA, Nieuwenhuis S (2004) The role of the medial frontal cortex in cognitive control. Science 306(5695):443–7

Rinne T, Alho K, Ilmoniemi RJ, Virtanen J, Naatanen R (2000) Separate time behaviors of the temporal and frontal mismatch negativity sources. Neuroimage 12(1):14–9

Rockstroh B, Elbert T, Birbaumer N, Lutzenberger W (1982) Slow brain potentials and behavior. Urban & Schwarzenberg, Baltimore

Rypma B, D'Esposito M (1999) The roles of prefrontal brain regions in components of working memory: Effects of memory load and individual differences. Proc Natl Acad Sci USA 96(11):6558–63

Sabri M, Liebenthal E, Waldron EJ, Medler DA, Binder JR (2006) Attentional modulation in the detection of irrelevant deviance: a simultaneous ERP/fMRI study. J Cogn Neurosci 18(5):689–700

Sammer G, Blecker C, Gebhardt H, Bischoff M, Stark R, Morgen K, Vaitl D (2007) Relationship between regional hemodynamic activity and simultaneously recorded EEG-theta associated with mental arithmetic-induced workload. Hum Brain Mapp 28(8):793–803

Scheffers MK, Coles MG (2000) Performance monitoring in a confusing world: error-related brain activity, judgments of response accuracy, and types of errors. J Exp Psychol Hum Percept Perform 26(1):141–51

Scheffers MK, Coles MG, Bernstein P, Gehring WJ, Donchin E (1996) Event-related brain potentials and error-related processing: an analysis of incorrect responses to go and no-go stimuli. Psychophysiology 33(1):42–53

Schroger E, Wolff C (1996) Mismatch response of the human brain to changes in sound location. Neuroreport 7(18):3005–8

Shallice T (1988) From neuropsychology to mental structure. Cambridge University Press, Cambridge

Sohlberg M, Mateer CA (1989) Introduction to cognitive rehabilitation: theory and practice. Guilford, New York

Sokolov EN (1963) Higher nervous functions: the orienting reflex. Annu Rev Physiol 35:545–80

Stevens MC, Calhoun VD, Kiehl KA (2005) Hemispheric differences in hemodynamics elicited by auditory oddball stimuli. Neuroimage 26(3):782–92

Stuss DT, Levine B (2002) Adult clinical neuropsychology: lessons from studies of the frontal lobes. Annu Rev Psychol 53:401–33

Sutton S, Braren M, Zubin J, John ER (1965) Evoked potential correlates of stimulus uncertainty. Science 150:1187–88

Tan HY, Choo WC, Fones CS, Chee MW (2005) fMRI study of maintenance and manipulation processes within working memory in first-episode schizophrenia. Am J Psychiatry 162(10):1849–58

Tecce JJ (1972) Contingent negative variation (CNV) and psychological processes in man. Psychol Bull 77(2):73–108

Ullsperger M, von Cramon DY (2001) Subprocesses of performance monitoring: a dissociation of error processing and response competition revealed by event-related fMRI and ERPs. Neuroimage 14(6):1387–401

Ullsperger M, von Cramon DY (2004) Neuroimaging of performance monitoring: error detection and beyond. Cortex 40(4–5):593–604

van der Stelt O, Frye J, Lieberman JA, Belger A (2004) Impaired P3 generation reflects high-level and progressive neurocognitive dysfunction in schizophrenia. Arch Gen Psychiatry 61(3):237–48

Veltman DJ, Rombouts SA, Dolan RJ (2003) Maintenance versus manipulation in verbal working memory revisited: an fMRI study. Neuroimage 18(2):247–56

Watanabe J, Sugiura M, Sato K, Sato Y, Maeda Y, Matsue Y, Fukuda H, Kawashima R (2002) The human prefrontal and parietal association cortices are involved in NO-GO performances: an event-related fMRI study. Neuroimage 17(3):1207–16

Weinberger DR, Berman KF, Zec RF (1986) Physiologic dysfunction of dorsolateral prefrontal cortex in schizophrenia. I. Regional cerebral blood flow evidence. Arch Gen Psychiatry 43(2):114–24

Yancey SW, Phelps EA (2001) Functional neuroimaging and episodic memory: a perspective. J Clin Exp Neuropsychol 23(1):32–48

Special Topics

Neuronal Models for EEG–fMRI Integration 22

James M. Kilner and Karl J. Friston

1
EEG and fMRI Integration

It is now generally accepted that the integration of fMRI and electromagnetic measures of brain activity has an important role in characterising evoked brain responses. These two measures are both related to the underlying neural activity, but whereas the electromagnetic measures are a direct measure and therefore capture the neuronal activity with millisecond temporal resolution, the fMRI measure is an indirect measure of the underlying neuronal activity and has poor temporal resolution, on the order of seconds. Conversely, the fMRI has excellent spatial resolution, on the order of millimetres, compared to EEG/MEG. Therefore, the obvious motivation for integrating these two measures is to provIDe a composite recording that has excellent temporal and spatial resolution. The possibility of integrating these two measures in humans is supported by the results of the study by Logothetis et al. (2001). In this study, the authors demonstrated that, within the macaque monkey visual cortex, intracortical recordings of the local field potential (LFP) and the BOLD signal were linearly correlated.

Approaches to integration can be classified into three schemes: integration through prediction; integration through constraints; and integration through fusion. These are depicted schematically in Fig. 1. Integration through prediction (Fig. 1, dotted line), uses the temporally resolved electroencephalography (EEG) signal as a predictor of changes in concurrently recorded fMRI. The ensuing region-specific haemodynamic correlates can then be characterised with high spatial resolution with conventional imaging methodology (Lovblad et al. 1999; Lemieux et al. 2001; Czisch M et al. 2004). Several studies of this type (Goldman et al. 2002; Laufs et al. 2003a, b; Martinez-Montes 2004) have focussed on correlating modulations in ongoing oscillatory activity measured by EEG with the haemodynamic signal. They have demonstrated that modulations in alpha rhythms

J. M. Kilner (✉)
The Wellcome Centre for Neuroimaging, Institute of Neurology, Queen Square, London WC1N 3BG, UK
e-mail: jkilner@fil.ion.ucl.ac.uk

C. Mulert and L. Lemieux (eds.), *EEG–fMRI*
DOI: 10.1007/978-3-540-87919-0_22, © Springer Verlag Berlin Heidelberg 2010

Fig. 1 Schematic showing the
approaches to EEG–fMRI
integration. (*i*) Integration
through prediction. (*ii*)
Integration through constraints.
(*iii*) Integration through fusion
with forward models

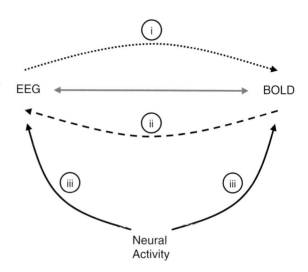

(oscillations at ~10 Hz) are negatively correlated with modulations in the BOLD signal (i.e. an increase in alpha power is associated with a decrease in the BOLD signal). Studies employing integration through constraints (Fig. 1, dashed line) have used the spatial resolution of focal fMRI activations to constrain equivalent dipole or distributed estimates of EEG or MEG sources (Dale et al. 2000; Phillips et al. 2002). However, neither of these schemes can be considered a true integration of multimodal data in the sense that there is no common temporal forward model that links the underlying neuronal dynamics of interest to measured haemodynamic and electrical responses (Fig. 1 solid black lines).

The characterisation of the relationship between the electrophysiology of neuronal systems and their slower haemodynamics in terms of their respective forward models is therefore crucial from a number of perspectives: not only for forward models of electrical and haemodynamic data, but also for the utility of spatial priors (derived from fMRI) in the inverse EEG/MEG source reconstruction problem, and for the disambiguation of induced (relative to evoked) brain responses using both modalities.

In the next section, we will describe perhaps the simplest of all models that helps to explain some empirical observations of EEG–fMRI integration using a dimensional analysis and a biophysical model.

2
Neuronal Model of EEG–fMRI Integration

2.1
Dimensional Analysis

Given the tenable assumption that haemodynamics reflect the energetics of underlying neuronal changes (Jueptner and Weiller 1995; Shulman and Rothman 1998; Hoge et al. 1999; Magistretti et al. 1999; Magistretti and Pellerin 1999; Shin 2000), we assume here that the BOLD signal b, at any point in time, is proportional to the rate of energy dissipation, induced by transmembrane currents. It is important to note that we are not assuming here that the increase in blood flow, which is the major contributor to the BOLD signal, is a direct consequence of the rate of energy dissipation, but rather that these two measures are proportional (see Hoge et al. 1999). Although recent work has suggested that the neurovascular coupling is driven by glutamate release (see Lauritzen 2001; Attwell and Iadecola 2002), in practice the measures of glutamate release, BOLD and energy usage, are correlated, and therefore the assumption here that the BOLD signal is proportional to the rate of energy dissipation is valid. This dissipation is expressed in terms of J/s and corresponds to the product of transmembrane potential (v, joules per coulomb) and transmembrane current (i, coulombs per second):

$$b \propto \left\langle v^{\mathrm{T}} i \right\rangle, \tag{1}$$

where the expectation is over time and $v = [v_1, \mathrm{K}, v_k]^{\mathrm{T}}$ corresponds to a [large] column vector of potentials for each neuronal compartment k within a voxel, similarly for i. Clearly, Eq. 1 will not be true instantaneously, because it may take some time for the energy cost to be expressed in terms of increased oxygen delivery, extraction and perfusion. However, over a suitable timescale, on the order of seconds, Eq. 1 will be approximately correct. Assuming a single-compartment model, currents are related to changes in membrane potential though their capacitance c, which we will assume is constant (see Dayan and Abbott 2001, pp 156). By convention, the membrane current is defined as positive when positive ions leave the neuron and negative when positive ions enter the neuron:

$$i = -c\dot{v}, \tag{2}$$

then

$$b \propto c\left\langle v^{\mathrm{T}} \dot{v} \right\rangle. \tag{3}$$

To relate changes in membrane potential to the BOLD signal, we need to adopt some model of a neuronal system and how it activates. A simple integrate-and-fire model of autonomous neuronal dynamics can be expressed in the form

$$\dot{v}_k = -v_k/\tau_k + u_k$$
$$= f_k(v) \tag{4}$$

for the kth compartment or unit. We have assumed here that synaptic currents are caused by some nonlinear function of the depolarisation status of all units in the population: i.e. $u_k = g_k(v)$. For a system of this form we can approximate the dynamics of perturbations with the first-order system

$$\dot{v}(t) = -Jv$$
$$J = \frac{\partial f}{\partial v}. \tag{5}$$

The Jacobian J summarises the functional or causal architecture of the neuronal system. The leading diagonal elements of J correspond to self-inhibition and play the role of effective membrane rates or conductances. In the absence of influences from any other units, the kth potential will decay exponentially to the equilibrium or resting potential ($v = 0$):

$$\dot{v}_k = -J_{kk} v_k. \tag{6}$$

It can be seen that $J_{kk} = 1/\tau_k$ has units of per second, and is the inverse of the effective membrane time constant. In fact, in most biophysical models of neuronal dynamics, this "rate" is usually considered the ratio of the membrane's conductance to its capacitance. Conductivity will reflect the configuration of various ion channels and the ongoing post-synaptic receptor occupancy. In a similar way, the off-diagonal elements of the Jacobian characterise the effective connectivity or intrinsic coupling among units, where $J_{kj} = \partial f_k / \partial v_j = \partial \dot{v}_k / \partial v_j$. Effective connectivity is simply the influence one neuronal system exerts over another. It is interesting to note that plausible neuronal models of ensemble dynamics suggest a tight coupling between average spiking rate and decreases in effective membrane time constants (e.g. Chawla et al. 2000). However, as we will see below, we do not need to consider spikes to close the link between BOLD and frequency profiles of ongoing EEG or MEG dynamics.

From Eqs. 3 and 5 we have

$$\begin{aligned} b &\propto c < v^T J v > \\ &\propto ctr(J < vv^T >) \\ &\propto ctr(J \, \mathrm{Cov}\{v\}). \end{aligned} \tag{7}$$

This means that the metabolic response is proportional to the trace of the product of the Jacobian (i.e. effective connectivity) and the temporal covariance of the transmembrane potentials.

2.2
Modelling Activations

At this point we have to consider how "activation" is mediated; in other words, how the dynamics over an extended period of time could change. If we treat the units within any voxel as an autonomous system, then any extrinsic influence must be mediated by changes in the Jacobian; for instance, changes in conductance or coupling among neurons induced by afferent input. The attending changes in potential are secondary to these changes in the functional architecture of the system and may, or may not, change their covariances $\mathrm{Cov}\{v\}$. According to Eq. 7, a metabolic cost is induced through changes in J, even in the absence of changes in the covariance. To link BOLD and EEG responses, we need to model the underlying changes in the Jacobian that generate them. This is accomplished in a parsimonious way by introducing an activation variable, α, that changes J. Here, α is a parameter that changes the effective connectivity (i.e. synaptic efficacies) and, implicitly, the dynamics of neuronal activity. In this model, different modes of brain activity are associated with the Jacobian

$$J(\alpha) = J(0) + \alpha \partial J / \partial \alpha. \tag{8}$$

We will assume that $\partial J/\partial \alpha = J(0)$. In other words, the change in intrinsic coupling (including self-inhibition), induced by activation, is proportional to the coupling in the "resting" state when $\alpha = 0$. The motivations for this assumption include:

- Its simplicity.
- Guaranteed stability, in the sense that if $J(0)$ has no unstable modes (positive eigenvalues) then neither will $J(\alpha)$. For example, it ensures that activation does not violate the "no-strong-loops hypothesis" (Crick and Koch 1998).
- It ensures the intrinsic balance between inhibitory and excitatory influences that underpins "cortical gain control" (Abbot et al. 1997).
- It models the increases in membrane conductance associated with short-term increases in synaptic efficacy.

2.3
Effect of Neuronal Activation on BOLD

These considerations suggest that the coupling J_{kj} among neurons (positive and negative) will scale in a similar way and that these changes will be reflected in changes to effective membrane time constants J_{kk}. Under this model for activation, the effect of α is to accelerate the dynamics and increase the system's energy dissipation. This acceleration can be seen most easily by considering the responses to perturbations around v_0 under $J = J(0)$ and $\tilde{J} = J(\alpha) = (1 + \alpha)J$:

$$v(t) = e^{-Jt}v_0$$
$$\tilde{v}(t) = e^{-\tilde{J}t}v_0 = v((1+\alpha)t).$$

(9)

In other words, the perturbation under $J(\alpha)$ at time t is exactly the same as that under $J(0)$ at $(1 + \alpha)t$. This acceleration will only make dynamics faster; it will not change their form. Consequently, there will be no change in the co-variation of membrane potentials, and the impact on the fMRI responses is mediated by (and only by) changes in J.

$$\frac{\tilde{b}}{b} \propto \frac{tr(\tilde{J}\,\mathrm{Cov}\{v\})}{tr(J\,\mathrm{Cov}\{v\})} = (1+\alpha).$$

(10)

In other words, the activation, α, is proportional to the relative increase in metabolic demands. This is intuitive from the perspective of fMRI, but what does an activation look like in terms of the EEG?

2.4
Effect of Neuronal Activation on EEG

From the point of view of the fast temporal activity reflected in the EEG, activation will cause an acceleration of the dynamics, leading to a "rougher" looking signal with loss of lower frequencies relative to higher frequencies. A simple way to measure this effect is in terms of the roughness r, which is the normalised variance of the first temporal derivative of the EEG. From the theory of stationary processes (Cox and Miller 1965), this is mathematically the same as the negative curvature of the EEG autocorrelation function evaluated at zero lag. Thus, for an EEG signal e:

$$r = \frac{\text{Var}(\dot{e})}{\text{Var}(e)} = -\rho(0)''.$$

Assuming that e (measured at a single site) is a linear mixture of potentials, i.e. $e = lv$, where l is a lead-field row vector, its autocorrelation at lag h is:

$$\rho(h) = \langle v(t)^T l^T l v(t + h) \rangle. \tag{11}$$

From Eqs. 9 and 11, we have:

$$\begin{aligned} \tilde{\rho}(h) &= \rho((1+\alpha)h) \\ \tilde{\rho}(h)'' &= (1+\alpha)^2 \rho(h)''. \end{aligned} \tag{12}$$

It follows that the change in r is related to neuronal activation by

$$\frac{\tilde{r}}{r} = \frac{\tilde{\rho}(0)''}{\rho(0)''} = (1+\alpha)^2. \tag{13}$$

As the spectral density of a random process is defined to be the Fourier transform of its autocorrelation function, $g(\omega) = \int \rho(h)e^{-iwh}dh$, the equivalent relationship in the frequency domain obtained from the "roughness" expressed in terms of spectral density $g(\omega)$ is:

$$r = \frac{\int \omega^2 g(\omega)d\omega}{\int g(\omega)d\omega}.$$

From Eq. 12, the equivalent of the activated case in terms of the spectral density is:

$$\tilde{g}(\omega) = \frac{g((1+\alpha)\omega)}{(1+\alpha)}. \tag{14}$$

Here, the effect of activation is to shift the spectral profile toward higher frequencies with a reduction in amplitude (see Fig. 2). The activation can be expressed in terms of the "normalised" spectral density

$$\frac{\tilde{r}}{r} = \frac{\int \omega^2 \tilde{p}(\omega)d\omega}{\int \omega^2 p(\omega)d\omega} = (1+\alpha)^2$$

$$p(\omega) = \frac{g(\omega)}{\int g(\omega)d\omega}, \tag{15}$$

$p(\omega)$ could be treated as an empirical estimate of probability, rendering roughness equivalent to the expected or mean square frequency. Gathering together the above equalities, we can express relative values of fMRI and spectral measures in terms of each other:

Fig. 2 Schematic showing the effect of activation on the spectral profile

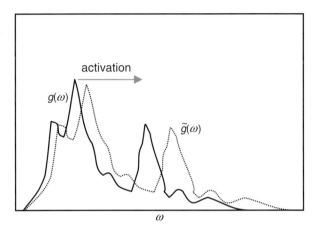

$$\left[\frac{\tilde{b}}{b}\right]^2 \propto (1+\alpha)^2 \propto \frac{\int \omega^2 \tilde{p}(\omega)\mathrm{d}\omega}{\int \omega^2 p(\omega)\mathrm{d}\omega}. \tag{16}$$

Equation 16 means that as neuronal activation increases, there is a concomitant increase in the BOLD signal and a shift in the spectral profile to higher frequencies. High-frequency dynamics are associated with small effective membrane time constants and high (leaky) transmembrane conductances. The ensuing currents and fast changes in potential incur an energy cost to which the BOLD signal is sensitive. Such high-frequency dynamics have also been shown to be dependent upon the firing patterns of inhibitory interneurons (Traub et al. 1996; Whittington and Traub 2003). The conjoint effect of inhibitory and excitatory synaptic input is to open ion channels, rendering the postsynaptic membrane leaky with high rate constants. The effect is captured in the model by the scaling of the leading diagonal elements of the Jacobian. This suggests that the changes in the temporal dynamics to which the BOLD signal is sensitive are mediated by changes in the firing patterns of both excitatory and inhibitory subpopulations.

Critically, however, the predicted BOLD signal is a function of the frequency profile as opposed to any particular frequency. For example, an increase in alpha (low frequency), without a change in total power, would reduce the mean square frequency and suggest deactivation. Conversely, an increase in gamma (high frequency) would increase the mean square frequency and speak to activation (see Fig. 3).

3
Empirical Evidence for the Model

The model described in this chapter ties together expected changes in BOLD and EEG measures and makes a clear prediction about the relationship between the different frequency components of ongoing EEG or MEG activity and the expected BOLD response.

Fig. 3 Schematic showing the effect of deactivation on mean square frequency

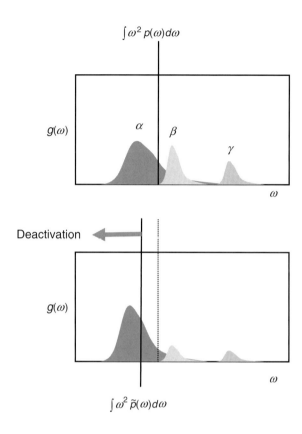

According to the model, any modulations in the degree of low-frequency relative to high-frequency components in the EEG signal will be inversely correlated with the BOLD signal. This is largely in agreement with the empirical data available. It is now generally accepted that modulations in the ongoing alpha rhythm, 8–12 Hz, when the eyes are shut, are inversely correlated with the BOLD signal at voxels within the parietal, parieto-occipital and frontal cortices (Goldman et al. 2002; Laufs et al. 2003a, b; Moosmann et al. 2003; Martinez-Montes 2004). Furthermore, during low-frequency visual entrainment using a periodic checkerboard stimulus, the BOLD signal is reduced compared to an aperiodic stimulus (Parkes et al. 2004). The model presented here also predicts that a shift in the frequency profile of the EEG to high-frequency components should be correlated with an increase in the BOLD signal. Although there is a much less literature on high-frequency EEG-BOLD correlations, what has been published is broadly in agreement with this prediction. Laufs et al. (2003a) report predominantly positive correlations between the BOLD signal and the EEG power in the 17–23 Hz and the 24–30 Hz bandwidth, and Parkes et al. (2004) demonstrate that an aperiodic checkerboard stimulus induces a greater BOLD signal than a low-frequency periodic stimulus. However, perhaps the most convincing empirical data that support the prediction of the model described here comes not from a human study but from a study on anaesthetised adult cats by Niessing et al. (2005). In this study,

Niessing et al. recorded a measure of the electrical activity, the LFP (the LFP is analogous to the EEG signal), directly from primary visual cortex using implanted electrodes, whilst simultaneously recording a measure of the BOLD signal using optical imaging. These measures were recorded whilst the cats were visually stimulated by moving whole-field gratings of different orientations. Niessing et al. showed that in trials in which the optical signal was strong, the neural response tended to oscillate at higher frequencies. In other words, an increase in the BOLD signal was associated with a shift in the spectral mass of the electrical signal to higher frequencies, in total agreement with the prediction of the model described here.

However, there are a number of observations that are not captured by the model. Firstly, the model does not address very slow changes in potentials, <0.1 Hz, that are unlikely to contribute to the event-related response. As such, it does not capture the very slow modulations in LFP that have previously been shown to be related to the BOLD response (Leopold et al. 2003). Secondly, and most notably, it does not explain the positive correlation of the BOLD signal with alpha oscillations in the thalamus (Goldman et al. 2002; Martinez-Montes 2004). This discrepancy could reflect the unique neuronal dynamics of the thalamus. Thalamic neurons are characterised by complex intrinsic firing properties, which may range from the genesis of high-frequency bursts of action potential to tonic firing (Steriades et al. 1993).

There are other shortcomings that could be invoked and that would have to be considered if the model failed to predict BOLD-EEG relationships. Having briefly deconstructed the model, it is worth noting that it highlights some conceptual issues that might be useful. These include the following:

- First, it reframes the notion of "activation" in dynamic terms, suggesting that activation is not simply an excess of spikes, or greater power in any particular EEG frequency band. Activation may correspond to an acceleration of dynamics, subserving more rapid computations. This sort of activation can manifest with no overall change in power but a change in the frequencies at which power is expressed. Because more rapid or dissipative dynamics are energetically more expensive, it may be that they are reserved for "functionally" adaptive or necessary neuronal processing.

- Second, under the generative model of activation, a speeding up of the dynamics corresponds to a decrease in the width of the cross-correlation functions between all pairs of units in the population. (At the macroscopic level of EEG recordings, considered here, the synchronisation between pairs of units, as measured by the cross-correlation function, is captured in the width of the autocorrelation of the EEG signal, because the EEG signal is a measure of synchronous neural activity). This width is a ubiquitous measure of synchronisation that transcends any frequency-specific changes in coherence. In short, activation as measured by fMRI is caused, in this model, by increased synchronisation and, implicitly, a change in the temporal structure of neuronal dynamics.

- Third, our analysis suggests that the underlying "activation" status of neuronal systems is not expressed in any single frequency but is exhibited across the spectral profile. This has implications for the use of classical terms like "event-related desynchronisation". If one only considered modulations in spectral density at one frequency, as in the classical use of the term desynchronisation, one would conclude that the effect of activation was a desynchronisation of low-frequency components. According to the model, however, the effect of activation is a shift in the entire spectral profile to higher frequencies with a concomitant attenuation in the amplitudes of all frequencies. This general conclusion does not preclude the selective expression of certain frequencies during specific cognitive operations (e.g. increases in theta oscillations during mental arithmetic; e.g. Mizuhara et al. 2004). However, the model suggests that the context in which these frequencies are expressed is an important determinant of the BOLD response. In other words, it is not the absolute power of any frequency but the profile that determines expected metabolic cost.

- Fourth, as introduced above, one of the assumptions treats neuronal systems as autonomous, such that the evolution of their states is determined in an autonomous fashion. This translates into the assumption that the presynaptic influence of intrinsic connections completely overshadows extrinsic inputs. This may seem an odd assumption. However, it is the basis of nonlinear coupling in the brain and may represent, quantitatively, a much more important form of integration than simple linear coupling. We have addressed this issue both empirically and theoretically in Friston (2000). In brief, if extrinsic inputs affect the excitability of neurons, as apposed to simply driving a response, the coupling can be understood in terms of changes in the system parameters, namely the Jacobian. This means the response to input will be nonlinear. Quantitative analyses (a simple form of bicoherence analysis) of MEG data suggest that this form of nonlinear coupling can account for much more variation in power than linear coupling, i.e. coherence (Friston 2000).

4
Summary

The integration of EEG and fMRI data is likely to play an important role in our understanding of brain function. Through such multimodal fusion it should be possible to harness the temporal resolution of EEG and the spatial resolution of fMRI in characterising neural activity. The majority of the studies integrating EEG and fMRI to date have focussed on directly correlating the two measures, after first transforming the data so that they are on the same temporal scale (usually by convolution of the EEG time series with a canonical haemodynamic response function). This approach has proved successful in demonstrating that multimodal fusion is feasible and that regionally specific dependencies between the two measures exist. However, this approach to characterising the relationship between the EEG and the fMRI is limited, as it does not characterise the integration in terms of the underlying neuronal activity. We will only be able to fully harness the benefits of EEG–fMRI integration by understanding the relationship between the underlying neuronal activity and the BOLD and EEG signals through their respective forward models. Although the current model falls a long way short of this, it can explain the nature of some of the previously reported correlations between EEG and fMRI by considering the integration in terms of the underlying neuronal dynamics.

We have proposed a simple model that relates BOLD changes to the relative spectral density of an EEG trace and the roughness of the EEG time series. Neuronal activation affects the relative contributions of high and low EEG frequencies. This model accommodates the observations that BOLD signal correlates negatively with the expression of alpha power and positively with the expression of higher frequencies. Clearly, many of the assumptions are not correct in detail, but the overall picture afforded may provide a new perspective on some important issues in neuroimaging.

References

Abbot LF, Varela JA, Sen K, Nelson SB (1997) Synaptic depression and cortical gain control. Science 275:220–223

Attwell D, Iadecola C (2002) The neural basis of functional imaging brain signals. Trends Neurosci 25(12):621–625

Chawla D, Lumer ED, Friston KJ (2000) Relating macroscopic measures of brain activity to fast, dynamic neuronal interactions. Neural Comput 12:2805–2821

Cox DR, Miller HD (1965) The theory of stochastic processes. Chapman and Hall, London

Crick F, Koch C (1998) Constraints on cortical and thalamic projections: the no-strong-loops hypothesis. Nature 39:245–250

Czisch M, Wehrle R, Kaufmann C, Wetter TC, Holsboer F, Pollmacher T, Auer DP (2004) Functional MRI during sleep: BOLD signal decreases and their electrophysiological correlates. Eur J Neurosci 20(2):566–574

Dale AM, Liu AK, Fischl BR, Buckner RL, Belliveau JW, Lewine JD, Halgren E (2000) Dynamic statistical parametric mapping: combining fMRI and MEG for high-resolution imaging of cortical activity. Neuron 26:55–67

Dayan P, Abbot LF (2001) Theoretical neuroscience. Computational and mathematical modelling of neural systems. MIT Press, CambrIDge

Friston KJ (2000) The labile brain I. Neuronal transients and nonlinear coupling. Phil Trans R Soc London B 355:215–236

Goldman RI, Stern JM, Engel J Jr, Cohen MS (2002) Simultaneous EEG and fMRI of the alpha rhythm. Neuroreport 13(18):2487–2492

Hoge RD, Atkinson J, Gill B, Crelier GR, Marrett S, Pike GB (1999) Linear coupling between cerebral blood flow and oxygen consumption in activated human cortex. Proc Natl Acad Sci USA 96(16):9403–9408

Jueptner M, Weiller C (1995) Review: does measurement of regional cerebral blood flow reflect synaptic activity? Implications for PET and fMRI. Neuroimage 2(2):148–156

Laufs H, Kleinschmidt A, Beyerle A, Eger E, Salek-Haddadi A, Preibisch C, Krakow K (2003a) EEG-correlated fMRI of human alpha activity. Neuroimage 19(4):1463–1476

Laufs H, Krakow K, Sterzer P, Eger E, Beyerle A, Salek-Haddadi A, KleinschmIDt A (2003b) Electroencephalographic signatures of attentional and cognitive default modes in spontaneous brain activity fluctuations at rest. Proc Natl Acad Sci USA 100(19):11053–11058

Lauritzen M (2001) Relationship of spikes, synaptic activity, and local changes of cerebral blood flow. J Cereb Blood Flow Metab 21(12):1367–1383

Lemieux L, Krakow K, Fish DR (2001) Comparison of spike-triggered functional MRI BOLD activation and EEG dipole model localization. Neuroimage 14(5):1097–1104

Leopold DA, Murayama Y, Logothetis NK (2003) Very slow activity fluctuations in monkey visual cortex: implications for functional brain imaging. Cereb Cortex 13(4):422–433

Logothetis NK, Pauls J, Augath M, Trinath T, Oeltermann A (2001) Neurophysiological investigation of the basis of the fMRI signal. Nature 412(6843):150–157

Lovblad KO, Thomas R, Jakob PM, Scammell T, Bassetti C, Griswold M, Ives J, Matheson J, Edelman RR, Warach S (1999) Silent functional magnetic resonance imaging demonstrates focal activation in rapID eye movement sleep. Neurology 53(9):2193–2195

Magistretti PJ, Pellerin L (1999) Cellular mechanisms of brain energy metabolism and their relevance to functional brain imaging. Philos Trans R Soc Lond B Biol Sci 354(1387):1155–1163

Magistretti PJ, Pellerin L, Rothman DL, Shulman RG (1999) Energy on demand. Science 283(5401):496–497

Martinez-Montes E, Valdes-Sosa PA, Miwakeichi F, Goldman RI, Cohen MS (2004) Concurrent EEG/fMRI analysis by multiway partial least squares. Neuroimage 22(3):1023–1034

Mizuhara H, Wang LQ, Kobayashi K, Yamaguchi Y (2004) A long-range cortical network emerging with theta oscillation in a mental task. Neuroreport 15:1233–1238

Moosmann M, Ritter P, Krastel I, Brink A, Thees S, Blankenburg F, Taskin B, Obrig H, Villringer A (2003) Correlates of alpha rhythm in functional magnetic resonance imaging and near infrared spectroscopy. Neuroimage 20(1):145 158

Niessing J, Ebisch B, Schmidt KE, Niessing M, Singer W, Galuske RA (2005) Hemodynamic signals correlate tightly with synchronized gamma oscillations. Science. 309(5736):948–951

Parkes LM, Fries P, Kerskens CM, Norris DG (2004) Reduced BOLD response to periodic visual stimulation. Neuroimage 21(1):236–243

Phillips C, Rugg MD, Friston KJ (2002) Anatomically informed basis functions for EEG source localization: combining functional and anatomical constraints. Neuroimage 16(3 Pt 1): 678–695

Shin C (2000) Neurophysiologic basis of functional neuroimaging: animal studies. J Clin Neurophysiol 17(1):2–9

Shulman RG, Rothman DL (1998) Interpreting functional imaging studies in terms of neurotransmitter cycling. Proc Natl Acad Sci USA 95(20):11993–11998

Steriade M, McCormick DA, Sejnowski T (1993) Thalamocortical oscillations in the sleeping and aroused brain. Science 262:679–685

Traub RD, Whittington MA, Stanford M, Jefferys JG (1996) A mechanism for generation of long-range synchronous fast oscillations in the cortex. Nature 383(6601):621–624

Whittington MA, Traub RD (2003) Interneuron diversity series: inhibitory interneurons and network oscillations in vitro. Trends Neurosci 26(12):676–682

BOLD Response and EEG Gamma Oscillations **23**

Gregor Leicht, Christoph S. Herrmann, and Christoph Mulert

1
Introduction

The rhythmic activities in the resting or "spontaneous" EEG are usually divided into several frequency bands (delta: <4 Hz; theta: 4–8 Hz; alpha: 8–12 Hz; beta: 12–30 Hz; and gamma: 30–70 Hz or higher, centred at 40 Hz), which are associated with different behavioural states, ranging from sleep to relaxation, heightened alertness and mental concentration (Lindsley 1952; Niedermeyer and Lopes Da Silva 2004; Nunez 1995). High-frequency EEG oscillations such as gamma oscillations with relatively small amplitudes can be measured on the scalp due to the fact that scalp EEG recording sensors are physically separated from intracranial activities by the resistive skull tissue, which acts as a low-pass filter. Since the amplitudes of the EEG oscillations decrease with increasing frequency, the importance of high-frequency EEG oscillations like gamma oscillations with respect to cognitive functions and disorders is often underestimated compared to slower oscillations. However, in recent years, a special interest in oscillations in the gamma frequency range has emerged in neuroscience, because there is a lot of evidence for a close correlation between gamma activity and cognitive functions (Engel and Singer 2001).

Evidence from neuropsychological and physiological studies suggests that consciousness and its different aspects, like sensory awareness for example, can be understood as a cooperating system involving several different brain regions, such as structures responsible for sensory perception, memory functions, executive control, or manipulation of emotion and motivation (Delacour 1997; Young and Pigott 1999). Theories about the neural correlates of consciousness must explain how multiple component processes can be integrated and which mechanisms underlie the dynamic selection of specific components of neuronal responses that gain access to consciousness from all available information. For both aspects, so called "neuronal binding" seems to play an important role (Crick and

G. Leicht (✉)
Department of Psychiatry and Psychotherapy, Clinical Neurophysiology and Functional Brain Imaging, Ludwig-Maximilians-University Munich, Nußbaumstr. 7, 80336 Munich, Germany
e-mail: gregor.leicht@med.uni-muenchen.de

C. Mulert and L. Lemieux (eds.), *EEG–fMRI*,   **465**
DOI: 10.1007/978-3-540-87919-0_23, © Springer Verlag Berlin Heidelberg 2010

Koch 1990; Engel and Singer 2001). The concept of dynamic binding by synchronising neuronal discharges has developed mainly in the context of perceptual processing and was first introduced in the context of feature integration (Gray et al. 1989; Treisman 1996) and perceptual segmentation (von der Malsburg 1994). The synchronisation of activity in neuronal assemblies appears to support specific processes during neural communication, whereas the behavioural specificity of synchronisation phenomena suggests a functional role of synchronised activity in neural information processing (Fries 2005). Meanwhile, the concept of binding has been applied to many different domains and is now employed in theories on object recognition (Hummel and Biederman 1992), arousal (Struber et al. 2000), attention (Fell et al. 2003; Niebur 1993; Pantev et al. 1991; Tiitinen et al. 1993), memory formation and recall (Damasio 1990; Herrmann et al. 2004), motor control (Murthy and Fetz 1992), sensorimotor integration (Roelfsema et al. 1997) and language processing (Eulitz et al. 1996; Pulvermuller 1999; Pulvermuller et al. 1995).

In the context of the theory of neuronal binding, the synchronous firing of neurons in the gamma band was proposed to represent an important integration mechanism of the brain (Gray et al. 1989). The gamma frequency range is defined quite differently across various studies. Whereas some human studies have mostly focused on activity around 40 Hz (Eckhorn et al. 1988; Tallon-Baudry et al. 1996), others have explicitly investigated activity in higher frequency ranges (Crone et al. 2001; Lachaux et al. 2005; Muller and Keil 2004). Animal studies have even considered gamma activity in still higher frequency ranges, up to 120 Hz (Bragin et al. 1995; Neuenschwander and Singer 1996).

2
Methodical Issues

Different methods have been suggested in order to investigate the relationship between fMRI and special oscillatory EEG components. Compared to the analysis of EEG components with slower frequencies, the investigation of high-frequency oscillations such as gamma oscillations produces additional difficulties. Since the skull tissue acts as a low-pass filter, high-frequency EEG oscillations measured on the scalp show relatively small amplitudes can be measured on the scalp. Therefore, the signal-to-noise ratio for these subtle EEG rhythms is usually low, especially in the MRI environment with high artefact contamination. Moreover, the clear separation of high-frequency activity from other frequency components is difficult, as it is often masked by more prominent, slower oscillatory EEG components. Statistical methods like principal component analysis (PCA) or independent component analysis (ICA) seem to present possible solutions to this problem. Additionally, functional modulation of individual rhythm strength (e.g. via experimental tasks) should facilitate the identification of subtle EEG rhythms as individual components (Ritter and Villringer 2006).

While investigating the EEG alpha rhythm, several studies have correlated the BOLD signal (electrode- and voxelwise) with the power time courses of this spectral band calculated by wavelet analysis and convolved with an assumed haemodynamic response function (Goldman et al. 2002; Laufs et al. 2003; Moosmann et al. 2003). Martinez-Montes et al. presented an alternative data-driven approach for the analysis of concurrent

EEG–fMRI recordings, especially in relation to high-frequency EEG oscillations like gamma activity. They used multiway partial least squares (N-PLS) analysis to identify the coherent systems of neural oscillators that contribute to the spontaneous EEG. Using this method, first, EEG data are decomposed in the space–frequency–time domain and fMRI data are decomposed in the space–time domain into a set of components (termed "atoms"). Second, the relationship between these EEG and fMRI components is examined, and the sources of the EEG atoms are analysed (Martinez-Montes et al. 2004).

Concerning technical problems, a sufficient analysis of EEG gamma activity recorded in the MRI scanner during simultaneous EEG–fMRI measurement may sometimes be impossible due to EEG artefacts caused by the MRI environment. One example is an EEG artefact in the frequency range between 30 and 60 Hz, which is generated by the helium pump of the MRI scanner. Switching this pump off some of the time during the simultaneous EEG–fMRI recording can solve this problem (Mulert et al. 2007a) (see Fig. 1).

In order to improve the quality of EEG data in simultaneous EEG–MRI experiments, especially regarding high-frequency EEG components, Anami et al. introduced the "stepping-stone sampling" method (Anami et al. 2003). By modifying a blip-type echo-planar sequence, they were able to perform EEG sampling at a digitisation rate of 1,000 Hz exclusively during the period in which the artefact resided around the baseline level. This

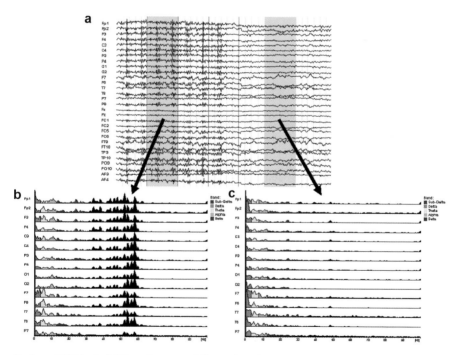

Fig. 1a–c EEG in the MRI environment. Effects of artefacts caused by the fMRI scanner's helium pump on the EEG frequency spectrum shown in an FFT analysis. **a** *Left*: Helium pump switched ON; *right*: helium pump switched OFF. **b** FFT analysis with pump artefacts that can be clearly seen in the frequency range between 40 and 60 Hz. **c** FFT analysis without pump artefacts. Data were recorded on a Siemens Sonata 1.5 T MRI scanner (Mulert et al. 2007a)

method was able to substantially attenuate the amplitude of the imaging artefact. Here, periodically artefact-free interspaces emerged that allowed EEG sampling with a high signal-to-artefact ratio. Analyses with a fast Fourier transform showed, apart from the successful retrieval of physiological α-activity, that the high-frequency EEG during scanning had a very similar power distribution to that of data recorded outside the MRI scanner (Anami et al. 2003). Therefore, it can be assumed that the availability of the high-frequency band—including gamma activity—is enhanced by using the stepping-stone sampling method in synchronous measurements of EEG and MRI.

Mandelkow et al. (2006) reported improved EEG quality, increasing the usable bandwidth of the EEG signal to higher frequencies, after synchronisation of the MRI sequence with the sampling pattern of the EEG. This was done by synchronising the internal clocks of both the MRI and the EEG acquisition systems and setting the TR of the MRI sequence to a multiple of the EEG sampling interval. In this way, the variability of the notorious MRI artefact was reduced and its removal by the common mean template subtraction method was facilitated. A direct comparison of EEG spectra from recordings done with and without synchronisation showed that the usable bandwidth of the EEG signal was increased to about 150 Hz, thus covering the full gamma-frequency range (Mandelkow et al. 2006). In the main, investigations of the gamma-frequency range may benefit from this innovation.

3
Gamma Activity and BOLD Response

3.1
Co-variation of High-Frequency Oscillations and the BOLD Signal

In a seminal study, Logothetis et al. simultaneously recorded the BOLD signal and intracranial recordings of single-unit activity, multiunit activity, and local field potentials (LFPs) in monkeys (Logothetis 2002; Logothetis et al. 2001). They reported that the time course of the LFPs correlated best with that of the BOLD signal for rotating checkerboard stimuli of variable durations. Such LFPs typically show discharges at frequencies in the gamma-frequency range (approximately 30–80 Hz). Subsequently, recordings in cats revealed that correlations between LFPs and BOLD signal are especially high in the gamma-frequency range (Niessing et al. 2005).

Similar results were found in studies combining fMRI and intracranial EEG recordings in human epilepsy patients, for instance by correlating intracortical electrophysiological recordings in the auditory cortex of two neurosurgical patients and BOLD responses from 11 healthy subjects during the presentation of an identical movie segment (Mukamel et al. 2005). A predicted fMRI signal derived from the spiking activity of single neurons of the patients and the measured fMRI signal from the auditory cortex of the healthy subjects showed a highly significant correlation, especially for high-frequency LFPs (see Fig. 2).

By investigating three patients with epilepsy in separate measurements of intracranial EEG recordings and fMRI, Lachaux et al. found spatially congruent patterns of BOLD

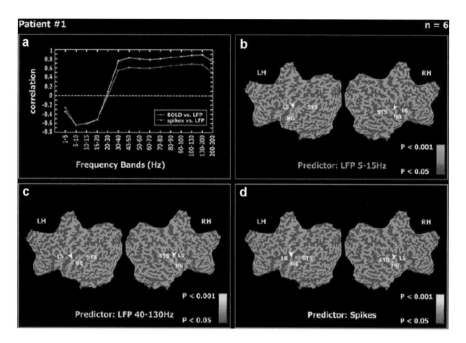

Fig. 2a–d   Correlation maps between the fMRI BOLD signal and different EEG frequency components. **a** The correlation of the different local field potential (LFP) predictors for one patient with the average fMRI BOLD signal in Heschl's gyrus (*orange trace*) and with the spike predictor calculated from the sum of auditory responses of 20 single neurons convolved with a standard haemodynamic response function (*cyan trace*) as a function of frequency band. Note the strong negative correlations between the BOLD activation and the low-frequency LFPs (5–15 Hz), and the strong positive correlation with the high-frequency LFPs (40–130 Hz). **b–d** Multisubject random-effect GLM map correlating the BOLD signals from six participants with the low-frequency (5–15 Hz) LFP predictor (**b**), the high-frequency (40–130 Hz) LFP predictor (**c**), and the spike predictor (**d**). *LS*, lateral sulcus; *STS*, superior temporal sulcus; *HG*, Heschl's gyrus; *RH* and *LH*, right and left hemispheres, respectively. *Arrowheads* point to regions of highly significant correlation in Heschl's gyrus. From Mukamel, R., Gelbard, H., Arieli, A., Hasson, U., Fried, I., and Malach, R. Coupling between neuronal firing, field potentials, and FMRI in human auditory cortex. Science (2005) 309(5736):951–4. Reprinted with permission from AAAS

responses and gamma activations in a visual cognitive task while trying to answer the question of whether fMRI has any predictive value regarding the anatomical location of cross-condition gamma-band modulations (Lachaux et al. 2007) (see Fig. 3).

In intracranial EEG recordings of a single patient with epilepsy, Brovelli et al. found that it was possible to differentiate ERPs as well as beta-frequency (15–30 Hz) and gamma-frequency (60–200 Hz) activity during processes of spatial attention and memory in contrast to motor intention processes. However, concerning the localisation of intracranial electrodes, ERPs and beta-frequency activity showed only weak or no spatial correlation with the BOLD response measured in a fMRI study in the same conditional visuomotor task, whereas the high-gamma frequency activity did colocalise with fMRI regions of interest (Brovelli et al. 2005).

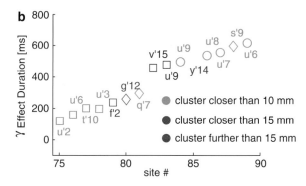

Fig. 3 In a contrast between two experimental conditions, intracranial EEG sites with stronger gamma energy increases were significantly closer than other sites to fMRI activation clusters. Fifteen intracranial EEG sites for which the maximal duration of a significant gamma (40–150 Hz) energy difference between the two experimental conditions was longer than 100 ms (= strong gamma energy increase) are shown. For each site, this value corresponds to the duration of the longest time window, across all frequencies in the gamma band, during which the p value for the Mann–Whitney comparison between the two conditions stays lower than 1×10^4. The shapes of the markers indicate which of the three patients was recorded. Sites closer than 10 mm (15 mm) from a fMRI activation cluster (i.e. sets of contiguous voxels above the significance threshold) in the same contrast between the two conditions are shown in *green* (*blue*). By contrast, the three "distant" EEG sites (shown in *red*, >15 mm away from an fMRI activation cluster) showed a later inversion of the earlier gamma energy increase, causing the total gamma energy during the whole response window to be equivalent in the two conditions. This analysis revealed that 12 out of these 15 (80%) sites with significant gamma energy increases were located <15 mm away from an fMRI activation cluster documenting an increase in BOLD response. In comparison, only 35 out of the 74 (47%) non-gamma sites (not displayed here) were <15 mm away from an fMRI activation cluster. From Hum Brain Mapp Vol. 28, No. 12, 2007, 1368-75. Copyright 2007 Wiley-Liss, Inc. Reprinted with permission of Wiley-Liss, Inc., a subsidiary of John Wiley & Sons, Inc

Foucher et al. tried to find an answer to the question of why auditory evoked P300 and fMRI activations differ in response to the presentation of two kinds of rare events (i.e. target and novel stimuli in an oddball task). It was reported that the auditory evoked P300 has a lower amplitude when a target stimulus has to be detected compared to when a novel stimulus that is unrelated to the task is presented. On the other hand, there are fMRI studies in which no novel stimulus-related activation was reported but where activations were elicited by targets (Clark et al. 2001; Kirino et al. 2000). These findings of differential reactivities of event-related potentials (ERPs) and the BOLD signal were replicated by Foucher et al. using combined measurements of EEG and fMRI. Additionally, in accordance with fMRI results, target-related gamma oscillations were more intense than their novel stimulus-related counterparts (Foucher et al. 2003) (see Fig. 4). The authors propounded a physiological hypothesis suggesting that the discrepancy between ERPs and the fMRI signal as well as gamma oscillations support evidence demonstrating that the BOLD signal is better correlated with high- than with low-frequency oscillations. Searching for reasons for this observation, the authors discuss the fact that, as opposed to ERPs reflecting the synchronous activity of synapses within milliseconds (Baillet et al. 2001; Speckmann and Elger 1999), event-related gamma oscillations do not need to be time-locked to the

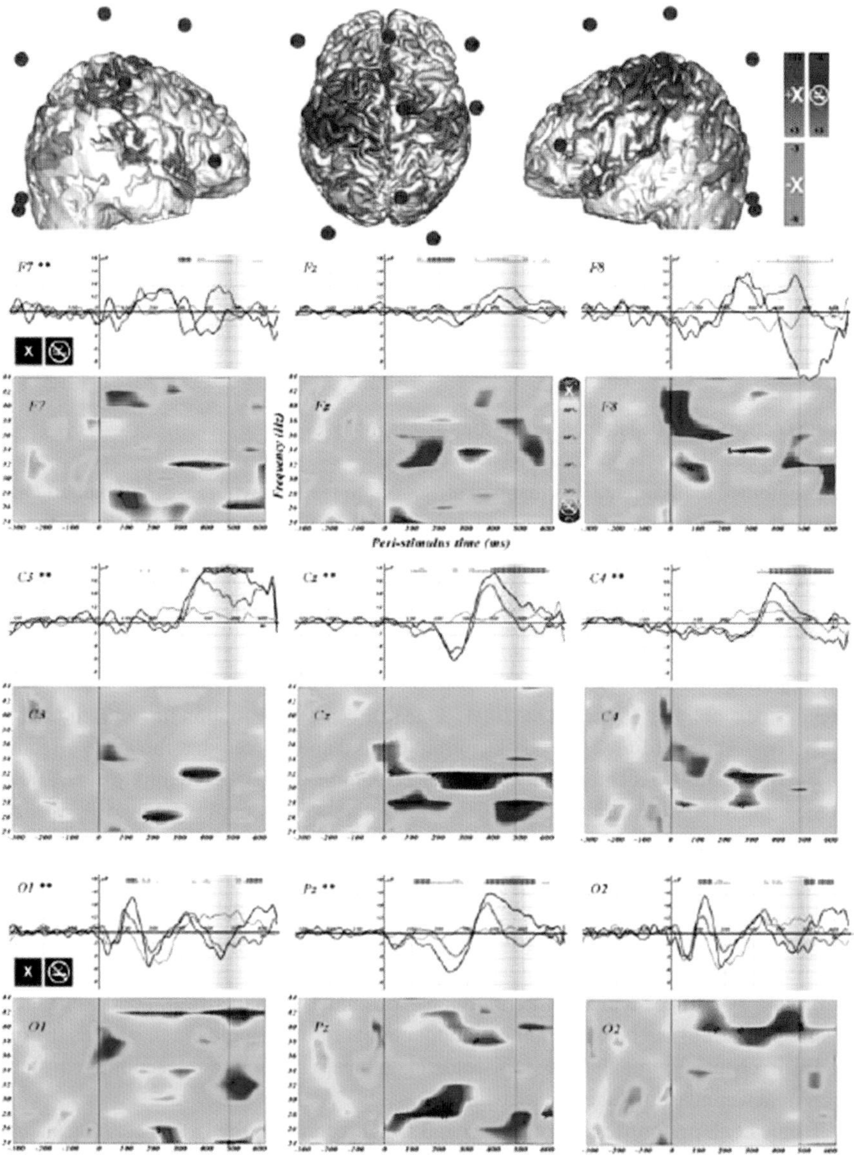

Fig. 4 FMRI results, evoked potentials (ERPs, P300) and event-related oscillations (EROs, gamma activity) calculated over all subjects ($n = 5$). The *upper part* presents three different views of the average electrode position relative to the areas with BOLD activation (threshold $p \leq 0.001$, 100 voxels; target stimulus-related activation in *red*; target stimulus-related deactivation in *green*; novel stimulus-related (rare distractor) activation in *blue*). The *lower part* displays ERPs and EROs for each electrode (targets in *red* and "X" marks; novels in *blue* and "no smoking" symbol; frequent distractor in *grey*). On the one hand, for C3, Cz, C4 and Pz, novel stimuli (*blue*) yielded larger ERPs than target stimuli (*red*). On the other hand, for all of the electrodes, the EROs showed significantly more oscillations in the gamma frequency range around 300–400 ms for target stimuli (*red*) in comparison to novel stimuli (*blue*), in line with stronger fMRI BOLD responses in the target condition. Reprinted from Foucher et al. (2003) with permission from BioMed Central

stimulus that precisely, and so they are less dependent on the small jitter of the neuronal response relative to a stimulus (Tallon-Baudry and Bertrand 1999), as the BOLD signal is. Furthermore, the authors mention the fact that ERPs reflect the synaptic input function of pyramidal cells only (Baillet et al. 2001; Speckmann and Elger 1999), whereas fMRI reflects the synaptic activities of all neural cells, including inhibitory interneurons (Logothetis et al. 2001; Mathiesen et al. 2000; Matsuura and Kanno 2001), which are involved in the synchronisation of gamma oscillations (Traub et al. 1996) too. A third possible reason could be related to the assumption that ERPs might correspond to the simple phase resetting of ongoing cerebral activity (Makeig et al. 2002), which should not consume much energy (Foucher et al. 2003).

3.2
Gamma Activity and BOLD Response: Variation Across Subjects

In a combined experiment, Herrmann et al. set out to test the hypothesis that human EEG gamma-band responses (GBRs) correlate with the BOLD responses. Since oscillatory activity in the gamma-band range is of very low amplitude (a fraction of a microvolt) and within the frequency range of the MR gradient switching, which results in EEG artefacts, the EEG and fMRI measurements were carried out separately.

Both GBRs and BOLD responses have repeatedly been shown to vary across subjects. For example, oscillatory gamma responses show interindividual variations both in frequency and amplitude (Busch et al. 2004). One source of this variation lies with the different polymorphisms of the subjects. Demiralp et al. demonstrated that the more effective variant of the DRD4 receptor results in enhanced gamma responses (Demiralp et al. 2007). At the same time, such variations correlate with differences in cognitive processes. Strüber et al. showed that subjects with high-amplitude gamma oscillations switch more often between two alternative percepts of an ambiguous figure (Struber et al. 2000). Also, the BOLD response shows variance across subjects. For example, spatial variations of BOLD activity can stem from anatomical variations, since even monozygotic twins have slightly different brain anatomies (Lohmann et al. 1999). Recent findings have shown that even early sensory cortices underlie interindividual variations (Amunts et al. 2000). For these reasons, atlases of the human brain are no longer based on a single brain, such as the one by Talairach and Tournoux (1988). Instead, anatomical variations are taken into consideration in newer atlases (Rademacher et al. 2001).

Zaehle et al. performed separate EEG and fMRI recordings for 18 subjects (mean age: 23.9 years, eight male) (Zaehle et al. 2009). The subjects had to view circular moving gratings that moved either outward ($p = 0.75$) or inward ($p = 0.25$). The gratings had a spatial frequency of 0.67 cycles per degree visual angle and were presented for 600 ms. During these 600 ms, one full cycle of movement occurred. The direction of movement had to be indicated by a button press (inward = right). In run 1, a static grating remained visible during the interstimulus interval (ISI). Thus, at the onset of a stimulus, only a motion onset was visible. In run 2, a grey screen was presented during the ISI. Thus, at stimulus onset, both the stimulus and the motion set in. The fMRI recording was carried out as a rapid event-related fMRI design. Identical timing was used for the EEG recording. Based on the

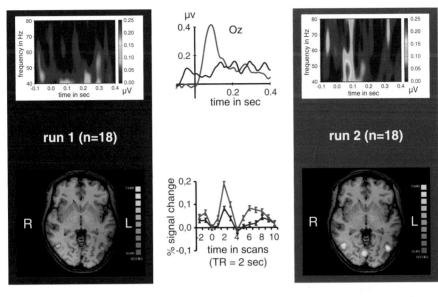

Fig. 5 Gamma-band responses (GBRs) and BOLD responses from the comparison between the two runs. Both response types were significantly stronger in run 2, where motion onset was preceded by a blank screen. *Top row*: Time–frequency representations (*left and right*) show the GBRs. A prominent response is visible for run 2 between 40 and 50 Hz shortly before 100 ms after stimulus onset (*right*). The difference between the two runs is most prominent in the time courses of the GBR (*middle*), which were computed from individual best response frequencies (roughly 45 Hz). *Bottom row*: The BOLD response is also stronger for run 2 (*right*) than for run 1 (*left*). The time course (*middle*) averaged across five regions of interest again shows this difference most prominently

amplitudes of their evoked GBRs, subjects were assigned to either a low- or a high-gamma group.

Comparison of run 1 and run 2 revealed that gamma responses were significantly stronger in run 2, where motion onset was preceded by a blank screen ($t = 5.042, p < 0.001$). This contrast also yielded more activated voxels in posterior brain regions ($t = 6.668, p < 0.001$), and a higher percentage signal change ($t = 4.744, p < 0.001$) (see Fig. 5).

Comparing the groups of the low-gamma and the high-gamma subjects for run 2 yielded no differences in BOLD response for either the number of activated voxels ($t < 1, p > 0.3$) or for the percentage signal change ($t < 1, p > 0.6$). Of course, the gamma responses were significantly stronger in the high-gamma group ($t = 5.190, p < 0.001$), since this was the criterion for assigning subjects to the groups (see Fig. 6).

The results obtained from comparing different runs are in line with the notion that BOLD and GBRs co-vary (Logothetis et al. 2001; Mukamel et al. 2005; Niessing et al. 2005). However, comparing subjects that showed either high- or low-gamma responses in their EEGs yielded no differences in their BOLD responses. The latter result was unexpected, and one can only offer a speculative explanation. It was demonstrated that the BOLD response shows interindividual variations (Aguirre et al. 1998). Sources of

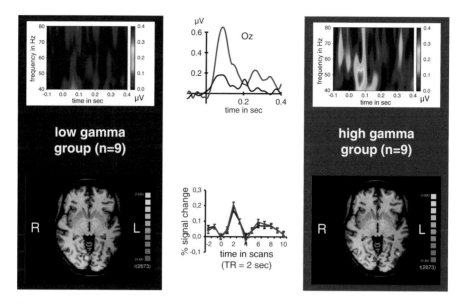

Fig. 6 GBRs and BOLD responses comparing the low-gamma group (*left*) vs. the high-gamma group (*right*). While the GBRs were, of course, significantly different between groups (*top row*), no differences could be found for the BOLD responses (*bottom row*)

variation have been identified in genetic polymorphisms (Goldberg and Weinberger 2004). At the same time, GBRs are influenced by a number of parameters that vary interindividually, such as age (Bottger et al. 2002), dopamine polymorphisms (Demiralp et al. 2007), and the individual rate at which the two percepts of bistable figures switch (Struber et al. 2000). Interestingly, dopamine polymorphisms modulate gamma and BOLD responses. However, while the VNTR polymorphism of DRD4 modulates GBRs, the Val158Met polymorphism of COMT does not (Demiralp et al. 2007). By contrast, the COMT polymorphism does modulate the BOLD response (Winterer et al. 2006). One difference between the two is the locus of effect. While the COMT polymorphism influences the amount of dopamine in the synaptic cleft, the DRD4 polymorphism affects the dopamine receptor but not the amount of dopamine. Thus, it seems plausible to assume that the amount of extracellular dopamine affects the BOLD but not the GBR, whereas the dopaminergic activation of neurons affects the GBR but not the BOLD response.

3.3
Gamma Activity and BOLD Response: Further Reports

Performing simultaneous measurements of EEG and fMRI, Giraud et al. showed that functional brain asymmetries in speech processing were the cause of different intrinsic sampling properties in each auditory cortex. Time courses of power from certain EEG bands calculated with a short-time Fourier transform were convolved with haemodynamic response function and used as regressors in a general linear model. As a result of this investigation, the authors report that, in line with the asymmetric sampling in time theory (Poeppel 2003), spontaneous power fluctuations of 3–6 Hz and intrinsic oscillations of 28–40 Hz (which are tuned to the major acoustic temporal characteristics of speech) are paralleled by specific modulations of neural activity in auditory/temporal cortices. The auditory activity in regions overlapping Heschl's gyrus is more prominently associated with the 3–6 Hz band in the right hemisphere and the 28–40 Hz band in the left hemisphere. Moreover, ventral premotor cortex activity is correlated with spontaneous neural oscillations at the syllabic rate of natural speech (Giraud et al. 2007).

Research in the field of resting-state networks (RSNs) raised the question of whether the analysis of the modulation of the whole EEG frequency spectrum could help to find electrophysiological signatures of such networks. In the EEG of the resting human brain, spontaneous rhythms that show different oscillatory signatures and are unrelated to any external or internal event are detectable. Simultaneous measurement of EEG and fMRI is necessary to investigate the haemodynamic correlates of these phenomena, because data fusion is not possible after separate recordings of electrical and haemodynamic measures (Ritter and Villringer 2006). Mantini et al. used a data-driven approach to investigate the relationship between neuronal oscillatory processes in different EEG frequency bands and coherent fMRI fluctuations. BOLD signal time courses corresponding to each of the independent components, identified using ICA, were correlated with the EEG reference waveforms of the power time series of the various frequency bands. In general, more than one rhythm was associated with the same network, whereas RSNs could be separated on the basis of their specific EEG power profiles. Regarding observations of gamma activity, the authors report a strong weighting of EEG power spectra associated with the ventromedial prefrontal cortex (RSN 6) towards gamma power (see Fig. 7), whereas the rest of the default network (RSN 1) was more strongly associated with alpha and beta powers (Mantini et al. 2007).

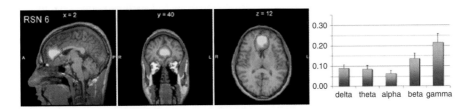

Fig. 7 Association between EEG rhythms and fMRI resting-state network (RSN) 6. *Left*: Sagittal, coronal, and axial spatial maps of RSN 6. *Right*: Bar plot of the average correlations between the brain oscillatory activities in the delta, theta, alpha, beta and gamma bands, and the RSN 6 time course. In general, more than one rhythm was associated with the same network, confirming that neurons oscillating at different frequencies may contribute to the same functional system. RSNs 1 (default) and 2 (dorsal attention) had stronger relationships with alpha and beta rhythms, RSN 3 (visual) with all rhythms except gamma rhythm, RSN 4 (auditory) with delta, theta and beta rhythms, and RSN 5 (somatomotor) with beta rhythm. The RSN 6 shown here (including the medial ventral prefrontal cortex, the pregenual anterior cingulate, the hypothalamus and the cerebellum, putatively related to self-referential mental activity; D'Argembeau et al. 2005) was mainly associated with gamma rhythm. From Mantini et al. (2007); copyright (2007) National Academy of Sciences, USA

In general, methods like the one used in the abovementioned investigation may be helpful in creating spatiotemporally resolved maps of the brain and correlating coherent neuronal, non-event-related activity to different behavioural and cognitive states (Ritter and Villringer 2006). The identification of those EEG signals and related cognitive states should be the domain of the integration of EEG and fMRI information, whereas very slow activity fluctuations in the EEG are particularly suitable for relating to the BOLD signal (Leopold et al. 2003).

The examination of five healthy subjects with MEG and fMRI using a simple visual task supplied evidence of event-related synchronisation in the gamma band that co-varied spatiotemporally with the BOLD effect in the occipital cortex (Brookes et al. 2005) (see Fig. 8).

A possible link between induced gamma activity and haemodynamic response was found in a work investigating spatiotemporal correlates of repetition priming in cortical word-recognition networks and their modulation by stimulus familiarity. The repetition of familiar stimuli (real words) led to reduced activation for repeated words in occipitotemporal cortical regions and significant reduction of induced GBRs and phase synchrony between electrode positions. By contrast, the repetition of unfamiliar stimuli (pseudowords) results in increased activation in the same areas, increased GBRs, and increased phase coupling (Fiebach et al. 2005).

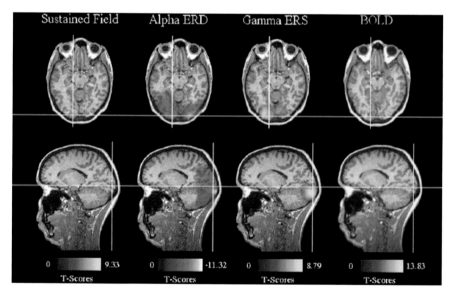

Fig. 8 Spatial distributions of the MEG sustained field, alpha-band power change, gamma-band power change and BOLD signals for a single subject. *Left*: MEG sustained field. *Inside left*: Event-related desynchronisation (ERD) in the alpha band (8–13 Hz). *Inside right*: Event-related synchronisation (ERS) in the gamma band (55–70 Hz). *Right*: fMRI BOLD signal ($p < 0.05$, corrected for multiple testing). Functional images are overlaid onto axial and sagittal slices of a high-resolution anatomical MRI. For the alpha- and gamma-band images (probability maps, $p < 0.001$, uncorrected), the *red* overlay represents an increase in power, whereas the *blue* overlay represents a decrease. The sustained field image represents the spatial distribution of a significant sustained response. Reprinted from Brookes et al. (2005). Copyright (2005), with permission from Elsevier

Combining the results from two studies investigating the effects of working memory load with human intracranial recordings and fMRI, Meltzer et al. concluded that gamma oscillatory power tends to increase with greater working-memory load, preferentially in occipital cortex. However, the oscillatory reactivity is not necessarily colocalised with fMRI activation observed consistently in normals performing the same task (Meltzer et al. 2008).

3.4
Outlook: Single-Trial Coupling of Gamma Activity and BOLD Response

With regard to the findings that BOLD and GBRs co-vary (Logothetis et al. 2001; Niessing et al. 2005; Mukamel et al. 2005), the direct fusion of information about the power of gamma activity and BOLD response following external stimulation in simultaneous measurements by single-trial coupling seems to be promising. Regarding evoked gamma activity, both in terms of phase and latency strictly triggered to stimulus onset, several authors have described its role in the context of attentional processes (Fell et al. 2003; Gurtubay et al. 2004; Senkowski et al. 2007). One example of early evoked gamma activity is the "transient" GBR to auditory stimulation (between 25 and 100 ms after stimulus presentation), which is known to be closely related to selective attention (Debener et al. 2003; Tiitinen et al. 1993). In preparation for a study simultaneously measuring EEG gamma activity and BOLD response in order to investigate a possible anterior cingulate cortex (ACC) generator of the early auditory evoked GBR and its functional role in auditory information processing, Mulert et al. showed a significant influence of the task difficulty on this evoked GBR and the auditory evoked N1 component (Mulert et al. 2007b) (see Fig. 9a-e). Generators of the early evoked GBR were found in the auditory cortex (primary and secondary auditory cortex) and in the dorsal ACC as well as the medial frontal gyrus in the whole-head LORETA analysis. Mulert et al. suggested that the early auditory evoked GBR might represent an early synchronisation of sensory and supervisory or monitoring brain areas in terms of a process of early top–down influence on information processing in the sensory area (Busch et al. 2006; Herrmann et al. 2004).

In order to gain more precision concerning localisation and the possibility of investigating subcortical structures (e.g. the thalamus), these findings were transferred to a study simultaneously measuring EEG and fMRI. Mulert et al. explored the specific BOLD response corresponding to the auditory evoked GBR using single-trial coupling of EEG and fMRI after matrix decomposition of the specific GBR information using Gram–Schmidt orthogonalisation. Distinct "GBR-specific" activations were found in the auditory cortex, the ACC and the thalamus (Mulert et al. 2007a) (see Fig. 9f).

4
Conclusions

In this chapter we discussed problems, recent developments and research findings regarding the relationship between EEG gamma activity and fMRI BOLD signal, and possible applications of the integration of EEG and fMRI in this field. Based on several investiga-

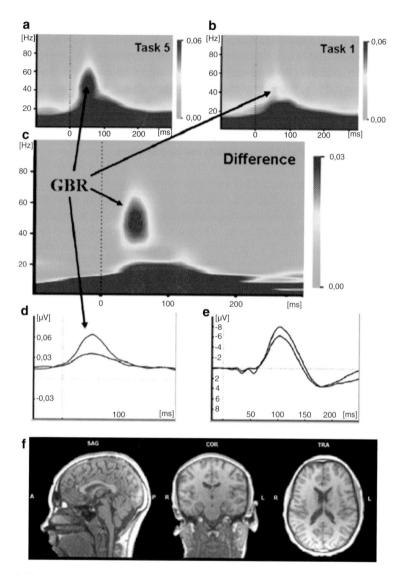

Fig. 9a–f Time–frequency analyses of the timeframe 0–200 ms after stimulus presentation averaged over all subjects for task one (**a**), the control condition, involving the lowest difficulty among the six auditory choice reaction tasks of varying difficulty presented, and task five (**b**), involving the highest difficulty among the tasks; the difference in activity obtained by subtracting the results of task one from the results of task five are also shown (**c**). Scaling was uniform for **a**, **b** and **c**. As indicated (*black arrows*), the evoked GBR can be seen as increased activity at about 50 ms at around 40 Hz. **d** GBR displayed as the results from the wavelet analysis (complex Morlet wavelet), focussing on 40 Hz, for task one (*black*) and task five (*red*). **e** N1 amplitude for task one (*black*) and task five (*red*). (**f**) Single-trial coupling of the GBR amplitude and the corresponding BOLD signal (random effects analysis, $n = 10$, $p < 0.0005$); GBR-related activations can be seen in the ACC, left auditory cortex and thalamus. Reprinted from Mulert et al. (2007b). Copyright (2007), with permission from Elsevier

tions, there seems to be a stronger correlation between the high-frequency components of the EEG signal (e.g. the gamma band) and the BOLD response than between lower frequency components of the EEG and the BOLD response (Brovelli et al. 2005; Foucher et al. 2003; Lachaux et al. 2007; Logothetis et al. 2001; Logothetis 2002; Mukamel et al. 2005; Niessing et al. 2005). Some problems emerge with the simultaneous recording of fMRI and gamma activity, since the amplitudes of high-frequency EEG fractions are small and the handicap presented by the artefact carries more weight. Statistical methods like PCA or ICA as well as various innovations in EEG- and fMRI-recording techniques may provide solutions to some of these technical challenges. The first attempts at directly fusing simultaneously recorded gamma activity and BOLD response via single-trial coupling have shown promising results.

References

Aguirre GK, Zarahn E, D'Esposito M (1998) The variability of human, BOLD hemodynamic responses. Neuroimage 8(4):360–369

Amunts K, Malikovic A, Mohlberg H, Schormann T, Zilles K (2000) Brodmann's areas 17 and 18 brought into stereotaxic space: where and how variable? Neuroimage 11(1):66–84

Anami K, Mori T, Tanaka F, Kawagoe Y, Okamoto J, Yarita M, Ohnishi T, Yumoto M, Matsuda H, Saitoh O (2003) Stepping stone sampling for retrieving artifact-free electroencephalogram during functional magnetic resonance imaging. Neuroimage 19(2 Pt 1):281–295

Baillet S, Mosher JC, Leahy RM (2001) Electromagnetic brain mapping. IEEE Signal Proc Mag 18:14–30

Bottger D, Herrmann CS, von Cramon DY (2002) Amplitude differences of evoked alpha and gamma oscillations in two different age groups. Int J Psychophysiol 45(3):245–251

Bragin A, Jando G, Nadasdy Z, Hetke J, Wise K, Buzsaki G (1995) Gamma (40–100 Hz) oscillation in the hippocampus of the behaving rat. J Neurosci 15(1 Pt 1):47–60

Brookes MJ, Gibson AM, Hall SD, Furlong PL, Barnes GR, Hillebrand A, Singh KD, Holliday E, Francis ST, Morris PG (2005) GLM-beamformer method demonstrates stationary field, alpha ERD and gamma ERS co-localisation with fMRI BOLD response in visual cortex. Neuroimage 26(1):302–308

Brovelli A, Lachaux JP, Kahane P, Boussaoud D (2005) High gamma frequency oscillatory activity dissociates attention from intention in the human premotor cortex. Neuroimage 28(1): 154–164

Busch NA, Debener S, Kranczioch C, Engel AK, Herrmann CS (2004) Size matters: effects of stimulus size, duration and eccentricity on the visual gamma-band response. Clin Neurophysiol 115(8):1810–1820

Busch NA, Schadow J, Frund I, Herrmann CS (2006) Time-frequency analysis of target detection reveals an early interface between bottom-up and top-down processes in the gamma-band. Neuroimage 29(4):1106–1116

Clark P, Fannon S, Lai S, Benson R (2001) Paradigm-dependent modulation of event-related fMRI activity evoked by the oddball task. Hum Brain Mapp 14(2):116–127

Crick F, Koch C (1990) Towards a neurobiological theory of consciousness. Semin Neurosci 2:263–275

Crone NE, Hao L, Hart J Jr., Boatman D, Lesser RP, Irizarry R, Gordon B (2001) Electrocortico-graphic gamma activity during word production in spoken and sign language. Neurology 57(11):2045–2053

Damasio AR (1990) Synchronous activation in multiple cortical regions: a mechanism for recall. Semin Neurosci 2:287–296

D'Argembeau A, Collette F, Van der Linden M, Laureys S, Del Fiore G, Degueldre C, Luxen A, Salmon E (2005) Self-referential reflective activity and its relationship with rest: a PET study. Neuroimage 25(2):616–624

Debener S, Herrmann CS, Kranczioch C, Gembris D, Engel AK (2003) Top-down attentional processing enhances auditory evoked gamma band activity. Neuroreport 14(5):683–686

Delacour J (1997) Neurobiology of consciousness: an overview. Behav Brain Res 85(2):127–141

Demiralp T, Herrmann CS, Erdal ME, Ergenoglu T, Keskin YH, Ergen M, Beydagi H (2007) DRD4 and DAT1 polymorphisms modulate human gamma band responses. Cereb Cortex 17(5):1007–1019

Eckhorn R, Bauer R, Jordan W, Brosch M, Kruse W, Munk M, Reitboeck HJ (1988) Coherent oscillations: a mechanism of feature linking in the visual cortex? Multiple electrode and correlation analyses in the cat. Biol Cybern 60(2):121–130

Engel AK, Singer W (2001) Temporal binding and the neural correlates of sensory awareness. Trends Cogn Sci 5(1):16–25

Eulitz C, Maess B, Pantev C, Friederici AD, Feige B, Elbert T (1996) Oscillatory neuromagnetic activity induced by language and non-language stimuli. Brain Res Cogn Brain Res 4(2): 121–132

Fell J, Fernandez G, Klaver P, Elger CE, Fries P (2003) Is synchronized neuronal gamma activity relevant for selective attention? Brain Res Brain Res Rev 42(3):265–272

Fiebach CJ, Gruber T, Supp GG (2005) Neuronal mechanisms of repetition priming in occipito-temporal cortex: spatiotemporal evidence from functional magnetic resonance imaging and electroencephalography. J Neurosci 25(13):3414–3422

Foucher JR, Otzenberger H, Gounot D (2003) The BOLD response and the gamma oscillations respond differently than evoked potentials: an interleaved EEG–fMRI study. BMC Neurosci 4:22

Fries P (2005) A mechanism for cognitive dynamics: neuronal communication through neuronal coherence. Trends Cogn Sci 9(10):474–480

Friston K (2002) Beyond phrenology: what can neuroimaging tell us about distributed circuitry. Annu Rev Neurosci 25:221–250

Giraud AL, Kleinschmidt A, Poeppel D, Lund TE, Frackowiak RS, Laufs H (2007) Endogenous cortical rhythms determine cerebral specialization for speech perception and production. Neuron 56(6):1127–1134

Goldberg TE, Weinberger DR (2004) Genes and the parsing of cognitive processes. Trends Cogn Sci 8(7):325–335

Goldman RI, Stern JM, Engel J Jr, Cohen MS (2002) Simultaneous EEG and fMRI of the alpha rhythm. Neuroreport 13(18):2487–2492

Gray CM, Konig P, Engel AK, Singer W (1989) Oscillatory responses in cat visual cortex exhibit inter-columnar synchronization which reflects global stimulus properties. Nature 338(6213): 334–337

Gurtubay IG, Alegre M, Labarga A, Malanda A, Artieda J (2004) Gamma band responses to target and non-target auditory stimuli in humans. Neurosci Lett 367(1):6–9

Herrmann CS, Munk MH, Engel AK (2004) Cognitive functions of gamma-band activity: memory match and utilization. Trends Cogn Sci 8(8):347–355

Hummel JE, Biederman I (1992) Dynamic binding in a neural network for shape recognition. Psychol Rev 99(3):480–517

Kirino E, Belger A, Goldman-Rakic P, McCarthy G (2000) Prefrontal activation evoked by infrequent target and novel stimuli in a visual target detection task: an event-related functional magnetic resonance imaging study. J Neurosci 20(17):6612–6618

Lachaux JP, Fonlupt P, Kahane P, Minotti L, Hoffmann D, Bertrand O, Baciu M (2007) Relationship between task-related gamma oscillations and BOLD signal: New insights from combined fMRI and intracranial EEG. Hum Brain Mapp 28(12):1368–1375

Lachaux JP, George N, Tallon-Baudry C, Martinerie J, Hugueville L, Minotti L, Kahane P, Renault B (2005) The many faces of the gamma band response to complex visual stimuli. Neuroimage 25(2):491–501

Laufs H, Kleinschmidt A, Beyerle A, Eger E, Salek-Haddadi A, Preibisch C, Krakow K (2003) EEG-correlated fMRI of human alpha activity. Neuroimage 19(4):1463–1476

Leopold DA, Murayama Y, Logothetis NK (2003) Very slow activity fluctuations in monkey visual cortex: implications for functional brain imaging. Cereb Cortex 13(4):422–433

Lindsley DB (1952) Psychological phenomena and the electroencephalogram. Electroencephalogr Clin Neurophysiol 4(4):443–456

Logothetis NK (2002) The neural basis of the blood-oxygen-level-dependent functional magnetic resonance imaging signal. Philos Trans R Soc Lond B Biol Sci 357(1424):1003–1037

Logothetis NK, Pauls J, Augath M, Trinath T, Oeltermann A (2001) Neurophysiological investigation of the basis of the fMRI signal. Nature 412(6843):150–157

Lohmann G, von Cramon DY, Steinmetz H (1999) Sulcal variability of twins. Cereb Cortex 9(7): 754–763

Makeig S, Westerfield M, Jung TP, Enghoff S, Townsend J, Courchesne E, Sejnowski TJ (2002) Dynamic brain sources of visual evoked responses. Science 295(5555):690–694

Mandelkow H, Halder P, Boesiger P, Brandeis D (2006) Synchronization facilitates removal of MRI artefacts from concurrent EEG recordings and increases usable bandwidth. Neuroimage 32(3):1120–1126

Mantini D, Perrucci MG, Del G ratta C, Romani GL, Corbetta M (2007) Electrophysiological signatures of resting state networks in the human brain. Proc Natl Acad Sci USA 104(32): 13170–13175

Martinez-Montes E, Valdes-Sosa PA, Miwakeichi F, Goldman RI, Cohen MS (2004) Concurrent EEG/fMRI analysis by multiway partial least squares. Neuroimage 22(3):1023–1034

Mathiesen C, Caesar K, Lauritzen M (2000) Temporal coupling between neuronal activity and blood flow in rat cerebellar cortex as indicated by field potential analysis. J Physiol 523(Pt 1): 235–246

Matsuura T, Kanno I (2001) Quantitative and temporal relationship between local cerebral blood flow and neuronal activation induced by somatosensory stimulation in rats. Neurosci Res 40(3):281–290

Meltzer JA, Zaveri HP, Goncharova II, Distasio MM, Papademetris X, Spencer SS, Spencer DD, Constable RT (2008) Effects of working memory load on oscillatory power in human intracranial EEG. Cereb Cortex 18(8):1843–1855

Moosmann M, Ritter P, Krastel I, Brink A, Thees S, Blankenburg F, Taskin B, Obrig H, Villringer A (2003) Correlates of alpha rhythm in functional magnetic resonance imaging and near infrared spectroscopy. Neuroimage 20(1):145–158

Mukamel R, Gelbard H, Arieli A, Hasson U, Fried I, Malach R (2005) Coupling between neuronal firing, field potentials, and FMRI in human auditory cortex. Science 309(5736):951–954

Mulert C, Hepp P, Leicht G, Karch S, Lutz J, Moosmann M, Reiser M, Hegerl U, Pogarell O, Möller HJ, Jäger L (2007a) High frequency oscillations in the gamma-band and the corresponding BOLD signal: trial-by-trial coupling of EEG and fMRI reveals the involvement of the thalamic reticular nucleus (TRN). 13th Annual Meeting of the Organization for Human Brain Mapping, Neuroimage 36(Suppl 1):S1–S125

Mulert C, Leicht G, Pogarell O, Mergl R, Karch S, Juckel G, Moller HJ, Hegerl U (2007b) Auditory cortex and anterior cingulate cortex sources of the early evoked gamma-band response: relationship to task difficulty and mental effort. Neuropsychologia 45(10):2294–2306

Muller MM, Keil A (2004) Neuronal synchronization and selective color processing in the human brain. J Cogn Neurosci 16(3):503–522

Murthy N, Fetz EE (1992) Coherent 25- to 35-Hz oscillations in the sensorimotor cortex of awake behaving monkeys. Proc Natl Acad Sci USA 89(12):5670–5674

Neuenschwander S, Singer W (1996) Long-range synchronization of oscillatory light responses in the cat retina and lateral geniculate nucleus. Nature 379(6567):728–732

Niebur E, Koch C, Rosin C (1993) An oscillation-based model for the neuronal basis of attention. Vision Res 33:2789–2802

Niedermeyer E, Lopes Da Silva F (2004) Electroencephalography: basic principles, clinical applications and related fields, 5th edn. Lippincott, Williams & Wilkins, Philadelphia

Niessing J, Ebisch B, Schmidt KE, Niessing M, Singer W, Galuske RA (2005) Hemodynamic signals correlate tightly with synchronized gamma oscillations. Science 309(5736):948–951

Nunez PL (1995) Neocortical dynamics and human EEG rhythms. Oxford University Press, New York

Pantev C, Makeig S, Hoke M, Galambos R, Hampson S, Gallen C (1991) Human auditory evoked gamma-band magnetic fields. Proc Natl Acad Sci USA 88(20):8996–9000

Poeppel D (2003) The analysis of speech in different temporal integration windows: cerebral lateralization as "asymmetric sampling in time". Speech Commun 41:245–255

Pulvermuller F (1999) Words in the brain's language. Behav Brain Sci 22(2):253–279; discussion 280–336

Pulvermuller F, Lutzenberger W, Preissl H, Birbaumer N (1995) Spectral responses in the gamma-band: physiological signs of higher cognitive processes? Neuroreport 6(15):2059–2064

Rademacher J, Morosan P, Schormann T, Schleicher A, Werner C, Freund HJ, Zilles K (2001) Probabilistic mapping and volume measurement of human primary auditory cortex. Neuroimage 13(4):669–683

Ritter P, Villringer A (2006) Simultaneous EEG–fMRI. Neurosci Biobehav Rev 30(6):823–838

Roelfsema PR, Engel AK, Konig P, Singer W (1997) Visuomotor integration is associated with zero time-lag synchronization among cortical areas. Nature 385(6612):157–161

Senkowski D, Talsma D, Grigutsch M, Herrmann CS, Woldorff MG (2007) Good times for multisensory integration: effects of the precision of temporal synchrony as revealed by gamma-band oscillations. Neuropsychologia 45(3):561–571

Speckmann EJ, Elger CE (1999) Introduction to the neurophysiological basis of the EEG and DC potentials. In: Niedermeyer E, Lopes da Silva F (eds) Electroencephalography, basic principles, clinical applications and related fields. Lippincott Williams & Wilkins, Baltimore, pp 15–27

Struber D, Basar-Eroglu C, Hoff E, Stadler M (2000) Reversal-rate dependent differences in the EEG gamma-band during multistable visual perception. Int J Psychophysiol 38(3):243–252

Talairach J, Tournoux P (1988) Co-planar stereotaxic atlas of the human brain. Thieme, New York

Tallon-Baudry C, Bertrand O (1999) Oscillatory gamma activity in humans and its role in object representation. Trends Cogn Sci 3(4):151–162

Tallon-Baudry C, Bertrand O, Delpuech C, Pernier J (1996) Stimulus specificity of phase-locked and non-phase-locked 40 Hz visual responses in human. J Neurosci 16(13):4240–4249

Tiitinen H, Sinkkonen J, Reinikainen K, Alho K, Lavikainen J, Naatanen R (1993) Selective attention enhances the auditory 40 Hz transient response in humans. Nature 364(6432):59–60

Traub RD, Whittington MA, Colling SB, Buzsaki G, Jefferys JG (1996) Analysis of gamma rhythms in the rat hippocampus in vitro and in vivo. J Physiol 493 (Pt 2):471–484

Treisman A (1996) The binding problem. Curr Opin Neurobiol 6(2):171–178

von der Malsburg C (1994)The correlation theory of brain function. In: Domany E, et al. (eds) Models of neural networks II. Springer, Berlin, pp 95–119

Winterer G, Musso F, Vucurevic G, Stoeter P, Konrad A, Seker B, Gallinat J, Dahmen N, Weinberger DR (2006) COMT genotype predicts BOLD signal and noise characteristics in prefrontal circuits. Neuroimage 32(4):1722–1732

Young GB, Pigott SE (1999) Neurobiological basis of consciousness. Arch Neurol 56(2):153–15

Zaehle T, Fründ I, Schadow J, Thärig S, Schoenfeld MA, Herrmann CS (2009) Inter- and intra-individual covariations of hemodynamic and oscillatory gamma responses in the human cortex. Front Hum Neurosci. 3:8

EEG–fMRI in Animal Models

24

Damien J. Ellens and Hal Blumenfeld

1
Introduction

Neuroscientists have long sought techniques for investigating the neuronal mechanisms of normal behaviour and disease. The uniquely enigmatic nature of the brain and the difficulties inherent to its study limited early physiological investigations of brain function. For example, although able to provide great insight into the localisation of brain function, lesion studies are inherently destructive, and thus reveal limited information about brain functioning in situ. Techniques for the noninvasive monitoring of brain function were needed. The advent of recording electrical brain activity via electroencephalography (EEG) opened up new avenues for the noninvasive study of brain activity (Berger 1929). For many years, neuroimaging lagged behind electrophysiological techniques. However, early studies of cerebral haemodynamic responses showed that brain function could be related to measurements of blood flow. Seizures occurring during neurosurgery have long been known to produce a focal blood flow increase in the cerebral cortex (Horsley 1892; Penfield 1933), and early measurements using intracarotid sensors likewise demonstrated increased cerebral blood flow (CBF) during seizures (Gibbs et al. 1934). Advancements in electrical recording and functional imaging technology in recent decades have now made it possible to noninvasively study the brain at sufficiently high temporal and spatial resolutions to reveal fundamental neuronal processes in great detail.

EEG measures extracellular electrical field potentials generated by populations of cortical neurons, and can capture brain electrical activity with excellent temporal resolution. Although EEG provides high temporal resolution, it is limited in its spatial sampling and cannot completely characterise neuronal activity throughout the entire brain. The spatial resolution of EEG is not sufficient to reveal the contribution of individual

H. Blumenfeld (✉)
Yale Departments of Neurology, Neurobiology, Neurosurgery, 333 Cedar Street, New Haven, CT 06520–8018, USA
e-mail: hal.blumenfeld@yale.edu

C. Mulert and L. Lemieux (eds.), *EEG–fMRI*
DOI: 10.1007/978-3-540-87919-0_24, © Springer Verlag Berlin Heidelberg 2010

brain regions to neuronal function. The electrical signal recorded in the EEG reflects a spatial summation of the underlying cortical electrical activity, and does not sample subcortical areas; thus, EEG with scalp electrodes may not detect deeply originating discharges (Gloor 1985).

Functional neuroimaging techniques offer a comprehensive spatial sampling of the brain and can look deep into subcortical structures noninvasively. Blood oxygen level dependent (BOLD) functional magnetic resonance imaging (fMRI) is a powerful tool, with excellent spatial resolution, for the noninvasive study of haemodynamic and metabolic changes during brain activity. BOLD–fMRI signals depend on blood oxygenation and CBF, the specific implications of which we will discuss below, and can therefore provide useful information about neuronal activity (Ogawa et al. 1990, 1993, 1998).

The advent of fMRI has generated an enormous interest in utilising the technique to study normal and abnormal brain function in *humans*. Studies combining multimodal data acquired in different (single modality) sessions allow the correlation of session-averaged effects across modalities, and therefore are indirect. Sequential EEG–fMRI has been employed to study epilepsy in the rat model of pentylenetetrazol (PTZ)-induced seizures (Keogh et al. 2005; Brevard et al. 2006), visual processing in the cat (Kayser et al. 2004) and the relationship between haemodynamic and EEG changes in the resting state (Lu et al. 2007). These studies are based on the assumption that the EEG–fMRI are acquired in the same brain state. Sequential measurements are not ideal for the study of animal models where the neuronal function under investigation is variable, and where the variability is an important aspect of the phenomenon being studied.

Simultaneous EEG–fMRI whereby signals from both modalities are recorded synchronously allows the interdependent neuronal, neuroenergetic and haemodynamic changes to be studied more directly. Importantly, simultaneous acquisitions are necessary for the study of individual events and are greatly advantageous for the study of spontaneous brain activity such as brain rhythms and epileptic discharges. However, human fMRI studies of pathological brain processes have been limited for several reasons. First, because fMRI techniques are highly sensitive to motion, many human studies are limited to the study of neuronal processes with limited movement, such as the spike-wave seizures associated with absence epilepsy, the interictal (between seizures) period of other epilepsy syndromes, or purely cognitive tasks. Second, human studies are inherently less well controlled than animal models due to intersubject variability, while consistent experimental methods and invasive techniques can be used in animal models.

Animal models offer the opportunity to fully utilise the power of EEG–fMRI methods to noninvasively record normal and abnormal activity throughout the brain. For example, the ictal (during seizure) activity of multiple seizure types can be investigated using animal models, and these studies are not limited by movement, as animals can be studied under anaesthetised, paralysed and ventilated conditions. Variables affecting brain activity can be better controlled in animals, such as the onset and type of seizure, and the induction and type of anaesthesia. Furthermore, invasive studies of electrical, haemodynamic, and histological properties can be performed in animals to relate fMRI signals to underlying neuronal activity. Thus, simultaneous EEG–fMRI studies of animal models can provide an important contribution to the understanding of many types of neuronal activity, including epilepsy, sleep, and sensory-motor processing. Additionally, studies of animal models can contribute to our knowledge of fMRI interpretation, thereby informing our understanding of neuroimaging studies in humans, and the neuronal basis of human pathology.

Many animal MRI studies are highly relevant for investigating changes in functional and structural anatomy and exploring physiology (Blumenfeld 2007; Grohn and Pitkanen 2007; Hiremath and Najm 2007). In this chapter we will focus on studies that have employed *simultaneous* EEG–fMRI methods in the same preparation.

2
Advantages of EEG–fMRI in Animal Models

Animal models offer a number of distinct advantages, compared to human subjects, in utilising simultaneous EEG–fMRI to study neuronal function. Animal models allow the investigator to exert greater control over the timing and conditions of neurological events, including seizures, sleep and sensorimotor processing. Animal models also allow for the invasive monitoring and control of anaesthesia and physiological parameters that may influence neuronal activity and fMRI signal changes. Small animal models allow for the use of higher magnetic field strengths, as the energy required to maintain a homogeneous magnetic field at a given strength is directly related to its size. Studying the haemodynamic response to neural activity at higher field strengths is desirable as it increases the sensitivity to BOLD contrast mechanisms (Menon et al. 1993; Turner et al. 1993; Yang et al. 1999). Additionally, the use of paralysed animals allows for the near elimination of movement artefact, which is important for all fMRI studies and particularly so for studying events associated with excessive muscle activity, such as partial or generalised motor seizures. Finally, the pulse-related artefact, a common problem in human fMRI (see the chapter "EEG Quality: Origin and Reduction of the EEG Cardiac-Related Artefact"), is comparatively small in small animals (Sijbers et al. 2000).

Animals also provide an excellent model for studying the relationship between neuronal activity and cerebral haemodynamic and metabolic responses. These fundamental relationships can be studied with invasive electrophysiological measurements and multiple imaging techniques (Logothetis et al. 2001; Schwartz and Bonhoeffer 2001; Smith et al. 2002; Hyder and Blumenfeld 2004; Nersesyan et al. 2004b; Shmuel et al. 2006; Maandag et al. 2007; Schridde et al. 2008; Englot et al. 2008). Simultaneous EEG and fMRI acquisitions allow the investigation of the relationship between neuronal and haemodynamic responses during individual events, whether the result of an experimental trigger or spontaneously occurring, and in relation to event features beyond experimental control such as amplitude or duration. Simultaneous EEG–fMRI investigations can guide tissue studies to specific brain regions of interest, and contribute to elucidating molecular mechanisms related to seizure susceptibility or other disorders. Finally, animal models with genetic variants can be studied with simultaneous EEG–fMRI to examine the neurophysiological changes associated with these genes.

3
Limitations and Technical Challenges of EEG–fMRI in Animal Models

Animal models are constrained by the same limitations inherent to any model system, namely that models are only an approximation of human disease, and need to be interpreted with appropriate caution. There are also several technical challenges to simultaneous EEG–fMRI studies of animals related to their size and the spatial constraints due to using relatively high magnetic fields (Blumenfeld 2007; Mirsattari et al. 2007). Anaesthesia must be carefully considered; as we will discuss, many anaesthetic agents can alter the cerebral haemodynamic response and may alter the neurophysiological behaviour under investigation. Guaranteeing the quality of the MR image can be a formidable challenge, as the imaging signals are sensitive to small amounts of movement, and to magnetic susceptibility differences, especially at air–tissue interfaces, that can introduce unwanted distortions. Animal movement in the scanner must be restricted, either by chemical muscular blockade (curarisation) or through habituation to a restraining device. Electrodes must be carefully chosen to avoid unwanted interactions with magnetic fields and with the tissue (e.g. scalp, subdermal, brain) they contact. Lastly, animal physiology must be carefully monitored during experiments utilising anaesthesia (Mirsattari et al. 2005a).

Investigations of particular brain processes will present their own unique challenges. Animal studies of epilepsy often encounter additional complications, as seizure activity is prone to alteration by commonly used anaesthetic agents, seizures may be difficult to induce in anaesthetised animals, and motion can occur during seizures (Blumenfeld 2007).

4
Anaesthesia

Choosing an appropriate anaesthetic agent is crucial in simultaneous EEG–fMRI studies; considerations of the agent's effects on the EEG data, fMRI signal intensity, long-term physiology, and on the neurological event being studied must all be carefully considered. Furthermore, anaesthetic agents are known to induce changes in the EEG (Winters 1976; Sloan 1998; Hudetz 2002), and different experimental designs may be best served by different combinations of anaesthetic agents.

Inhaled anaesthetic agents may be ideal for some designs because of the swiftness with which the depth of anaesthesia can be adjusted (Makiranta et al. 2005; Mirsattari et al. 2005b). However, these agents can alter the haemodynamic response. Isoflurane has been found to greatly diminish the BOLD signal changes seen in the gamma-butyrolactone (GBL)-induced spike-and-wave discharge (SWD) rat model (Tenney et al. 2003). Conversely, the use of both fentanyl and haloperidol does not block the occurrence of SWDs in two rat genetic models of absence epilepsy (Pinault et al. 1998; Nersesyan et al. 2004b). Furthermore, haloperidol can actually increase the frequency of SWDs (Coenen and Van Luijtelaar 1987; Midzianovskaia et al. 2001). Fentanyl in combination with haloperidol has also been used successfully to produce anaesthesia without blocking tonic-clonic seizures in a rat model (Nersesyan et al. 2004b; Schridde et al. 2008).

A change in the signal strength of the BOLD–fMRI signal compared to the awake state can be seen with anaesthetic agents such as alpha-chloralose (Shulman et al. 1999; Peeters et al. 2001; Hyder et al. 2002a; Smith et al. 2002), propofol (Lahti et al. 1999) and halothane (Maandag et al. 2007). In a porcine model, sudden deepening of thiopental anaesthesia in nonepileptic animals produced significant signal changes in the fMRI response (Makiranta et al. 2002). High-dose morphine and the sedating antihistamine acepromazine was found to provide adequate anaesthesia in a sheep model of penicillin induced focal epilepsy with minimal EEG suppression (Opdam et al. 2002). Alpha-chloralose with urethane has been successfully used in a rat model of PTZ-induced seizures (Keogh et al. 2005). Ketamine and xylazine produces adequate anaesthesia without blocking limbic seizures studied by fMRI (Englot et al. 2008).

In a rat model, halothane was found to have no effect on the BOLD response at doses that showed a clear reduction in the baseline neuronal activity on EEG, while a transition from halothane to alpha-chloralose showed an immediate reduction in the spatial extent of the BOLD response without a change in the peak signal change, which evolved over several hours to an increase in both the spatial extent and peak signal change of the BOLD signal (Austin et al. 2005; Maandag et al. 2007). Halothane has been successfully used to induce temporary anaesthesia in rodent models during subject preparation, with data acquired from paralysed unanaesthetised animals treated with mivacurium (Van Camp et al. 2003); however, special training is needed for unanaesthetised preparations, as discussed shortly. Inhalation anesthetic agents are commonly used as induction agents to allow rapid anaesthesia of an animal for placement of intravascular lines, tracheostomy, electrodes and placement in a holding apparatus for positioning of the surface coil (Nersesyan et al. 2004b; Schridde et al. 2008). A 1-h period has been used to allow complete washout of the inhalation anesthetic (Keogh et al. 2005).

Limiting the use of general anaesthesia to the period of preparing the animal with reversal of the anaesthesia during simultaneous EEG–fMRI acquisition has also been accomplished with the combination of the anaesthetic medetomidine (alpha 2 adrenoreceptor agonist) and the reversal agent atipamezole (alpha 2-adrenergic antagonist) in rats (Tenney et al. 2003), or with ketamine and medetomidine reversed with atipamezole in rats (Tenney et al. 2004a; Brevard et al. 2006), or with the combination of medetomidine, ketamine and isoflurane reversed with atipamezole in marmoset monkeys (Tenney et al. 2004b).

In situations where significant movement does not occur, such as during spike-wave seizures, the study of unanaesthetised animals may be feasible (Tenney et al. 2003; Van Camp et al. 2003). This raises additional technical challenges, as lengthy training of animals is necessary to habituate them to the recording procedures (Khubchandani et al. 2003; Sachdev et al. 2003). Recording from awake animals can further be facilitated by the use of a topical anaesthetic (e.g. lidocaine gel) at any pressure points from restraint devices or needle electrodes (Tenney et al. 2004a, b). Performing simultaneous EEG–fMRI studies in awake animals is an important technical challenge to overcome, as these studies more closely resemble human studies of conscious subjects. The wide variety of successful protocols illustrates the importance of tailoring the experimental design to the specific animal model and research question being investigated.

5
Movement: Curarisation and Habituation

As in human studies, subject movement must be addressed in studies with animal models to limit the creation of artefact in the MR images. As previously discussed, anaesthetic agents must be carefully considered for possible interference with the neurological event being studied, and for possibly altering the haemodynamic response. Lightly anaesthetised preparations or unanaesthetised preparations are advantageous for preserving the normal electrophysiology and neurovascular response but will increase the likelihood of movement by the subject. This has been overcome by curarisation with nondepolarising neuromuscular blockers, such as mivacurium (Van Camp et al. 2003), pancuronium (Opdam et al. 2002; Makiranta et al. 2005), D-tubocurarine (Nersesyan et al. 2004b; Schridde et al. 2008; Englot et al. 2008), or vecuronium (Mirsattari et al. 2006). Curarisation requires the animal be ventilated and their physiology monitored throughout the experiment.

Habituation to the restraint device and the noise of the MRI scanner is required for the study of awake and conscious animals. This has been accomplished through the use of habituation to a custom-designed restraint devices in rats (Khubchandani et al. 2003; Sachdev et al. 2003). Habituation to a restraint device may be facilitated by positive reinforcement (e.g. chocolate milk) combined with diazepam administered 1 h prior to data acquisition to minimise stress (Sachdev et al. 2003).

It is critical to review data carefully after acquisition for movement artefact using methods such as cine review and centre of mass analysis (Nersesyan et al. 2004b) and to reject data in which significant movement occurs, since even tiny movements can result in large fMRI signal changes.

6
Physiology

Physiological stability is crucial in the study of animals during simultaneous EEG–fMRI. Animal models are commonly studied using inhaled anaesthetic agents, which require that the animal undergo a tracheostomy and be ventilated. Animals require physiological stabilisation for the duration of the experiment (Wood et al. 2001). Monitoring of heart rate, blood pressure, temperature and ventilation rate can be done continuously (Nersesyan et al. 2004b; Schridde et al. 2008). Arterial blood gas measurements of pH, pCO_2, and pO_2 can be performed to monitor the physiological state of the animal, as these parameters will affect the haemodynamic response and may affect neuronal function (Jones et al. 2005; Mirsattari et al. 2005a). Mechanical ventilation may be required for some anaesthesia regimens or when muscle paralysis is used (Nersesyan et al. 2004b; Tenney et al. 2004a; Schridde et al. 2008). Mechanical ventilation, blood pressure monitoring and anaesthesia delivery machinery should be kept far from the imaging field to avoid disturbances in the images. This equipment is preferably kept outside of the room containing the magnet, which ideally is itself magnetically shielded.

Hypercapnia can alter the cerebral haemodynamic response, causing vasodilatation of veins and microcapillaries in rat cortex at even mild levels (Nakahata et al. 2003). Hypercapnia has also been shown to reduce blood flow and volume changes during whisker stimulation, and may also affect changes in the BOLD–fMRI signal (Jones et al. 2005). Furthermore, hypercapnia can alter neuronal activity in rats (Kida et al. 2007) possibly by inducing periods of cortical desynchronisation that may be associated with changes in oxidative metabolism (Martin et al. 2006).

7
MR-Compatible Electrodes

MRI-compatible electrodes and EEG recording equipment have been developed and utilised in multiple studies using simultaneous EEG–fMRI (Mirsattari et al. 2007). EEG electrodes commonly contain metals that are affected by an external magnetic field; silver-silver chloride (Ag/AgCl), gold-plated silver, platinum, stainless steel, and tin. While silver and copper electrodes have desirable properties for use in the MR environment, they are not appropriate for invasive recording that may involve direct contact of the electrode with brain tissue due to possible toxicity (Babb and Kupfer 1984). Gold and platinum electrodes have been found to be nontoxic to living tissue (Tallgren et al. 2005). Custom-made gold electrodes were found to be superior compared to both custom-made carbon and commercial platinum-iridium alloy electrodes in size and affect on image quality (Jupp et al. 2006). However, gold and platinum may cause artefacts in MR images due to differences between their magnetic susceptibly and that of brain tissue (Mirsattari et al. 2007). The choice of appropriate MRI-compatible EEG recording equipment will depend on whether they are for scalp, subdermal, or intracranial recordings.

Scalp and subdermal electrodes have the advantage of leaving the brain intact and will theoretically introduce the least amount of artefact in the MR images. Carbon fibre electrodes are the most widely used material for EEG with simultaneous MRI for scalp (Van Audekerkea et al. 2000) and subdermal recordings (Nersesyan et al. 2004b; Makiranta et al. 2005; Schridde et al. 2008), and when directly overlying the cortex via insertion through burr holes (Mirsattari et al. 2006). Carbon fibre electrodes can also be used for intracranial recordings (Opdam et al. 2002; Mirsattari et al. 2005b). Teflon-coated silver-silver chloride (Ag/AgCl) electrodes can be used alone or in combination with carbon fibre electrodes (Mirsattari et al. 2005b; Young et al. 2006). fMRI-compatible electrodes designed for human use, such as conductive plastic cups and gold-plated silver disc electrodes attached to copper wires can be used in larger animal studies (Mirsattari et al. 2007).

Intracranial EEG recordings with simultaneous fMRI have the advantage of recording neuronal activity from specific areas of the brain, such as the occipital cortex (Logothetis et al. 2001; Shmuel et al. 2006) and deep structures, or from the site of seizure induction in animal models of focal epilepsy (Opdam et al. 2002; Englot et al. 2008). However, intracranial electrode placement increases the risk of damaging the cerebral cortex and may cause artefact in the MR images if there is bleeding under the burr holes or at the craniotomy site (Mirsattari et al. 2007). Burr holes should be made with a drill that is compatible with MRI; for example, one coated with titanium or made of diamond to avoid artefacts from any metallic particles the drill may leave (Mirsattari et al. 2007).

Intracranial electrodes may also be used to stimulate brain regions during fMRI experiments. Electrical stimulation has been accomplished in the rat, including in the motor cortex with carbon fibre electrodes (Austin 2003), in the amygdala kindling model with custom-made carbon and gold electrodes, and commercial platinum-iridium electrodes (Jupp et al. 2006), in rat medial thalamus with glass-coated carbon fibre microelectrodes (Shyu et al. 2004), and in perforant pathway (Angenstein et al. 2007) and dorsal hippocampus using bipolar tungsten electrodes (Englot et al. 2008). Precise electrical stimulation of the macaque monkey visual cortex using custom glass-coated iridium microelectrodes during fMRI signal acquisition has also been done (Tolias et al. 2005).

8
EEG Artefacts and Artefact Removal

As discussed in the chapters "EEG Instrumentation and Safety", "EEG Quality: Origin and Reduction of the EEG Cardiac-Related Artefact", "EEG Quality: The Image Acquisition Artefact" and "Image Quality Issues", the simultaneous acquisition of EEG and fMRI is hindered by fMRI equipment causing artefacts in the EEG, and particularly during image acquisition (Ives et al. 1993), and EEG equipment can cause artefacts in the fMRI images (Krakow et al. 2000). Gradient coil-induced magnetic field variations and radiofrequency pulses associated with image acquisition can cause high voltages in the EEG recording electrodes that obscure EEG signals. Revealing the full EEG signal may require removal of the MRI artefact through offline digital filtering, including simple low-pass frequency filtering (Fig. 1) (Nersesyan et al. 2004b), or using methods such as temporal principal component analysis (Negishi et al. 2004). Care must be taken when placing the EEG electrodes on the animal skull to do this in such a way as to minimise unwanted magnetic field inhomogeneity and image distortion (Nersesyan et al. 2004b).

Movement-related artefact has already been discussed, and any runs containing significant movement may be considered for rejection from the analysis. Low-frequency (approximately $f < 1/60 \text{ s}^{-1}$) drift can also occur, especially during prolonged fMRI acquisitions, which may be related to a number of physiological or technical factors (e.g. as can be demonstrated by scanning a phantom, or a nonliving perfused brain), and can be a source of bias, particularly when comparing scans acquired a long time apart. It is important to limit these at the source and to take them into consideration when planning data analysis.

9
Data Analysis

Analysis of simultaneously acquired EEG–fMRI data generally aims at correlating fMRI with neuronal signals (see the chapter "Experimental Design and Data Analysis Strategies" for a general discussion of the analysis strategies employed in human studies). In animal

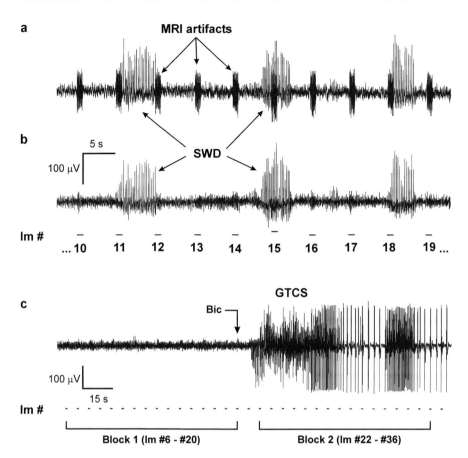

Fig. 1a–c EEG recordings from a simultaneous EEG–fMRI study of spike-wave discharges (SWD) and generalised tonic clonic seizures (GTCS) in the rat. **a** EEG acquired from the Wistar Albino Glaxo rats of Rijswijk (WAG/Rij) showing intermittent episodes of SWD. Large high-frequency artefacts produced by the MRI gradient coils appear every 5 s during the MRI data acquisitions, partially obscuring the EEG. **b** Digital low-pass filter with a 30 Hz cut-off eliminates most of the MRI-related artefacts. Image acquisition numbers (Im #) for this data run are seen below the EEG tracing. To analyse SWD images vs. baseline, *t*-maps were constructed that compared pairs of consecutive images, each consisting of a quiet baseline image just before a given SWD, followed immediately by an image acquired during or within 2 s after the same SWD. In the example shown here, pairs of consecutive baseline and SWD images, respectively, would include images #11 and 12, 14 and 145, 18 and 19, and other similar pairs from this data run. Baseline images Bi (images 11, 14, 18, etc.) were then contrasted with SWD images Ai (images 12, 15, 19, etc.) to construct *t*-maps. Scale bar in **b** applies to EEG traces in both **a** and **b**. **c** EEG (after filtering to remove artifact) acquired during a bicuculline-induced GTCS. The seizure onset is predictable and occurred approximately 5 s after the bolus injection of 0.2 mg intravenous bicuculline (Bic, *arrow*). Average BOLD signal changes can be calculated by comparing two blocks of images (*n* = 15 per block) corresponding to baseline (*Block 1*), and the initial portion of the seizure (*Block 2*) on the EEG. Baseline images Bi (images 6–20 in the example) were contrasted with seizure images Ai (images 22–36 in the example) to construct the *t*-map. Reproduced with permission from Nersesyan et al. (2004b)

models, the availability of prior knowledge of the time course of CBF changes during the neuronal activity being studied can have an important impact on the analysis of the fMRI signal. For example, when analysing fMRI signals during rodent SWD, prior measurements using LDF showed that CBF peaked 3–4 s after SWD onset began on EEG, and then decreased back to baseline after 3–4 s (Nersesyan et al. 2004a). Pixel-based measurements of the BOLD change showed a similar time course (Fig. 2) (Nersesyan et al. 2004b). Therefore, when constructing functional maps of BOLD signal changes during SWD compared to baseline, it was first assumed that each BOLD image acquisition should be related mainly to SWD occurring in the preceding 5 s EEG interval. Pairs of consecutive images and associated pairs of consecutive EEG intervals were selected where the first EEG interval contained a quiet EEG baseline and the second contained SWD (Fig. 1a, b) (Nersesyan et al. 2004b). t-maps were then constructed by contrasting the set of baseline images to SWD images on a pixel-by-pixel basis (Fig. 2) (Nersesyan et al. 2004b). t-maps can also be combined with region of interest analysis to evaluate differences in BOLD signal change and time course limited to specific brain regions (Englot et al. 2008; Tenney et al. 2003, 2004a, b; Schridde et al. 2008).

Generalised tonic-clonic seizures (GTCS) begin with an abrupt onset of sustained, high-frequency neuronal firing during the tonic phase, followed by rhythmic high-frequency firing in the clonic phase (Matsumoto and Marsan 1964; Avoli et al. 1990), with a total duration of several minutes. Therefore, analysis of more prolonged events such as tonic-clonic seizures requires a different approach to analysis. Comparison of bicuculline-induced tonic-clonic seizures to baseline activity has been done by comparing a set of baseline images before bicuculline injection to a set of images after seizure onset (Fig. 1c) (Nersesyan et al. 2004b; Schridde et al. 2008). t-maps can then be constructed by comparing the set of baseline images to the set of images during the beginning of seizure activity (Figs. 3 and 4) (Nersesyan et al. 2004b; Schridde et al. 2008).

Hierarchical clustering algorithms can also be used to identify voxels of interest in the fMRI data (Keogh et al. 2005). The clustering analysis utilises a t-test applied independently to each voxel, comparing a chosen baseline period to a period of signal activity; voxels without significant changes are discarded. Voxels with signal changes that match those of

Fig. 2a–b fMRI changes at 7 T in cortex, thalamus and primary visual cortex during SWD in the WAG/Rij rat with corresponding EEG recording. Note that only fMRI signal increases are shown here, and that decreases have been investigated in subsequent studies (data not shown). **a** Example of BOLD activations during SWD. fMRI signal increases can be seen during SWD. t-maps were calculated from 23 pairs of images, with one image in each pair acquired at baseline and the other during SWD. Results were overlaid onto corresponding high-resolution anatomical images. Eight coronal slices were acquired from back to front (numbered 1–8) at 1 mm intervals, with the first slice at approximately −7.04 and the last slice at +0.40 mm relative to bregma (Paxinos and Watson 1998). Bilateral and relatively symmetrical increases in BOLD signal are present mostly in frontoparietal (somatosensory and motor) cortex, thalamus, and brainstem nuclei, whereas temporal and occipital regions do not show significant changes. t-maps display threshold = 2. **b** Time course of BOLD–fMRI signal changes with simultaneous EEG during SWD. Increases in the BOLD–fMRI signal ($\Delta S/S$) occur in barrel cortex (*purple line*, SIBF) and thalamus (*blue line*, Thal) with the onset of most SWD episodes, particularly those lasting more than 3 s. No significant changes related to seizure activity were observed in primary visual cortex (*green* line, V1M). Reproduced with permission from Nersesyan et al. (2004b)

brain regions can be identified by applying a further test requiring that each voxel is correlated with two other voxels. This has been applied in the study of PTZ-induced seizures in rats (Keogh et al. 2005).

Finally, changes in $CMRO_2$ can be estimated for individual brain regions using the known general relationship between oxygen consumption and BOLD, CBV, and CBF data at steady state (Kida et al. 2007; Schridde et al. 2008). This can be done using CBF values obtained from ASL-MRI or from LDF, together with separate measurements of BOLD and CBV (Fig. 5) (Schridde et al. 2008).

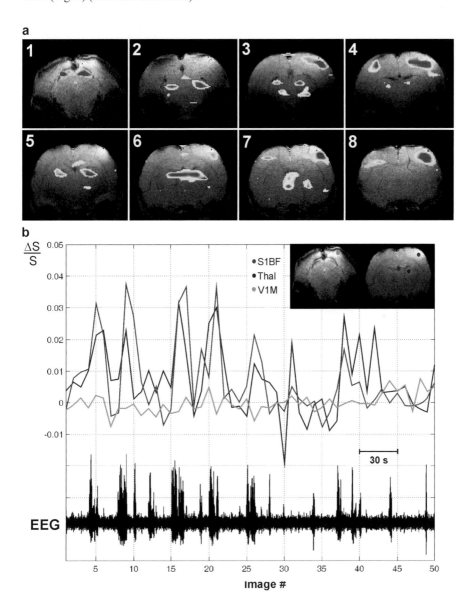

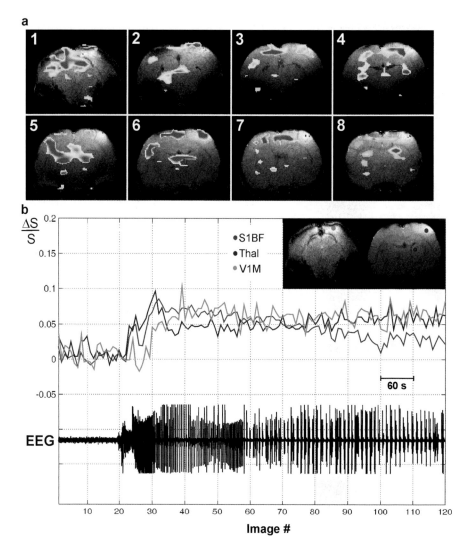

Fig. 3a–b BOLD–fMRI activations at 7 T during a bicuculline-induced GTCS in the WAG/Rij rat with corresponding EEG recording. Note that only fMRI signal increases are shown here, and that decreases have been investigated in subsequent studies (e.g. see Fig. 4). **a** fMRI increases in a WAG/Rij rat during a bicuculline-induced tonic-clonic seizure. *t*-maps were calculated from 16 baseline images compared to the first 16 images after seizure onset, with images acquired every 5 s (see Fig. 1c), and overlaid onto corresponding high-resolution anatomic images. Eight coronal slices were acquired from back to front (numbered 1–8) at 1 mm intervals, with the first slice at approximately −7.04 and the last slice at +0.04 mm relative to bregma (Paxinos and Watson 1998). Bilateral and relatively symmetrical increases in BOLD signal are present in most major brain regions, although some spatial heterogeneity is evident. t-map display threshold = 6. **b** Time course of BOLD–fMRI signal changes with simultaneous EEG during the same tonic clonic seizure as in **a**. On seizure onset, the BOLD–fMRI signal (ΔS/S) increases in barrel cortex (*purple line*, SIBF) and thalamus (*blue line*, Thal), as well as in primary visual cortex (*green line*, V1M). Increases in SIBF and Thal are approximately twice as large as during SWD in the same regions and the same animal (see Fig. 2). Reproduced with permission from Nersesyan et al. (2004b)

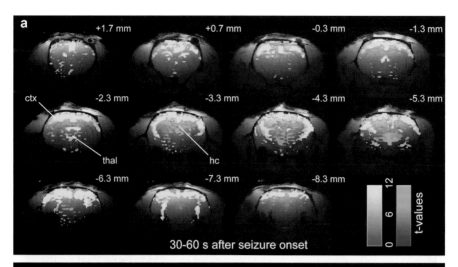

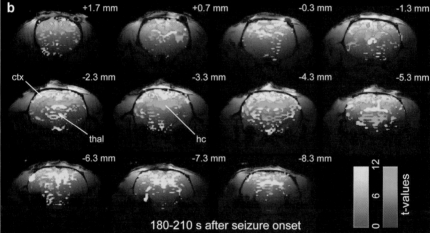

Fig. 4a–b BOLD–fMRI increases and decreases at 9.4 T during bicuculline-induced GTCS in Wistar rats. **a** BOLD–fMRI signals during the beginning of the seizure show not only a mixed pattern of widespread increases across the whole brain, including cortex (*ctx*) and thalamus (*thal*), but also prominent focal decreases, especially in hippocampus (*hc*). **b** Toward the end of the seizure, BOLD increases became less prevalent, though still prominent, whereas decreases became more widespread throughout the brain. In **a** and **b**, *t*-maps are shown for 30 s of data (ten consecutive fMRI images acquired every 3 s) during seizure compared with 30 s baseline. Maps are superimposed on high-resolution anatomical images. Slices are shown from anterior to posterior, with approximate coordinates relative to bregma (Paxinos and Watson 1998). *Colour bars* indicate *t*-values for increases (*warm colours*) and decreases (*cool colours*). Reproduced with permission from Schridde et al. (2008)

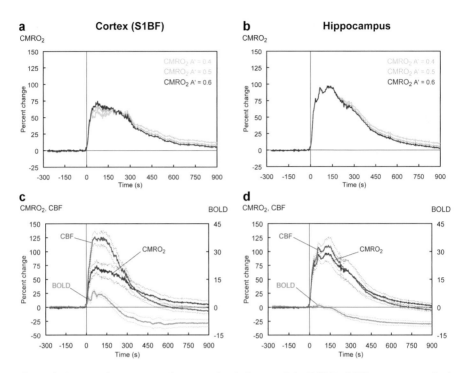

Fig. 5a–d Average time courses of percent signal change of the BOLD–fMRI response, cerebral blood flow (CBF), and cerebral metabolic rate of oxygen consumption (CMRO$_2$) over time during bicuculline-induced tonic-clonic seizures. The changes show that blood supply exceeds oxygen consumption in the barrel field cortex but not the hippocampus. In all graphs, the straight vertical line at time = 0 marks seizure onset. **a, b** Time courses of mean signal change in CMRO$_2$ over time, calculated for three different values of the BOLD calibration parameter A' (0.4, 0.5 and 0.6), for the barrel field cortex (S1BF) (**a**) and hippocampus (**b**). In all cases CMRO$_2$ showed a pronounced increase in both structures during seizures but was higher in hippocampus compared with cortex, independent of A'. **c, d** Relationship between the mean percent signal changes for BOLD, CBF, and estimated CMRO$_2$ (A' = 0.6) for cortex (SIBF) (**c**) and hippocampus (**d**). In the cortex, the increase in CBF during seizures was nearly double the increase in CMRO$_2$, and was accompanied by an increase in the BOLD signal. In the hippocampus, however, increases of CBF and CMRO$_2$ during seizures nearly matched, and no signal changes were observed in the BOLD signal on average, despite strong neuronal activity in both structures. Reproduced with permission from Schridde et al. (2008)

10
Applications of Simultaneous EEG–fMRI in Animals

Simultaneous EEG recording with MRI was first performed in a rat cortical spreading depression model in 1995 (Busch et al. 1995). Here, we will review EEG–fMRI animal studies of epilepsy, including generalised and partial seizures, sleep, and studies where electrical stimulation was applied during signal acquisition. We will also discuss animal studies where the primary aim was to investigate the relationship between neuronal activity and the BOLD signal response.

11
Epilepsy

The first animal model studies of epilepsy with simultaneous EEG–fMRI were performed in 2000 (Van Audekerkea et al. 2000). Animal models provide a means of studying the ictal activity of all seizure types with superior experimental control compared to human studies, and invasive studies can be done to relate fMRI signals to underlying neuronal activity (Blumenfeld 2007).

12
Absence Seizure Models

Human studies of SWD in absence epilepsy patients (Archer et al. 2003; Salek-Haddadi et al. 2003; Aghakhani et al. 2004) have revealed a great deal regarding the neural networks involved in SWD formation and propagation. However, additional information is needed to correctly interpret fMRI signal increases and decreases in this disorder. Animal models can be used to study in depth the relationship of fMRI signal changes to underlying neuronal activity, and molecular mechanisms during SWDs (Blumenfeld 2005a). The Wistar Albino Glaxo rats of Rijswijk (WAG/Rij) have spontaneous SWDs, and are an established model of human absence epilepsy (Coenen and Van Luijtelaar 2003). fMRI studies in this model have shown BOLD signal increases in focal bilateral regions of the cortex and thalamus (Fig. 2a) (Nersesyan et al. 2004b). Interestingly, although considered a generalised seizure disorder, focal anterior regions of the brain are most intensely involved in both fMRI and electrical recordings of SWD, while other brain regions are relatively spared (Fig. 2b) (Meeren et al. 2002; Nersesyan et al. 2004b). Although human fMRI studies of SWD have shown both increases and decreases in the cortex (Archer et al. 2003; Salek-Haddadi et al. 2003; Gotman et al. 2005; Labate et al. 2005; Aghakhani et al. 2006; Hamandi et al. 2006; Laufs et al. 2006), studies in WAG/Rij rats have so far shown mainly increases in the cortex (Fig. 2) (Nersesyan et al. 2004b; Tenney et al. 2004a). However, recent studies have shown that the basal ganglia show prominent fMRI signal decreases during SWD in rodent models (David et al. 2008; Mishra et al. 2007).

GBL is a precursor of gamma-hydroxybutyrate, and produces robust SWD in rats, resembling petit mal status epilepticus (Snead et al. 1999; Tenney et al. 2003). A simultaneous EEG–fMRI study, using epidural electrodes, of SWD in rats treated with GBL showed thalamic increases and mixed cortical increases and decreases in fMRI signals (Tenney et al. 2003). However, a similar study in marmoset monkeys given GBL showed only fMRI increases during SWD (Tenney et al. 2004b).

13
Generalised Tonic-Clonic Seizure Models

GTCS in animal models can be induced by pharmacologic means, allowing the researcher control over the timing of seizures. The first investigation of GTCS using fMRI was performed over 15 years ago (Ogawa and Lee 1992). Simultaneous EEG–fMRI studies of GTCS in animals face the challenge of constraining movement in the scanner (Van Camp et al. 2003; Nersesyan et al. 2004b; Schridde et al. 2008).

Kainic acid, a potent central nervous system stimulant, has been used to induce GTCS in animals (Ben-Ari et al. 1979). A distinct change in the BOLD-fMRI signal has been seen following the injection of kainic acid (Ogawa and Lee 1992). Another proconvulsive agent, PTZ, an antagonist of GABA, has also been used to induce GTCS in rats (Van Camp et al. 2003; Keogh et al. 2005; Brevard et al. 2006). Finally, bicuculline, another GABA receptor antagonist, has also been used to induce rat GTCSs, showing widespread cortical BOLD-fMRI increases (Figs. 3 and 4) (Nersesyan et al. 2004b; Schridde et al. 2008).

Studies of bicuculline-induced GTCS using multiple techniques to investigate neuronal activity, CBF, CBV, $CMRO_2$, and BOLD signal changes indicate that these parameters all increase in parallel in the cortex during bicuculline-induced GTCS. In contrast, some regions such as the hippocampus may show variable BOLD signal changes or even BOLD decreases (Fig. 4), even though direct recordings of neuronal activity from the hippocampus showed consistent large increases in neuronal activity during GTCS (Schridde et al. 2008). Interestingly, the CBF increase exceeded the $CMRO_2$ increase in the cortex, producing the expected consistent increase in BOLD (Fig. 5a, c). However, in the hippocampus, CBF increases did not on average exceed $CMRO_2$ (Fig. 5b, d), so that mismatch between metabolism and CBF can lead to apparent paradoxical BOLD decreases in some cases (Fig. 4) (Schridde et al. 2008).

14
Partial Seizure Models

Simultaneous EEG–fMRI in animal models of focal epilepsy necessitates additional operative techniques to induce localised seizure activity. Where genetic and systemic pharmacological models allow the study of generalised seizure disorders, direct focal introduction of seizure-inducing drugs, commonly penicillin, or electrical stimulation is required to cause focal seizures. One such early study used focal penicillin infusion into the prefrontal cortex of sheep (Opdam et al. 2002). Localised increases in the fMRI signal were identified in the sheep cortex during seizures (Fig. 6) (Opdam et al. 2002). Penicillin has also been applied to the somatosensory cortex in a porcine model, showing regional signal increases during interictal spikes (Makiranta et al. 2005), and to the occipital cortex in rats, showing regional signal increases during seizures (Mirsattari et al. 2006).

Electrical stimulation of the hippocampus has recently been performed during simultaneous depth electrode and fMRI (Englot et al. 2008). Following electrical stimulation,

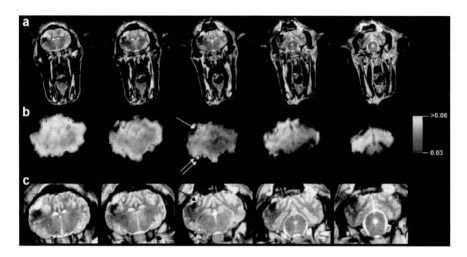

Fig. 6a–c fMRI activations during penicillin-induced focal seizures in sheep. **a** Anatomical images of the brain and head. **b** Corresponding segmented fMRI signal changes (greyscale: mean of within-brain voxels scaled to 1.0) with thresholded time-course variance map overlaid (colour: variance > 0.03). **c** fMRI map overlaid onto anatomical images. *Single* and *double arrows* point to the injection site of penicillin and to the amygdala, respectively, and to corresponding functional activations. The intensity scale is standardised such that each slice time series is scaled by a constant factor such that the mean within-brain voxels of the time series mean image is 1.0. Reproduced with permission from Opdam et al. (2002)

neuronal electrical activity increased intensely in the hippocampus. BOLD signal increases were also observed in the hippocampus, as well as in the thalamus and septal nuclei during seizures. Separate experiments also showed neuronal electrical activity increases in the thalamus and septal nuclei in this model. In addition, BOLD decreases were seen in the orbital frontal cortex (Englot et al. 2008), which may resemble decreases in neocortical function seen during human limbic seizures (Blumenfeld et al. 2004a, b).

See the chapters "EEG–fMRI in Adults with Focal Epilepsy", "EEG–fMRI in Idiopathic Generalised Epilepsy (Adults)" and "EEG–fMRI in Children with Epilepsy" for discussions of human epilepsy studies.

15
Sleep

Simultaneous EEG–fMRI has been used to investigate sleep in rodent models (Khubchandani et al. 2005). Simultaneous EEG allows for the determination of sleep and wake cycles in the animal while scanning. fMRI signal increases were shown in the medial preoptic area during sleep, corroborating other work indicating the importance of this area in maintaining slow-wave sleep (Khubchandani et al. 2005). Simultaneous EEG–fMRI has been used primarily in epilepsy research, but the potential exists for much additional work in other fields, including sleep. See the chapter "Sleep" for a review of human studies of sleep.

16
Sensorimotor Stimulation Models

Simultaneous EEG–fMRI can be used to study the haemodynamic changes that occur during sensorimotor stimulation. Electrical forepaw stimulation has been used to compare cortex activation during fully conscious curarisation compared to during alpha-chloralose anaesthesia (Peeters et al. 2001). Simultaneously acquired EEG data was used to identify the awake and anaesthetised states, showing BOLD decreases under alpha-chloralose anaesthesia, compared to the awake state (Peeters et al. 2001). Simultaneous EEG–fMRI has also been used to study the interaction between simultaneous and sequential electrical forepaw stimulations in the rat and the effects on the associated stimulation-evoked potentials and BOLD signal responses (Ogawa et al. 2000) showing fMRI signal modification in response to two stimuli directly following another, although on EEG the changes associated with the second stimulation was extinguished.

Studies investigating fMRI changes during anaesthesia with parallel electrophysiology recordings during forepaw stimulation are ongoing, and have recently shown differences in the strength of fMRI changes under different types of anaesthesia (Hyder et al. 2002a; Smith et al. 2002; Maandag et al. 2007).

17
The Electrophysiological Substrates of the BOLD Effect: Simultaneous Microelectrode EEG Recordings and fMRI

One of the major goals of animal studies in this field is to relate neuroimaging signals to underlying electrical neuronal activity. Simultaneous recordings of single neurons, local field potential and BOLD–fMRI signals has been accomplished in anaesthetised monkeys (Logothetis et al. 2001; Tolias et al. 2005; Shmuel et al. 2006), but this method remains a significant challenge technically. These experiments provide the opportunity to study the relationship between BOLD and electrophysiology during spontaneous brain events and, in the case of evoked responses, beyond effects averaged across events or sessions, by measuring signal changes during individual events. See the chapter "Locally Measured Neuronal Correlates of Functional MRI Signals" for further discussion of this work.

The relationship between fMRI signals and electrophysiology can be successfully investigated by parallel bench-top electrophysiology and fMRI experiments performed under identical conditions (Hyder et al. 2002b; Smith et al. 2002). Recent work has also allowed the investigation of short-lasting dynamic events (Sanganahalli et al. 2009). Studies designed to investigate both modalities in the same animal model have shown good correspondence between fMRI increases and physiological measurements (Nersesyan et al. 2004a; Schridde et al. 2008). In epilepsy models, anterior brain regions such as the somatosensory cortex where fMRI signals are increased during SWD show increased neuronal firing and CBF, while posterior areas such as visual cortex spared by fMRI signal changes show few changes in physiological measurements (Fig. 2) (Nersesyan et al.

2004b). Direct physiological measurements during GTCS, on the other hand, show increases in both anterior and posterior brain regions, in agreement with fMRI measurements in the same areas (Fig. 3) (Nersesyan et al. 2004b). Interestingly, in the somatosensory cortex, the magnitude of BOLD–fMRI, neuronal firing, and CBF changes were greatest for GTCS, less for normal whisker stimulation, and even less for SWD (Nersesyan et al. 2004a, b). Understanding the relationship between fMRI signal increases and decreases in other regions will be the subject of future investigations, as will understanding the neuroenergetic mechanisms of fMRI signal changes.

18
Future Directions

The use of fMRI as a research tool in animal models of epilepsy is still in its early stages, and there is tremendous potential for additional future work in this field. Simultaneous EEG–fMRI is now a reality and has contributed greatly to our understanding of haemodynamic changes that precede, accompany and follow epileptiform discharges, and to our understanding of haemodynamic and metabolic responses to neuronal activity. Additionally, the use of simultaneous EEG–fMRI will open up many lines of investigation and will continuously refine our understanding of the temporal and spatial characteristics of neuronal activity. BOLD signal acquisition is only one of many promising MRI modalities, and it will become increasingly feasible to fully investigate the neuroenergetic basis of activity changes in the brain using multimodal techniques. The integration of measurements of BOLD–fMRI, CBV, and CBF can be used to obtain estimates of the $CMRO_2$, thereby allowing a full investigation of neuronal energetics (Davis et al. 1998; Hyder et al. 2002b; Smith et al. 2002; Hyder and Blumenfeld 2004; Shulman and Rothman 2004; Stefanovic et al. 2004; Maandag et al. 2007; Sanganahalli et al. 2009).

Further technical advances in fMRI acquisition and analysis, combined with advances in combining the EEG data, will allow for a better signal-to-noise ratio and improved spatial and temporal resolution. Future studies will be able to perform detailed investigations of the time course of the haemodynamic response to varying neuronal events. Intracranial electrical recording during fMRI is magnifying the resolution with which we can measure the activity of individual brain regions. Additionally, intracranial electrical stimulation is opening up new avenues of investigation with the development of models of partial seizures, and into the fundamental relationship between neuronal activity and the cerebral haemodynamic and metabolic response. Crucial questions regarding the fMRI changes during epileptiform events, and other neuronal processes, remain unanswered. Which region(s) are involved in seizure onset and propagation? Which regions of the brain are involved in sensorimotor processing? How do different regions of the brain vary in their haemodynamic and metabolic responses regarding temporal and amplitude characteristics from varying stimuli or processes? How do these haemodynamic and metabolic responses relate to electrical activity before, during and after neuronal events? Answering these questions will contribute to our understanding of neuronal function, and to the development of targeted investigations of molecular and genetic changes associated with abnormal brain function.

19
Conclusions

We have reviewed the technical challenges related to animal preparation, data analysis, signal acquisition and study design, and the innovative solutions to these problems have been highlighted. EEG–fMRI studies in animals can contribute to our understanding of epilepsy, sensorimotor processing and other neuronal events, and the relationship between fMRI signals and neuronal activity.

The animal model studies discussed here have yielded important data, elucidating specific cortical and subcortical network changes during epileptiform events, and will guide future studies of this disorder. More work is needed to map the anatomical distribution of the changes, and to fully investigate the physiology of brain responses using modalities that measure changes in CBV, CBF, and $CMRO_2$, and electrical neuronal activity throughout the brain. Interpretations of human studies will be improved by a better understanding of the relationship between neuronal activity and the fMRI signal in animal models. A better understanding of the local networks and brain regions involved in specific seizure disorders may help to design improved focal resective surgery, and could provide targets for deep brain stimulation, medication or even gene therapy. Finally, animal studies may also improve our understanding of functional brain impairment and cognitive dysfunction.

Acknowledgements   We thank Dario Englot, Asht Mishra and Michael Purcaro for helpful comments on the manuscript. This work was supported by NIH R01 NS049307, P30 NS052519, and by the Loughridge family. Damien Ellens is supported by the Howard Hughes Medical Institute as a Medical Fellow.

References

Aghakhani Y, Bagshaw AP, et al. (2004) fMRI activation during spike and wave discharges in idiopathic generalized epilepsy. Brain 127(Pt 5):1127–44

Aghakhani Y, Kobayashi E, et al. (2006) Cortical and thalamic fMRI responses in partial epilepsy with focal and bilateral synchronous spikes. Clin Neurophysiol 117(1):177–91

Angenstein F, Kammerer E, et al. (2007) Frequency-dependent activation pattern in the rat hippocampus, a simultaneous electrophysiological and fMRI study. Neuroimage 38(1):150–63

Archer JS, Abbott DF, et al. (2003) fMRI "deactivation" of the posterior cingulate during generalized spike and wave. Neuroimage 20(4):1915–22

Austin VC, Blamire AM, et al. (2005) Confounding effects of anesthesia on functional activation in rodent brain: a study of halothane and alpha-chloralose anesthesia. Neuroimage 24(1):92–100

Austin VC, Blamire AM, et al. (2003) Differences in the BOLD fMRI response to direct and indirect cortical stimulation in the rat. Magn Reson Med 49(5):838–47

Avoli M, Gloor P, et al. (Eds.) (1990) Generalized Epilepsy. Boston, Birkhauser

Babb TL, Kupfer (1984) Phagocytic and metabolic reactions to chronically implanted metal brain electrodes. Exp Neurol 86(2):171–82

Behar K, Petroff OA, et al. (1986) Detection of metabolites in rabbit brain by 13C NMR spectroscopy following administration of [1–13C]glucose. Magn Reson Med 3(6):911–20

Ben-Ari Y, Lagowska J, et al. (1979) A new model of focal status epilepticus: intra-amygdaloid application of kainic acid elicits repetitive secondarily generalized convulsive seizures. Brain Res 163(1):176–9

Berger H (1929) Ueber das Elektrenkephalogramm des Menschen. Arch Psychiat 87:527

Blumenfeld H (2005a) Cellular and network mechanisms of spike-wave seizures. Epilepsia 46(Suppl 9):21–33

Blumenfeld H (2005b) Consciousness and epilepsy: why are patients with absence seizures absent? Prog Brain Res 150:271–86

Blumenfeld H (2007) Functional MRI studies of animal models in epilepsy. Epilepsia 48(Suppl 4): 18–26

Blumenfeld H, McNally KA, et al. (2004a) Positive and negative network correlations in temporal lobe epilepsy. Cereb Cortex 14(8):892–902

Blumenfeld H, Rivera M, et al. (2004b) Ictal neocortical slowing in temporal lobe epilepsy. Neurology 63:1015–21

Blumenfeld H, Taylor J (2003) Why do seizures cause loss of consciousness? Neuroscientist 9(5): 301–10

Brevard ME, Kulkarni P, et al. (2006) Imaging the neural substrates involved in the genesis of pentylenetetrazol-induced seizures. Epilepsia 47(4):745–54

Busch E, Hoehn-Berlage M, et al. (1995) Simultaneous recording of EEG, DC potential and diffusion-weighted NMR imaging during potassium induced cortical spreading depression in rats. NMR Biomed 8(2):59–64

Coenen AM, Van Luijtelaar EL (2003) Genetic animal models for absence epilepsy: a review of the WAG/Rij strain of rats. Behav Genet 33:635–55

Coenen AM, Van Luijtelaar EL (1987) The WAG/Rij rat model for absence epilepsy: age and sex factors. Epilepsy Res 1(5):297–301

David O, Guillemain I, Saillet S, Reyt S, Deransart C, Segebarth C, Depaulis A. 2008. Identifying neural drivers with functional MRI: an electrophysiological validation. PLoS Biol. 6(12): 2683–97.

Davis TL, Kwong KK, et al. (1998) Calibrated functional MRI: mapping the dynamics of oxidative metabolism. Proc Natl Acad Sci USA 95(4):1834–9

Detre JA, Leigh JS, et al. (1992) Perfusion imaging. Magn Reson Med 23(1):37–45

Detre JA, Wang J (2002) Technical aspects and utility of fMRI using BOLD and ASL. Clin Neurophysiol 113(5):621–34

Englot DJ, Mishra AM, Mansuripur PK, Herman P, Hyder F, Blumenfeld H. (2008). Remote effects of focal hippocampal seizures on the rat neocortex. Journal of Neuroscience, 28(36): 9066–9081.

Gibbs FA, Lennox WG, et al. (1934) Cerebral blood flow preceding and accompanying epileptic seizures in man. Arch Neurol Psychiatry 32:257–72

Gloor P (1985) Neuronal generators and the problem of localisation in electroencephalography: application of volume conductor theory to electroencephalography. J Clin Neurophysiol 2(4): 327–54

Gotman J, Grova C, et al. (2005) Generalized epileptic discharges show thalamocortical activation and suspension of the default state of the brain. Proc Natl Acad Sci USA 102(42):15236–40

Grohn O, Pitkanen A (2007) Magnetic resonance imaging in animal models of epilepsy-noninvasive detection of structural alterations. Epilepsia 48 (Suppl 4):3–10

Gruetter R, Novotny EJ, et al. (1994) Localized 13C NMR spectroscopy in the human brain of amino acid labeling from D-[1–13C]glucose. J Neurochem 63(4):1377–85

Gruetter R, Seaquist ER, et al. (1998) Localized in vivo 13C-NMR of glutamate metabolism in the human brain: initial results at 4 Tesla. Dev Neurosci 20(4–5):380–8

Hamandi K, Salek-Haddadi A, et al. (2006) EEG–fMRI of idiopathic and secondarily generalized epilepsies. Neuroimage 31(4):1700–10

He J, Devonshire M, et al. (2007) Simultaneous laser doppler flowmetry and arterial spin labeling MRI for measurement of functional perfusion changes in the cortex. Neuroimage 34(4):1391–404

Hiremath GK, Najm IM (2007) Magnetic resonance spectroscopy in animal models of epilepsy. Epilepsia 48(Suppl 4):47–55

Horsley V (1892) An address on the origin and seat of epileptic disturbance. Br Med J 1:693–6

Hudetz AG (2002) Effect of volatile anesthetics on interhemispheric EEG cross-approximate entropy in the rat. Brain Res 954(1):123–31

Hyder F (2004) Neuroimaging with calibrated FMRI. Stroke 35(11 Suppl 1):2635–41

Hyder F, Blumenfeld H (2004) Relationship between CMRO2 and neuronal activity. In: Shulman RG, Rothman DL (eds) Brain energetics and neuronal activity: applications to fMRI and medicine. New York, Wiley, pp 173–94

Hyder F, Rothman DL, et al. (2002a) Total neuroenergetics support localized brain activity: implications for the interpretation of fMRI.[comment]. Proc Natl Acad Sci U S A 99(16):10771–6

Hyder F, Kida I, et al. (2002b) Quantitative fMRI of rat brain by multi-modal MRI and MRS measurements. Int Symp Brain Activat CBF Control Int Congr Ser 1235:57–71

Hyder F, Kida I, et al. (2001) Quantitative functional imaging of the brain: towards mapping neuronal activity by BOLD fMRI. NMR Biomed 14(7–8):413–31

Ives JR, Warach S, et al. (1993) Monitoring the patient's EEG during echo planar MRI. Clin Neurol 87:417–20

Jones M, Berwick J, et al. (2005) The effect of hypercapnia on the neural and hemodynamic responses to somatosensory stimulation. Neuroimage 27(3):609–23

Jupp B, Williams JP, et al. (2006) MRI compatible electrodes for the induction of amygdala kindling in rats. J Neurosci Methods 155(1):72–6

Kayser C, Kim M, et al. (2004) A comparison of hemodynamic and neural responses in cat visual cortex using complex stimuli. Cereb Cortex 14(8):881–91

Kennan RP, Zhong J, et al. (1994) Intravascular susceptibility contrast mechanisms in tissue. Magn Reson Med 31:9–21

Keogh BP, Cordes D, et al. (2005) BOLD-fMRI of PTZ-induced seizures in rats. Epilepsy Res 66(1–3):75–90

Khubchandani M, Jagannathan NR, et al. (2005) Functional MRI shows activation of the medial preoptic area during sleep. Neuroimage 26(1):29–35

Khubchandani M, Mallick HN, et al. (2003) Stereotaxic assembly and procedures for simultaneous electrophysiological and MRI study of conscious rat. Magn Reson Med 49:962–7

Kida I, Rothman DL, et al. (2007) Dynamics of changes in blood flow, volume, and oxygenation: implications for dynamic functional magnetic resonance imaging calibration. J Cereb Blood Flow Metab 27(4):690–6

Kida I, Kennan RP, et al. (2000) High-resolution CMR(O2) mapping in rat cortex: a multiparametric approach to calibration of BOLD image contrast at 7 Tesla. J Cereb Blood Flow Metab 20(5):847–60

Krakow K, Allen PJ, et al. (2000) EEG recording during fMRI experiments: image quality. Hum Brain Mapp 10(1):10–15

Labate A, Briellmann RS, et al. (2005) Typical childhood absence seizures are associated with thalamic activation. Epileptic Disord 7(4):373–7

Lahti KM, Ferris CF, et al. (1999) Comparison of evoked cortical activity in conscious and propofol-anesthetized rats using functional MRI. Magn Reson Med 41(2):412–6

Laufs H, Lengler U, et al. (2006) Linking generalized spike-and-wave discharges and resting state brain activity by using EEG/fMRI in a patient with absence seizures. Epilepsia 47(2):444–8

Logothetis NK, Pauls J, et al. (2001) Neurophysiological investigation of the basis of the fMRI signal. Nature 412(6843):150–7

Lu H, Zuo Y, et al. (2007) Synchronized delta oscillations correlate with the resting-state functional MRI signal. Proc Natl Acad Sci USA 104:18265–9

Maandag NJ, Coman D, et al. (2007) Energetics of neuronal signaling and fMRI activity. Proc Natl Acad Sci USA 104(51):20546–51

Makiranta MJ, Jauhiainen JP, et al. (2002) Functional magnetic resonance imaging of swine brain during change in thiopental anesthesia into EEG burst-suppression level–a preliminary study. Magma 15(1–3):27–35

Makiranta M, Ruohonen J, et al. (2005) BOLD signal increase preceeds EEG spike activity—a dynamic penicillin induced focal epilepsy in deep anesthesia. Neuroimage 27(4):715–24

Mandeville JB, Marota JJ, et al. (1999) MRI measurement of the temporal evolution of relative CMRO(2) during rat forepaw stimulation. Magn Reson Med 42(5):944–51

Martin C, Jones M, et al. (2006) Haemodynamic and neural responses to hypercapnia in the awake rat. Eur J Neurosci 24(9):2601–10

Mason GF, Behar KL, et al. (1992) NMR determination of intracerebral glucose concentration and transport kinetics in rat brain. J Cereb Blood Flow Metab 12(3):448–55

Mason GF, Gruetter R, et al. (1995) Simultaneous determination of the rates of the TCA cycle, glucose utilization, alpha-ketoglutarate/glutamate exchange, and glutamine synthesis in human brain by NMR. J Cereb Blood Flow Metab 15(1):12–25

Matsumoto H, Marsan CA (1964) Cortical cellular phenomena in experimental epilepsy: ictal manifestations. Exp Neurol 9:305–26

Meeren HK, Pijn JP, et al. (2002) Cortical focus drives widespread corticothalamic networks during spontaneous absence seizures in rats. J Neurosci 22(4):1480–95

Menon RS, Ogawa S, et al. (1993) Tesla gradient recalled echo characteristics of photic stimulation-induced signal changes in the human primary visual cortex. Magn Reson Med 30(3):380–6

Midzianovskaia IS, Kuznetsova GD, et al. (2001) Electrophysiological and pharmacological characteristics of two types of spike-wave discharges in WAG/Rij rats. Brain Res 911:62–70

Mirsattari SM, Bihari F, et al. (2005a) Physiological monitoring of small animals during magnetic resonance imaging. J Neurosci Methods 144(2):207–13

Mirsattari SM, Ives JR, et al. (2005b) Real-time display of artifact-free electroencephalography during functional magnetic resonance imaging and magnetic resonance spectroscopy in an animal model of epilepsy. Magn Reson Med 53(2):456–64

Mirsattari SM, Ives JR, et al. (2007) EEG monitoring during functional MRI in animal models. Epilepsia 48(Suppl 4):37–46

Mirsattari SM, Wang Z, et al. (2006) Linear aspects of transformation from interictal epileptic discharges to BOLD fMRI signals in an animal model of occipital epilepsy. Neuroimage 30(4):1133–48

Mishra AM, Schridde U, et al. (2007) Physiology and imaging of increases and decreases in BOLD signals during spike-wave seizures in WAG/Rij rats. http://web.sfn.org/

Nakahata K, Kinoshita H, et al. (2003) Mild hypercapnia induces vasodilation via adenosine triphosphate-sensitive K+ channels in parenchymal microvessels of the rat cerebral cortex. Anesthesiology 99(6):1333–9

Negishi M, Abildgaard M, et al. (2004) Removal of time-varying gradient artifacts from EEG data acquired during continuous fMRI. Clin Neurophysiol 115(9):2181–92

Nersesyan H, Herman P, et al. (2004a) Relative changes in cerebral blood flow and neuronal activity in local microdomains during generalized seizures. J Cereb Blood Flow Metab 24(9):1057–68

Nersesyan H, Hyder F, et al. (2004b) Dynamic fMRI and EEG recordings during spike-wave seizures and generalized tonic-clonic seizures in WAG/Rij rats. J Cereb Blood Flow Metab 24(6):589–99

Ogawa S, Lee T (1992) Blood oxygen level dependent MRI of the brain: effects of seizure induced by kainic acid in the rat. Proc Soc Magn Reson Med 1:501

Ogawa S, Lee TM, et al. (2000) An approach to probe some neural systems interaction by functional MRI at neural time scale down to milliseconds. Proc Natl Acad Sci USA 97(20):11026–31

Ogawa S, Lee TM, et al. (1990) Brain magnetic resonance imaging with contrast dependent on blood oxygenation. Proc Natl Acad Sci USA 87(24):9868–72

Ogawa S, Menon RS, et al. (1993) Functional brain mapping by blood oxygenation level-dependent contrast magnetic resonance imaging. Biophys J 64:803–12

Ogawa S, Menon RS, et al. (1998) On the characteristics of functional magnetic resonance imaging of the brain. Annu Rev Biophys Biomol Struct 27:447–74

Opdam H. I, Federico P, et al. (2002) A sheep model for the study of focal epilepsy with concurrent intracranial EEG and functional MRI. Epilepsia 43(8):779–87

Paxinos G, Watson C (1998) The rat brain in stereotaxic coordinates. Academic, San Diego

Peeters RR, Tindemans I, et al. (2001) Comparing BOLD fMRI signal changes in the awake and anesthetized rat during electrical forepaw stimulation. Magn Reson Imaging 19(6):821–6

Penfield W (1933) The evidence for a cerebral vascular mechanism in epilepsy. Ann Int Med 7:303–10

Pinault, D, Leresche N, et al. (1998) Intracellular recordings in thalamic neurones during spontaneous spike and wave discharges in rats with absence epilepsy. J Physiol 509(Pt 2):449–56

Ritter P, Villringer A (2006) Simultaneous EEG–fMRI. Neurosci Biobehav Rev 30(6):823–38

Rothman DL, Sibson NR, et al. (1999) In vivo nuclear magnetic resonance spectroscopy studies of the relationship between the glutamate-glutamine neurotransmitter cycle and functional neuroenergetics. Philos Trans Royal Soc Lond B 354(1387):1165–77

Sachdev RN, Champney GC, et al. (2003) Experimental model for functional magnetic resonance imaging of somatic sensory cortex in the unanesthetized rat. Neuroimage 19(3):742–50

Salek-Haddadi A, Lemieux L, et al. (2003) Functional magnetic resonance imaging of human absence seizures. Ann Neurol 53(5):663–7

Salek-Haddadi A, Merschhemke M, et al. (2002) Simultaneous EEG-correlated ictal fMRI. Neuroimage 16(1):32–40

Sanganahalli BG, Herman P, Blumenfeld H, Hyder F. (2009). Oxidative Neuroenergetics in Event-Related Paradigms. Journal of Neuroscience, 29(6):1707–1718.

Schridde U, Khubchandani M, et al. (2008) Negative BOLD with large increases in neuronal activity. Cereb Cortex 18(8):1814–27

Schwartz TH, Bonhoeffer T (2001) In vivo optical mapping of epileptic foci and surround inhibition in ferret cerebral cortex. Nat Med 7(9):1063–7

Shmuel A, Augath M, et al. (2006) Negative functional MRI response correlates with decreases in neuronal activity in monkey visual area V1. Nat Neurosci 9(4):569–77

Shulman RG, Rothman DL, et al. (1999) Stimulated changes in localized cerebral energy consumption under anesthesia. Proc Natl Acad Sci USA 96(6):3245–50

Shulman RG, Rothman DL, et al. (2004) Energetic basis of brain activity: implications for neuroimaging. Trends Neurosci 27(8):489–95

Shulman RG, Hyder F, et al. (2001) Cerebral energetics and the glycogen shunt: neurochemical basis of functional imaging. Proc Natl Acad Sci USA 98(11):6417–22

Shulman RG, Hyder F, et al. (2002) Biophysical basis of brain activity: implications for neuroimaging. Q Rev Biophys 35(3):287–325

Shulman RG, Rothman DLE (2004) Brain energetics and neuronal activity: applications to fMRI and medicine. Wiley, New York

Shyu BC, Lin CY, et al. (2004) A method for direct thalamic stimulation in fMRI studies using a glass-coated carbon fiber electrode. J Neurosci Methods 137(1):123–31

Sijbers J, Vanrumste B, et al. (2000) Automatic localisation of EEG electrode markers within 3D MR data. Magn Reson Imaging 18(4):485–8

Sloan TB (1998) Anesthetic effects on electrophysiologic recordings. J Clin Neurophysiol 15(3):217–26

Smith AJ, Blumenfeld H, et al. (2002) Cerebral energetics and spiking frequency: the neurophysiological basis of fMRI. Proc Natl Acad Sci USA 99(16):10765–70

Snead OC 3rd, Depaulis A, et al. (1999) Absence epilepsy: advances in experimental animal models. Adv Neurol 79:253–78

Stefanovic B, Warnking JM, et al. (2004) Hemodynamic and metabolic responses to neuronal inhibition. Neuroimage 22(2):771–8

Tallgren P, Vanhatalo S, et al. (2005) Evaluation of commercially available electrodes and gels for recording of slow EEG potentials. Clin Neurophysiol 116(4):799–806

Tenney JR, Duong TQ, et al. (2003) Corticothalamlic modulation during absence seizures in rats: a functional MRI assessment. Epilepsia 44(9):1133–40

Tenney JR, Duong TQ, et al. (2004a) fMRI of brain activation in a genetic rat model of absence seizures. Epilepsia 45(6):576–82

Tenney JR, Marshall PC, et al. (2004b) fMRI of generalized absence status epilepticus in conscious marmoset monkeys reveals corticothalamic activation. Epilepsia 45(10):1240–7

Tolias AS, Sultan F, et al. (2005) Mapping cortical activity elicited with electrical microstimulation using FMRI in the macaque. Neuron 48(6):901–11

Turner R, Jezzard P, et al. (1993) Functional mapping of the human visual cortex at 4 and 1.5 Tesla using deoxygenation contrast EPI. Magn Reson Med 29(2):277–9

Van Audekerkea J, Peeters R, et al. (2000) Special designed RF-antenna with integrated non-invasive carbon electrodes for simultaneous magnetic resonance imaging and electroencephalography acquisition at 7 T. Magn Reson Imaging 18(7):887–91

Van Camp N, D'Hooge R, et al. (2003) Simultaneous electroencephalographic recording and functional magnetic resonance imaging during pentylenetetrazol-induced seizures in rat. Neuroimage 19:627–36

Weisskoff RM, Zuo CS, et al. (1994) Microscopic susceptibility variation and transverse relaxation: theory and experiment. Magn Reson Med 31:601–10

Winters WD (1976) Effects of drugs on the electrical activity of the brain: anesthetics. Annu Rev Pharmacol Toxicol 16:413–26

Wood AK, Klide AM, et al. (2001) Prolonged general anesthesia in MR studies of rats. Acad Radiol 8(11):1136–40

Yang Y, Wen H, et al. (1999) Comparison of 3D BOLD Functional MRI with spiral acquisition at 1.5 and 4.0 T. Neuroimage 9(4):446–51

Young GB, Ives JR, et al. (2006) A comparison of subdermal wire electrodes with collodion-applied disk electrodes in long-term EEG recordings in ICU. Clin Neurophysiol 117(6):1376–9

EEG–fMRI Information Fusion: Biophysics and Data Analysis

25

Jean Daunizeau, Helmut Laufs, and Karl J. Friston

1
Introduction

Cerebral activity has many attributes: bioelectrical, metabolic, haemodynamic, hormonal, endogenous, exogenous, specialised, integrated, pathological, stable, dynamic, to mention but a few. The diverse nature of biological processes has been recognised for centuries. It seems obvious that moving from unimodal recordings to multimodal measurements will allow neuroscientists to better understand the nature and structure of cerebral activity. This means that fusing electrophysiological data and BOLD-related measurements represents an important methodological challenge.

The realisation of any cognitive, motor or sensory process rests on cerebral dynamics and creates order in the bioelectric and haemodynamic signals measured with EEG and fMRI, respectively. To detect and interpret the relevant features of these signals, one typically describes processes at their own temporal and spatial scales. The main sources of scalp EEG signals are postsynaptic cortical currents associated with large pyramidal neurons, which are oriented perpendicular to the cortical surface (Nunez 1981). However, the scalp topology of measured electrical potentials does not, without additional (prior) information, uniquely specify the location of underlying bioelectric activity. This issue is referred to as the ill-posed nature of the EEG/MEG inverse problem. Conversely, even though fMRI discloses complementary features of neuronal activity (Nunez and Silberstein 2000; Mukamel et al. 2005), it is only an indirect measure, through metabolism, oxygenation and blood flow, where these slow mechanisms provide temporally smoothed correlates of neuronal activity.

Standard unimodal EEG (fMRI) data analysis relies on the specificity of a given bioelectric (haemodynamic) feature of neuronal activity. The vast majority of existing EEG–fMRI integration strategies attempt to enhance the spatial or temporal resolution of the combined EEG–fMRI data set. But can we exploit their complementary nature to infer the

J. Daunizeau (✉)
Wellcome Trust for Neuroimaging, Institute of Neurology UCL, WC1N 3BG 12 Queen Square, London, UK
e-mail: j.daunizeau@fil.ion.ucl.ac.uk

C. Mulert and L. Lemieux (eds.), *EEG–fMRI*
DOI: 10.1007/978-3-540-87919-0_25, © Springer Verlag Berlin Heidelberg 2010

underlying neuronal activity and its dynamics? This chapter focuses on the alternative approaches to integrating EEG and fMRI information, from a biophysical modelling and signal analysis perspective. We have tried to represent state-of-the-art knowledge and know-how in this important neuroimaging challenge. We will identify promising research directions in EEG–fMRI fusion and the sorts of scientific questions that this approach can address.

2
EEG–fMRI Information Fusion: Limitations

Observed mismatches between EEG and fMRI can be interpreted as: (a) a *decoupling* between the electrophysiological and the haemodynamic activity or (b) a signal detection failure (i.e. false-positive/negative results). This distinction is important, because decoupling itself might be very informative. For example, in clinical applications (e.g. neuroimaging investigations of epilepsy), evidence for a decoupling between electrophysiological and metabolic activity might be a feature of the pathology itself. The question is whether one can reliably distinguish between a neurovascular decoupling and a signal detection failure. In the following, we will try to list the potential physiological and experimental confounds that constitute the main limitations of any EEG–fMRI information fusion procedure.

2.1
Neurovascular Coupling and Decoupling

Despite the increasing amount of literature in the field of neurovascular coupling (see, for a recent example, Riera et al. 2006), none of the existing biophysical models specify precisely what is meant by "neural activity" that drives haemodynamic responses. Therefore, these models cannot tell us what aspect of neural information processing is reflected in the BOLD signal. Neural information processing within a cortical unit can be described in many different ways, and its relationship to neurophysiological processes can be characterised on different scales; for example, local field potentials versus spiking activity, excitatory versus inhibitory postsynaptic potentials, or different types of receptor activation (Stephan et al. 2004).

Sophisticated animal studies that combine invasive multielectrode recordings with fMRI (Puce et al. 1997; Logothetis et al. 2001, 2004; Jones et al. 2004; Patel et al. 2004, 2005; Shmuel et al. 2006; Ureshi et al. 2004) or with optical imaging techniques (Mathiesen et al. 1998; Martindale et al. 2003) have started to address these issues. A significant correlation between the time courses of haemodynamic and electrophysiological signals has been established by these studies. These encouraging results, at the mesoscopic scale, confirm what had already been suggested by noninvasive studies at the macroscopic scale; the latter essentially comparing locations of EEG and fMRI sources for a given subject and task. For example, these studies have shown a good concordance for primary sensorimotor (Korjenova et al. 1999) and visual (Mangun et al. 1998) sources. Similar conclusions emerge when using more complex cognitive tasks; e.g. the motor response to visual stimulation (Kawakami et al. 2002), decision-making tasks (Thees et al. 2003) and face perception (Horovitz et al. 2004). However, a similar number of studies have shown significant differences between the regions implicated by EEG and in fMRI, respectively. Gonzales (2001) list many of these case reports (mostly involving sensorimotor and auditory cortices), as well as ambiguous multimodal identifications of epileptogenic foci (see also Laufs et al. 2008). Using a bilateral auditory stimulation with ten subjects, Stippich et al. (1998) found an average distance of 14 mm between the MEG dipole and the centre of the fMRI activation.

In brief, the principal limitations on multimodal EEG–fMRI integration are imposed by physiology. One reason why EEG and fMRI sources may be dislocated is the distance between the neuronal population whose electrical activity is generating the EEG signal and the vascular tree, which provides the blood supply to these neurons, since BOLD signal changes are essentially haemodynamic (Beisteiner et al. 1997). Similarly, in addition to pre- and postsynaptic electrochemical dynamics, a number of physiological processes also require energetic support; for example, neurotransmitter synthesis (Patel et al. 2004), glial cell metabolism (Lauritzen 2005), maintenance of the steady-state transmembrane potential (Kida et al. 2001), etc. These phenomena may cause haemodynamic BOLD changes without EEG correlates (Arthurs and Boniface 2003). This differential sensitivity to neuronal activity and energetics can also arise whenever haemodynamic activity is caused by unsynchronised electrophysiological activity, or if the latter has a closed source configuration that is invisible to EEG. Conversely, if the electrophysiological activity is transient, it might not induce any significant (i.e. detectable) metabolic activity changes (Nunez and Silberstein 2000).

2.2
Experimental Limitations

Another important potential source of bias in EEG–fMRI fusion is experimental variability. In some situations, it might be necessary to acquire the EEG and fMRI data in separate sessions. In this case, habituation effects, variations in the stimulation paradigm, or any other difference between sessions may lead to differential activity of neural networks (Gonzales 2001; Rosen et al. 1998; Wagner et al. 2001).

Simultaneous EEG–fMRI acquisition techniques have been developed specifically to address these issues[1]. Nevertheless, and despite advances in simultaneous EEG–fMRI hardware and software, the signal-to-noise ratio (SNR) of these signals is still significantly lower than the corresponding unimodal paradigms (but see Liston et al. 2006). This is mainly due to reciprocal electromagnetic perturbations (Kruggel et al. 2000; Krakow 2000). For the EEG signal, this SNR degradation can be catastrophic: the most important artefacts in the raw data can completely mask the signal of interest. These are due to a complex combination of factors, including the MR field strength (and thus frequency) and the orientation/positioning of the EEG recording equipment relative to the RF coil and the

---

[1]This technical challenge has been largely pioneered by neuroimaging groups focussing on pharmacoresistant epilepsy (Ives et al. 1993; Warach et al. 1996; Lemieux 2001).

MR gradients. All of these unavoidable artefacts manifest themselves as induced voltages that add linearly to the EEG signal and obscure the biological signal of interest; see the chapters "EEG Instrumentation and Safety", "EEG Quality: Origin and Reduction of the EEG Cardiac-Related Artefact" and "EEG Quality: The Image Acquisition Artefact". Although denoising algorithms have been reasonably successful in gradient artefact correction (Allen et al. 2000; Garreffa et al. 2003), the pulse-related artefact remains a challenge (Nakamura et al. 2006; Ellingson et al. 2004), as described in the chapter "EEG Quality: Origin and Reduction of the EEG Cardiac-Related Artefact".

3
EEG–fMRI Information Fusion: Solutions

Since the main potential limitations of EEG–fMRI information fusion are well established, many data analysts have argued that dedicated modelling and signal processing tools should be used to combine the advantages of EEG and fMRI (Dale and Halgren 2001; Hallett 2002; Mulert et al. 2004; Liu et al. 2006).

3.1
Information Fusion: Definition

Reconstructing the spatial deployment of current density from EEG measurements is an intrinsically ill-posed problem. On the other hand, estimating neuronal activity from the haemodynamic response is a difficult temporal deconvolution problem. Critically, the dual fitting of the bioelectric and haemodynamic responses does not necessarily circumvent the difficulties of the inverse problems that attend each modality. So what exactly *do* we expect to gain from EEG–fMRI information fusion? What does "information fusion" mean? The *Collins Concise Dictionary* gives the following definitions: "information: knowledge acquired through experience or study" and "fusion: the act or process of fusion or melting together". Although we may be able to reconcile these two notions, intuitions about information fusion can be finessed using psychoacoustics[2] and the link between "consonance" and "auditory sensation of fusion".

In music, a consonance (Latin *consonare*, "sounding together") is a harmony, chord or interval that is considered stable, as opposed to a dissonance, which is considered unstable. The strict definition of consonance may relate to sounds that are pleasant, while the more general definition includes any sounds that are used freely. An example of perfect consonance is the octave interval. The correlation between consonance and fusion has been known since the mid-nineteenth century: the more the interval is consonant, the more we tend to perceive only one sound; the more the interval is dissonant, the more we can tease apart the different sounds that comprise the chord.

---

[2]Psychoacoustics is the study of auditory sensations as a psychophysical response to some acoustic attributes of a sound.

This characteristic is an essential aspect of information fusion procedures, which rely on the coherence of information, in the context of uncertainty. In other words, optimal information fusion should be framed in information-theoretic terms. Bayesian inference furnishes a probabilistic framework that allows one to formalise the propagation of both information and uncertainty from observations (the data) to unknown causes. This framework requires a so-called *generative model* (or forward model) that specifies the (possibly uncertain) relationships between the data and what caused them. In this context, data analysis entails specifying an appropriate model, with a set of unknown parameters, and then looking for parameter distributions that explain the data. This is called *model inversion* and involves extracting information from data by quantifying the uncertainty associated with a model of the system generating data. If the model can generate multimodal data, its inversion corresponds to fusion. Not all approaches to multimodal integration rely on a multimodal generative model. In what follows, we will reserve the term fusion for inference on multimodal models and their parameters. Because the inversion depends bilaterally on multimodal data, fusion is inherently symmetric. However, there are other (asymmetric) approaches, where one modality is treated as a cause or predictor of the other. We now consider the distinction between symmetrical and asymmetrical procedures.

3.2
Asymmetrical vs. Symmetrical Approaches

As noted above, the quantitative contribution of neurophysiological processes in "active" areas to electromagnetic and haemodynamic signals is largely unknown (Gonzales et al. 2001; Stefan et al. 2004; Daunizeau et al. 2005). Nevertheless, one can define "neuronal activity" operationally as the state of nodes in a network responding to specific events (e.g., cognitive, sensorimotor or spontaneous changes in brain activity) (Friston 2005b). This allows one to consider event-related (ER) EEG and fMRI data as measures of "neuronal activity", since the ER response is a reproducible EEG or fMRI signature that can be elicited systematically (Friston 2005a). However, electromagnetic and metabolic responses, as detected by EEG and fMRI, are not necessarily caused by the same underlying neuronal processes.

"Neuronal activity" ζ can be decomposed into two overlapping subspaces, ζ_{EEG} and ζ_{fMRI}, that correspond to the parts of ζ that contribute to EEG and fMRI signals, respectively (Pieger and Greenblatt 2001). The intersection ζ_1 (see Fig. 1) defines a "common substrate" of neuronal activity. Conversely, ζ_2 (ζ_3) denotes the subspace of neuronal activity detected by EEG (fMRI) that does not contribute to fMRI (EEG) measurements. This decomposition formalises the apparent coupling–uncoupling between bioelectrical and haemodynamic responses.

What should we expect to learn about neuronal activity by combining EEG and fMRI? Since no information about ζ_2 (ζ_3) is available from the fMRI (EEG), no multimodal procedure will provide a better characterisation of this activity subspace than a unimodal EEG (fMRI) analysis. However, a multimodal approach should benefit from the complementary nature of EEG and fMRI by providing different perspectives on the common subspace, ζ_1.

During the past decade, many reports have focused on analytical techniques devoted to EEG–fMRI integration. Here we classify them as (i) asymmetrical EEG to fMRI

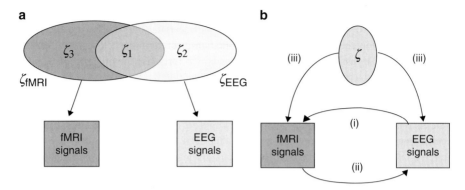

Fig. 1a–b Formalisation of the EEG–fMRI coupling–uncoupling (**a**) and EEG–fMRI fusion approaches (**b**) (adapted from Daunizeau et al. 2007 and Kilner et al. 2005). Any multimodal information fusion approach will be beneficial for inferring common neuronal states, ζ_1. This means that asymmetrical EEG–fMRI approaches systematically bias their estimate of ζ_1 by introducing information from ζ_{EEG} [(*i*): EEG to fMRI approaches, i.e. integration through prediction] or ζ_{fMRI} [(*ii*): fMRI to EEG approaches, i.e. integration through constraints]. In contrast, symmetrical EEG–fMRI fusion approaches rely on a joint EEG–fMRI generative model, which allows the estimation of ζ_1 to be derived from an optimal balance between EEG- and fMRI-derived information [(*iii*): integration through forward models]

approaches, (ii) asymmetrical fMRI to EEG approaches, and (iii) symmetrical fusion approaches (see Fig. 1).

3.3
EEG to fMRI Approaches

The objective of these techniques is to localise, using fMRI, brain regions whose response is temporally correlated with a given EEG-defined event or feature. In other words, temporal information from the EEG signal is used as a constraint or predictor variable in the fMRI time-series model. This type of EEG–fMRI integration is necessarily implemented within a simultaneous EEG–fMRI acquisition paradigm.

This pioneering work has been pursued largely by functional imaging groups focussing on presurgical planning for pharmacoresistant epilepsy (Warrach et al. 1996; Lazeyras et al. 2000; Krakow et al. 2001; Lemieux et al. 2001; Boor et al. 2003; Archer and Briellmann 2003; Salek-Haddadi 2003; Asmi et al. 2003; Aghakani et al. 2004; Grova et al. 2008); see the chapter "EEG–fMRI in Adults with Focal Epilepsy" for an overview. After artefact correction, the epileptiform activity is identified by an expert on the EEG traces. These events are then convolved with a haemodynamic response function (HRF), and used as a regressor in standard GLM analysis (Lemieux 2001; Bagshaw et al. 2005); as described in the chapter "Experimental Design and Data Analysis Strategies".

Other EEG to fMRI asymmetrical approaches have investigated the neuronal correlates of spontaneous cerebral activity occurring when the subject is not exposed to any extrinsic stimulation or pathological activity (i.e., at "rest", hence term "default mode" network; see e.g.

Gotman et al. 2005; Lauf et al. 2003). After simultaneous EEG–fMRI acquisition, spontaneous fluctuations of power in specific frequency bands are quantified in the EEG traces. Time-dependent power in each of these frequency bands is used to form a regressor in the GLM of fMRI. This type of exploratory analysis tends to confirm observations made using invasive recordings looking at frequency-dependent correlates in fMRI (Luck 2000; Benar et al. 2002; Bagshaw et al. 2004). Some multivariate extensions of this type of approach have also been proposed. Essentially, these techniques try to find a linear decomposition of fMRI data that co-varies with a time-frequency decomposition of the EEG (Martinez-Montes 2004; Moosmann et al. 2008).

3.4
fMRI to EEG Approaches

The aim of these techniques is to finesse the study of fast dynamics of neuronal activity as measured by EEG by using fMRI-derived spatial priors in the EEG source reconstruction problem. Again, this has been the subject of many reports in the past decade. The conceptual framework that dominates in this field rests on functional integration or coupling among sources (Lin et al. 2004; Liu et al. 2006). Going beyond functional specialisation (Friston et al. 1996), evoked responses are understood as arising in an interacting network of connected "nodes" (the localised regions); these interactions are referred to as "arcs" or "edges" in graph theory. Interactions are expressed in the temporal dynamics of neuronal activity, since they shape the influence of one neuronal population on another. It is thought that characterising these connections requires the use of EEG, since this is the only neuroimaging modality whose temporal resolution is similar to that of the underlying neuronal processes. However, the EEG spatial inverse problem induces uncertainty about the number and deployment of nodes in the network, which is why fMRI constraints are potentially useful.

This approach can be divided into two classes, associated with the EEG source model employed: (a) the equivalent current dipole (ECD) model (Kiebel et al. 2008) and (b) the distributed source model (Friston et al. 2008). Dipolar fMRI to EEG approaches simply associate each fMRI focus with an ECD, whose position lies a priori at the centre of the activation (Wagner et al. 2001). This type of a priori constraint is *hard*, in the sense that the results of the fMRI analysis are not questioned (e.g. the number of active regions). In addition, since the ECD model does not accommodate the spatial extent of underlying active regions, it is difficult to assess the relevance of the fMRI constraint (Liu 2006). For example, it has been shown that many ECDs are required to model spatially extended regions correctly (Shiraishi et al. 2005).

Distributed fMRI to EEG approaches rely on "weighted regularisation techniques". In these techniques, the model uses the fMRI activation as a prior on the spatial profile of cortically distributed sources. As a consequence, the estimation penalises sources whose fMRI-derived activation probability is low. This approach has been shown to estimate the position and extent of underlying sources robustly whenever the fMRI-derived constraints are valid (Ahlfors 2004). However, when some sort of decoupling occurs, the EEG source reconstruction is strongly biased, which is why many variants of the fMRI penalty term have been proposed (Liu et al. 1998; Babiloni et al. 2003; Halchenko et al. 2005). Furthermore, these techniques require the tuning of a "hyperparameter" that regulates the weight of the penalty term in relation to accuracy or model fit. This hyperparameter is critical because it determines the balance between the effects of the fMRI prior and the EEG data on the estimation. Therefore, some authors (Mattout et al. 2006; Daunizeau et al. 2005) have proposed principled Bayesian techniques for optimising standard regularisation procedures by estimating this hyperparameter from the EEG data. Finally, the plausibility of the inverse reconstruction should depend on the relevance of the prior information. However, given solutions constrained or unconstrained by fMRI, which should be chosen? In Daunizeau et al. (2005), we proposed a Bayesian model comparison method to decide whether one should use the fMRI constraint or not. This approach has been applied successfully to clinical epilepsy data (Grova et al. 2008).

3.5
Towards Symmetrical EEG–fMRI Approaches

As noted above, divergences between the anatomical localisation obtained by functional techniques and those obtained from electrocortical stimulations are not infrequent. This has insidious consequences for asymmetrical EEG–fMRI approaches, since the relative importance of EEG and fMRI is not evaluated. For instance, in Dale and Liu (2000), the authors recognised that when fMRI was considered the "truth" for spatial information, serious biases could occur in fMRI-regularised EEG source reconstruction when the actual electrophysiological activity did not induce significant variations in the BOLD signal. Therefore, it has been observed that the "integration of functional modalities into the solution of the neuroelectromagnetic inverse problem should be cautiously considered until a tighter coupling between BOLD effects and electrophysiological measurements could be established" (Gonzales-Andino et al. 2001).

Given this, an outstanding modelling effort has focussed on designing forward models of neurovascular coupling that are neurophysiologically grounded. This has been done for the healthy brain (Shulman and Hyder 2001; Attwell et al. 2002; Aubert et al. 2005; Lauritzen 2005; Riera et al. 2006, 2007; Babajani 2006; Sotero and Trujillo 2007; Sotero and Trujillo-Barreto 2007) and in the context of neurological pathology (see e.g. Iadecola 2004; Lu et al. 2004). Despite the lack of established neurovascular coupling models, the main link between electrophysiological activity and energy consumption is invariably modelled through glucose metabolism. This assumes a monotonic mapping between excitatory activity and energy budget, and thus the BOLD signal (through blood flow). The last part of this metabolic-haemodynamic cascade (i.e. the mesoscopic relationship between blood flow and measured BOLD signal) is relatively well established, and forms the basis of the "balloon model" (see Buxton et al. 1998 for seminal work, and Friston et al. 2000 for its extension).

Despite these advances, three major issues regarding the neurovascular coupling at the level of the mapping between energy budget and blood flow changes remain unresolved: (a) some authors emphasise the potentially important role of interplay between neuronal and glial metabolisms in neurovascular coupling–decoupling (see e.g. Pellerin and Magistretti 1994; Aubert et al. 2005); (b) whether or not the energy consumption drives cerebral blood flow directly or is flow modulated by independent fast neurotransmitters (Attwell et al.

2002; Riera et al. 2006); (c) so far, the quantitative contribution of inhibitory neuronal activity to energy consumption remains unclear (Kida et al. 2001; Chatton et al. 2003; Sotero and Trujillo-Barreto 2007); (d) the contribution of physiological noise to the variability of induced electroencephalographic and haemodynamic responses may have been overlooked (Kruger and Glover 2001; Buckner and Vincent 2007; Fukunaga et al. 2008).

Figure 2 summarises the key components of a neurophysiologically and biophysically grounded generative model of both EEG and fMRI data, considering state-of-the-art modelling on both the anatomofunctional and the neurovascular coupling. This model would ideally involve many levels of description, including (a) the macroscale, i.e., the

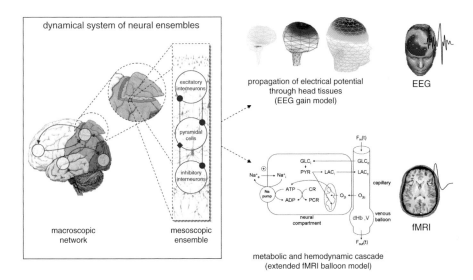

Fig. 2 Integrative EEG–fMRI symmetrical fusion. Recent advances in understanding physiological mechanisms at different spatiotemporal scales have provided a framework within which sophisticated biophysical models for integrating different imaging modalities can be developed. More precisely, evolution and observation equations encoding the relationship between bioelectric and haemodynamic mesostates can be developed based on both physiological and physical evidence. An increasing amount of experimental evidence shows that the dynamical behaviour of a source depends on both its intrinsic and extrinsic connectivity. Dynamic causal models (Friston et al. 2003) based on neural mass models may be an appropriate framework for models of bioelectric and metabolic activity in neural populations (Kiebel et al. 2008). In this sort of model, the EEG scalp data is assumed to be an instantaneous measure of the electrical potential generated by the activity of a subpopulation or neural mass (e.g., pyramidal cells), which has been propagated through the head tissues (Baillet et al. 2001). On the other hand, the fMRI data are modelled as a temporally smoothed response to mostly presynaptic neuronal activity (Logothetis et al. 2001) that results from a slow cascade of metabolic–haemodynamic events (Aubert et al. 2005, Friston et al. 2000, Riera et al. 2006). A first step towards such an integrated EEG–fMRI generative model was proposed by Sotero and Trujillo-Barreto (2007). This biophysically informed model couples neuronal activity, cerebral metabolic rates of glucose and oxygen consumption, and finally cerebral blood flow in order to predict both electroencephalographic and BOLD responses. Inversion of these integrative dynamic causal models for EEG and fMRI may provide us with the key insights into the genesis of neuronal activity and how it is mediated by intrinsic-extrinsic connections

relationship among active brain regions, shaping the dynamics of local (mesoscale) neuronal populations (Friston et al. 2003); (b) the mesoscale, i.e., the interplay of local excitatory and inhibitory neuronal populations (see e.g. Kiebel et al. 2008); and (c) the microscale, where neurovascular coupling is mediated through cellular mechanisms (see e.g. Riera et al. 2006).

Until such a model and its associated inversion are available, the objectives of any symmetric fusion of multimodal EEG–fMRI information should be twofold. First, the approach should be able to identify the parts of EEG and fMRI signals that convey complementary information about the common substrate underlying these signals (i.e. ζ_1 in Fig. 1). Second, it should exploit such information to decrease uncertainty when inferring on this common subspace. As a consequence, a symmetrical fusion approach requires the explicit definition of the common neuronal states that engenders both EEG and fMRI measurements. This entails building a model that encompasses our knowledge about the link between bioelectrical and haemodynamic activities and being able to invert that model, given the joint EEG–fMRI data. In practice, very few fusion approaches (i.e. data analysis techniques) have relied on realistic neurophysiological models (see e.g. Riera et al. 2006). This is because the complexity of real metabolic–haemodynamic cascades renders the estimation of their parameters an intractable problem (see discussion in Sotero and Trujillo-Barreto 2007).

In contrast, other researchers have relied on simplified variants of the neurovascular coupling model by restricting its parameters to model some common properties exhibited by "active" areas contributing to both event-related EEG and fMRI measurements. For example, Kilner et al. (2005) recently applied dimensional analysis to relate haemodynamic changes (as monotonically mapped from rates of energy dissipation) to the spectral profile of EEG activity. The analysis suggests that increases in BOLD signal should be associated with a shift in the EEG spectral profile to higher frequencies. The predictions of this phenomenological model have been partially experimentally verified in a single-subject case study (Laufs et al. 2006), but have not been included in any symmetrical EEG–fMRI fusion approach so far. As another example, in Daunizeau et al. (2007), the authors restricted common parameters to the spatial profile (i.e. the position and extent) of the EEG and fMRI sources. In other words, the only parameters affecting both bioelectrical and haemodynamic responses were those defining the spatial support of the signal generators. Despite its somewhat heuristic aspect, this fusion approach is not confounded by the lack of detailed information about neurovascular coupling (see Fig. 3). Other approaches have simply included the balloon model itself as a surrogate for the neurovascular coupling (Trujillo 2004; Deneux et al. 2006), but have not, so far, included any estimation of the haemodynamic parameters.

These techniques, any of which can be framed in Bayesian terms, represent the first attempts to bridge the gap between EEG and fMRI signals in a symmetrical, physiologically rigorous and optimum way. No doubt the next decade will bring increasingly sophisticated models and inversion methods that will extend the validity and accuracy of EEG–fMRI information fusion (see Fig. 3).

However, any EEG–fMRI fusion procedure that is necessarily "model based" will suffer from the usual limitation of modelling: refutability. Whether the assumptions of the model are satisfied or not in a given experimental context will remain a question in itself. There is a subtle balance between the plausibility of the assumptions and the efficiency of

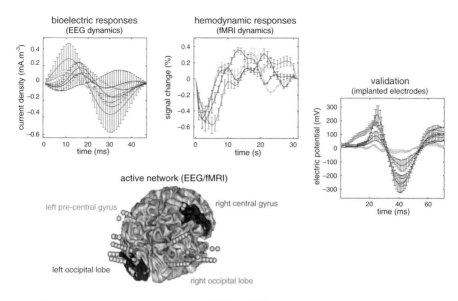

Fig. 3   Bayesian spatiotemporal event-related EEG–fMRI fusion approach (adapted from Daunizeau et al. 2007). Symmetrical multimodal EEG–fMRI information fusion has been applied to the analysis of event-related bioelectric and haemodynamic responses. In this work, the spatial profile of EEG–fMRI sources was introduced as an unknown hierarchical prior on cerebral activity. A bespoke variational Bayesian (VB) learning scheme is derived in order to infer sources from a joint EEG–fMRI dataset. This yields an estimate of the common spatial profile, which embodies a trade-off between information harvested from the EEG and fMRI data. Furthermore, the spatial structure of the EEG–fMRI coupling–uncoupling is elucidated from the data. The figure shows (*left*) the application of the fusion approach to EEG–fMRI recordings from a patient with epilepsy in order to identify areas involved in the generation of epileptic spikes, and (*right*) intracranial EEG data. In all graphics, the colour code is as follows: *green*, right occipital region; *blue*, left occipital region; *red*, right postcentral gyrus; *turquoise*, left postcentral gyrus. Both the measured intracranial EEG and estimated cortical sources seem to exhibit a similar temporal response: the epileptiform activity starts in the right occipital region and spreads to left occipital and right postcentral regions, the latter being temporally coherent. In contrast, the estimated haemodynamic responses did not conform to the same chronology. Since haemodynamic responses are driven partly by biophysical processes that are independent of the underlying neuronal activity (e.g. glial cell processes), one might be inclined to favour EEG-related analysis in any inference regarding causal relations within the active network

any model to make precise inferences. The tighter the prior belief regarding the underlying causes of our observations, the more precise our interpretations of the data. However, these inferences become increasingly constrained by our priors and indeed the space of models examined. Therefore, theoretical neurobiology, experimental evidence and dedicated statistical data analysis may have to make significant progress before any robust information fusion technique is adopted by the neuroimaging community (see Wan et al. 2006 and Riera et al. 2007 for the most recent insights from complementary invasive recordings and sophisticated metabolic modelling).

4
Conclusion

We have reviewed the advances and issues relating to EEG–fMRI information fusion. We have emphasised the importance of neurovascular coupling for generative models, which are the key to any balanced fusion procedure. This issue underlies many of the challenges to fusion, and has been a source of much debate: "it is far from trivial to suppose, for instance, that a statistically significant Z-score in the left inferior frontal gyrus and a large left anterior negativity at 200 ms after stimulus presentation correspond to the same thing" (Horwitz and Poepple 2002). In this chapter, we tried to identify those features of cerebral activity that could form the basis of models of electromagnetic and haemodynamic markers of neuronal activity and are required for EEG–fMRI multimodal fusion. We have emphasised the importance of developing statistical methods for model inversion, given EEG and fMRI signals.

Finally, gathering the knowledge and know-how necessary for EEG–fMRI fusion has proven to be a challenging exercise for the neuroimaging community. However, very few rational criticisms have questioned the intrinsic motivation of EEG–fMRI fusion. In short: what is the type of scientific question (apart from established diagnostic applications, e.g. epilepsy) that really requires EEG–fMRI fusion? This potentially controversial question must be addressed before we can finesse our scientific strategy in this challenging area.

Acknowledgements The Wellcome Trust and a Marie Curie Fellowship to Dr. Daunizeau funded this work.

References

Aghakani Y, Bagshaw A, et al. (2004) fMRI activation during spike and wave discharges in idiopathic generalized epilepsy. Brain 127:1127–1144

Ahlfors, SP, and Simpson GU, Geometrical interpretation of fMRI-guided MEG/EEG. Neuroimage, 22:323–332, 2004

Allen PJ, Josephs O, et al. (2000) A method for removing imaging artefact form continuous EEG recorded during functional MRI. Neuroimage 12:230–239

Archer JS, Briellmann RS (2003) Spike-triggered fMRI in reading epilepsy. Neurology 60:79–93

Arthurs OJ, Boniface SJ (2003) What aspect of the fMRI BOLD signal best reflects the underlying electrophysiology in humans somatosensory cortex? Clin Neurophysiol 114:1203–1209

Asmi A, Benar CG, et al. (2003) MRI activation in continuous and spike-triggered EEG–fMRI studies of epileptic spikes. Epilepsia 44:1328–1339

Attwell D, Iadecola C, et al. (2002) The neural basis of functional brain imaging signals. Trends Neurosci 25:621–625

Aubert A, Costalat R, et al. (2005) Interactions between astrocytes and neurons studied using a mathematical model of compartmentalized energy metabolism. J Cereb Blood Flow Metab 12:23–41

Babajani A, Soltanian-Zadeh H (2006) Integrated MEG/EEG and fMRI model based in neural masses. IEEE Trans Biomed Eng 53:1794–1801

Babiloni F., Babiloni C., Carduci F., Romani G. L., Rossini P. M., Angelone L., and Cincotti F. Multimodal integration of high-resolution EEG and functional magnetic resonance imaging data: a simulation study. Neuroimage, 19:1–15, 2003

Bagshaw A, Aghakhani Y, et al. (2004) EEG–fMRI of focal epileptic spikes: analysis with multiple hemodynamic functions and comparison with gadolinium-enhanced MR angiograms. Hum Brain Mapp 22:179–192

Bagshaw A, Hawco AP, et al. (2005) Analysis of the EEG–fMRI response to prolonged bursts of interictal epileptiform activity. Neuroimage 24:1099–1112

Baillet S, Leahy RM, et al. (2001) Supplementary motor area activation preceding voluntary finger movements as evidenced by magnetoencephalography and fMRI. IJBEM 3:1

Beisteiner R, Erdler M, et al. (1997) Magnetoencephalography may help improve function MRI brain mapping. Eur J Neurosci 9:1072–1077

Benar CG, Aghakhani Y, et al. (2002) The BOLD response to interictal epileptiform discharges. Neuroimage 17:1182–1192

Boor S, Vucurevic G, et al. (2003) EEG-related functional MRI in benign childhood epilepsy with centrotemporal spike. Epilepsia 44:688–692

Buckner RL, Vincent JL (2007) Unrest at rest: default activity and spontaneous network correlations. Neuroimage 37:1091–1096

Buxton RB, Wong EC, Frank LR (1998) Dynamics of blood flow and oxygenation changes during brain activation: the balloon model. MRM 39:855–864

Chatton JY, Pellerin L, et al. (2003) GABA uptake into astrocytes is not associated with significant metabolic cost: implications for brain imaging of inhibitory transmissions. Proc Natl Acad Sci USA 100:12456–12461

Dale AM, Halgren E (2001) Spatiotemporal mapping of brain activity by integration of multiple imaging modalities. Curr Opin Neurobiol 11:202–208

Dale AM, Liu AM (2000) Dynamic statistical parametric mapping: combining fMRI and MEG for high-resolution imaging of cortical activity. Neuron 26:55–67

Daunizeau J, Grova C, et al. (2005) Assessing the relevance of fMRI-based prior in the EEG inverse problem: a Bayesian model comparison approach. IEEE Trans Sign Process 53:3461–3472

Daunizeau J, Grova C, et al. (2007) Symmetrical event-related EEG–fMRI information fusion in a variational Bayesian framework. Neuroimage 3:69–87

Deneux T, Faugeras O, et al. (2006) EEG–fMRI fusion of non-triggered data using Kalman filtering. In: Third IEEE Int Symp On Biomed Imag (ISBI), Arlington, VA, USA, 6–9 April 2006, pp 1068–1071

Ellingson ML, Liebenthal E, et al. (2004) Ballistocardiogram artefact reduction in the simultaneous acquisition of auditory ERPS and fMRI. Neuroimage 22:1534–1542

Fukunaga M, Horovitz SG, et al. (2008) Metabolic origin of BOLD signal fluctuations in the absence of stimuli. J Cereb Blood Flow Metab 28:1377–1387

Friston KJ (2005a) Models of brain function in neuroimaging. Annu Rev Psychol 56:57–87

Friston KJ (2005b) A theory of cortical responses. Phil Trans Roy Soc 360:815–836

Friston KJ, Price CJ, et al. (1996) The trouble with cognitive subtraction. Neuroimage 4:97–104

Friston KJ, Mechelli A, Turner R, Price CJ (2000) Nonlinear responses in fMRI: the balloon model, Volterra kernels and other hemodynamics. Neuroimage 12:466–477

Friston KJ, Harrison L, et al. (2003) Dynamic causal modelling. Neuroimage 12:466–477

Friston KJ, Harrison LM, et al. (2008) Multiple sparse priors for the M/EEG inverse problem. Neuroimage 39:1104–1120

Garreffa G, Carni M, et al. (2003) Real-time artefact filtering during continuous EEG–fMRI acquisition. Magn Reson Imag 21:1175–1189

Gonzales-Andino ASL, Blanke O, et al. (2001) The use of functional constraints for the neuromagnetic inverse problem: alternatives and caveats. Int J Bioelectromag 3:103–114

Gotman J, Grova C, et al. (2005) Generalized epileptic discharges show thalamocortical activation and suspension of the default state of the brain. Proc Natl Acad Sci USA 102:15236–15240

Grova C, Daunizeau J, et al. (2008) Assessing the concordance between distributed EEG source localization and simultaneous EEG–fMRI studies of epileptic spikes. Neuroimage 39:755–774

Halchenko YO, Hanson SJ, et al. (2005) Multimodal integration: fMRI, MRI, EE, MEG. In: Landini L, Santarelli MF, Posatino V (eds) Advanced image processing in magnetic resonance maging. Marcel Dekker, New York

Hallett M (2002) Multimodality brain imaging. Int Cong Ser 1226:17–26

Horovitz SG, Rossion B, et al. (2004) Parametric design and correlational analyses help integrating fMRI and electrophysiological data during face processing. Neuroimage 22:1587–1595

Horwitz B, Poeppel D (2002) How can EEG/MEG and fMRI/PET data be combined? Hum Brain Mapp 17:1–3

Iadecola C (2004) Neurovascular regulation in the normal brain and in Alzheimer's disease. Nat Rev Neurosci 5:347–360

Ives JR, Warach S, Schmitt F, Edelman RR, Schomer DL (1993) Monitoring the patient's EEG during echo planar MRI. Electroenceph Clin Neurophysiol 87:417–420

Kida I, Hyder F, et al. (2001) Inhibition of voltage-dependent sodium channels suppresses the functional magnetic resonance imaging response to forepaw somatosensory activation in rodent. J Cereb Blood Metab 21:585–591

Jones M, Hewston-Stoate N, et al. (2004) Nonlinear coupling of neural activity and CBF in rodent barrel cortex. Neuroimage 22:956–965

Kawakami O, Kanaoke Y, et al. (2002) Visual detection of motion speed in humans: spatiotemporal analysis by fMRI and MEG. Hum Brain Mapp 16:104–118

Kiebel SJ, Garrido M, et al. (2007) Dynamic causal modelling of evoked responses: the role of intrinsic connections. Neuroimage 36:332–345

Kilner KM, Mattout J, Henson R, Friston KJ (2005) Hemodynamic correlates of EEG: a heuristic. Neuroimage 28:280–286

Korjenova A, Huttunen J, et al. (1999) Activation of multiple cortical areas in response to somatosensory stimulation: combined magnetoencephalography and function magnetic resonance imaging. Hum Brain Mapp 10:10–15

Krakow K, Allen PJ, et al. (2001) EEG recordings during fMRI experiments: image quality. Hum Brain Mapp 10:10–15

Krakow K, Allen PJ, Lemieux L, Symms MR, Fish DR (2000) Methodology: EEG-correlated fMRI. Adv Neurol 83:187–201

Kruggel F, Wiggins CJ, et al. (2000) Recording of the event-related potentials during functional MRI at 3.0 Tesla field strength. Magn Reson Med 44:277–282

Kruger G, Glover GH (2001) Physiological noise in oxygenation-sensitive magnetic resonance imaging. Magn Res Med 46:631–637

Laufs H, Krakow K, et al. (2003) Electroencephalographic signatures of attentional and cognitive default modes in spontaneous brain activity fluctuations at rest. Proc Natl Acad Sci USA 100: 11053–11068

Laufs H, Holt JL, Elfront R, Krams M, Paul JS, Krakow K, Kleinschmidt A (2006) Where does the BOLD signal goes when alpha EEG leaves. Neuroimage 31:1408–1418

Laufs H, Daunizeau J, et al. (2008) Recent advances in recording electrophysiological data simultaneously with magnetic resonance imaging. Neuroimage 40:515–528

Lazeyras F, Blanke F, et al. (2000) EEG-triggered functional MRI in patients with pharmacoresistant epilepsy. J Magn Reson Imaging 12 177–185

Lauritzen M (2005) Reading vascular changes in brain imaging: is dendritic calcium the key? Nat Rev Neurosci 6:77–85

Lemieux L, Krakow K, Fish DR (2001) Comparison of spike-triggered functional MRI BOLD activation and EEG dipole model localization. Neuroimage 5:1097–1104

Liu AK, Belliveau JW, and Dale AM. Spatiotemporal imaging of human brain activity using functional MRI constrained magnetoencephalographic data: Monte Carlo simulations. Proc. Natl. Acad. Sci. USA, 95:8945–8950, 1998

Liu Z, Ding L, et al. (2006) Integration of EEG/MEG with MRI and fMRI in functional neuroimaging. IEEE Eng Med Biol Mag 25:46–53

Lin F, Witzel T, et al. (2004) Spectral spatiotemporal imaging of cortical oscillations and interactions in the human brain. Neuroimage 23:582–595

Liston AD, Lund TE, et al. (2006) Modelling cardiac signal as a confound in EEG–fMRI and its application in focal epilepsy studies. Neuroimage 30:827–834

Logothetis NK, Wandell BA (2004) Interpreting the BOLD signal. Annu Rev Physiol 66:8945–8950

Logothetis NK, Pauls J, et al. (2001) Neurophysiological investigation of the basis of the fMRI signal. Nature 412:150–157

Lu H, Golay X, et al. (2004) Sustained poststimulus elevation in cerebral oxygen utilization after vascular recovery. J Cereb Blood Flow Metab 24:764–770

Luck SJ (2000) Direct and indirect integration of event-related potentials, functional magnetic resonance images, and single-unit recordings. Hum Brain Mapp 8:115–201

Martindale J, Matthew J, et al. (2003) The hemodynamic impulse response to a single neuronal event. J Cereb Blood Flow Metab 23:546–566

Martinez-Montes E, Valdes-Sosa PA, Miwakeichi F, Goldman RI, Cohen MS, 2004. Concurrent EEG/fMRI analysis by multiway partial least squares. Neuroimage 22 (3), 1023–1034

Mathiesen C, Caesar K, et al. (1998) Modification of activity-dependent increases of cerebral blood flow by excitatory synaptic activity and spikes in rat cerebellar cortex. J Physiol 512:555–566

Mattout J, Phillips C, et al. (2006) MEG source localization under multiple constraints: an extended Bayesian framework. Neuroimage 30:753–767

Mangun GR, Buonocore MH, et al. (1998) ERP and fMRI measures of visual spatial selective attention. Hum Brain Mapp 6:383–389

Moosmann M, Eichele T, et al. (2008) Joint independent component analysis for simultaneous EEG–fMRI: principle and simulation. Int J Psychophysiol 67:212–221

Mukamel R, Gelbard H, et al. (2005) Coupling between neuronal firing, field potentials, and fMRI in human auditory cortex. Science 5:951–954

Mulert C, Jager L, et al. (2004) Integration of fMRI and simultaneous EEG: towards a comprehensive understanding of localization and time-course of brain activity in target detection. Neuroimage 22:83–94

Nakamura W, Anami K, Mori T, Saitoh O, Cichocki A, Amari S (2006) Removal of ballistocardiogram artefacts from simultaneously recorded EEG and fMRI data using independent component analysis. IEEE Trans Biomed Eng 53:1294–308

Nunez PL (1981) Electric fields of the brain. Oxford University Press, New York

Nunez PL, Silberstein RB (2000) On the relationship of synaptic activity to macroscopic measurements: does co-registration of EEG with fMRI make sense? Brain Topogr 13:79–96

Patel AB, de Graaf RA, et al. (2004) Glutamatergic neurotransmission and neuronal glucose oxidation are coupled during intense neuronal activation. J Cereb Blood Flow Metab 24:972–985

Patel AB, de Graaf RA, et al. (2005) The contribution of GABA to glutamate/glutamine cycling and energy metabolism in the rat cortex in vivo. Proc Natl Acad Sci USA 102:5588–5593

Pellerin L, Magistretti PJ (1994) Glutamate uptake into astrocytes stimulates aerobic glycolysis: a mechanism coupling neuronal activity to glucose utilization. Proc Natl Acad Sci USA 25: 10625–10629

Pflieger PJ, Greenblatt RE (2001) Nonlinear analysis of multimodal dynamic brain imaging data. Int J Bioelectromag 3:1

Pflieger PJ, and Greenblatt RE. Nonlinear analysis of multimodal dynamic brain imaging data. Int. J. Bioelectromag., 3, 2001. Available at http://www.ijbem.org/volume3/number1/toc.htm

Puce A, Allison T, et al. (1997) Comparison of cortical activation evoked by faces measured by intracranial field potentials and functional MRI: two case studies. Hum Brain Mapp 5: 298–305

Riera J, Wan X, et al. (2006) Nonlinear local electro-vascular coupling: part I. A theoretical model. Hum Brain Mapp 27:896–914

Riera J, Jimenez JC, Wan X, Kawashima R, Ozaki T (2007) Nonlinear local electro-vascular coupling. Part II. From data to neural masses. Hum Brain Mapp 28:335–345

Rosen BR, Buckner RL, et al. (1998) Event-related functional MRI: past present and future. Proc Natl Acad Sci USA 895:773–780

Salek-Haddadi A, Lemieux L, Merschhemke M, Friston KJ, Duncan JS, Fish DR (2003) Functional magnetic resonance imaging of human absence seizures. Ann Neurol; 53(5): 663–667

Shiraishi H, Ahlfors S, et al. (2005) Application of magnetoencephalography in epilepsy patients with widespread spike or slow-wave activity. Epilepsia 46:1264–1272

Shulman RG, Hyder F (2001) Cerebral energetics and the glycogen shunt: neurochemical basis of functional imaging. Proc Natl Acad Sci USA 98:6417–2704

Shmuel A, Augath M, et al. (2006) Negative functional MRI response correlates with decrease in neuronal activity in monkey visual area V1. Nat Neurosci 9:569–577

Sotero RC, Trujillo NJ (2007) Modelling the role of excitatory and inhibitory neuronal activity in the generation of the BOLD signal. Neuroimage 35:149–165

Sotero RC, Trujillo-Barreto NJ (2007) Biophysical model for integrating neuronal activity, EEG, fMRI and metabolism. Neuroimage 39:290–309

Stephan K, Harrison L, et al. (2004) Biophysical models of fMRI responses. Curr Opin Neurobiol 14:629–635

Stippich C, Freitag P, et al. (1998) Motor somatosensory and auditory cortex localization with fMRI and MEG. Neuroreport 9:1953–1957

Thees S, Blankenburg F, et al. (2003) Dipole source localization and fMRI of simultaneously recorded data applied to somatosensory categorization. Neuroimage 18:707–719

Trujillo NJ, Aubert-Vasquez E, et al. (2001) Bayesian model for fMRI and EEG/MEG NeuroImage fusion. Int J Bioelectromag 3:1

Ureshi M, Matsuura T, et al. (2004) Stimulus frequency dependence of the linear relationship between local cerebral blood flow and field potential evoked by activation of rat somatosensory cortex. Neurosci Res 48:147–153

Wagner M, Fuchs M, et al. (2001) Integration of functional MRI, structural MRI, EEG and MEG. Int J Bioelectromag 3:1

Wan X, Riera J, Iwata K, Takashashi M, Wakabayashi T, Kawashima R (2006) The neural basis of the hemodynamic response nonlinearity in human primary visual cortex: implications for neurovascular coupling mechanism. Neuroimage 32:616–625

Warach S, Ives JR, Schlaug G, Patel MR, Darby DG, Thangaraj V, Edelman RR, Schomer DL (1996) EEG-triggered echo-planar functional MRI in epilepsy. Neurology 47:89–93

Outlook

Our main aim in putting this book together was to give the reader an overview of EEG–fMRI: its technical aspects, the basic physiology of the mechanisms that give rise to those signals, the principles that underlie its optimal application, and the technique's main applications to date.

While we feel that the book has broadly achieved this aim, we cannot claim to have covered the field in its entirety. For example, the relationship between neuronal spiking activity and the BOLD signal could have been explored further, as could the relationship between subtle vigilance changes and the BOLD signal (to give examples in the field of basic physiology) and applications of EEG–fMRI in psychiatry (to give an example in the field of applications).

Throughout the book, we have underlined the notion that *simultaneous* multimodal measurements are optimal for the study of signal variations beyond experimental control. In practice this means the study of the relationship between haemodynamic and electrophysiological signals during spontaneous ("resting state") brain activity and the study of residual interevent response variability for stimulus-driven brain activity. It also guarantees that the multimodal data is free of the type of intersession bias that can arise in serial, unimodal experiments. The potential downsides to simultaneous measurements are additional cost and signal degradation.

EEG and ERPs reflect mainly synchronised postsynaptic potentials. This is basically an advantage for the combination of EEG and fMRI, since synaptic activity can be assumed to be highly energy consuming and therefore responsible for a large proportion of BOLD signal changes. But what about the efferent activity of neurons: the "spiking"? In the last few years it has been suggested that high-frequency bursts in the range of 600 Hz represent population spikes. Accordingly, the idea emerged of using these high-frequency oscillations in combination with simultaneous fMRI measurements to detect fMRI activations related to action potentials/spiking activity of neurons emerged. First results suggest that this strategy can be applied successfully, for example in the investigation of somatosensory thalamocortical pathways.

Although the concept of the awake resting brain is somewhat nebulous, functional imaging has revealed interesting patterns of baseline metabolic activity. These observations have created a lot of interest in the study of the brain left to its own devices. Although the experimental paradigm ("controlled experimentation") remains dominant in the field of neuroimaging, pure observation ("natural experimentation") has recently gained increased importance, partly as a result of the availability of simultaneous EEG–fMRI. While this is a relatively new perception in the context of functional brain imaging, neurophysiologists have observed spontaneous changes in brain activity as reflected in the EEG. In fact, EEG can be used to differentiate between very subtle changes in the vigilance levels of subjects. These vigilance changes might well influence the majority of fMRI results presented today, and EEG–fMRI might help to distinguish, for example, between brain regions specifically involved in a task and regions that are found to be activated due to their role in an arousal or vigilance fluctuation. In epilepsy, the attraction of EEG–fMRI is clear: it is absolutely without rival as a technique for studying spontaneous epileptic discharges. While its clinical potential remains to be properly assessed, it has already provided important new information on focal and generalised epilepsies, and has become an important new research tool. We envisage that it will continue to provide crucial new data on the networks that underlie epileptic activity, as well as those that are affected by the said activity. The availability of high-resolution EEG with fMRI in larger and better-characterised patient groups, combined with other data such as MR tractography and further modelling developments in multimodal data fusion and connectivity, will offer great scope for new discoveries.

While the EEG is an important tool in clinical epilepsy, today it is worth mentioning that a psychiatrist, Hans Berger, thought that EEG would be helpful in gaining a deep understanding of psychiatric disorders. At present, reduced amplitudes of P300 are among the most robust findings of biological psychiatry. ERPs have a strong genetic background and therefore can be used as intermediate phenotypes in the search for specific genes involved in psychiatric diseases. Moreover, a number of authors suggest that distinct oscillation patterns (such as the gamma-band oscillation) may play a crucial role in the pathophysiology of psychiatric disorders. Since, for example, gamma-band oscillations rely on intact circuitry between pyramidal cells and fast spiking interneurons, findings of disturbed gamma bands may reflect the basic pathophysiology in diseases such as schizophrenia. In addition, fMRI has provided the psychiatrist with great insight into the biological nature of pathological mental phenomena, such as auditory hallucinations or depressive mood states, for example. EEG–fMRI can therefore be expected to link direct measurements of neural activity with a close relationship to underlying (patho)physiological mechanisms with knowledge about the brain structures involved.

The above examples of "missing chapters" are representative of what we think the near future will be about, although we are also excited about the prospect of other unforeseen topics that will no doubt soon emerge in the fast-developing field of EEG–fMRI.

Louis Lemieux and Christoph Mulert

Index

Printing and Binding: Stürtz GmbH, Würzburg